Textbook of

Microbiology

An Integrated and Clinical Case Based Approach

V.S. Randhawa MD, FIMSA
Director Professor, Department of Microbiology
Lady Hardinge Medical College, New Delhi
Formerly: Dr. R.M.L. P.G.I.M.S., New Delhi
J.N. Medical College, Aligarh
S.G.P.G.I.M.S., Lucknow
M.A.M.C. and Associated Hospitals, New Delhi

Co-Editor
Gagandeep Singh MD, MAMS
Consultant, Department of Microbiology
A.I.I.M.S., New Delhi

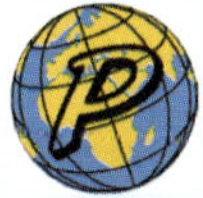

Peepee Publishers and Distributors (P) Ltd.®

Textbook of Microbiology

Published by
Pawaninder P. Vij and Anupam Vij

Peepee Publishers and Distributors (P) Ltd.
Head Office: 160, Shakti Vihar, Pitam Pura, Delhi-110 034 (India)

Correspondence Address:

7/31, First Floor, Ansari Road, Daryaganj
New Delhi-110 002 (India)

Ph: 41512412, 23246245, 9811156083

e-mail: peepee160@yahoo.co.in

e-mail: peepee160@gmail.com

www.peepeepub.com

join us on facebook.com/pp.publishers

First Edition: 2019

ISBN: 978-81-8445-249-5

Dedicated to

My Guru

and

My Parents (Late) Jaswant Kaur and Prof. H.S. Randhawa

PREFACE

Medical Microbiology plays a key role in the diagnosis and management (including prevention) of infectious diseases. However, majority of the medical students fail to grasp that essence, while studying the subject. They struggle with the vast microbiological information available in the microbiology textbooks. They are unable to see the relevance of the vast microbiological information, besides find difficulty in its recapitulation and integration with the medical curriculum. The current book is not a compilation of facts but comprises meaningful integrated clinical data. Such a style also encourages application of microbiological information.

The microbiological, pathological and clinical data of the ever changing diverse microbes is phenomenal and to present direction and organization amongst it to the undergraduates is a challenge. The MCI recommends integration of the medical microbiology, to make the subject relevant to the medical curriculum. Passionate discussion on revamping of the medical microbiology curriculum has been deliberated upon in the IAMM national conferences of Mumbai in 2003 and Chennai in 2005. But nothing significant has occurred, as partly there is no resource material for the medical teachers and students along these directions.

To meet these challenges, the current book has been designed. All key chapters in this book start with an opening vignette/clinical case; often with relevant quotations to convey the theme of the topic. Subsequently the topic is worked out systematically in Q-A format. This is done, so that the study becomes exciting and the relevance of the subject matter becomes clear to the student. All the main chapters with clinical cases have been provided with linkages for providing comprehensive grasping of topics. Linkages in other areas have also been provided. Numerous bacterial/viral agents have diverse microscopic, metabolic features, colony characteristics, media requirements, varying laboratory diagnosis profiles, treatment profiles and vaccines. To understand them and to recall them, there is no better way than to tabulate them on a mega scale covering entire topics. This approach has been followed comprehensively for these parameters.

The book has been divided into 17 sections for the organization purpose. Section I and II deal with General Microbiology and Immunology, respectively. Both the sections are opening vignette/integrated clinical case based in Q-A format. The systemic bacteriology portion has been divided into eight independent sections; from III-X. In a section, before the integrated clinical case based studies are depicted, there are chapters devoted to the bacterial and disease characteristics, so that these can be applied and understood in the clinical cases. The laboratory diagnosis and treatment profiles are provided towards the end part of each of the sections.

The virology section has four sections from XI to XIV. The section XI deals with General Virology. Section XII and XIII deals with DNA and RNA Viruses, respectively. The latter two sections begin with overview of clinical profile, followed by integrated clinical based studies in Q-A format and end with outline of the laboratory diagnosis. Section XV deals with Mycology. It has been divided into six chapters for easy understanding of the mycological aspects. In it, chapters 2 to 5 deal with the clinical units of mycoses. Each of this chapter starts with a clinical based case study to highlight the key aspects to be followed by other aspects related to case theme/examination assessment. Section XVI deals with Clinical Microbiology. In it, chapters 2 to 8 deal with the infectious diseases of various anatomical system of the body. Each chapter starts with relevant quotation and has clinical based integrated studies in Q-A format. Section XVII deals with Applied Microbiology and has 11 chapters. Each chapter starts with opening vignette/integrated clinical case based studies in Q-A format and has relevant quotations.

At places it appears that information is getting duplicated, this is a deliberate attempt to reinforce some important information to the undergraduates, so that they remember it! The author has seen that many times students are not able to understand and retain the basic information, the material has been so arranged and depicted, that the student overcomes this difficulty and develops confidence. To ensure that the novice student does not get lost in the sea of microbiological information, all chapters have question and answer format (except those tabulating key microbiological information) and all sections are referenced with a list of key examination/assessment questions (to which references/answers are provided). This approach would be helpful especially to students, who lack command on the English language, but have to clear the examination in the English language.

The key features of the book are:

- General Bacteriology presented as integrated opening vignette based studies, primarily in Q-A format.
- Immunology section based as more than 18 integrated clinical case based studies, in Q-A format.
- A major chunk of Bacteriology, Virology, Mycology and Clinical Microbiology presented in the form of more than 51, 25, 5 and 11 integrated clinical case based studies, respectively.
- Bacterial and viral outbreaks that have actually occurred in S.E. Asia are incorporated. Besides the coverage of the microbiological facts, the economic and the social implications involved in these episodes have also been highlighted.
- All bacteriology sections have separate section for Outline/Classification of organisms, Metabolic and microscopic features, Media requirements and colonial characters (including diagnostic), clinical profile, laboratory diagnosis (of important bacteria) and treatment. This is organized in an integrated tabular format.
- Molecular biology aspects highlighted.
- Some original classical experiments described to maintain touch with history.
- Clinical Microbiology section organized anatomical systemwise, with 11 exclusive integrated clinical case based studies in Q-A format. Includes relevant quotations. Special emphasis on sample collection, transportation and principles of choosing the right specimen.
- Applied Microbiology section is integrated opening vignette based including more than 9 clinical case based studies in Q-A format. Includes relevant quotations.
- All biochemical reactions/bacterial/viral vaccines covered in a compact tabular format.
- For examination purpose at places, short notes incorporated separately.
- Space is provided to incorporate new and changed concepts in the book.
- More than 50 quotations to inspire the student.
- Varying font size to grade varying importance of information.
- Footnotes provided for difficult terms.
- Separate section on Internet resources for Microbiology.
- Complimentary teaching resource for medical teachers.

Studying with understanding may be time consuming initially, but is a sound investment in the student's long medical career. It is with this in mind, the book has been presented. Mr. P.P. Vij, the publisher wanted to have a very basic book of Microbiology, but I could convince him of the importance of presentation in opening vignette based/integrated clinical case format, even though it was becoming comprehensive and exhaustive. The author is confident that the student will retain more information, score well in the examination, develop a rational approach to the subject, be able to analyze microbiological data in clinical cases rationally in his medical career and continue to learn throughout his medical career, studying the current book.

A textbook should not merely provide information but should make it meaningful and realistic.

"A teacher...who has no living traffic with his knowledge but merely repeats his lesson to his students, can only load their minds, he cannot quicken them..."

—Rabindranath Tagore

I hope the challenges are met and the subject reclaims its importance both amongst the teachers and students. Any feedback or criticism would be welcome at my email–vsrandh@gmail.com

V.S. Randhawa

ACKNOWLEDGEMENTS

I am grateful to my teachers who have made me reach my present position.The notable amongst them include Dr D.S. Agarwal (Ex-Dean, Maulana Azad Medical College), Late Dr K.B. Sharma (formerly; Regional WHO adviser), Dr V.K. Sharma, Dr Usha Baveja, Dr Preena Bhalla (HOD, MC; Hindu Rao), Dr Beena Uppal, Dr Krishan Prakash, Dr Anita Chakravarty (HOD at SGT) and Dr Mridu Dudeja (Jamia Hamdard MC). I am also indebted to Dr T.D. Chugh (Formerly, Kuwait Medical School) and Dr Anuj Sharma (Consultant WHO), who constantly prodded me to portray the clinical component, as the core component in the text of microbiology for medical students.

I am also indebted to my colleagues in the Lady Hardinge with whom I regularly interacted namely Dr Geeta Mehta, Dr M. Deb, Dr Renu Dutta (HOD, Sharda University), Dr R. Kaur, Dr B.L. Sherwal (currently Director, RGSH), Dr V.L. Malhotra (Currently faculty at SGT, Gurugram), Dr Manoj Jais, Dr Sonal Saxena, Dr A. Lakshmy, Dr Deepti Rawat, Dr Manoj Kumar and Dr Yogita Rai. I am also grateful to Dr Charu Jain for contributing the websites in Internet resources chapter and Dr Meenakshi Singh for troubleshooting.

I am grateful to all the students of various institutions with whom I have interacted till date notably of Maulana Azad Medical College, New Delhi, SGPGIMS Lucknow, J.N. Medical College, Aligarh, Dr RML PGIMS and LHMC, New Delhi. A special mention of 5th semester students of LHMC 2017, 2018, and Nikhita Goyal (MAMC) whose caricatures/cartoons poems/mnemonics have been incorporated in this text.

We are obliged to Public Health Image Library (public domain),CDC, Atlanta and other sites for the use of images. In medical textbook writing you are helped by many experts, besides being inspired by various personalities and learn in ones interaction with numerous luminaries. It would not be fair, if they are not acknowledged. These include: Dr Samant Ray (ex-HOD, AIIMS), Dr Shobha Broor, Dr Gita Satpathy (HOD, AIIMS), Dr P. Sugandhi Rao, Dr Rama Chaudhary, Dr Arti Kapil, Dr Lalit Dar, Dr B.R. Mirdha, Dr Bimal Das, Dr Seema Sood, Dr Immaculata, Dr Z.U. Khan, Dr H.C. Gugnani, Dr Iqbal Kaur (HOD, ESI MC, Faridabad), Dr Ashwani Kumar, Dr N.P. Singh (HOD, UCMS), Dr Rama Chandran, Dr Rajni Gaind (HOD, VMMC), Dr Manju Bala, Dr Balvinder Singh, Dr Malini Capoor, Dr Deepthi, Dr C.P. Baveja (HOD, MAMC), Dr Surender Kumar, Dr Vikas Manchanda, Dr Rohit Chawla, Dr Dakshina Bisht (HOD, Santosh Medical College), Dr Ajoy Kumar, Dr Malini Sharif (HOD, VPCI), Dr Indu Shukla, Dr Harris M Khan, Dr Meher Rizvi, Dr Nandini Duggal (HOD, Dr RML PGIMS), Dr Rakesh Mahajan, Dr Nirmaljeet, Dr Shalini, Dr Archana Thakur (HOD, G.B.P.H.), Dr. Chand Wattal (SGRH), Dr Poonam Sood, Dr Sanjay Singhal (HOD ESI-PGIMSR, Basaidarapur), Dr R. Agarwal (Delhi Govt. Secretariat), Dr Jagdish Chander (HOD, GMC, Chandigarh), Dr Varsha Gupta, Dr Anil Kanga, Dr Digvijay Singh (HOD,GMC, Shimla), Dr Poonam Gupta, Dr Rajeev Thakur (HOD, IBHAS), Dr Renu Goyal, Dr Sunil Gupta (HOD, NCDC), Dr Partho Ganguli, Dr Somenath, Dr Charu Prakash, Dr Mala Chaabra, Dr Mayank Dwivedi, Dr T. N. Dhole (HOD, SGPGIMS), Dr K.N. Prasad, Dr J. Kishore, Dr Bharti Arora (HOD, MAMC, Agroha), Dr J. Singh, Dr Sanjib Gogoi, Dr Sudesh Sharma (GMC, Jammu), Dr B.N. Harish, Dr Mannu Jain (HOD, SMIMER, Surat), Dr Summaiya A. Mulla (HOD, GMC, Surat), Dr Berry (CMC, Ludhiana), Dr Ciraj, Dr Chitra Pai (Antigua, West Indies), Dr Hem Lata, Dr S. Sharma (HOD, SGRDIMS, Amritsar), Dr K.D. Singh, Dr M.M. Vegad (BJMC, Ahmedabad), Dr Neelam Khanna (HOD, Batra Hospital), Dr Sanjay Jain, Dr Radha Rani (Consultant, Indo–American Institute), Dr Namita Jaggi, Dr Ramesh Ranganathan (Gulf Medical Institute, UAE), Dr Nitya Vyas, Dr R. Maheshwari (HOD, SMS, Jaipur), Dr R.K. Mishra, Dr Gautam (PGIMER, Chandigarh), Dr R. Sehgal (HOD,PGIMER), Dr R.K. Ratho (HOD,Virology, PGIMER), Dr S. Gautam (HOD, BARC), Dr Shabbir Simjee (Technical Advisor, Eli Lily), Dr Kamlesh Thakur (HOD, RPGMC, Tanda), Dr Manoj Kumar (HOD, RIMS, Ranchi), Dr Camilla Rodrigues (Consultant, P.D. Hinduja, Mumbai), Dr Pranay K. Shah (BJMC, Ahmedabad), Dr Sharmila Sengupta, Dr M.K. Sen (HOD, Safdarjang Hospital), Dr Pratima Gupta (HOD, AIIMS, Rishikesh), Dr R. Ravi Kumar (HOD, NIMHANS), Dr Umesh (HOD, MC Haldwani), Dr Shahriar Roushani (PMC, Loni), Dr G. Viswanath (HOD,

JJMC, Davangere), Dr V.C. Kallia (Chief, CSIR-IGIB), Dr Jugal Kishore (HOD,VMMC), Dr Ranjana Khuraijam (JNH, Imphal), Dr Ameeta Joshi (HOD, J.J.M.C., Mumbai), Dr Shyamal Bhattacharya, Dr Basudha Khanal (HOD, BPKIHS, Nepal), Dr Uma Choudhry, Dr Madhu Sharma (PGIMS, Rohtak), Dr P.S. Gill and Dr Kiran.

I am also obliged to many of my students and residents, who currently occupy key faculty positions, Dr Neelam Taneja (PGIMER, Chandigarh), Dr Mandira (VPCI), Dr Anuradha Choudhary (VPCI), Dr Neeraj Goel (SGRH, New Delhi), Dr Nishant Verma, AIIMS,New Delhi), Dr Rakesh Singh (JIPMER), Dr Neelam Gulati (GMC, Chandigarh), Dr Anuradha (PGIMER, New Delhi), Dr Jyotsna (SMIMS), Dr Prafulla Sonagara (MGMMC, Indore), Dr Pankaj Lal (Consultant, Liverpool Clinical Labs.), Dr Lavanya J. (PSGIMSR, Coimbatore), Dr Mala Vinayak (LBSH), Dr Suchitra (Hi-Tech MC, Rourkela), Dr Ritu Singh Chauhan (WHO), Dr Ritu Singhal (LSR-TB Centre), Dr Sarika (CDC projects), Dr Surraiya (MC, Kanpur), Dr Shweta Bhagat (LHMC), Dr Gaurav Dhaka (MAMC), Dr Meenakshi, Dr Suruchi, Dr Harman, Dr Vineet Khanna, Dr Priyam, Dr Nidhi (NCDC), Dr Madhulika, Dr Shivani Satia, Dr Trishla, Dr Debjani, Dr. Anju (MGMMS, Indore), Dr Nupur (ESI, DC), Dr Kanika, Dr Monica, Dr Anchan, Dr Kamaldeep, Dr Charu, Dr Shipra, Dr Sonam, Dr Bhawna (NACO), Dr Madhumita, Dr Nivedita, Dr Neha, Dr Sikander and Dr Imsen. I also acknowledge the inputs of my current postgraduates, Dr Nisha, Dr Suresh, Dr Snigdha, Dr Priyanka, Dr Yogita, Dr Garima, Dr Larinpari, Dr Indira, Dr Masoom, Dr Fathima, Dr Srestha, Dr Anusha and Dr Shweta.

Mr Shankar Sharma of Computer shop, AIIMS for preparing the draft.

Mr Pawan Sharma, Mr Satnam and Mr Sanjeev Kumar for the final formatting of the text. Mr S.K. Sharma for proof reading.

Ms Gurpreet for the illustrations and figures.

Mr P.P. Vij and Mr Anupam Vij for a positive attitude on the project and ensuring that the project completed on time.

Lastly Mrs Rominder my wife and son Jasmeet for bearing with me during the work.

V.S. Randhawa

LIST OF CONTENTS

NB: Figure/Table are denoted by three numbers, in which the first number refers to section, second number refers to chapter and third number refers to sequence, for e.g., **Fig. 2.3.3** implies the figure is from section 2, chapter 3 and sequence is 3.

DETAILED CONTENTS

SECTION I: GENERAL BACTERIOLOGY

Opening Vignette/Integrated Clinical Case Based Q&A Studies

SECTION II: IMMUNOLOGY

Opening Vignette/Integrated Clinical Case Based Q&A Studies

SYSTEMIC BACTERIOLOGY
(Section III–X)

SECTION III: GRAM POSITIVE COCCI

SECTION IV: GRAM NEGATIVE COCCI

SECTION V: GRAM POSITIVE RODS/BACILLI

SECTION VI: GRAM NEGATIVE BACILLI–ENTEROBACTERIACEAE

SECTION VII: GRAM NEGATIVE BACILLI–NON FASTIDIOUS, OXIDASE +ve

SECTION VIII: GRAM NEGATIVE BACILLI–CURVED/SPIRAL SHAPED

SECTION IX: GRAM NEGATIVE BACILLI–FASTIDIOUS

SECTION X: ATYPICAL/UNCONVENTIONAL/OBLIGATE INTRACELLULAR BACTERIA

VIROLOGY
Section XI – XIV

SECTION XI: GENERAL VIROLOGY

Opening Vignette/Integrated Clinical Case Based Q&A Studies

SECTION XII: DNA VIRUSES

Section I: General Bacteriology

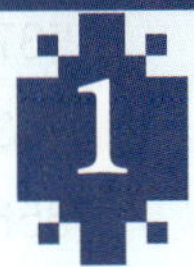

1 Historical Perspectives

Science is an attempt, largely successful to understand the world, to get a grip on things, to get hold of ourselves and to steer to safe course..microbiology and meterology now explain what only a few centuries ago was considered sufficient cause to burn women to death.
— Carl Sagan

Infectious diseases comprise a leading cause of morbidity and mortality of the human diseases (Fig. 1.1.1a). Most of these infectious diseases can be easily diagnosed, treated and prevented. Lack of effective control measures may lead to outbreaks. New diseases and etiologic agents continue to appear.

Let's make a beginning of this critical area of medical science.

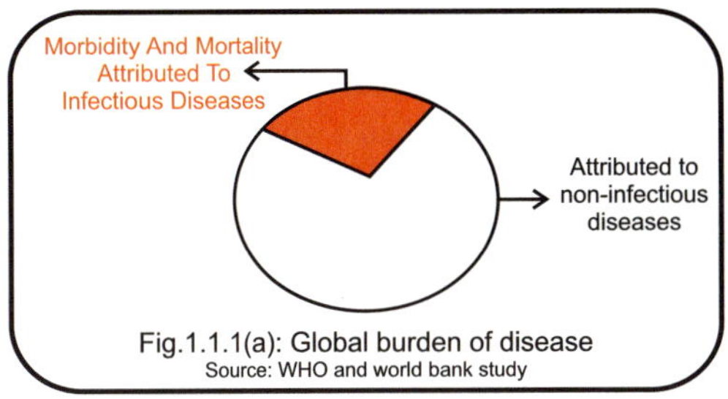

Fig.1.1.1(a): Global burden of disease
Source: WHO and world bank study

What are the basic divisions in the field of microbiology?

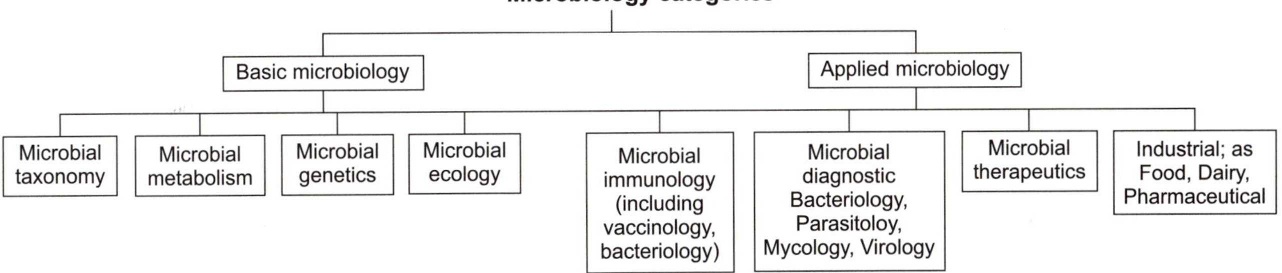

A.1 Numerous branches of microbiology exist as soil microbiology, agriculture microbiology, industrial microbiology, dairy microbiology, space microbiology and others. *Medical Microbiology* concerns with medical aspects in the field of microbiology. It deals with microbes that cause human infection, their pathogenicity, diagnosis, treatment and prevention.

What benefits does the study of medical microbiology provide?

A.2 It helps in:

(i) Studying the role of microbes in human health (it is estimated that the human body has about 10^{14} cells, of which 90% are microbes and only 10% are of human origin).

(ii) Making earlier and specific diagnosis, thereby initiating earlier treatment.

(iii) Sensitive and specific tests help to clearly delineate these diseases from some non-infectious diseases, which they may resemble and require different management.

(iv) Perform antimicrobial susceptibility tests, which help in deciding the dose and type of the antimicrobial drug to be administered.

(v) Helping in initiating control measures to prevent further spread of the infection and preventing outbreaks.

(vi) Useful in making vaccines and in initiating other preventive strategies.

(vii) More diseases may be found to have an infectious aetiology, as currently some viruses are implicated in some psychiatric disorders and *Chlamydia trachomatis* has been implicated in coronary artery disease and stroke.

What was the concept in medical microbiology till the eighteenth century that prevented the development of this discipline, as it is practised today?

A.3 The theory of spontaneous generation prevalent in that period, hampered development in microbiology. According to this theory, microorganisms could arise from non-living substance (as it had vital characters) by spontaneous generation although the larger organisms could not. As long as this thought prevailed the need to study the epidemiology, pathogenesis, treatment and control of diseases could not arise.

A theory was proposed in the eighteenth century, which laid the foundation for the development of microbiology; as known today. Describe briefly.

A.4 **(a)** The proposal of *germ theory* of disease was critical in laying the foundation of microbiology. According to this theory, microbes arose only from their like and not 'de novo'. These microbes could invade others organisms and cause disease.

The germ theory though in the current time appears simple, but it took about two hundred years of experimental work of several scientists to root out the deeply entrenched concept in many biologists that non-living organic matter had a vital force that could yield microbes 'de novo'. The scientists with this thought demonstrated that boiled extracts of meat or hay would turn turbid after some time, due to growth of microbes in the solution.

Describe the early events in the development of Microbiology.

A.4 **(b)** Work by Italian biologist, Francesco Redi in late 17th century (1668), Italian anatomist; Lazzaro Spallanzani in 18th century (1776) and Louis Pasteur in nineteenth century (1861) led the theory of spontaneous generation to rest. F. Redi proved that maggots from eggs laid by flies arose only on pieces of meat, that had not been protected by gauge piece. The gauze piece would prevent the flies to come, sit and lay eggs on the meat. L. Spallanzani demonstrated that sterile nutrient broth in flask would not yield any microbes, if it had been sealed initially. Louis Pasteur's experiments with famous 'swan necked' flask with which he organized a competition in 1859, silenced all his critics. The longs curved tubes of the flask prevented the outside microbes to enter the main part of the vessel with broth, though the contents of vessel remained in contact with the outside air. The early events are depicted in table 1.1.1.

Table 1.1.1: Early events in development of Medical Microbiology

Date/period	Event and its significance
1361-1380	First use of quarantine to control the spread of epidemic plague (bubonic)
1590	*Zacharias Janssen*, a Dutch spectacle maker, invented the first compound microscope
1660	*Robert Hooke*, an English scientist explore various living and non-living matter with a compound microscope (that used reflected light)
1676 [1623-1723]	*Antony van Leeuwenhoek*, a Dutch cloth merchant, devised simple microscope to observe microbes including protozoa. He came from a family of businessmen. He received no formal education and the only language known to him was Dutch. With his open mind and curiosity, be discovered bacteria, free -living parasites, sperm cells, blood cells and many more living organisms.
1838	A French physician, *Philippe Ricord*, inoculated 2,500 human subjects to demonstrate that syphilis and gonorrhoea were two different diseases
1839	*Theodor Schwann*, A German zoologist and *Matthias Schleiden* a botanist, formalized the theory of all living organisms being composed of cells
1847-1850	*Ignaz Semmelweis*, a Hungarian physician, proposed the theory of childbed fever to be a contagious once and transmitted to women by their obstetricians during childbirth
1853-1854	A London physician *John Snow*, demonstrates the spread of human cholera in the city through a water supply contaminated with human sewage
1857	*Louis Pasteur*, a French microbiologist, demonstrated that fermentation is due to microbes, originated a process to control it and coined the term 'pasteurization' for it
1858	A German pathologist, *Rudolf Virchow*, introduced the concept of all living cells originating from pre-existing cells
1876	*Robert Koch*, a German bacteriologist, identified *Bacillus anthracis* as a causative agent of Anthrax
1879	*Hansen* discovered *Mycobacterium leprae* to be a causative agent of leprosy
1880	*Ogston* discovered *Staphyloccous aureus*
1880	*Neisser* disovered *Neisseria gonorrhoeae* to be a cause of gonorrhoea *Laveran and Ross* identified malarial life cycle in red blood cells of infected man
1882	*Robert Koch* identified/discovered *M. tuberculosis* to be the cause of tuberculosis
1883	*Robert Koch* discovers *V. cholerae* to be cause of cholera
1884	*Loeffler* discovered diphtheria bacillus *Robert Koch* outlined his postulates *Hans Christian Gram* devised the gram stain (the most frequently used stain in bacteriology)

Contd.

Contd.

1885	*Nicolaier* discovered tetanus bacillus *Bumm* isolated *N. gonorroheae* by culturing it
1886	*Escherich* discovers *E. coli* *Frankel* discovers pneumococci
1887	*Julius Petri* a German bacteriologist discovered pneumococci, invented culture dish (petri dish, used world over for cultivating and isolating microbes) *Weichselbaum* discovers meningococci *Bruce* discovers brucella (*Brucella melitensis*), as a causative agent of brucellosis in cattle.
1892	*Welch-Nuttall* discovered *Clostridium welchii.*
1894	*Pfeiffer* identifies *Haemophilus influenzae* (Pfeiffer bacillus, mistaken to be cause of the influenza pandemic/epidemic in nineteenth century) *Yersin and Kitasato* discovered plague bacillus
1896	*Shiga* discovered shigella bacillus
1897	*van Ermengem* discovered *Clostridium botulinum,* which causes botulism
1898	*Shiga* discovered *Shigella dysentriae* as cause of dysentery
1905	*Schaudinn and Hoffman* identified *Treponema pallidum,* as causative agent of syphilis

Describe the contributions of Louis Pasteur and discuss their significance.

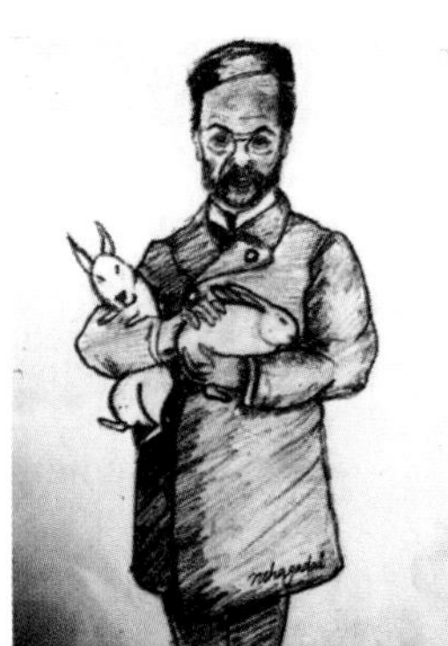

Fig. 1.1.1(b): Louis Pasteur

A.5

- Showed that fermentation of various organic fluids is always associated with microbes
- Different types of fermentation are associated with different microbes (boost to wine industry)
- Discovered fermentation and found that selective/specific yeast made good wine. But other microbes could produce acids and other products, which could alter the taste of good wine for worse
- Disproved spontaneous generation theory – Devised narrow, 'swan-necked' flasks
- Proposed germ theory of disease – all forms of life arise from their like and not 'de novo'. Showed that diseases could arise, when microbes interacted with tissue.
- Introduced techniques of sterilization as:
  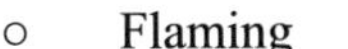
  - Flaming
  - Pasteurization: Recommended heating wine at 96°C for half an hour to kill undesired organisms, later technique modified for other fluids; as milk etc.
  - Hot air oven
  - Autoclave
- Studied Pebrine (silk worm disease): While studying silkworms identified three different microbes, which caused unique diseases, this was a boost to the silk industry.
- Suggested that etiological agent of rabies was ultramicroscopic in form.
- Coined this term 'Vaccine' (from 'vacca'-cow). Developed several vaccines (live attenuated), namely:
  - Chicken cholera[Δ]. Attenuated by ageing and repeated subculture.
  - Anthrax – Attenuated *B. anthracis* (1881) by incubating at higher temperature (42-43°C). Success of anthrax vaccine was demonstrated in public experiment on a farm in France (Pouilly-le Fort) in 1881, in which vaccinated animals, when challenged with virulent anthrax culture survived the challenge. Whereas the unvaccinated animals challenged with the virulent anthrax microbes, succumbed to the infection.
  - Rabies (1888) – Attenuated strain was obtained by serial intracerebral passage in rabbits and then drying pieces of spinal cord of such rabbits. Interestingly the vaccine was first tried on a 9 year old Joseph Meister (after testing in animals), who was severely bitten by a rabid dog and was doomed to die. Luckily the boy survived, grew and became the caretaker of the famous *Pasteur Institute*. He was later killed by the German forces during World War II for refusing to give the keys of the Pasteur Institute.
  - Pasteur institute was built by him with money from various sources.
- Trained several scientists and gifted several students.

[Δ] 'Chicken Cholera' – is a disease of chicken, which resembles human cholera.

- Most important application of his work was introduction of aseptic techniques in surgery by Lister (1867).

Describe the contributions of Robert Koch and discuss their significance

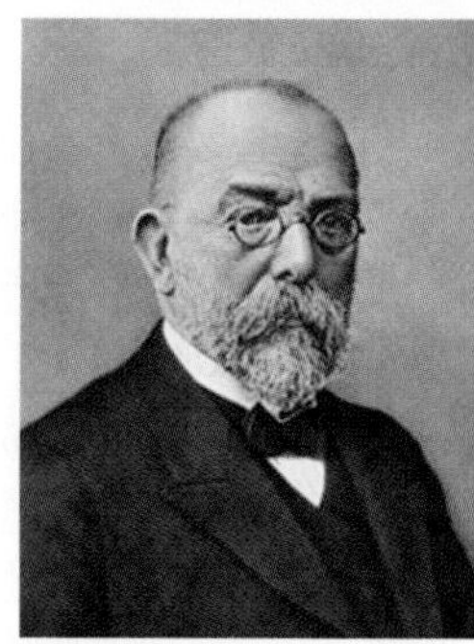

Fig. 1.1.2: Robert Koch

A.6
- Robert Koch (1843-1910)
- Germany physician by training
- Regarded by many as – 'Father of bacteriology'
- Introduced staining technique to demonstrate bacteria
- Introduced solid media to isolate organisms. He realized that study of bacteria would require separating organisms from each other and growing them in culture.

Work in bacteriology could not progress until organisms could be isolated on solid media, so the importance of this work can not be underestimated.

He initially introduced gelatin (which melts at room temperature), later potato slices and then 'agar-agar' (suggested by an American wife of an colleague, who used it in the kitchen as a thickening agent) as media.

- Discovered
  - *B. anthracis* – found out its life cycle, which involves mainly animals, but man is accidentally infected. Identified spore stage involved in it and cultured it.
  - *M. tuberculosis* (1882) – Identified organism that causes TB. Devised complex staining method and cultured it.
  - *Vibrio cholerae* (1883) – Studied epidemic in Egypt (demonstrated by histopathological studies in 1883) and showed that organism is confined to intestine. Showed its characteristic comma shape, worked in Bengal on this agent and could culture it
- Epidemiology – showed that both 'cholera' and 'typhoid' are water borne, which is an important aspect in control of these diseases.
- Discovered old tuberculin (hoping to make good vaccine, although not helpful for this purpose), it became a useful agent for skin test to diagnose TB.
- Described Koch's phenomenon (p 237, A7)
- Nobel prize in physiology in 1905 for studies in Tuberculosis media
- Introduced Koch's Postulates*
  - His postulates resulted in discovering causative agents of twenty diseases in last quarter of 19th century
  - His postulates are standard for identifying role of different pathogen; even today
- Gifted Many students
- Invented many techniques of microscopic examination, media preparation, inoculation, pure culture maintenance and isolation.

*Koch's Postulates

Introduction:

After the spontaneous generation theory was disproved, etiological agents, started getting reported; so much that it became necessary to introduce criteria for accepting the claim, that a microbe isolated from a disease was causally related to it. The criteria enunciated by Robert Koch that should exist before a microbe can be accepted; as a causative agent of an infectious disease are:

1. The microbe should be constantly associated with the lesion of the disease
2. It should be possible to isolate the microbe in pure culture from the lesion
3. Inoculation of the isolated (pure) microbe into an appropriate animal should reproduce the disease
4. It should be possible to reisolate the same microbe from the characteristic lesion of the laboratory animal
5. An additional criterion; subsequently introduced required demonstration of specific antibodies in serum of the patient.

Exceptions

- *N. gonorrhoeae* (no animal model, though can grow 'in vitro')
- *M. leprae* – has animal model, but unable to grow in artificial media.
- *Treponema pallidum* ⎫ Unable to grow on
- Rickettsiae ⎬ artificial media
- Viruses ⎭ (cell free media)
- Multiorganism infection

Limitations of this concept

1. All exposures to a known human pathogen does not always result in infection of human/animals. All infections in the human don't result into disease
2. Suitable animal models for many human diseases don't exist
3. Many human pathogen cannot be cultivated on inanimate artificial media
4. Pathogen of one species can tremendously vary in its virulence
5. All postulates may not be proved in some diseases
6. Same pathologic or clinical state can be produced by different etiological agents.

Example of recent applications of Koch's postulates:

Lyme disease, Legionnaire's disease, toxic shock syndrome, AIDS, all emerging diseases

Nb: Implied in Koch's postulates, are one microbe one disease concept.

How are the Koch's postulates currently understood, i.e., molecular form of Koch's postulates?

A.7 The advancement in molecular biology has created the current scenario, where genes are associated with microbial pathogenicity. With this perspective, the postulates could be described as:

1. The pathogenic members of the microbe (genus/species) should be (significantly) associated with the pathogenic lesion. The non-pathogenic strains should not have the gene in question.
2. Specific inactivation of the gene/genes associated with the virulence of the microbe, should lead to significant decrease in the virulence of the microbe.
3. Restoration of the normal functioning of all the genes of the microbe, should lead to revival of the virulence of the microbe.

The Koch's postulates are useful reference point but should not be treated as rigid criteria. If these criteria are not fulfilled, then the etiological agent can not be eliminated as the cause of the disease.

Tabulate the developments in Immunology/Molecular Biology.

A.8 (see Section II, A3a, Pg 94)

Tabulate developments in Chemotherapy/Antiseptics

A.9

1481-89	• Elemental mercury given; as a treatment for syphilis
1847-1850	• *Ignaz Semmelweiss* initiated the first use of antiseptics to control (reduce) hand borne diseases (childbed fever)
1867	• *Joseph Lister* an English surgeon, introduced aseptic surgical techniques (known as the father of antiseptic surgery)
1908	• *Paul Ehrlich*, a German scientist, developed Salvarsan an arsenic based drug to treat syphilis (also known as *Father of chemotherapy*). Also worked on the staining of the animal tissue with aniline dyes and further classified the dyes. Discovered the technique of staining the tubercle bacillus. Also worked in Immunology; especially the haemolysins, toxin-antitoxin reactions including standardization of sera.
1928	• *Sir Alexander Fleming* accidentally discovered penicillin
1935	• *Gerhard Domagh* discovered Sulpha drug (Prontosil)
1940	• Englishman *Ernst Chain* and an Australian *Howard Florey* developed safe and stable preparations of penicillin and commercialized its production
1944	• *Selman Waksman*, a Russian, discovered the antibiotic streptomycin

Tabulate the developments in Virology

A.10 (scc Scction XI)

Nobel laureates (for CONTRIBUTION in the field of microbiology)

A.11

Year	Laureate and contribution
1901	*Emil A Von Behring* for diphtheria serum therapy
1902	*Ronald Ross*–Transmission/life cycle of MP
1905	*Robert Koch*–Tuberculosis discovery
1907	*Charles L. A. Laveran*–Discovery of malarial parasite in unstained blood preparation
1908	*Paul Ehrlich and Elie Metchinikoff*–Role of humoral antibody and phagocytes in immunity
1913	*Charles Richet*–Discovery and characterization of anaphylaxis
1919	*Jules Bordet*–Role of complement and complement fixation text
1928	*Charles Nicolle*–Typhus exanthematicus
1930	*Karl Landsteiner*–Blood group types
1939	*Gerhard Domagk*–Antibacterial effect of first type "Prontosil" sulphonamide
1945	*Alexander Fleming*, E. B. Chain and H. W. Florey–Discovery of penicillin and its commercialization
1951	*Max Theiler*–Vaccine for yellow fever
1952	*Selman Abraham Waksman*–Discovery of streptomycin
1954	*John F. Enders, Frederick C. Robbin and Thomas H. Weller*-cultivation of polio virus in tissue culture (landmark study, which showed that even neurotropic viruses could be cultivated on cell lines)
1958	*Joshua Lederberg, Edward L. Tatum and George W. Beadle-genes* act by regulating specific chemical processes and gene arrangement in bacteria including genetic recombination in bacteria
1959	*Ochoa and Kornberg*–Isolation and synthesis of RNA and DNA – the basis for this was laid down by Avery and colleagues in 1944 by pneumococcal transformation experiments. Showed that DNA carries genetic information
1960	*F. Macfarlane Burnet and Peter B. Medawar*–Acquired immunological tolerance (Medwar), clonal selection theory (Burnet).
1962	*Francis H. Crick, James, D. Watson and Maurice H. F, Wilkins*-Molecular structure of DNA (Double helix model)
1965	*Francis Jacob, Jacques Monod and Lwoff Andre* (Operon hypothesis and protein synthesis) – Regulatory mechanisms in microbial genes.
1966	*Peyton Rous*–Viral oncogenesis (avian sarcoma) for his work in Sarcoma virus, which he discovered in 1911)
1968	*H. G. Khorana, Nirenberg and Holley*–defined genetic code (they used microbes as tools)
1969	*Max Delbruck, Alfred D Hershey, Salvodar D Luria*–mechanism of viral infection in living cells
1972	*G. M. Edelman and R. Porter*–chemical structure of antibody
1974	*Albert Claude, C. de Dure, G.E. Palade*–structural and functional organization of cell
1975	*Renato Dulbecco, David Baltimore and H. M. Temin*–interactions between tumor viruses and genetic material of cell, discovered reverse transcriptase.
1976	*Carleton Gajdusek and B. S. Blumberg (Australia Antigen)*–new mechanisms for the origin of dissemination of infectious diseases
1977	*Rosalyn Yalow, Roger Guillemin and Andrew Schally*–developed Radioimmunoassay
1978	*Warner Arber, Hamilton Smith and Daniel Nathans*–discovered restriction enzymes
1980	*Jean Dausset, Baruj Benacerraf, George Snell*–MHC, transplantation and genetic control of immune response
1981	*Frederick Sanger*–Nucleotide sequencing
1983	*Barbara McClintock*–Jumping genes (transposons/mobile genetic elements)
1984	*G. Kohler and C. Milstein*–monoclonal antibodies and hybridoma – technology *Niels Jerne*–idiotype network hypothesis
1987	*Susumu Tonegawa hypothesis*–genetics of antibody diversity
1989	*J. Michael Bishop and Hanold E. Varmus*–identified first cellular oncogene and characterized it
1990	*J Murray and ED Thomas*–transplantation techniques and immunosuppressant drugs (Performed first successful transplant of living donor kidney)
1993	*Kary Mullis*–development of PCR technology
1993	*Sharp and Roberts*–split genes/gene splicing discovery
1996	*PC Doherty and RM Zinkernagel*–recognition of viruses by immune system. Cell mediated responses.
1997	*Stanley and Pruisner*–discovery of prions
2005	*Barry J. Marshall (auto-infected) and J. Robin Warren* – discovery of **H. pylori** and role in gastritis and peptic ulcer disease
2007	*Mario Capechi, Martin Evans an Oliver Smithies* – creation of 'designer mice' and forged a new science termed 'Gene targetting'
2008	*Luc Montagnier (Pasteur Institute)* – HIV discovery *Francoise Barre – Sinoussi, Herald Hausen* – Role of Human Papilloma virus in cervical cancer
2011	*Ralph Steinman, Bruce Beutler and Jules Hoffmann* – role of dendritic cells in defense and activation of innate immunity
2012	*John B Gurdon and Shinya Yamanaka* – mature cells can be reprogrammed to become pluripotent
2013	*James E. Rothman, Randy W. Schekman and Thomas C. Sudof* – discovery of machinery regulating vesicle traffic, a major transport system in cells
2015	*William Campbell and Satoshi Omura* – Discovery of avermectin, a drug that kills roundworms *Youyou Tu* – Discovery of artemisinin, a drug effective against malaria
2016	*Yoshinori Ohsumi* for discoveries of mechanisms for autophagy

What is the future of medical microbiology?

A.12 The science as currently practised may change to a speciality like Infectious diseases. Individuals who practise this speciality are designated as I.D. [Infectious disease] specialists. In India, the places where it is practised in this form include Hinduja Hospital, Mumbai; CMC, Vellore; Sri Ramachandra Medical Centre, Chennai. Diploma/certificate courses in this area are offered by some institutes in India; as SGPGIMS, Lucknow; School of Tropical medicine, Calcutta and Hinduja Hospital. A D.M. (Infectious diseases) course has recently been started in AIIMS, New Delhi.

In many hospitals of UK, the clinical microbiologist accompanies in the clinical rounds, participates actively in making the diagnosis and initiating the treatment of the cases afflicted with infectious diseases.

Staining Techniques and Microscopy

"The selectivity of the stains was demonstrated in the classic Tulip experiments of Paul Ehrlich"

The relative size of various objects including microbes is depicted in Fig. 1.2.1. For many centuries the existence of the microbes was a mystery. Their existence started unfolding with the use of simple microscope by Antony van Leeuwenhoek in the 1600s. The development in the microscopy continues till date with the invention of the scanning tunnelling microscope in 1981 by two scientists in Switzerland. One challenge in the study of the microbes is the transparent and motile character of many microbes. This challenge is partly overcome by the staining techniques. The selectivity of the stains was demonstrated in the Paul Ehrlich's classic 'Tulip experiment' and mice experiments. The development in this field continues with new specific stains getting developed till date ! Let's study these two technologies.

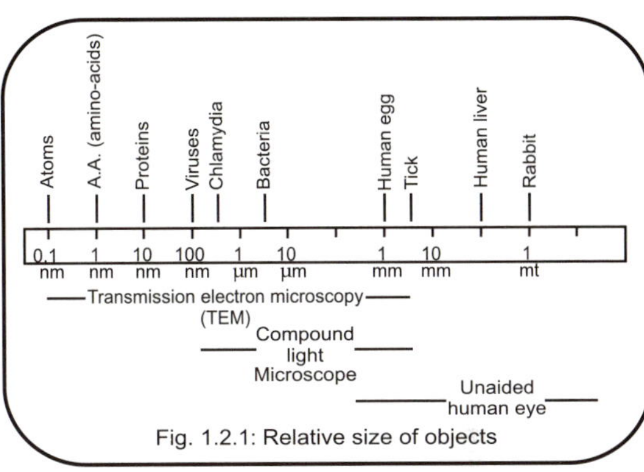

Fig. 1.2.1: Relative size of objects

What is the conventional specialized microbiological technique, used to study microorganisms; especially bacteria?

A.1 Staining the bacteria to be followed by microscopic examination.

STAINING TECHNIQUES

How does staining help in the visualization of microorganisms?

A.2 Bacteria are colourless and have same refractive index of the surrounding liquid, so light microscopic examination with unstained preparations have difficulty in providing much information, about the organism.

What is the principle of staining?

A.3 Stains carry colored cations or anions, which can stain the various structures in a microorganism.

What do you understand by positive and negative stains?

A.4 Positive stains have a strong affinity for one or more components of the microorganisms, whereas negative stains cannot penetrate the microorganisms and make them visible by providing a dark contrast or background.

What are acidic dyes? Give their examples and mention their role.

A.5 Acidic dyes have a colored anion and colorless cation, e.g., nigrosin, India Ink, acid fuschin and congo red. They can be used to stain background; for example in negative staining. They stain basic compounds in cell, primarily proteins with positive charge (mainly basic amino-acids).

What are basic dyes and their role in clinical microbiology?

A.6 Basic dyes consist of colored cation with a colorless anion, e.g., methylene blue+ chloride-. These stain the bacterial cell, which is rich in nucleic acid bearing negative charges; as phosphate groups, DNA and RNA.

Give other examples of basic dyes.

A.7 Crystal violet, safranin and malachite green

What is the difference between vital and supravital staining?

A.8 In vital staining, the organisms are not killed; whereas in supravital staining, the organisms are killed. Most of the staining techniques belong to the latter category

What are the common staining techniques employed?

A.9 (i) Simple staining; as by methylene blue

(ii) Differential staining (commonly Gram's staining)

(iii) Negative staining

(iv) Acid fast staining; as India Ink

(v) Impregnation staining (for instance; to increase the thickness of the flagella by silver stains).

What is the principle of simple staining? Give example.

A.10 Staining in which a single stain is used for staining and all the structures are stained with the same color, e.g., Methylene blue

Gram Staining

What information does gram staining confer?

A.11 It gives information on the shape and arrangement of the organism and classifies the bacteria on the basis of the gram stain.

Categorize the organisms on the basis of gram reaction.

A.12 Broadly the organisms can be categorized into Gram positive and Gram negative (Fig. 1.2.2).

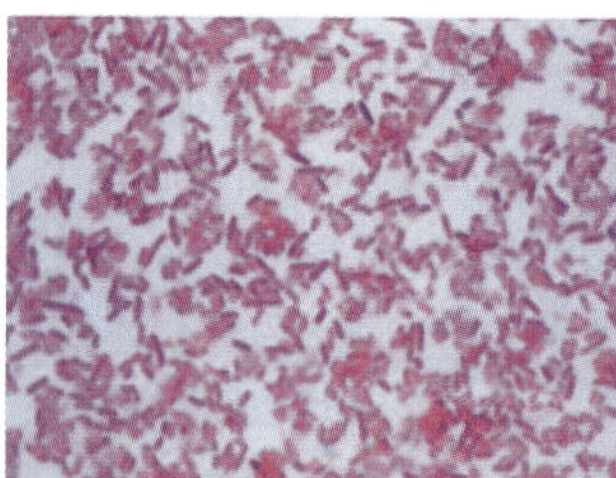

Fig. 1.2.2: Gram stained smear demonstrating Gram negative bacilli

Classify bacteria on the basis of gram stain.

A.13

<table>
<tr><th>Gram positive Bacteria</th><th colspan="2">Gram negative bacteria</th></tr>
<tr>
<td>• All Staphylococci
• All Streptococci
• Pneumococci
• Corynebacterium spp
• Bacillus (Gram +ve or variable)
• All spore forming anaerobes
• Non-sporing anaerobes
Cocci
– Peptococci
– Peptostreptococci
– Sarcina
Rods
– Lactobacillus
– Bifidobacterium
– Propionibacterium
– Actinomyces
• All acid-fast bacilli
– Mycobacterium tuberculosis (difficult to stain)
– Nocardia
• Actinomyces
• Coxiella
• Erysipelothrix
• Streptomyces</td>
<td>• Neisseria
• Non-sporing anaerobes
Cocci
– Veillonella spp.
Rods
– Bacteroides
– Fusobacterium
– Dialister
– Sphaerophorus
• Enterobacteriaceae
• Vibrio
• Pseudomonas
• Pasteurella multocida
• Francisella tularensis
• Haemophilus spp.
• Bordetella spp.
• Brucella spp.
• Borrelia spp.
• Leptospira spp.
• Mycoplasma spp.
• Rickettsiae
• Chlamydiae
• Alcaligenes faecalis</td>
<td>• Bartonella bacilliformis
• Campylobacter fetus, C. pyloridis
• Chromobacterium violaceum
• Klebsiella granulomatis
• Legionella pneumophila
• Spirillum minus
• Streptobacillus moniliformis</td>
</tr>
</table>

What are the organisms, which are stained with difficulty with Gram's stain?

A.14 Spirochaetes and 'atypical' organisms. Also organisms as *M. tuberculosis,* sometimes designated as gram 'neutral' organisms.

What is the common stain used for organisms, which are difficult to stain with Gram's stain?

A.15 Giemsa stain.

Can bacteria give variable results with Gram's stain?

A.16 Yes, certain category of bacteria called 'gram variable' organism do so, e.g., *H. influenzae*, they sometimes get stained as gram positive and sometimes as gram negative

What are the common conditions, when gram positive organisms may appear as gram negative? How do you explain this phenomenon and what is the clinical implication of it?

A.17 Staining of the organisms, after they have been exposed to antimicrobials given during treatment and old age of the culture. The administered antimicrobial can damage the thick cell wall of the gram positive organism; making it lose the iodine complex, rendering the organism gram negative in appearance. Treatment administered provisionally on basis of gram staining of the clinical sample with incorect result, may result in poor outcome.

ZIEHL NEELSEN (Z.N.) STAINING

What are the indications of performing Ziehl Neelsen staining (acid fast) staining?

A.18 Clinical sample likely to be infected with Mycobacteria and Nocardia should be stained with the technique, as the organisms are most likely to be missed, if stained with conventional methods.

What are the conventional categories of organisms stained by the ZN stain and mention the basis of the staining?

A.19
- Acid fast organisms-*M. tuberculosis, M. leprae,* Nocardia spp.
- Acid fast organisms (Fig. 1.2.3) retain the basic fuschin dye after decolorization, whereas the non-acid fast organisms lose the basic fuschin dye after decolorization.

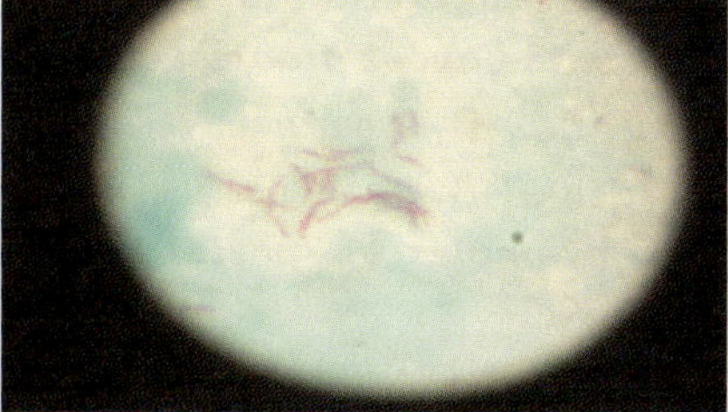

Fig. 1.2.3: Z.N. stained smear demonstrating acid fast bacilli

What is the limitation of studying bacteria after staining them?

A.20 Most of the stains come in the category of supravital staining. So these organisms cannot be studied in the living state, hence functions as motility, metabolism etc cannot be studied.

MICROSCOPY

Why does the study of bacteria require the help of a microscope?

A.21 It increases the resolution of objects, as bacteria, which are in the range of 0.1-10 µm. The unaided human eye can resolve objects more than 40 µm apart (i.e., eye can detect two points, if they are more then 40 µm apart). The organisms are usually in this range – Bacteria from 0.1-10 µm, viruses from 0.03-0.3 µm and Protozoa 4-40 µm

NB: Only bacterium that can be seen with human eye is *Epulopiscium fishelsoni* (600 µm long, lives symbiotically in fish's intestine in reefs of Australia).

Which is the microscope commonly employed in the clinical microbiology laboratory?

A.22 Light (bright field) microscope.

What is the magnification range of this microscope and how can the magnification of this microscope be determined?

A.23 Commonly the range varies between 50-500X (if the magnification of the eye piece is 5X).

The magnification is found by multiplying the magnification of the eyepiece with that of the objective.

NB: 1000 µm = 1 mm

What is the main limitation of the classical light (bright field) compound microscope?

A.24 Resolution is limited.

What do you understand by resolution?

A.25 It is the ability the eye (aided or unaided) to separate close objects to each other, as distinct and separate entities.

On what factors does the resolution of the microscope depend on?

A.26 The relationship of the resolution can be expressed as:

$$\text{Resolution } (\alpha) = \frac{\text{Wavelength of light}}{\text{Numerical aperature of microscope}}$$

What is the usual resolution of a light (bright field) microscope?

A.27 0.2 µm (which means, that it can separate objects more than 0.2 µm apart)

What does increasing the resolution of a microscope mean?

A.28 It means that the microscope should be able to separate object very close to each other (so resolution value should in fact, fall for increase of magnification)

(Numerical aperture indicates the light gathering power of the microscope)

How can resolution of the microscope be increased?

A.29 It can be increased by using light of shorter wavelength or increasing the numerical aperture of the microscope. The former principle is used in electron microscope, where electrons with wavelength of approximately 0.005 nm is used (0.5 µm is approximately wavelength of the bright light). An electron microscope can magnify (about 1000 times a light microscope) 1000,000 times an object.

What are the limitations of studying wet mount (organisms in liquid) in bright field microscope?

A.30 Organism are usually transparent (and) colorless, so despite being big; cannot be demonstrated, unless stained.

How is the above problem overcome?

A.31 (i) By staining the cells
(ii) By using special kinds of microscope

Give examples of special kinds of light microscope used to overcome the problem of transparency of organisms.

A.32 (i) Dark-field microscope
(ii) Phase contrast microscope

Can a light microscope be converted into a the dark ground microscope? Mention its principle.

A.33 Yes. A bright field microscope can be converted into a dark ground microscope, by installing a special dark-field condenser with a central circular stop. Thus, the object gets illuminated with only scattered light rays instead of the transmitted light falling directly on the specimen through the objective lens. So in this microscope, the field is completely dark except for the objects being viewed. This technique makes it possible to observe organism at lower magnification than that would have been possible with ordinary light microscope (of same magnification).

What are the common clinical uses of dark ground microscopy?

A.34 (i) To view extremely thin (slender) organisms; as spirochaetes (not demonstrable) under ordinary light microscope
(ii) To demonstrate microfilaria, vibrio, campylobacter and leptospires in clinical specimens and cultures.

What is the principle of phase contrast microscope?

A.35 A bright field microscope can be converted into a phase contrast microscope by attaching accessories including a special type of condenser. These devices improves the contrast of structure within the organism and the surroundings. Light passing through denser objects are slowed more than the surroundings. The different structures with different densities slow down the light in varying degrees. These differences are converted into differences in intensity of light, producing varying contrast in the image. Thus; though this microscope has almost the similar magnification as a bright field microscope, it makes possible the visualization of organisms and structures that would not be demonstrable otherwise under the same magnification.

What are the clinical uses of the phase contrast microscope?

A.36 (i) To observe living organisms and their movement in unstained preparation, e.g., trophozoites of *E. histolytica, V. cholerae*
(ii) To study the internal structures of large organisms

What is the role of fluorescent microscope in clinical microbiology?

A.37 It facilitates the detection of many microorganisms, as the incriminating pathogen becomes fluorescent and is easily visible to the observer (microbiologist), as a fluorescent structure against a non-fluorescent background.

This facility is often used in laboratories, where the load of slides to be screened is large; as for acid fast bacilli.

What is the principle of fluorescent staining technique?

A.38 The specimen is stained with fluorescent dyes tagged to specific antibodies (which attach to specific antigen) and then observed under UV microscope, where instead of normal light, UV light, illuminates the object. These dyes have a unique property of absorbing U.V. light but emitting a light of higher wavelength in the visible range. The structures are detected by the specific color the fluorescent dyes impart them. Two types of immunofluorescent antibody tests (details in chapter section 2, A9, Pg. 130) are used, namely. Direct and Indirect IFAT are available.

NB: A special filter blocks the passage of any UV light from the stage of the microscope to the observer (which can be harmful).

What is the role of electron microscopy in classical microbiology?

A.39 It does not have much role in the clinical microbiology; as in identification of bacteria, fungi and parasite but is helpful in detection of viruses and in studying the ultra-structural details of all microorganisms.

What are the two common types of electron microscopy?

A.40 One is called transmission electron microscopy (TEM) in which resolution upto 0.5 nm is possible (light microscopy can have resolution of 0.2 μm) The second is the scanning electron microcopy (SEM), in which the surface details of the microorganisms can be studied to give a three dimensional image of the object.

What is the basic principle of an electron microscope.

A.41 In this microscope, instead of ordinary light, a beam of electrons is used to target the specimen. The tungsten filament generates the electrons, which are directed by the magnetic coils. The wave length of electrons is approximately 0.05 nm as compared to 500 nm of visible light. This implies a theoretical 1000 times greater resolution than a light field microscope, but in reality the resolution is 0. 1nm. Here magnetic lens focuses the beam of electron and the specimen is mounted on a metal grid instead of glass slide.

Is there a microscope, which is superior in resolution, in comparison to the electron microscope?

A.42 Yes, in 1981, Gerd Binning and Heinrich Rohrer invented a scanning tunnelling microscope that can map the atoms of a sample. These two scientists received a Nobel prize in 1986 in physics for their invention.

What do you understand by autoradiography?

A.43 It is a technique in which biological material incorporated with radioactive substances is placed on a slide. On X-ray film, a pattern is imaged that is dependent on the pattern of decay emissions.

Section I: General Bacteriology

Morphology of Bacteria

- *Morphology is to function, as geography is to history; it is the backbone.*
- *That one rule #133*
  In biology, you will never truly understand it, until its anatomy is clear.

The small size of bacterium appears to be a disadvantage for its survival. It is not so, as the microbes have colonized most parts of the animate and inanimate world and have existed for millions of years. In fact their small size may provide unique opportunities, for instance their large surface area to volume ratio in comparison to eukaryotes; implies no part of the bacterium is very far from the surface, so nutrients can easily reach all parts of the cell and the toxic substances easily exit the organism. Numerous biochemical and electron microscope studies have revealed their intricate structure and functional complex nature.

The bacterium parts can be categorized into envelope and its appendages and internal core, consisting of nucleus and cytoplasm (Fig. 1.3.1). Let's study them.

Hey son! don't eat so much we are rods and you are looking like a coccus!
Rosy Sinha

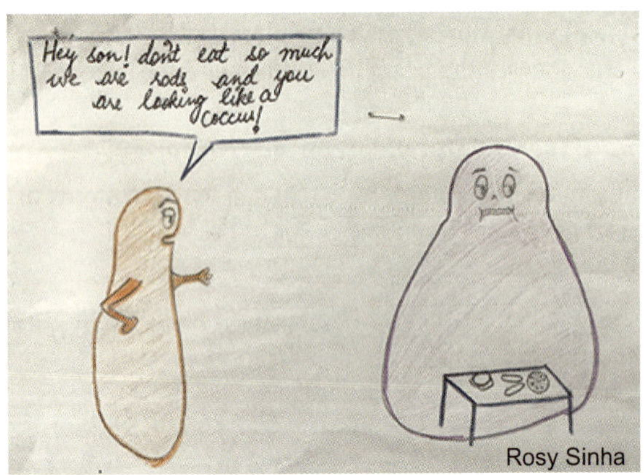

Student cartoon 1A

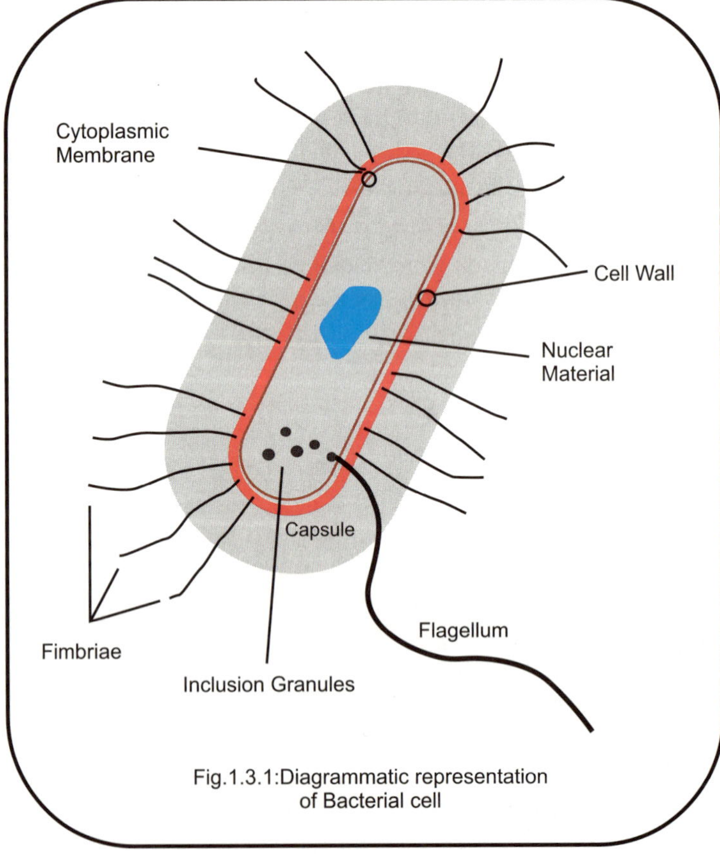

Fig.1.3.1:Diagrammatic representation of Bacterial cell

Tabulate the structural features and functions of different components of bacterium.

A.1

Table 1.3.1(a): A comparison of the structure and function of the bacterial components

	Structure	Demonstration	Function	Importance
CAPSULE or SLIME LAYER	About 0. 2 μm wide, is amorphous, viscid material which surrounds cell wall of some bacteria, when organized in definite structure is *capsule* and when remains loosed, undemarcated secretion in Leuconstoc is known as *slime*	• Gram stain - Not visible(as less affinity for basic dyes) • Negative staining: eg. India-Ink it appears as clear halo around bacterium (Fig. 1.3.2) • Quellung reaction by mixing with specific antisera, becomes swollen	• Protection against bacteria, phagocytes & enzymes • Capsular antigen - haptene in nature and specific • Lost on repeated subculture	• Micropeptide component of cell wall possesses target sites for antibiotics, lysozymes & bacteriophage • Protects bacterium
OUTER MEMBRANE	Seen primarily in gram negative bacteria, consists of lipopolysaccharide molecules	Electron microscopy	Acts as sieve,access is provided by special membrane channels,the porin proteins that span completely across the membrane	Has some antigens and receptor. Vancomycin a bulky antibiotic cannot penetrate this membrane, hence ineffective in GNBs
CELL WALL	• Is a tough rigid structure surrounding bacterium like a shell • Is elastic & freely permeable to solute molecules of <10,000 MW	• Microdissection • Electron microscopy • Antigen- Antibody reaction • Plasmolysis (place in solution with high solute concentration)	• Protects from environment • Protects against osmotic damage • Takes part in cell division by forming ingrowths from cell wall • Forms & other cell wall deficient forms can be responsible for antibiotic resistance and chronicity of disease	Cell wall defective forms can be: • Mycoplasma (display plasticity) • L-form • Spheroplasts (derived from gram negative bacteria) • Protoplast (derived from gram positive bacteria)
	Structural differences between			
	Gram +ve bacteria	In Gram -ve bacteria		
	• **Layers** • Peptidoglycan with teichoic acid • Cytoplasmic membrane	• Outer membrane with surface of lipopolysaccharide • Periplasmic space • Peptidoglycan • Cytoplasmic (Inner) membrane	• Has sites for phages,colicins, complement,antibiotics,antibodies • Has components which, when released into the circulation e.g. lipopolysaccharide are toxic (endotoxaemia) *NB:* Lipopolysaccharide (endotoxin) consists of polysaccharide and lipld A, the latter portion is responsible for toxic properties of gram negative bacilli, which include fever, hypotension etc.	Defective forms can also be responsible for: • Pleomorphism (variation in size and shape) • Involution form • Aberrant form Many antimicrobials for their action act by inhibiting cell wall synthesis Lysozyme destroys bacteria by dissolving peptidoglycan, Predominant lipid cell wall composition of acid fast bacilli make them resistant to conventional dyes Lipids also has protective activity against acids and alkalis Some disinfectants; as alcohols act by action at the cell wall
	• **Thickness:** Thicker	• Thinner		
	• **Lipids:** Absent/Scanty	• Present		
	• **Teichoic acid:** Present	• Absent		
	• **Variety of amino acids:** Few	• More		
	A diagrammatic representation of cell wall of gram positive and gram negative bacteria is depicted in *Fig. 1.3.3, page 16*			
	Peptidoglycan is composed of alternate glycan molecules of N-acetyl muramic acid and N-acetyl glucosamine molecules alternating in chains cross linked by peptide subunits. *(Fig. 1.3.4), page 18.*			

	Structure	Demonstration	Function	Importance
CELL MEMBRANE Internal	• Semi-permeable layer, beneath cell wall, which separates if from cytoplasm • Is composed of 3 layers, central is of protein & on either side are lipid molecules (Fig. 1.3.5), p. 19 The outer ends of phospholipids are charged and hydrophobic in contrast to inner ends which are polar and hydrophilic One of the models to explain the function of cell membrane is the *fluid mosaic model* in which the proteins are dispersed among the phospholipids in fluid forming a mosaic,the proteins can move within the membrane	- Electron microscopy	• Osmotic barrier,actively transports material in and out of cell • Synthesis of cell wall components • Synthesis of numerous enzymes as permease, oxidase involved in active transport of selective nutrients • Respiratory activity (analogous to mitochondria) • Assist in DNA replication	
FIMBRIA (pilus)	• Fine, hair like appendages (0.1-1.5 µm long & 4-8 nm thick) extruding from cell membrane • Composed of protein subunits	• Electron microscopy • Negative staining by phosphotungstic acid • Haemgglutination: Certain fimbriated bacteria strongly agglutinated by RBC's of different species & in some haemagglutination is inhibited by D-mannose	• Common fimbriae: Anchoring of bacterium to nutritional favourable environment, for some part in virulence • Sex fimbriae transfer genetic material from male to female by conjugation	Antisera prepared for bacterial agglutination should be prepared from non fimbriate phase cultures, as sera containing fimbrial antibodies may cause cross reaction
		Differences		
		Common Fimbriae	*Sex Fimbriae*	
	Length	Shorter	Longer	
	Number	40-1000	Few	
	Presence determined by	Chromosome	Episome	
	Role in conjugation	No	Yes	
CYTOPLASM	Colloidal system containing both organic as well as inorganic solutes in a viscous watery solution	Stain	Contains important structures as; nuclear material, plasmids, ribosomes, granules, mesosomes, Inclusions, vacuoles etc.	
FLAGELLUM	Filamentous, cytoplamic long thread like appendages protruding through cell-wall are unbranched, 5-20 µm in length and 0.01 µm diameter • Composed of protein(flagellin) • Has 3 distinct parts (Fig. 1.3.6), p.19 • Filament(lies external to cell) • Hook • Basal body	• Dark ground illumination(some instances) • Electron microscopy • Special staining techniques, in which thickness of flagellum increased by agents; as phosphotungstic acid	Motility: Speed of flagellated bacterium is usually phenomenal, e.g., *E.coli* at rate of 20 body lengths per second Function similar to propeller of a ship	

	Structure	Demonstration	Function	Importance
	Filament is attached to the hook,which is in turn fastened to the basal body,thus anchoring the cell wall and the cytoplasmic membrane • Arrangement (Fig. 1.3.7), p. 19 • Monotrichous - e.g. *V. cholerae* (single flagellum) • Amphitrichous - e.g. *Alcaligenes faecalis* (single flagellum at each end) • Lophotrichous - e.g. Spirillum (tufts of flagellum at both ends) • Peritrichous - e.g. S. Typhi (flagella all around the organism)			
		Flagellum	*Pilus (fimbra)*	
	Size	Longer(5-20μm)	0.1-1μm)	
	Thickness	+++	+	
	Attached to	Cytoplasmic membrane	Cell wall	
	Function	Movement	Adhesion, conjugation	
NUCLEAR MATERIAL	Thin fibril of double stranded DNA helix coiled (inside cytoplasm) about 2 mm long, when straightened Does not possess nuclear membrane, nucleolus. deoxyribonucleoprotein	• Electron microscopy • Acid or ribonuclease hydrolysis & subsequent staining for nuclear material by Feulgen stain(specific for DNA) **Note :** • Since it is not bound to protein, it does not stain like a eukaryotic chromosome • Basic dyes stain whole bacterial cell without any nuclear cytoplasmic differentiation	• Contain all the genetic information of the cell • Undergoes semiconservative replication	Laboratory based diagnostic tests based on detection of specific sequences exist as hybridization assays Nucleic acid used as vector for genetic engineering
PLASMID	• Extranuclear genetic element consisting of DNA (may be multiple)	• Cell lysis & then electrophoresis	Not essential to life of bacterium, unless property acquired gives the bacterium a survival advantage e.g. if plasmid confers resistance in a microbe to certain antibiotic or metal toxin, the microbe can to survive in that environment	Confers properties like • Toxigenicity • Drug resistance (transferable) etc. details see chapter 6, section 17, p. 609.
RIBOSOMES	Thousand of such units may be contained in a cell,appear under high magnification; as fine spherical specs dispersed throughout cytoplasm	Ultracentrifuge processing can isolate these units They are characterized by Svedberg units. Lighter structures are assigned lower S rating. High resolution electron micrography gives information on its shape		

Table 1.3.2: Differences between prokaryotes and eukaryotes

Structure	Characteristic	Prokaryotic cell	Eukaryotic cell
Size (μm)		1	2-100
Cell wall		+	-/+ [when present, then as cellulose/chitin]
	• Muramic acid and Peptidoglycan in cell wall	+	–
	• Sterols	–	+
Cytoplasmic membrane		Has enzymes for respiration, involved in active secretion of enzymes and is sit of phospholipid and DNA synthesis	• No such function
Lysosome		–	+
Pinocytosis		–	+
Nucleus	DNA	Circular	Linear
	Deoxyribonucleoprotein	–	+
	Chromosome number	One	More than one
	True nucleus	–	+
	Nuclear membrane	–	+
	Histones	–	+
	Genetic information on	Single chromosome	Paired chromosomes
Reproduction	Mitosis	–	+
	Production of sex cells	-/+	+
	Cell division	Binary division	Mitosis and/or Meiosis
Biosynthesis	Golgi apparatus	–	+
	Endoplasmic reticulum Ribosome	– +	+ +
		(70S)	(80S)
Respiration	Mitochondria	–	+
Photosynthesis	Site	Cell membrane	Chloroplast
Motility/locomotion	Amoeboid movements	–	+
	Cilia	–	+ / -

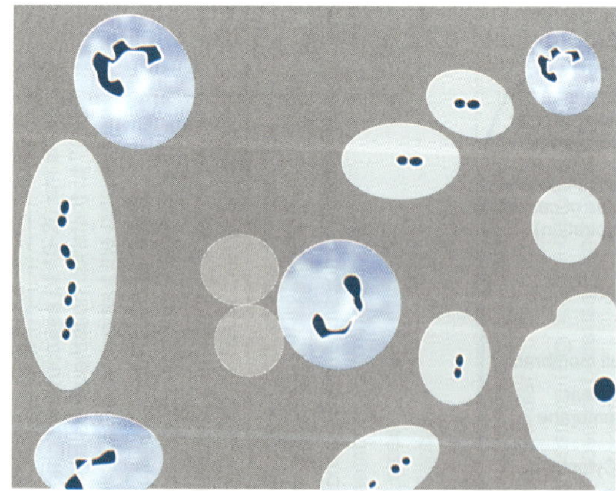

Fig. 1.3.2: A mount of pneumonoccus stained with India ink to demonstrate bacterial capsule

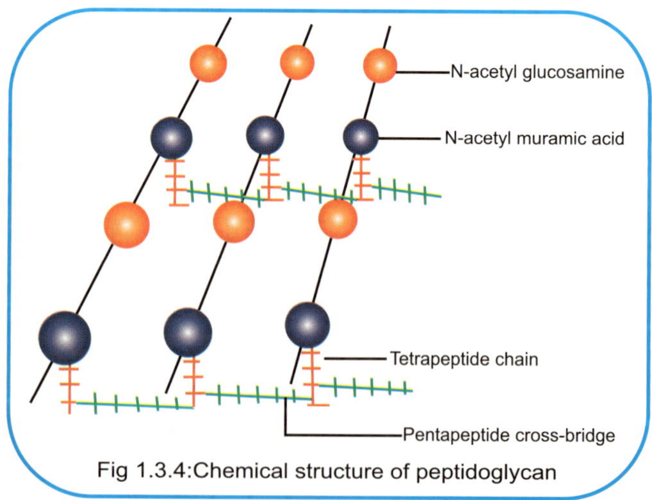

Fig 1.3.4:Chemical structure of peptidoglycan

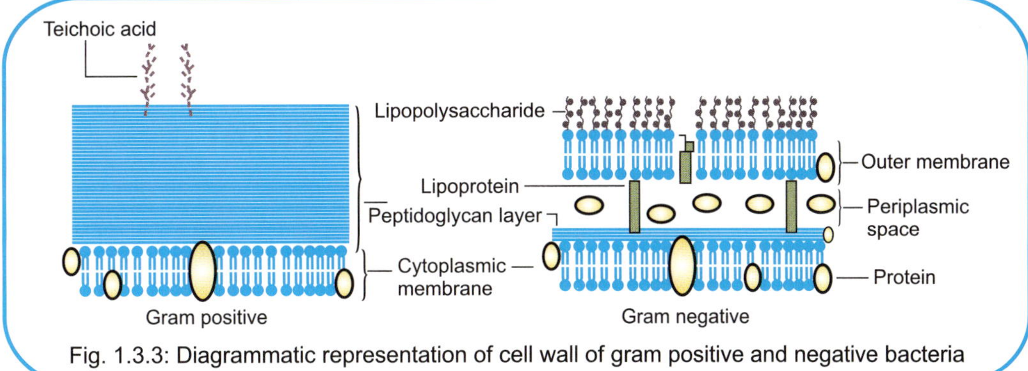

Fig. 1.3.3: Diagrammatic representation of cell wall of gram positive and negative bacteria

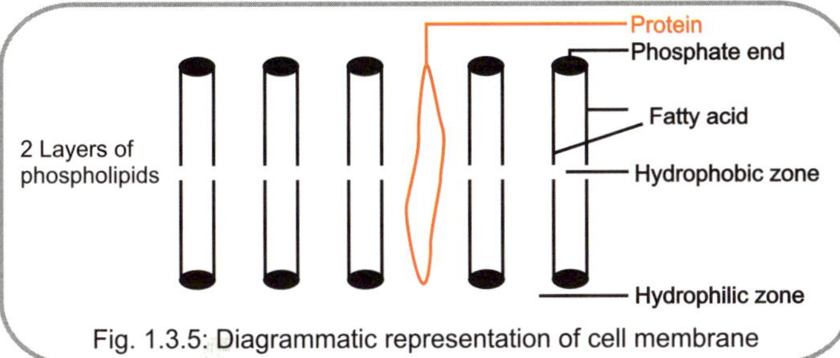

Fig. 1.3.5: Diagrammatic representation of cell membrane

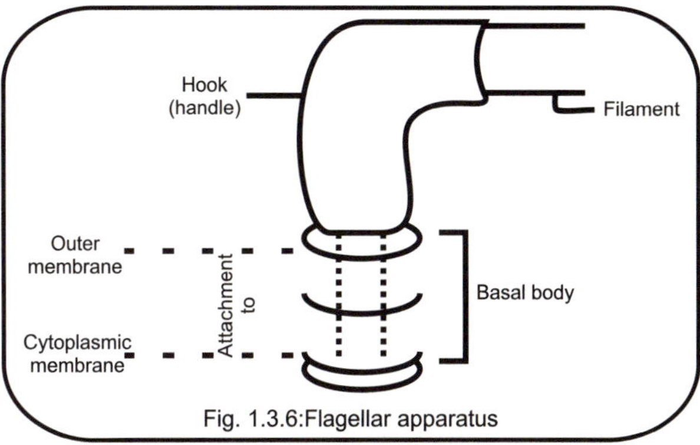

Fig. 1.3.6:Flagellar apparatus

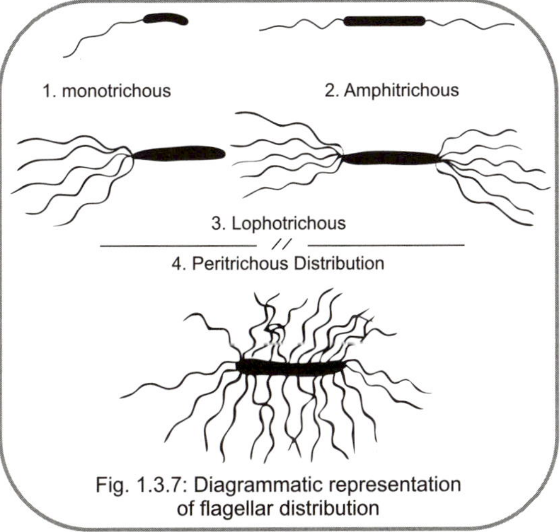

Fig. 1.3.7: Diagrammatic representation of flagellar distribution

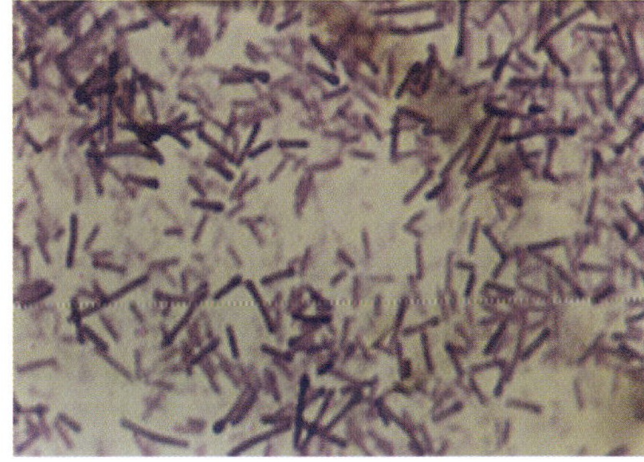

Fig. 1.3.8: Gram stained smear demonstrating gram positive bacilli having spores

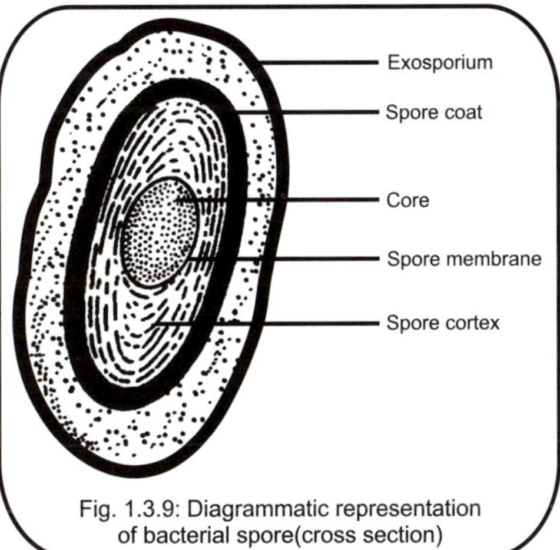

Fig. 1.3.9: Diagrammatic representation of bacterial spore(cross section)

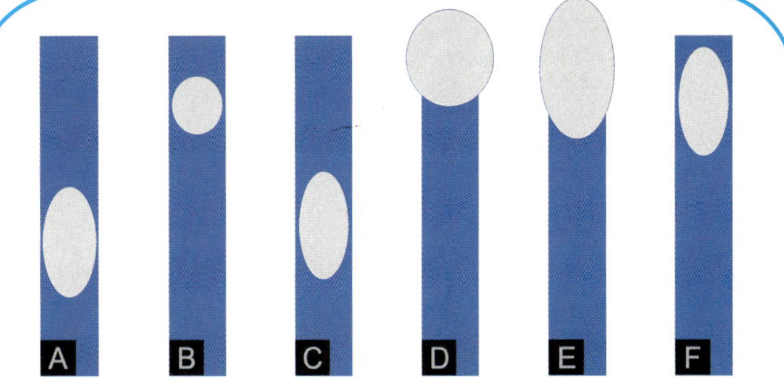

Fig. 1.3.10: Diagrammatic representation of the position and shape of spore A. Bulging, oval and central; B. Non-bulging, round and subterminal; C. Non-bulging, oval and central; D. Bulging, round and terminal; E. bulging, oval and terminal; F. Non-bulging, oval and terminal

Section I: General Bacteriology

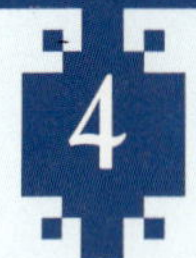

Sterilization and Disinfection

- *Male sterilization procedure-Vasectomy*
- *Autoclaving surgical items-Sterilization*
- *'Soap, water and common sense are the best disinfectants'* — *William Osler*

Let's study this challenging subject, as three integrated clinical based studies.

Integrated Clinical Case Based Study-1

There is an increase in number of cases of *surgical site infections, who got operated in the surgical OT of a leading hospital. Investigations revealed that there was a lapse in the sterilization technique, used to sterilize the drapes, used in preparing the cases in the OT.

***Are infections in the body following surgery**

What procedure is used to sterilize drapes used in the OT?

A.1 (a) Commonly, autoclave (steam sterilizer) is used to sterilize the drapes in a hospital setting (Fig. 1.4.1a). Such items are also available in packaged form, which have been sterilized by ionizing radiation; as gamma rays.

Define the terms: Sterilization, Disinfection and Asepsis.

A.1 (b)
- Sterilization is a process by which an article is made free of all microorganisms (including viruses and spores)
- Disinfection is a process by which an article is freed of all pathogenic organisms except spores.
- Asepsis is a technique to prevent infection gaining to an uninfected site.

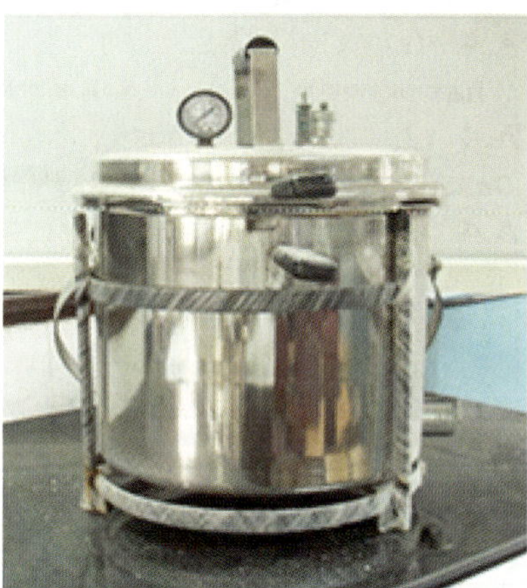

Fig. 1.4.1a: Autoclave

Mention briefly about Antiseptics, sanitation and sanitizer.

A.1 (c)
- Antiseptics are chemicals used on living tissue to prevent infection.
- Sanitation is a process by which bacterial contamination is brought to a 'safe' level (term used for inanimate objects)

  Sanitizer is an agent used during sanitation to reduce number of bacteria to a safe level.

Classify the methods used in sterilization and disinfection.

A.1 (d) Physical methods
- Heat*: (i) Natural-Sunlight
  - (ii) Dry Heat (oxidizes molecules)
  - (iii) Moist Heat (denatures proteins and disrupts hydrogen bonds)
- Filtration
- Radiation
- Gases (as ethylene oxide and formaldehyde)

Chemical methods:

(i) Alcohols (ii) Aldehydes (iii) Phenol (iv) Halogen

(v) Salts (vi) Surface active agents (vii) Dyes

* It is the preferred methods for sterilization, unless the article to be sterilized can get damaged by it.

Mention the broad uses of sterilization and disinfection techniques.

A.1 (e) (i) In surgical and diagnostic procedures (as asepsis)

(ii) In Microbiology for providing sterile media and reagents; besides techniques in processing clinical samples

(iii) In Food and Drug industry for dispensing food and drugs

(iv) In hospital waste management

What type of autoclaves is available to sterilize material of operation theaters?

A.2 They are of three types namely; *Simple, Steam jacketed* (Steam jacket heats side walls of the autoclave independently of the steam, so it facilitates the drying of the load) and *Prevaccum type* (air is removed from the autoclave by vaccum pump, so less time is required for the sterilization).

Commonly the 'Prevaccum' type is used for sterilizing the material used in operation theatre, as faster sterilization of load facilitates the critical working of the OTs.

How can the surgeon ensure that the material that the OT receives is sterile?

A.3 The surgeon/anaesthetist should ensure that the autoclave processing the supplies is having an appropriate indicator control 'test', which it must pass.

Autoclaves use three types of indicators namely:

(a) *Chemical:* Bowie Dick types are frequently used in which appropriate color or design change, indicates that appropriate temperature and conditions were used.

(b) Thermocouple is placed in articles inside the autoclave, with wire outside to the potentiometer to record the temperature.

(c) *Biological:* Ampoules containing spores of *Geobacillus stearothermophilus* are placed in the material to be sterilized. After sterilization, the ampoule is transferred to appropriate medium, incubated at appropriate temperature (55° C) for appropriate time. If growth occurs, it indicates failure of the sterilization process to kill the spores. Spores of this organism require an exposure of 121°C for 12 minutes to be killed.

What is the physical agent used for sterilization in autoclave and hot air oven?

A.4 (a) Moist heat is used in autoclave and dry heat is used in hot air oven

What is the mechanism of action of dry heat?

A.4 (b) Dry heat causes carbonization of the microbial material (destruction of microorganisms)

Describe the methods, which use dry heat for sterilization.

A.4 (c) (i) *Flaming:* It involves passing of an item in naked flame for a few seconds, few times. It is used during handling of glass slides, scalpels and mouth of culture tubes.

(ii) *Red heat:* It involves direct heating of an instrument in direct flame till it becomes red hot. It is a method to sterilize inoculating wires/loops, tips of forceps etc.

(iii) *Incineration.* It uses a high temperature of 800-1000°C for sterilizing and disposing contaminated material by direct burning. Incinerators are frequently installed in hospitals and results in safe destruction of infective material; as dressings, bandages, bedding and other infective material. Air pollution by this system is of concern and polystyrene material should not be fed into this system, as causes extreme pollution (black smoke).

(iv) **Hot air oven:**

Principle: It involves exposure of items at 160°C for 1 hour or 180°C for 30 minutes in an electrically operated oven.

Indications: For sterilizing of glassware such as flasks, pipettes, test tubes, glass petri dishes etc.

- Sterilization of surgical instruments*, forceps, scissors, scalpels.
- Sterilization of swabs
- Sterilization of pharmaceutical products; as liquid paraffin, dusting powder, fats etc.

* As those used in eye surgery (as cutting edge does not get dulled and no corrosion occurs)

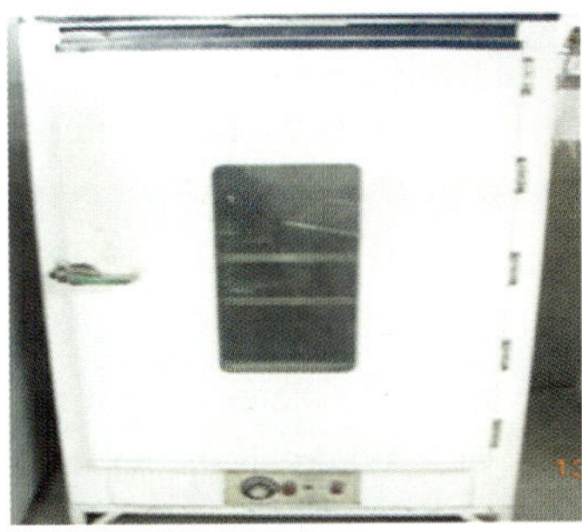

Fig. 1.4.2: Hot air oven

Procedure: Material to be sterilized should be dry and wrapped in paper, placed in a chamber such that free circulation occurs between objects.

- Appropriate temperature allowed to reach and then timing starts
- Material allowed to cool and taken out of the oven.

Precaution: Avoid sudden opening of oven before cooling, as it can result in burns and cracking of glassware.

Sterilization controls: Physical, Chemical and Biological (*Bacillus subtilis*) (see A3; above)

Describe the methods, which use moist heat for sterilization.

A.4 (d) (i) **Temperatures below 100°C**

- *Pasteurization:* This method was originally used for wines. Now it is most often used for milk but it is also used for beer and other items; as eggs. The three common techniques are:

Holder method-63°C for 30 minutes (*Coxiella burnetii* is resistant to this process)

Flash method-72°C for 20 seconds, followed by rapid cooling to 13°C or lower.

Ultra heat treated (UHT); It raises the temperature from 74°C to 140°C, followed by rapid cooling to 74°C in 5 seconds.

- Vaccine bath: Vaccines are exposed at 60°C for 1 hour in a vaccine bath.
- Water bath: Serum or body fluids are exposed at 56°C for 1 hour in water bath.

Inspissation: This process is used for sterilizing serum or egg media; such as Loeffler's medium and LJ medium. It involves heating in a water jacketed copper box at 80-85°C for 30 minutes for 3 consecutive days. The first exposure kills all vegetative forms and results in germination of spores, not killed. The second exposure kills the newly vegetative forms, resulting from the germination of the spores present on the first day of incubation. The third day incubation destroys any forms not destroyed on the second day of incubation.

(ii) **Temperature at 100°C**

- *Boiling at 100°C:* It is a technique often used at peripheral level health care settings to sterilize items; as glass syringes. The period of boiling varies between 10-30 minutes. The process can destroy most vegetative spores except some spores.
- *Tyndallization:* It is an intermittent sterilization technique in which an item is exposed at 100°C for 30 minutes on three successive days. The intervals between the days results in destruction of the spores not previously destroyed. This method is used in sterilization of serum, eggs or sugar containing media.
- Steam sterilizer at 100°C for 90 minutes

  This method is done in a Koch's/Arnold's sterilizer, in which articles are placed in a perforated tray, through which steam passes. It is used for media as containing sugars, which may get damaged at higher steam temperatures.

(iii) **Temperature above 100°C**

Autoclave: This is the most widely used method for sterilization. This method can be used for any material that is not damaged by heat and moisture. Most instruments, culture media, swabs, heat stable liquids and rubber gloves are sterilized by this method.

Describe the mechanism and principle of steam autoclave.

A.5 Steam acts by coagulating and denaturing enzymes and structural proteins. The technique requires the steam to be able to be in contact with all parts of the load. Ideally the steam should not be too dry or wet and should have less than 3% moisture (Dryness should be 0.9-0.95, value of 1 implying no moisture). The advantage of steam is that: it is economically generated, has great penetration abilty, immense energy in latent form and is clean, i.e., does not require purging from items; as in the case of ethylene oxide.

The principle of autoclave is that, when the pressure in a vessel increases, then the boiling temperature in it also increases (water boils, when its vapour pressure equals that of the surrounding atmosphere). Steam when it comes in contact with a cooler surface condenses to water liberating latent heat (1600 ml of steam at 100°C at atmospheric pressure condenses into 1 ml of water liberating 518 calories of heat). The large contraction of volume brings more steam to the same site and the process continues till the temperature of the article is that of steam.

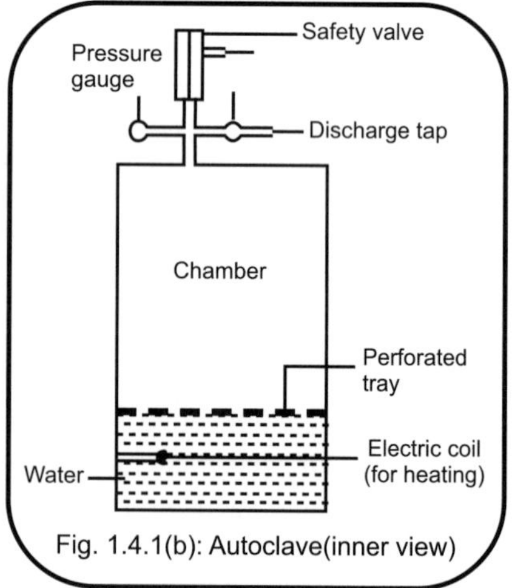

Fig. 1.4.1(b): Autoclave(inner view)

Describe the procedure and precautions in usage of simple autoclave.

A.6

- Water is put in the autoclave (Fig. 1.4.1b)
- The water is heated
- The steam and air mixture is allowed to escape from the valve
- When all the air escapes, the lid is closed (similar to weight in domestic pressure cooker)
- The pressure starts rising in the autoclave, the pressure/temperature is set.
- When the set pressure/temperature is reached, timer is started.

At the recommended temperature of 121°C (15psi/pounds per square inch) the holding time recommended is 15 minutes in contrast to 134°C (30 lb/square inch); the recommended temperature is 3 minutes.

- After the adequate time is reached, the autoclave heater is turned off and the system is allowed to cool till the pressure equals the atmospheric pressure.
- The steam tap is opened slowly and the steam is allowed to escape.
- The lid is opened and the sterilized items are taken out.

Precautions:

- All air should be allowed to escape, otherwise appropriate temperature would not be reached.
- The equipment should never be opened, till it cools down or steam burns can occur.
- The contents should be arranged loosely, so that steam can circulate easily inside the container.

Integrated Clinical Case Based Study-2

A gastroenterologist Dr J.S. Puri has given appointment to four patients in row in his endoscopy clinic in the evening. He has only one 'heat sensitive' endoscope. He wants a minimal waiting period for his cases, after he scopes one patient.

What are the challenges in disinfecting an endoscope? Mention about high level disinfection and decontamination techniques.

A.1 Most of the endoscopes are heat labile. They have narrow lumens and are difficult to disassemble, making cleaning of proteins and debris difficult.

High level disinfection is a process in which the usage of a germicide results in killing (elimination) of all pathogens excepting large number of bacterial endospores, when used according to specifications.

Decontamination is a cleaning process which results in reduction (not elimination) of pathogenic microbes to a level, where the items are 'safe to handle'. The importance of this simple cleaning process is that it results in greater than ≥1 log CFU (colony forming unit) reduction of microbes making a disinfection process easy and effective, as the biological burden has been reduced.

What process can the gastroenterologist subject the endoscope to, so that when the reuses the endoscope, there is no fear of infection being transmitted from one case to another?

A.2 Ideally (desirable) the gastroenterologist should use a sterilization process, but that may not be feasible on account of time constraint, he has. He can use a *high level disinfection* process, in which he can use a fast acting disinfectant, which is effective against most bacteria including tubercle, fungi and viruses. Glutaraldehyde is one such disinfectant that can be used. It is available commercially; as Cidex (2%) and must be activated before use.

How do you define critical and semicritical device according to 'Spaulding classification' of devices? Give example.

A.3 A *critical device* is one that is intended to enter a normally sterile environment, sterile tissue or the vasculature.
e.g., surgical instruments

A *semi critical device* is one that is intended to come in contact with mucous membranes or minor skin breaches.
e.g., flexible endoscope

A *non-critical device* is one which comes in contact with intact skin; as BP cuff and stethoscope.

What is the limitation of various processes in sterilizing the endoscope?

A.4 The technologies involving heat; as a steriliant cannot be used, as the instrument is heat sensitive. Gases; as ethylene oxide cannot be used, as the gas in mutagenic and removing all residual gas from the instrument is time consuming. Using disfinfectants as steriliants would require choosing that are non-deleterious to the delicate instrument and their lenses. The time they would take achieve sterilization would be very lengthy, as a 2% glutaraldehyde would take 10 hours at 25°C to achieve this level.

The gastroenterologist decides to use glutaraldehyde (2%) to achieve high level disinfection of his endoscope. In a hurry to finish his appointments, he just directly dips the endoscope into the disinfectant solution for the disinfection for a minute, before using it on the next case.

What important principle, is the gastroenterologist not aware of, while he follows the above technique?

A.5 (a) One, the gastroenterologist isn't reducing the bioburden (microbial contamination) on the endoscope by simple rinsing techniques, which would make the action of the disinfectant more effective. Secondly; the gastroenterologist is disregarding the duration, the endoscope must remain in contact with the disinfectant to have adequate action. In this case, the period should be about 20 minutes.

What additional step he should follow, before he dips the endoscope in the disinfectant?

A.5 (b) He must wash/rinse the endoscope, before dipping it in the disinfectant.

The next day the gastroenterologist uses the same glutaraldehyde solution to disinfect the endoscope.

What is the limitation of using this disinfectant to act as an sterilant?

A.6 Glutaraldehyde loses its activation after prolonged use. So glutaraldehyde must be dispensed fresh every day and must be activated everyday with alkali for activation. For this agent to act as a steriliant, the contact period has to be extended to many hours.

Aspects related to case theme/examination assessment

What is the broad indication for the usage of disinfectants?

A.7 The most common disinfectants are chemicals.

Indications:

(i) Reduction of microbial contamination of inanimate objects, e.g., room vacated by a TB infected patient, routine processing of wash basins, toilet seats (by hypochlorite solution)

(ii) Disinfection of skin of hand of surgeon and operation site of patient

(iii) Decontamination of objects before disposal, e.g., clinical samples, inoculated media and used slides.

What are the properties an ideal disinfectant should possess?

A.8

(i) Broad spectrum activity

(ii) Not affected by physical agents; as organic matter

(iii) Non toxic, odourless

(iv) Fast acting

(v) High penetration power

(vi) Economical

(vii) Possessing residual effect and should not damage surface of objects.

A disinfectant possessing all these properties is yet to be developed! Depending on the need in a situation, one has to choose a disinfectant.

What are the factors that can influence the potency of the disinfectants?

A.9 The factors include (i) Temperature (ii) pH (iii) Time of action (iv) Concentration of the disinfectant (v) Nature of the dilutant (vi) Nature of microbes in the article to be disinfected (vii) Presence of organic matter.

Classify and describe important disinfectants.

A.10 ALCOHOLS

Types: (i) Ethyl alcohol (ii) Isopropyl alcohol

Mechanism: Denatures bacterial protein

Action (Spectrum) – Acts on bacteria including *M. tuberculosis*

– Not sporicidal or virucidal

Uses: On skin, ethyl alcohol in concentration of 60-70% is used; as it is more effective than 100% concentration, as water is essential for its action.

Isopropyl alcohol is superior than ethyl alcohol; as it is a better fat soluble, more bactericidal and is less volatile.

ALDEHYDES – *Formaldehyde* (employed in both liquid and gaseous states)

– *Glutaraldehyde:* It is an alkylating agent (disrupts proteins).

Glutaraldehyde acts against bacteria, fungi and viruses and requires about 30 minutes for action. It is available as a 2% solution (Cidex) and requires an alkali to be activated, before use. (application A1, 2, 5 of case 2, pg 23-24).

It is an expensive agent. It has no deleterious effect on lenses, so used for disinfection (sterilization) of cystoscopes, endoscopes etc.

PHENOLS

It is bactericidal. In low concentrations, it causes precipitation of the proteins (including enzymes) and damage cell membrane resulting in cell damage.

It has low solubility in water, hence is formulated with soap (e.g., Cresol). At 1% concentration, it is readily adsorbed by skin and mucus membrane, so can cause toxicity.

Types:

(i) *Cresol:* It is toxic to skin and tissues, so used to sterilize glassware, excreta and cleaning floors of wards. It is available as Lysol, which is a solution of cresols in soap.

(ii) *Chloroxylenol:* It is an ingredient of Dettol. It is inactivated by organic matter and is inactive against *Pseudomonas aeruginosa*.

(iii) *Savlon:* It is a combination of chloroheximide and Cetrimide.

It is bactericidal for wide range of microbes including Pseudomonas spp.

It is used in burns, skin disinfection, for surgical instruments and bladder irrigation.

(iv) *Hexachlorophane:* It is used in soaps but because of skin absorption, can cause neurotoxicity. So, it should be used cautiously (with limited exposure) as skin disinfectant, as it has resulted in death of babies.

HALOGENS

(i) *Chlorine:* Is used as a water disinfectant.

Elemental chlorine (**Cl_2**): It is rapidly bactericidal and is an oxidizing agent. It forms hypochlorous acid with water. It is bactericidal and sporicidal but activity influenced by organic matter.

(ii) *Iodine:* Is used as an skin disinfectant.

(iii) *Bleaching powder* (sodium hypochlorite): It is bactericidal, sporicidal, fungicidal and virucidal. It acts rapidly but solution decays rapidly, so should be prepared daily.

It is used as 1% solution and often used for HIV disinfection. It is available and marketed as 3.5% solution. It is to be diluted with 2.5% volumes of water to give a dilution of 1%.

SALTS: e.g., Merthiolate in dilution of 1:10, 000 is used for preservation of sera.

DYES: (i) *Aniline*, e.g., Crystal violet, Malachite green

(ii) *Acridine*, e.g., Acriflavine, Euflavine, Proflavine

CATIONIC DISINFECTANT: e.g., Cetrimide (Cetavlon), Savlon

NB: For preserving cultures a technique known as Freeze drying (Lyophilzation), which involves fast freezing (e.g., putting in alcohol/dry ice) to be followed by drying (subjecting to vacuum) and finally sealing in vacuum. Some of the coffee brands available in the market are also processed by this technique (aroma gets preserved).

Describe tests for testing of disinfectants.

A.11 (i) *Rideal Walker test:* It is defined as a ratio of the dilution of test disinfectant, which sterilizes a test suspension of organism to the dilution of the phenol, which sterilizes the same suspension. This value is designated as the phenol coefficient of the disinfectant (Phenol = 1). So, a phenol coefficient of 1.0 for the disinfectant under testing, implies same effectiveness as phenol, whereas a coefficient of move than 1.0 indicates greater effectivity. The limitation of the technique is that it does not tell, how the disinfectant would function in the presence of organic matter.

(ii) *Chick Martin test:* This test minimizes the limitation of the above technique, as it is performed in the presence of a certain percentage of organic matter.

(iii) 'In Use' test: The 'use' dilution is determined during actual usage, which rarely yield growth.

(iv) *Capacity test (Kelsey and Sykes)*: In it, test organism is added in increments rather than at one time.

Mention about the usage of formalin (formaldehyde).

A.12 Forms: – Aqueous (10% often used)

– Gaseous (commercially gas in water, 40% w/v used)

Uses: (i) Preserve histological tissue

(ii) Sterilize bacterial vaccine

(iii) Killing bacterial culture

(iv) Disinfecting room/OT: Currently this method is not in vogue; as the agent is carcinogenic. For best action of this agent, the environment should have high humidity of 60-80%, at least 18°C and the contact period should be 1-2 days (post application, neutralization of irritant vapor is done by ammonia vapor). The formalin gas is generated by adding $KMnO_4$ to liquid formalin.

Enumerate vapour phase disinfectants.

A.13 (a) The common vapour phase disinfectants are ethylene oxide, formaldehyde gas (mentioned in A.12), Beta propiolactone and vapour phase hydrogen peroxide.

Describe the agent - ethylene oxide

A.13 (b) Ethylene oxide

- *Indication:* Sterilization of plastic and rubber articles; as heart-lung machines, respirators, syringes and dental equipment. This agent has the advantage of great penetrability.
- *Action:* Is effective against all bacteria, viruses and spores.

- *Mechanism of action:* It is an alkylating agent, so alkylates amino, carboxyl, hydroxyl and sulfydryl groups of proteins. It disrupts structure of nucleic acid and proteins.
- *Limitation:* It is an inflammable gas, so is mixed with carbon dioxide. It is also irritant and carcinogenic, so items sterilized with it are flushed with sterile air for 8-12 hours, before packaging the item.
- *Control:* A biological control as *Bacillus globigii* (a variant of *B. subtilis*) is used to test the effectiveness of the process.

Mention briefly about plasma sterilizer.

A.14 Plasma sterilizer: Plasma is the fourth state of matter, the other three being gases, solid and liquid. This sterilizer uses this state of matter, which is gas-like substance consisting of paricles; such as positive ions and electrons.

In a hydrogen peroxide gas Plasma sterilizer, ions are generated from vaporized hydrogen peroxide in a chamber by applying electric current, which generates the ions, electrons and free radicals. The latter agent, sterilizes the item placed in the container. Commercial plasma sterilizers are available in the market.

Integrated Clinical Case Based Study-3

Many households use water purification systems available in their places, as the quality of water supply has deteriorated and reliance on the efficacy of the municipality water treatment facility is not without risk.

What is the commonest principle on which the household water purification systems are based?

A.1 Filtration of water using filters.

What is the composition of the filters used for sterilizing water?

A.2 Candle filters in the form of hollow candles are used, available in different grades of porosity. Two types are commonly available, namely porcelain (hydrous aluminum silicate) and diatomaceous earth filters.

What are the other indications of using filtration sterilization technology?

A.3 Filtration is method used generally used for sterilizing heat labile liquids and air. The following are some of the applications:

Air sterilization (in biosafety cabinets, operation theatre), sterilization of solutions (containing sugar, sera, urea, antibiotics and pharmaceutical products), water purification, detection of small number of bacteria; as S Typhi by passing water through a filter, separating toxins and phages from solutions containing bacteria, obtaining bacteria free samples for virus isolation, sterilization of hydatid fluid (used in Casoni's test).

What is the mechanism by which filters act?

A.4 The fluid to be filtered is is sucked (passed) through a filter by negative pressure with the help of an exhaust pump. Often a filter with the pore size of 0.22 µm is used, i.e., with usage of this filter, particles larger than this get retained on the filter and smaller pass through to the filtrate. With a filter of this size, the bacteria get retained on the filter.

What type of filters are commonly used to sterilize sera or antibiotics for clinical use?

A.5 Membrane (Millipore) filters are commonly used for this purpose. They are made of cellulose esters and their pore size varies between 0.015 to 12 µm. As the name indicates they are in the form of a membrane, which can be placed in an appropriate attachment.

Commonly pore size of 0.22 µm is used. This pore size would hold back bacteria, but would allow viruses and Mycoplasma to pass through, so may not be safe for clinical use.

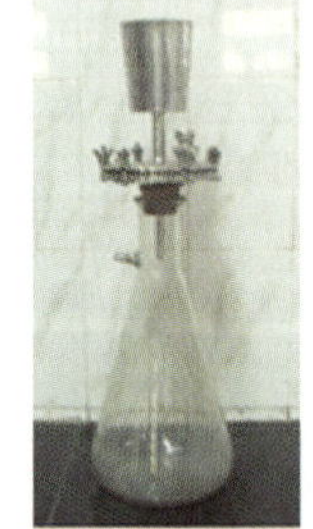

Fig. 1.4.3: Seitz filter

Mention types of filters, other than membrane category in common usage.

A.6
- Asbestos (Seitz) Fig. 1.4.3 – These are made of asbestos (magnesium trisilicate) and are available in different grades. They are put on a metallic disc (perforated) and put in a vacuum flask. After usage are discarded.
- HEPA filters (High efficiency particulate air) are used to sterilize air; as in operation theatre and biohazard safety cabinets in laboratories. It usually removes organisms >0. 3 µm in diameter.
- Sintered glass filters: As the name indicates are made of fine glass particles, which are fused together and graded according to pore size.

Some leading water purification manufacturers use another technology to doubly safeguard the drinking water that is processed by their system

What is the technology used by these manufacturers? Mention its other uses and limitations.

A.7 Ultraviolet light is commonly used to disinfect surfaces. The wavelength between 240-280 nm is most effective and applied for usually 30 minutes. The radiation is also used to disinfect wards, OTs, laboratories (inoculation hoods). The limitation of this light is that, it has limited effect on viruses, causes burns, injurious to eye and causes skin cancer.

Depict the components of the electromagnetic spectrum?

A.8 See Fig. 1.4.4

What method is commonly referred as 'cold' sterilization?

A.9 (a) Ionizing radiation with wavelength less than that of visible light; as X-rays and gamma rays usage is referred to as 'cold' sterilization; as there is no significant increase in temperature of the articles with this technique.

Ionizing radiation have high penetrative power and cause a breakdown of DNA and other cell constitutents.

What is the key indication of usage and indicator used in 'cold' sterilization?

A.9 (b) Ionizing radiation can be used to sterilize heat sensitive items and wherever the penetration potential of these rays may be necessary. The biological indicator used to assess the efficacy of ionizing radiation is *Bacillus pumilus*.

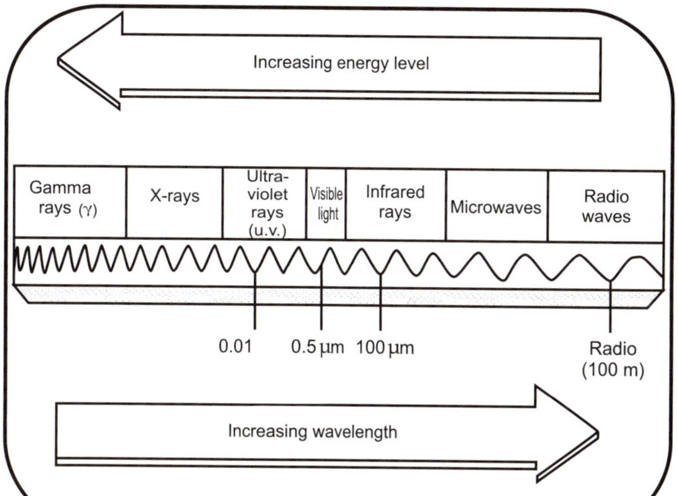

Increasing energy level

Gamma rays (γ) | X-rays | Ultra-violet rays (u.v.) | Visible light | Infrared rays | Microwaves | Radio waves

0.01 0.5 μm 100 μm Radio (100 m)

Increasing wavelength

Fig. 1.4.4:Depiction of the electromagnetic spectrum

What method is commonly referred as 'hot' sterilization?

A.10 (a) Non ionizing radiation with wavelength greater than that of visible light; as Infra red light is referred to as 'hot' sterilization. In this process heat is absorbed by the articles and results in rise of temperature. Ultraviolet rays also belong to the category of nonionizing radiation but its wavelength (approx 390 nm) is shorter than that of visible light.

What are the indications of usage of 'hot' sterilization?

A.10 (b) Infrared radiation is used for rapid sterilization of items; as syringes and catheters.

Tabulate the sterilization/disinfection techniques used for key items.

A.11

Table 1.4.1: Sterilization/Disinfection techniques used for key items

	Material	Method
1.	Metallic inoculating loop/wire	Red Heat
2.	Glassware, syringes	Hot air oven
3.	Gloves, aprons, dressings, catheters, surgical instruments except sharp instrument	Autoclaving
4.	Sharp instruments	5% Cresol
5.	Milk	Pasteurization
6.	Culture media containing serum, sugar or egg	Tyndallization
7.	Toxin, sugar, serum and antimicrobial solutions	Filtration
8.	Rubber, plastic and polythene tubes	Gamma radiation/ethylene oxide gas
9.	Faeces, vomitus, sputum	Disinfectants as bleaching powder, cresols
10.	Disposable syringes, bone and tissue grafts	Ionizing radiations (as infrared)
11.	Sera	Merthiolate
12.	OTs, wards and critical labs	Formaldehyde gas (not ideal)
13.	Polythene tubing, heart-lung machine	Ethylene oxide
14.	Water	Chlorine; as hypochlorite
15.	Skin	Tincture iodine, spirit (70%)
16.	Culture media (most)	Autoclaving
17.	Blankets and woolen material	Formaldehyde gas

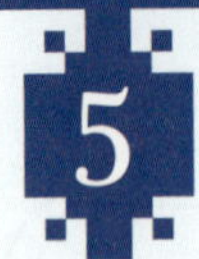

Bacterial Genetics

- *'Genetics is about how information is stored and transmitted between generations'.* — John Maynard Smith
- *'The capacity to blunder slightly is the marvel of DNA. Without this special attribute, we would still be anaerobic bacteria and there would be no music'.* — Lewis Thomas

Genetic engineering techniques has made possible to almost surgically!!! correct some of the cellular defects and cure the diseases at the genetic (molecular) level. One such disease, where success has been achieved is the cystic fibrosis disease, where a functional copy of the '*cftr*' gene is delivered to the human cell. To achieve such successes understanding of the bacterial genetics; including its replication and other related processes is essential. Let's study it in two steps. In the *first step*, the basics of DNA structure and function are analysed (p. 28-34). The second step discusses the processes related to variability in microbes (p. 34-44).

STEP ONE (Basics of DNA Structure and Function) p. 28-34

Mention milestones in the development of molecular biology and recombinant DNA technology.

A.1 Some milestones in the development of molecular biology and recombinant DNA technology.

1869: *Miescher* isolated DNA for the first time.

1944: *Avery* provided experimental evidence that DNA (not protein) carried the genetic information during the studies of bacterial transformation.

1953: *Watson and Crick* proposed the double-helix model for DNA structure, based on the X-ray diffraction studies.

1957: *Kornberg* discovered the enzyme DNA polymerase, which has numerous applications; as in producing labeled DNA probes.

1958: *Meselson* and *Stahl* demonstrated that DNA replicates semi conservatively.

1961:
- *Jacob* and *Monod* proposed the 'operon model' for gene regulation.
- *Marmur* and *Doty* discovered DNA renaturation, which is the basis of the specificity of the nucleic acid hybridization reaction.
- Messenger RNA is uncovered.

1962: *Arber* gave evidence of DNA restriction endonuclease enzyme, which play key role in recombinant DNA techniques.

1966: *H. Gobind Khorana* and *Marshall Nirenberg* elucidate the genetic code.

1967: *Gellert* discovered the DNA ligase enzyme, which participates in joining 'the nick' in DNA fragment.

1970: *Temin* and *Baltimore* report the discovery of reverse transcriptase in retroviruses

1970-73: Work in various laboratories led to a complete gene getting synthesized 'in vitro', first recombinant DNA molecule getting generated and the use of plasmid vector for gene cloning.

1974: Eukaryotic genes are cloned, in bacterial plasmids.

1975: *Southern* developed the southern blot technique for detecting specific DNA sequences.

1975-1977: Methods of rapid DNA-sequencing developed (by Sanger and Barrell & Maxam and Gilbert).

1978: Human genomic library constructed.

1979: Insulin synthesized using recombinant DNA technology, hepatitis B antigen cloned.

1981:
- *Palmiter* and *Brinster* produce transgenic mice.
- Foot and mouse disease viral antigen cloned

1982: Commercial production of genetically engineered human insulin in *E. coli*

1985: Kary Mullis invented the polymerase chain reaction, for which he got the Nobel prize in 1993.

1988:
- The first successful production of a crop of soya bean by recombinant DNA technology.
- Development of gene gun (an instrument that can generate high pressure to deliver an atomized mist of genetic material into skin and other tissues).

1991:
- Development of transgenic pigs which can manufacture proteins; as human hemoglobin.
- First test of gene therapy on man with malignancies.

1996: Yeast genome sequenced

1997: *E. coli* genome sequenced

1998: *M. tuberculosis* genome sequenced

Define the important terms used in molecular biology.

A.2 Terms:

- *Clone:* A population of identical cells, derived from a single ancestor by non-sexual means (especially those containing identical recombinant DNA molecules).
- *Antisense RNA:* An RNA that is the reverse complement of a naturally occurring mRNA, and which can be used to prevent translation of that mRNA in a transformed cell.
- *Auxotroph:* A mutant microorganism that will grow, only if supplied with a nutrient not required by the wild-type.
- *Avidin:* A protein that has a high affinity for biotin and is used in the detection of biotinylated probes.
- *Bacteriophage/phage:* A virus whose host is a bacterium.
- *Biotin:* A molecule that can be incorporated into dUTP and used as a non-radioactive label for a DNA probe.
- *Blunt/Flush end:* An end of a DNA molecule at which both strands terminate at the same nucleotide position with no single-stranded position.
- *Chimaera:* A recombinant DNA molecule made up of DNA fragments of more than one organism, named after the mythological beast.
- *Recombinant DNA molecule:* A DNA molecule created 'in vitro' by ligating together fragments that aren't normally contiguous.
- *Complementary:* It refers to two polynucleotides that can base-pair to form a double-stranded molecule.
- *Recombinant protein:* A polypeptide that is synthesized, as a result of expression of a cloned gene.
- *Cos site:* one of the cohesive single – stranded extensions present at the end of the DNA molecules of certain types of λ phage.
- *Cosmid:* A cloning vector consisting of the λ cos site inserted into a plasmid, which is used to clone DNA fragments up to 40 kb in size.
- *Dideoxynucleotide:* A modified nucleotide that lack the 3′ hydroxyl group and so prevents chain elongation when incorporated into a growing polynucleotide.
- *Endonuclease:* An enzyme that breaks, phosphodiester bonds within a nucleic acid molecule.
- *Exonuclease:* An enzyme that sequentially moves nucleotides from the end of a nucleic acid molecule.
- *Ethidium bromide:* A fluorescent chemical that intercalates between base pairs in a double stranded DNA molecule, used in the detection of DNA.
- *Fluorescence in situ hybridization (FISH):* A hybridization technique that uses fluorochromes of different colors to enable genes to be located (within a chromosome) in a tissue preparation.
- 'In situ' hybridization: A technique for gene mapping involving hybridization of a probe (labeled cloned gene) to a large DNA molecule, usually in a chromosome.
- *Gene:* A segment of DNA that codes for an RNA and/or polypeptide molecule (in RNA viruses, RNA segment would act as the gene).
- *Genetic engineering:* The use of experimental techniques to produce DNA molecules containing new! genes or new combinations of genes.
- *Genetic fingerprinting:* A hybridization technique that detects the organization of highly polymorphic target sequences and which can be produced to produce a banding pattern which is unique for each organism.
- *Horseradish peroxidase:* An enzyme that can be complexed to DNA and used, as a non-radioactive procedure for DNA labeling.

- *Ligase:* An enzyme that repairs single-stranded discontinuities in double-stranded DNA molecules of the cell. Purified form of this enzyme is used in gene cloning experiments.
- *M13:* A bacteriophage that infects *E. coli*, derivatives of which are extensively used in cloning.
- *Origin of replication:* The specific position on a DNA molecule where DNA replication begins.
- *Restriction analysis:* Determination of the number and sizes of DNA fragment produced when restriction endonuclease enzyme is used on a specific DNA molecule.
- *Restriction endonuclease:* An endonuclease that cuts DNA molecules at limited number of specific nucleotide sequences.
- *Primer:* A short single-stranded oligonucleotide, which can act the start point for complementary DNA strand synthesis, when attached by base-pairing to a single stranded DNA template molecule.
- *Promoter:* The nucleotide sequence, upstream of a gene, which acts as a signal for RNA polymerase binding.
- *Template:* A single-stranded polynucleotide able to direct synthesis of a complementary polynucleotide.
- *5′ terminus:* One of the two ends of polynucleotide, which carries the phosphate group attached to the 5′ position of the sugar.
- *3′ terminus:* One of the two ends of a polynucleotide, which carries the hydroxyl group attached to 3′ position of the sugar.
- *Yeast artificial chromosome:* A cloning vector comprising the structural components of a yeast chromosome and able to clone large pieces of DNA.
- *Vector:* A DNA molecule which is capable of replication in a host organism, into which a recombinant DNA molecule (having a gene of interest) is inserted.

Mention about the bacterial genome.

A.3 The bacterial genome consists of a single circular chromosome (excepting *V. cholerae* and *Leptospira icterohaemorrhagiae,* which have two chromosomes), consisting of double stranded DNA, which is approximately 1.6 mm in length; when straightened. It has no nuclear membrane or nucleolus. The bacterial division doesn't occur by mitosis but by binary fission. The study of bacterial genetics has undergone a revolution, since the availability of genomic sequences of many bacteria The first bacterium to be fully sequenced was *H influenzae*. The next challenge was deciphering the code.

Describe the structure of Deoxyribonucleic acid (DNA).

A.4 **DNA:** Each strand of DNA (Fig. 1.5.1) consists of a backbone of deoxyribose sugars, phosphate residues and bases (purine/pyrimidine) attached to the deoxyribose sugar in DNA. The 'double helix' which indicates a twisted ladder like structure was worked up by James Watson and Francis Crick. Two antiparallel polydeoxyribonucleotide chains are wound around each other with the purine and pyrimidine bases on the inside of the helix and the deoxyribose and phosphates on the outside. It is noteworthy to note that it wasn't a pure biological technique that led to the unravelling of the DNA structure but it was the result of interdisciplinary study, which depended essentially on X-ray diffraction studies.

One characteristic of the DNA structure is that the strands have a *polarity* i.e. one end of the strand is different from the other. One strand has a 5 prime (5′) end at the top and a 3 prime (3′) end at the bottom. The complementary strand is oriented in the opposite direction with the 3′ end at top and its 5′ end at the bottom of strand. So, the two strands can be described as being antiparallel. The 5 prime end has a phosphate molecule attached to it's fifth carbon, while the 3 prime end has a free hydroxyl group attached to the 3rd carbon of the deoxyribose sugar. The bases are read conventionally in the direction of 5 prime end to 3 prime end (5′ → 3′), i.e., from the five prime terminus at the left to the third prime end at the right.

The sugar-phosphate backbone consists of 5′-3′ *phosphodiester linkages*, as the 5′ position of one pentose sugar is connected to the 3′ position of the next pentose ring via a phosphate group. The bases of the two strands are linked by hydrogen bonds, which number three between G-C pair and two between A-T pair.

- A base (purine/pyrimidine) linked to a sugar is called a *nucleoside*.
- The combination of a phosphate group to a nucleoside is called a *nucleotide* (or a base-sugar-phosphate complex).
- DNA exists predominantly as a *right handed helix*, i.e., the turns run clock-wise looking along the helical axis.
- The two purine bases are adenine and guanine, whereas the two pyrimidine bases are cytosine and thymine.
- The sequence of the four purine and pyrimidine bases is specific and contains the genetic information for all the activities of the organism.

- Adenine (A) always pairs with thymine (T) and cytosine (C) always pairs with guanine (G). This is the basis for the *Chargaff's rule,* which state that in almost all DNA studied, the proportion of A equals the proportion of T, and the content of C equals the proportion of G. This is also the reason for the *A + T/C + G ratio* being used for classification (phylogenetic) studies, as the ratio is unique for each species. For the same reason, the composition of any DNA can be described by the proportion of it bases namely G + C, which ranges from 26-77% for different species.

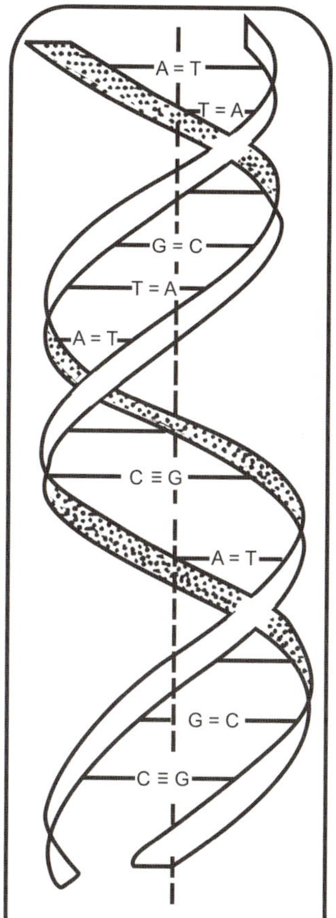

Supercoils are introduced into DNA, when a duplex is twisted in space around its own axis. To give a physical concept of it, you can imagine an already coiled cord of the old landline phone cord having further coils. The property of supercoiling makes the cellular DNA to have a highly compacted structure, yet being able to replicate and transcribe, when necessary by going into a relaxed state. Negative supercoils twists the DNA about its axis in the opposite direction from the clockwise turns of the right-handed double helix. When there is no net bending of the DNA axis upon itself, the DNA is said to be in a *relaxed state*. The double helical chains of DNA have a unique ability to *dissociate* (denature) from one another and to *reassociate* again. This property is necessary for the processes of DNA replication, transcription and the various assays performed in the diagnostic laboratories.

Denaturation implies the rupture of the hydrogen bonds between the bases resulting in the two strands to come apart, which can result from increasing the temperature or exposure to extreme pH. When heat is used to denature DNA, the dissociation of the two strands occurs at a specific temperature and this process is referred to as melting. The term *Tm* is used to denote the temperature at which 50% of the double helix is unwound. The *renaturation (reassociation)* of the DNA strands occurs, when they are exposed to and held at a temperature which is about 20-35°C below the Tm.

Fig. 1.5.1: Structure of DNA

The combination of DNA and proteins is called *chromatin*, as it can be stained by numerous microscopic stains. The DNA in eukaryotes (unlike prokaryotes) is associated with basic proteins called histones and with other proteins called nonhistone chromosomal protein.

Describe the structure of Ribonucleic acid.

A.5 Ribonucleic acid (RNA):

- RNA usually occurs as a single stranded chain and is not as long as DNA.
- RNA differs from DNA in having uracil base; instead of thymine and containing ribose sugar; instead of deoxyribose.
- Three types of RNA exists is a cell; namely messenger RNA (mRNA), ribosomal RNA (rRNA) and transfer RNA (tRNA).
- *Messenger RNA* carries information from DNA for the synthesis of a protein. It has triplets called *codons,* which constitutes the genetic code and it's molecules corresponds to one or more genes of the DNA.
- *Ribosomal RNA* combines with specific proteins to form ribosomes, which serve as sites for protein synthesis.
- *Transfer RNA* is found in the cytoplasm, whose function is to pick up amino acids and transfer them to mRNA. Each molecule has a cloverleaf shape with a specific site for attachment of a specific amino acid. Each molecule has a single triplet of bases called an *anticodon* which pairs complementarily with the corresponding codon in mRNA.

Describe the structural and functional aspects of gene.

A.6 Gene:

Definition: A segment of DNA that codes for a RNA and/or polypeptide or a functional product.

Units: It is expressed as number of base pairs *or* as kilo base pairs (kb), i.e., 1000 base pair units. It is also represented sometimes in Daltons.

Some related terms:

- *Operon*: Is a functioning unit of genomic DNA containing a cluster of genes under the control of a single promoter.
- *Codon:* It is a sequence of three bases storing information for one amino acid.
- *Nonsense codons:* These are codons, which don't code for any amino acids but act as 'stop codon', i.e., for terminating message for the synthesis of a polypeptide egs UAA, UGA and UAG.

- *Intron:* These are intervening regions of DNA between exons, which although are transcribed but not translated. They don't code for polypeptide synthesis. They may occur as depicted below:

Exon	Intron	Exon

Prokaryotes are haploid, as have only one chromosome.

Locus: Position of a gene on a chromosome is called locus.

Allele: Genes with different information at the same locus are called alleles or an alternative form of a gene occupying the same locus.

Homogygous: Both alleles at one locus are the same, e.g., in the ABO blood system, an AA complement represent homozygous character

Heterozygous: Both alleles are different, e.g., an AO complement represents heterozygous character

What is the central dogma of molecular genetics?

A.7 Central dogma of molecular genetics:

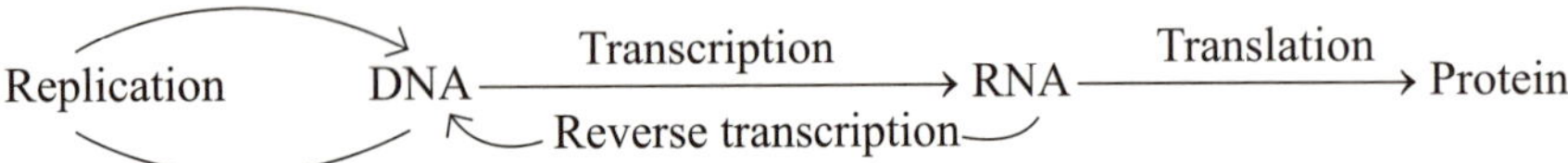

All the information for the cellular division and protein synthesis is stored in DNA (except RNA viruses and prions). The DNA can act as a template for its own replication and for the transcription process. Three major steps are involved in processing of the genetic information. The flow of information from DNA to RNA to protein is often referred to as the *central dogma of molecular biology*. It was once believed that information proceeded only in this direction. Now, we know that genetic information for RNA viruses exist in the form of RNA and for retroviruses the information can also flow from RNA to DNA by reverse transcriptase enzyme and then in the usual flow.

DNA is a master molecule that can control all metabolic processes. If DNA can finally synthesize only proteins (enzymes), then how can it control lipid or carbohydrate metabolism?

A.8 By synthesis of enzymes, which can control fat and carbohydrate metabolism.

Decsribe the process of bacterial DNA replication, transcription and translation.

A.9 DNA replication:

For bacterial division to occur, the event must be preceded by the division of the chromosome into two. In a fast growing bacterium like *E. coli*, the time taken for chromosomal replication would be about 20 minutes, although this process can be affected by several factors.

Before one goes in the details, one must recapitulate the antiparallel structure of the DNA and the fact that DNA synthesis occurs only in the 5′ → 3′ direction.

For understanding sake, the DNA replication can be divided into four stages. In the **first stage**, which is called the unwinding (or relaxation) stage, the supercoiled DNA unwinds, itself. This process is initiated by the enzymes called *topoisomerases*. The enzyme acts by nicking one strand of the DNA, allowing the DNA to become uncoiled in the region of the nick.

The **next stage** of the replication involves the unzipping of the complementary strands of the parental DNA, so that they can act as templates. This process is performed by the enzyme *helicase*. It must be appreciated that the structure of the DNA is quite stable and in the absence of specific enzyme, it takes temperatures close to boiling point to separate the strands. This property of tight and specific interaction between the two strands of DNA is the basis of various DNA and RNA hybridization assays performed in various diagnostic laboratories.

The **third stage** involves the synthesis of new DNA strands. This step is facilitated by the enzyme *DNA polymerase*. For the replication to begin, the DNA must have a special sequence called the replication origin, which must be recognized by the enzyme complex (primosome) that initiates DNA replication. The place where the replication begins; results in separation of the two DNA, which resemble a Y-shaped structure called the *replication fork*. Two replication forks are generated and DNA replication occurs in both directions and the fork moves until the entire DNA molecule strands separate.

For DNA polymerase to carry out synthesis or polymerization of the new strand, it requires a template, a DNA primer (which is hydrogen bonded to the template), a free 3′-hydroxyl on the growing strand and all four nucleoside triphosphates. As DNA polymerase can add nucleotides only to the 3′ end of the growing DNA strand, so only one strand of DNA can serve as a template, called the *leading strand* of the original DNA, It can serve as a template for the continuous synthesis of DNA in the 5′ to 3′ direction. The other strand of the original DNA is called the *lagging strand*, as in it continuous DNA synthesis can't occur. The DNA synthesis in it occurs in short segments, which are later joined by the enzyme *ligase*.

As the two DNA strands are getting synthesized, it is necessary that the supercoiling character of the DNA is restored, this aspect is performed by the enzyme, DNA* gyrase. This type of DNA replication is called semi conservative, as one DNA strand is always conserved.

The *final stage* is the termination of the replication, which results in release of two DNA molecules.

*Fluroquinolone group of antibiotics act by binding to DNA gyrase and preventing the right degree of supercoiling, which interferes with DNA synthesis and results in lysis of bacterium. Bacteria become resistant to fluoroquinolones by mutating their DNA gyrase, so that the fluoroquinolone can not bind to it.

TRANSCRIPTION

The bacterial cell has to continuously synthesize protein to carry out various processes; as growth, repair, reproduction and regulation of bacterial metabolism. For the bacterial ribosome to function, it must receive the genetic message in a format it can read. The ^ribosome can't read a direct template of DNA, it can only read a mRNA •form, which must reach to it.

^ It is a superstructure composed of proteins and ribosomal RNA.

Three types of RNA are synthesized during transcription using DNA, as a template; namely messenger RNA *(mRNA)*, ribosomal RNA *(rRNA)* and transfer RNA *(tRNA)*. Each RNA consists of a single strand of nucleotides.

For transcription to occur, the key *requirements* are a template of double-stranded (usually) DNA, DNA-dependent RNA polymerase (a complex enzyme), all four ribonucleoside triphosphates (i.e., adenosine triphosphate (ATP), guanosine triphosphate (GTP), uridine triphosphate (UTP), cytidine triphosphate and Mg^{2+} or Mn^{2+} ions.

•In eukaryote the mRNA must reach cytoplasm, where protein synthesis occurs; unlike in prokaryote, where no nuclear-cytoplasm differentiation exists.

The process of transcription involves namely, unwinding of DNA strand with binding of RNA polymerase at specific sites, initiation of RNA polymerization, RNA chain elongation and chain termination/release. It must be appreciated that only one strand of DNA can act as template for synthesis of mRNA for one specific gene, the other complementary strand can't perform this function. The central process in this pathway is the attachment of sigma factor at specific sites of DNA called *promoters*. Promoter sequences are found at sites before the start of the DNA, responsible for encoding protein. The sigma factor provides a docking site for the RNA polymerase. The RNA strand synthesis proceeds in the 5′ → 3′ direction with the process somewhat similar to DNA synthesis; except that UTP gets added instead of TTP. The RNA polymerase stops transcribing the DNA segment, when it detects a sequence in the DNA called a *terminator sequence*.

TRANSLATION

Once the gene has been transcribed into mRNA, the information contained in the mRNA is to be converted into a sequence of amino acids, i.e., polypeptide. This function in the bacterium is performed by a 70S ribosome, which is composed of two subunits, namely a large (50S) subunit and a small (30S) subunit. This process is called *translation*, which is a complex one and involves several different enzymes and two additional types of RNA, namely tRNA and rRNA. The latter two types of RNA are coded by DNA, transcribed by RNA polymerase but they don't code for any polypeptides. The *tRNA* is an important molecule which has 2 ends. *One end*, called the anticodon, has three nucleotides complementary to a specific codon (three nucleotides) in the mRNA. The *other end* has a specific amino acid covalently bonded to it. The tRNA is said to be 'charged', if it carries an amino acid and 'uncharged'; if it does not carry one. The number of different tRNA molecules that exist correspond to the number of codons in the genetic code.

The process of translation begins when the 5′ end of the mRNA binds to the ribosome at a special recognition site called the ribosome binding site. The process can be divided into four stages. The *first stage* is called the initiation of translation begins, when the mRNA becomes properly oriented on the ribosome and the reading of the first codon begins. Translation starts, when the first AA tRNA binds the ribosome-mRNA complex. The first AA-tRNA is usually a formyl-methionine in bacteria. So AUG is usually the start codon.

The *second stage* is called the elongation of the polypeptide chain. The assembled ribosome has two aminoacyl-tRNA binding sites, the A (aminoacyl or acceptor) site and the P (peptidyl) site. The first tRNA molecule charged with the amino acid binds to the 'P site', leaving the A site unoccupied. The second charged tRNA molecule, whose anticodon is complementary to the second codon binds to the A site, a reaction known as *transpeptidation*. The amino acid from the P site leaves it and forms a peptide bond with the amino acid on the A site. As the ribosome moves along the mRNA three nucleotides at a time (translocates), the A site comes over the next codon. A new charged tRNA comes at this site. In this fashion, as the mRNA moves, the polypeptide chain keeps growing.

The *third stage* is called the termination phase, which occurs when the ribosome on movement encounters a stop codon, (i.e., UAA, UAG, UGA) which don't code for any amino acid. The protein gets released, the ribosome leaves the mRNA and dissociates into the 30S and 50S subunits. The *fourth* or the *last stage* is the post-translation modification, in which the protein may undergo some folding or any other change.

Describe briefly the genetic code.

A.10 Genetic code: It is the correspondence between the triplet codon in DNA (or RNA) and the amino acids (proteins) they code for. The codon is a triplet of nucleotides that represents an amino acid or a termination signal.

The four bases can form 64 possible combinations from three bases, 61 of these have been assigned to the coding of amino acids and three to stop (chain termination) signals.

The triplet codes are represented in the 5′ to 3′ direction. Most amino acids are coded by more than one codon, i.e., the codon is *degenerate.*

STEP TWO (Variability in Microbes) p. 34-44

Changes in the bacterial genome do occur naturally and have important implications. Rifampicin is a key antituberculous drug used in the treatment of tuberculosis, however it can become ineffective, when *M. tuberculosis* undergoes a mutation in its lone gene coding for the RNA polymerase. Rifampicin acts by binding to beta unit of the RNA polymerase (enzyme participates in the bacterial transcription) present in the *M. tuberculosis* organism. However the change in the structure of the enzyme makes the drug ineffective, as it cannot bind to the enzyme. It is important to study the processes that can result in the variability of the microbial genome and phenotype.

Define the terms phenotype and genotype.

A.1 (a) *Genotype* is defined as the sum total of all the genes in an organism.

Phenotype is defined as the expression of all characters by an organisms in a given environment.

Is it important for the organism to undergo variability in its phenotype and the genotype? Discuss.

A.1 (b) Genetic variability is essential to a microbe for evolutionary purpose and to be able to adapt to changing environmental conditions. It should be realized that an organism must be able to maintain balance between variability and constancy, as the latter characteristic is also important.

Can a change in the organisms phenotype occur by environmental changes, without any change in the genotype? Give examples.

A.2 Yes. Phenotype represents the portion of the genetic potential that is actually expressed by the cell under defined conditions

It is essential to appreciate that the organism's phenotype can undergo changes with changes in the environment only (*without* any change in its genotype). The following are the examples:

(i) Ample amount of sugar in medium may cause some organisms to produce larger capsule.

(ii) Spore formation by *Bacillus anthacis* is unlikely to occur inside host tissue, unlike ample spore formation, when organism is present in outside environment.

(iii) Bacterial capsule usually does not form outside the host.

(iv) *Serratia marscescens* produces pigment at room temperature but mayn't do so at higher temperature.

(v) Pleomorphism usually is seen in an old culture but this character is lost, if the bacterium is freshly cultured.

(vi) S. Typhi; when grown in phenol agar usually loses its flagella and this character is regained, when regrown in an enriched medium.

(vii) Induction of galactosidase enzyme production in presence of lactose environment by *E. coli* (by lac operon).

What its the process by which change in the bacterial genotype occurs?

A.3 Changes in the genotype can result due to mutation, conjugation, transformation, transduction and, transposition. Genotypic changes are rare, usually stable may involve a single/few genes of few organisms in a large population of organisms. This contrasts with the phenotypic changes, which are reversible (revert as environment change back to the original).

Describe mutation.

A.4 MUTATION

It may be *defined* as any change in the structure of the genetic material or more precisely as a random, undirected, heritable change in the sequence of the nucleotides.

The organism carrying the altered gene is called the *mutant.*

An organism carrying the normal (unaltered) gene is called the *wild type.*

Rate: It is defined as 10^{-4}-10^{-12} per bacterium per division, i.e., one can expect any particular gene likely to be mutant in about one in a million cells.

It appears to be a very low mutation rate, but that doesn't mean that mutations are seen rarely. If one takes an agar plate full of bacterial colonies, it will have hundreds of mutations, as each colony has millions of bacteria. Cells in a single colony that contains millions of cells aren't identical because of generation of mutants. All these mutations mayn't be detectable or be of any consequence, is another matter. An 'in vivo' example of above situation would be an active tuberculous lung cavity lesion, which may have millions of acid fast bacilli, some of which may have mutants, that may make the antituberculous treatment ineffective.

It may be expressed as the probability that a mutation occurs in a given gene each time a cell divides and is usually expressed as a negative exponent per cell division.

Types of mutation:

The change in the base sequence of DNA can occur due to addition, deletion or substitution of one or more bases in the nucleotide sequence of DNA. The commonest type of mutation is the incorrect base substitution (i.e., purine or pyrimidine) during DNA synthesis. This may occur when hydrogen atom on the molecules of A, T, G or C change their location, which alters the hydrogen bonding capability of the base. The base substitutions can be of two types namely transition and transversion. In *transition* substitutions, a purine (A or G) replaces a purine and a pyrimidine (C or T) replaces a pyrimidine. In *transversion* substitutions, a purine replaces a pyrimidine or vice versa. A mutation in which a single base pair is changed is called as a *'point' mutation.* The addition or deletion of the bases results in a *frameshift mutation.*

Effects of Mutation:

The consequences of a base insertion or deletion are that it leads to a shifting of the reading frame of the ribosome, which can significantly alter the amino acid sequence or result in a production of a premature polypeptide, due to introduction of terminator codon in mRNA.

The consequences of the base substitution may be no effect, i.e., a 'silent' mutation, as no change in the amino acid sequence specified by the mRNA codon occurs. A different polypeptide may also get provided due to change in DNA resulting in different mRNA codon or even a production of a useless polypeptide, due to creation of a terminator codon in the mRNA.

These mutations can cause microscopic level effect in the bacteria. The gross effect could be manifested; as altered colonial morphology and pigment production. The microscopic effects include altered antigenic structure, drug susceptibility, capsular and flagellar characteristics. *Auxotrophs* (nutritional mutants) that grow only, when a specific (missing) nutrient is provided, also result from mutation.

The effects of the mutation can be silent or even be lethal. An example of the latter category could be a mutation that destroys the function of DNA polymerase, which is vital for the sustenance of the cell. There can be another category of mutants namely *conditional lethal mutants*, i.e., the mutant can be lethal to the cell, only under certain conditions. An example of this category is the temperature sensitive mutants, that as the name indicate can grow at certain temperature. These mutants are of tremendous medical importance, as are used in influenza vaccine. One of the influenza vaccine consists of a strain that can grow at lower temperature of 32°C, which exists in the nose but can't grow at 37°C, a temperature, which is present in the lungs, so pneumonia can't be caused by this strain. This could be explained by the mutation in the DNA polymerase causing this enzyme to be folded unnaturally at a higher temperature, making it ineffective in its functions.

Mutagenesis: It is a process by which a mutation is produced. As mutations occur rarely, organisms in which mutations are being sought for research purposes, need to be treated with mutagens to increase the frequency of mutations to a thousand fold or more.

Induced mutations are caused by many physical and chemical agents called *mutagens,* unlike spontaneous mutations which occur in the absence of any known mutagen and occur by errors in base pairing during DNA replication.

The inducing agents can be classified into two categories namely *physical agents* and chemical mutagens. The list in the former category includes various types of irradiation; as U.V. rays and high-energy ionizing radiations; as X-rays. UV rays attack DNA and result in the formation of pyrimidine dimers. Binding of pyrimidines to each other prevent base pairing during DNA replication, so that a gap is produced in the replicated DNA. X-rays and gamma rays are highly energetic; unlike UV rays and result in production of free radicals, which can damage DNA and result in deletion of bases. UV rays are only detrimental to human skin. These can easily, kill microbes. For this reason, UV light is used in labs and hospitals to kill airborne bacteria, however they lack penetrability.

The common *chemical mutagens* and their effects are depicted in table 1.5.1.

Table 1.5.1: Common chemical mutagens

Mutagen	Effect
Base analogs; as 5-bromouracil Caffeine□	These are chemical structures, which resemble purine or pyrimidine bases closely and get incorporated into the DNA in place of natural bases. These pseudo bases don't have the same hydrogen-bonding properties as the natural bases, so base pair with wrong complementary base
Alkylating agent; as Nitrosoguanidine, *Mustard gas	As name indicates, alkyl groups are added, which alter the shape of base pairing, resulting in error in base pairing
Deaminating agents; as ^Nitrates, nitrites, nitrous acid	As the name indicates, these remove an amino group ($-NH_2$) from bases; as adenine, which then resembles guanine and causes error in base pairing
Intercalating agents; as Acridine orange Quniacrine, Ethidium bromide	As the name indicates, these insert (intercalate) between two base pairs in both strands of the double helix. This results in widened space between bases, which could result in base additions and frame shift mutation. An antimalarial that was used in past Used in labs to isolate plasmids, the label on the container marks it as carginogenic.

^Nitrates (NO_3^-) and Nitrites (NO_2^-) are sometimes added to food; as coloring and flavouring agent, which can be harmful to health.

*Was used in trenches in the World War I and resulted in killing of thousands of soldiers.

□ Caffeine is a purine base analog, that can cause mutations in the unborn child and for this reason, pregnant women are advised to limit or stop their caffeine intake.

Tests for demonstration of mutations.

Mutational (genetic) studies of cells can be performed easily on organisms, that multiply rapidly on simple media and can produce billions of cells in less than 24 hours. In such a big population, every gene can have atleast one mutation.

To identify a mutant bacterium, it is essential to have an established standard for comparison. One should be familiar with two terms for this purpose namely 'wild type' and prototroph. The term '*wild type*', when it was originally used, indicated that it was an organism that could easily survive in the wild, but it could be any type that could be taken as the standard. The term '*prototroph*' would indicate an organism that can grow in a basal medium (minimal medium), whose only organic constituent; as a carbon source, may be only glucose. Such an organism can synthesize all organic substances they need; as amino acids, nucleotides, lipids etc. This is in contrast with '*auxotroph*' (auxo means increase), i.e., an increase in requirements (nutritional mutant), which arise when a prototrophic cell undergoes a mutation in any of its biosynthetic genes and results in the cell getting dependent on the presence of that nutrient in the medium for it's growth.

Laboratory demonstration of mutations:

- Sequencing
- Studying phenotypic changes

  - Gain mutation – synthesis of a new enzyme begins
  - Loss mutation – Synthesis of a functional enzyme stops*
- Qualitative screening for ^rare mutants
  - Drug resistance
  - Phage resistance
  - Fermentative change
- Technique for detecting #large number of mutants
  - Fluctuation test
  - Fermentative test
- Ames test (to detect mutagens)

^Usually spontaneously occurring mutants can be present in a proportion of about one in 10^6-10^7 in a population

#Mutagenic agents can increase the mutant formation 100-1000 fold (process can occur as an enrichment)

*Cell remains enzymatically active due to pre-existing enzyme. The level falls to < 1% after 7 generations.

Fluctuation test:

Mutation of a particular type, let's say drug resistance to streptomycin can occur by induction to this agent or occur independently of exposure to this agent. Making this distinction helps us to understand the microbial genetic mechanisms and metabolic pathways.

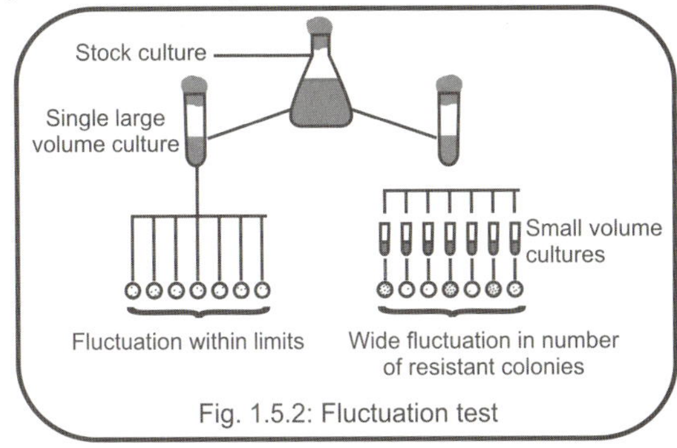

Fig. 1.5.2: Fluctuation test

Luria and Delbruck in 1943 devised an experiment to throw light on this aspect.

The experiment is depicted in Fig. 1.5.2. The number of resistant colonies to streptomycin was counted in a plate, which was subcultured from a large volume of culture fluid in a flask and from plates that were inoculated from small test tubes (none were exposed to streptomycin). There was a wide significant fluctuation seen in the number of strepyomycin resistant colonies in plates subcultured from test tubes. It indicated that drug resistant colonies could arise spontaneously at different times in incubation period and mutants arose *independently* of environmental selective agent, i.e., here of exposure to streptomycin.

Replica plating: (Fig. 1.5.3) This was another technique devised by the husband and wife team of Joshua and Esther Lederberg in 1952, which demonstrated that mutations could arise spontaneously without the need of exposure to the concerned substance. This technique also provides a technique of isolating the resistant organisms. The technique is depicted in the Fig. 1.5.3. The tiny threads of velveteen act like numerous tiny inoculating needles. Before the replicating technique was devised, one had to individually transfer colonies from one plate to another to study the growth characteristics of the colonies, which was a laborious task.

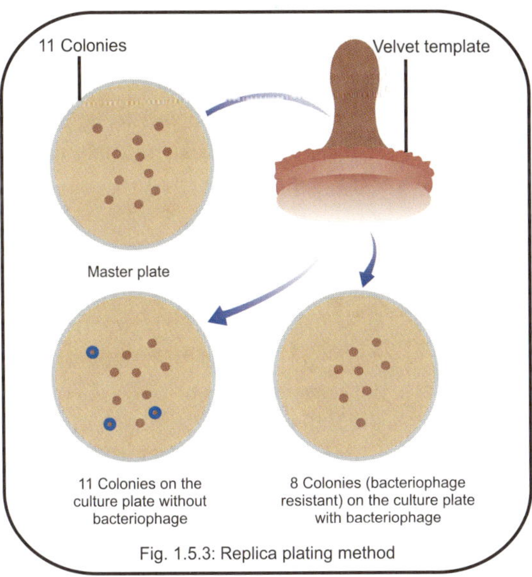

Fig. 1.5.3: Replica plating method

Ames test:

- Devised by Bruce Ames and his team in the 1960s.
- *Basis*: Many substances in the environment; as pesticides, herbicides can be potential carcinogenic substances. The test assumes that there is a relationship between mutagenesis and carcinogenesis. Carcinogens tend to be mutagenic and determining; if a substance is mutagenic could be the first step in labeling it as a carcinogen.

In the test, a mutant strain of a bacterium is used and it is assumed that the rate of its back conversion to the wild type will be significantly enhanced by the presence of a mutagen. The mutant strain could be one as of Salmonella Typhimurium, which requires histidine in the medium in order to grow.

Utility: This test is a good initial screening test. It is an easier and cheaper test than performing the similar test on laboratory animals, which is also time consuming and may take many months to get results.

The *limitation* of the test is that some mutagens mayn't be carcinogenic and further testing would be required; for instance tests in animals, before the agent labeled; as mutagenic by this test, could be labeled; as carcinogenic.

Repair of DNA damage:

Both prokaryotes (including bacteria) and eukaryotes have internal mechanism to repair the damaged cellular DNA, which may occur due to different reasons. Briefly the mechanism can be divided into three categories namely *light repair* (photoactivation), i.e., repair in presence of visible light, *recombinational repair* and *excision repair* (the defective segment is excised, synthesis of the affected part and finally ligation).

One should be aware of a human disease called *Xeroderma pigmentosum*, which is a genetic (transmitted as an autosomal recessive trait) disease, in which the enzymes that normally repair UV damage to DNA are defective and excessive exposure to sunlight; as during prolonged sunbathing can lead to multiple skin cancers.

NB: sunbathers on beaches have tendency to acquire dimers (pyrimidine), as a result of exposure to U.V. light.

NB: Cultures that have been irradiated with U. V. light to induce mutations, must be retained in dark for the mutations to be retained (to prevent light repair to occur).

Describe transformation.

A.5 TRANSFORMATION:

It is the process of uptake of naked DNA from the environment to a cell; as a bacterium. The process does not require cellular appendages and hence no need of the donor and the recipient cell, to be in contact.

Historical: Pioneering work was done by Frederick Griffith, an English microbiologist, while studying pneumococcal infections in mice. It may be recalled that pneumococci with capsule form smooth colonies on inanimate media. They are pathogenic (lethal) to the animal, as the capsule of the organism prevents the antibodies and white blood cells from interacting with the organism and destroying it. This is in contrast to the non-capsulate pneumococci, which form rough colonies, which are non-pathogenic and can't cause pneumonia.

The investigator had surprising results, when a mixture of heat killed capsulated and live non-capsulated bacteria were adminstered into mice. The results were shocking to the investigator, but he couldn't give any explanation to it.

Now we explain it as a process of transformation. The substance that was responsible for explaining the results of the experiment (in mice) in was found to be DNA in 1944 by Avery and McCarty and the process was described as *transformation* of pneumococci. They explained that DNA had the capability of transformation and DNA from encapsulated dead pneumococci could transform the live non encapsulated pneumococci into encapsulated pneumococci. This work laid the foundation to the birth of molecular genetics. At the time of this work, it was not known that DNA carried the genetic information.

NB:
- Mice are considered to be susceptible for pneumococcal infection, as few pneumococcal organisms; when injected into it can multiply in it and kill it.
- *Naked DNA*; is DNA that is not incoroporated into chromosome or other structures

Type of transformation:

1. *Natural:* This type is seen in nature. The natural transformation systems are uncommon in bacteria that inhabit the human or animals. Example of this type is seen in *S. pneumoniae*, *N. gonorrhoeae* (that causes gonorrhoea), *H. influenzae* and *Saccharomyces cerevisae*.
2. *Artificial:* This; as the name implies application of techniques to make organisms transformable that would not naturally accept DNA. The techniques employed include high voltage* electric field (electroporation) and alternate salt and heat shock to force the uptake of DNA. These techniques become necessary, when studying *E. coli,* which isn't naturally transformable, but often used in molecular biology work.

*The current apparently makes holes in the bacterial cell wall and membrane through which the DNA enters.

Mechanism: It is a unique (mysterious) process in which DNA with a high molecular weight can enter the cell wall and membrane of a bacterium. The ability of a cell to be transformed, depends on a transitory state of the cell that allows the foreign DNA to cross the cell membrane. A factor known as competent factor believed to be required for this step, which makes the cell able to be transformed (called competence). The uptake of DNA occurs probably only in a certain stage of cell's growth cycle prior to cell wall synthesis. The cell can apparently take only up to 10 DNA fragments. Some modifications in host cell wall and specific receptor sites on the plasma membrane are apparently required for the binding of the incoming DNA. The DNA of distantly related genera and species is rejected. At the entry sites, the endonucleases cut the double stranded DNA into numerous strands. The single strand invades the resident DNA, seeking a region of sequence homology. Once such a strand is found, the invading strand cuts (excises) the recipient DNA and replaces it with homologous strand of the incoming DNA. The leftover recipient DNA is subsequently broken down.

Importance: The transformation process is seen to occur in nature, but it's likely impact on production of genetic diversity of organisms in nature and other processes isn't completely known. By this process genes coding for capsule, antibiotic resistance and bacteriocin production have been seen to transfer naturally among bacteria.

The artificial transformation process has been used to do genetic mapping (studying location of genes in chromosome) and in gene cloning (as; introducing human gene into bacterial cell)/genetic engineering work.

NB:
- *Transfection*: Process of transfer of DNA into eukaryotic cell
- Another context of transformation implied by cancer biologist is a process; where normal cell gets transformed (immortalized) to malignant cell

Describe transposition (transposon).

A.6 TRANSPOSITION

In the past, it was believed that the arrangement of the genes in the genome of organisms (prokaryotes and eukaryotes) was stable and in the living organism, no change in sequence was possible. It was for this reason that when Barbara McClintock proposed the concept of 'jumping' genes, it was met with scepticism. In 1983, Barbara McClintok received Nobel prize for her work on transposons (also called 'jumping' genes) conducted in corn. Subsequently this process was discovered in Drosophilia. Now it has been detected in all organisms including viruses.

Transposition occurs uncommonly approximately once every 10^5 to 10^7 generation. Transposition can result in genetic recombinations; it can replace damaged DNA, result in change in antigenic characters, pili, pigmentation and colonial morphology and change in flagellar constitution of H1↔H2.

If transposition results in the insertion of a transposon into a functional gene, then it can result in the inactivation of that gene. In fact, it was this basis, by which transposons were discovered. However it can also result in an activation of a dormant function or an overexpression of a gene, if the promoter of the IS integrates with the promoter of that gene.

The transposons can result in bringing about mutations in chromosomes. For this reason, it has also been termed as an *internal mutagenic agent.* It has also resulted in transfer of antibiotic resistance amongst different genera. One of the important example is the spread of amp C gene that encodes a β-lactamase (that inactivates many β lactam antibiotics) in many strains of *Klebsiella pneumoniae.*

NB: ISs may be found; as multiple copies at end of large transposons

Insertion sequences (IS): These are DNA segments that are approximately about 1-2 kbp in size and can move from one site in the DNA of the bacterium and integrate into another site on the DNA. As IS contain only genes for transpositions, their presence is difficult to detect. The unique feature of the sequences is that they can integrate randomly and independently of homologous recombination. This feature is possible because of the presence of *Inverted repeats* numbering about 9-41 on both sides of inverted repeats and the presence of *enzyme transposase* in the middle, which mediates the excision, selection of the target area and integration of the IS. So in transposition one segment of DNA can transfer from one site to another, which has no genetic homology with transposon or recipient DNA.

The IS can duplicate itself, original copy remains at the original site and the new copy can go to the new site or the IS can just move to a new site without duplication.

A unique structure present in the IS is that near their ends, they often have promoters, that are pointing outward, this structure has the property of activating expression of adjacent genes.

Transposon: Fig. 1.5.4(a,b) It is a structure in which two ISs (left and right) flank a chromosomal DNA (which can be a antibiotic resistance gene) and the whole unit moves as a unit from one place to another.

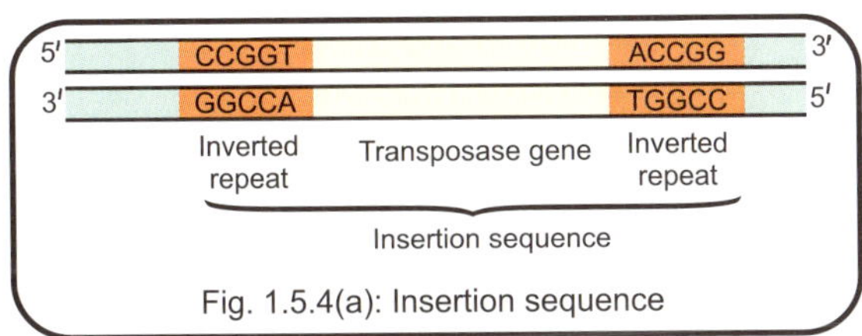

Fig. 1.5.4(a): Insertion sequence

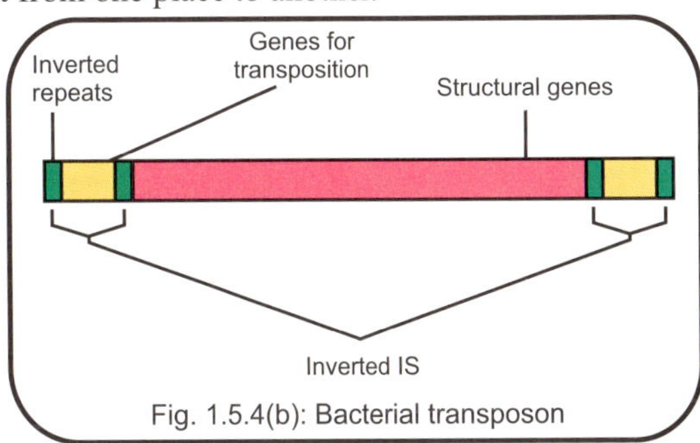

Fig. 1.5.4(b): Bacterial transposon

Integron: These are IS or transposons that have a big cluster of genes that move as a single unit. The uniqueness of the transposons is the ability to move from one site in the chromosome to another, from chromosome to plasmid and vice versa and within the different sites of the plasmid and phages. The mobility of the transposons between different cells increases tremendously, when it get associated with plasmids and especially viruses. Such movement can even occur across different species of prokaryotes and eukaryotes, although transposition is rare and detected with difficulty in eukaryotes.

Describe plasmids (in general).

A.7 (a) **PLASMIDS:** (see clinical problem two in Drug resistance, Pg 615, Section 17)

Are extrachromosomal circular, double stranded DNA molecules, consisting of about 10^3 to 10^5 kb and encoding not less than 50 genes (Fig. 1.5.4(c)).

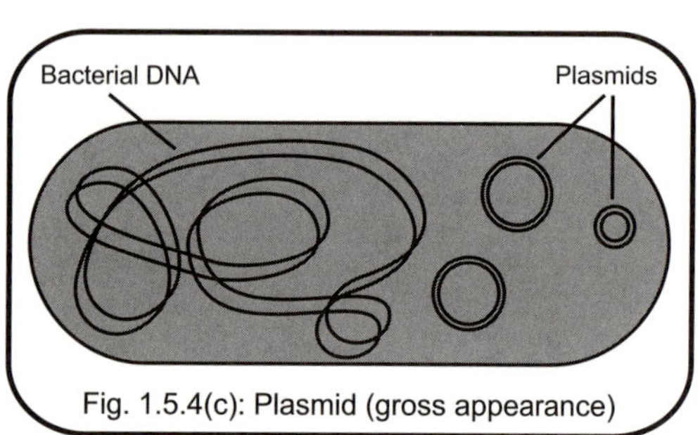

Fig. 1.5.4(c): Plasmid (gross appearance)

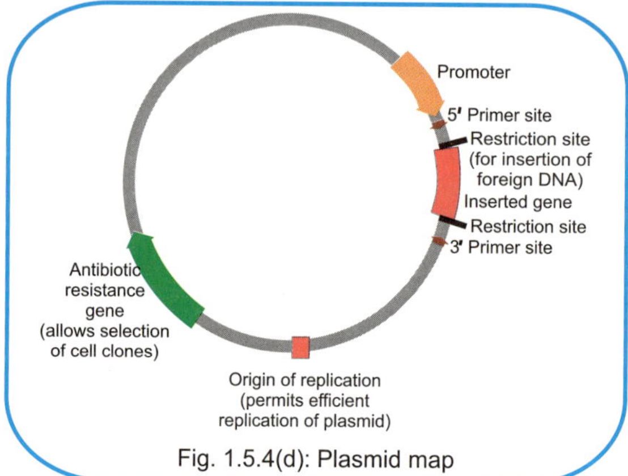

Fig. 1.5.4(d): Plasmid map

They can but do not replicate independently of the bacterial chromosome, as have genes for self replication (Fig. 1.5.4(d). They aren't essential to the survival of the organism, but can have function, that can aid the survival of the organism. Sometimes the plasmids can integrate with the host chromosomes, then they are termed as *episomes*. They are present in both gram positive and gram negative bacteria. An organism carrying plasmid may lose them naturally or when exposed to some agents, this process is called *curing,* e.g., Acridine orange, U. V. light.

Classification: They can be classified on several parameters:

1. Molecular basis
   - Small
   - Large

   This can help in molecular typing of organisms
2. Conjugation basis
   - Conjugative plasmids: if can be (transferred from one organism to another).
   - Non conjugative plasmid: Few copies of it (usually 1-2) are present per bacterium.
3. Functional basis:
   - 'R'-plasmids: named so as carry drug resistance (R) genes (see A7b, below)
   - 'F'-plasmids: named so, as possess a fertility factor, that mediates conjugation. (see A7c, below)
   - 'Col' plasmids carrying colicinogenic (Col) factor that encodes production of colicins, which have specific lethal activity for some organisms, e.g., colicins produced by *E. coli*, pyocyanin produced by *Pseudomonas aeruginosa* and diphthericin by *C. diphtheriae*.
   - Degradative plasmids: E.g., some enzymes secreted by some pseudomonas strain can clean oil spills.
4. Incompatibility basis: To be able to coexist in the same organism, the different plasmids must be compatible.

Role of plasmids:

1. Mediates drug resistance to many antibiotics
2. Production of colicin
3. Synthesis of pili that mediate the colonization (adherence) of bacteria to cell surfaces, e.g., K99 in uropathogenic *E. coli.*
4. Synthesis of exotoxins encoded by plasmids; as exfoliative toxin of *S. aureus*, tetanospasmin of *Clostridium tetani*), haemolysin of *Clostridium perfringens* enterotoxins (LT & ST) of *E. coli*.
5. Also mediates resistance of bacteria to heavy metals present in the environment; as silver and mercury, which helps in their survival in the toxic environment.
6. Production of enzyme urease by *Helicobacter pylori,* which plays part in the pathogenesis of peptic ulcer disease
7. As vector for gene cloning.

Laboratory detection:

The organisms containing plasmids are cultivated (grown) and a cell extract is prepared. The extract is deproteinized, the RNA removed and the DNA is concentrated by ethanol precipitation. Different techniques have to be employed to separate the plasmid DNA, from the large amount of bacterial chromosomal DNA. The separation of the two can be done on basis of size (DNA fragment are large) and conformation basis (most plasmids exist as supercoiled structure). Ethidium bromide caesium chloride density gradient centrifugation is a technique often employed, which is based on the latter principle.

Describe 'R' plasmids.

A.7 (b) 'R' plasmid:

History: They were discovered, when it was detected that common bacteria in gut acquire drug resistance to certain antibiotics. In Japan in 1959, drug resistance transfer between *E. coli* and Shigella was demonstrated.

Spectrum: The resistance has been seen to involve many important antibiotics and have been seen in many pathogenic and commensal bacteria.

Incidence: The prevalence of this plasmid in bacteria varies, but overall an increase in their prevalence has been recently observed.

Role and origin: Charles Darwin proposed selection to be play a major role in the survival of an organism. According to him, those organisms can survive, which can adapt to a changing environment and those that can't adapt to the changed environment, perish. An organism which has the capability of not succumbing to an antibiotic in an environment would have an advantage over those organisms that are sensitive to that antibiotic.

Organisms preserved have been shown to exhibit resistance to those antibiotics, to which they had never been previously exposed, so it was highly unlikely that antibiotic resistance was induced by exposure to those antibiotics. However, antibiotics in an environment contribute to selective survival of strains that contain resistance plasmids over the strains that don't have resistance plasmids (to the antibiotics in the environment).

Spread and structure of 'R' plasmid:

The spread of these plasmids to organisms, not having these plasmids is rapid, i.e. large number of strains not carrying the plasmid quickly acquire it, from the strain with the plasmid.

The transfer occurs readily 'in vitro' and 'in vivo' in intestine. The transfer of resistance plasmids occurs not only within a species but also between closely related genera, for instance 'R' plasmid within *E. coli* easily spreads to other members of enterobacteriaceae; as Klebsiella, Salmonella and Shigella.

The 'R' plasmid consists of two components, namely resistance transfer factors *(RTF)* and '*r*' determinants, which carry one or more resistance genes to antimicrobials or to toxic metals (mercury etc.). The DNA of the RTF resembles to that of the 'F' plasmid, which implies that the transfer of the 'R' plasmid to another organism occurs by the formation of conjugation tube between the donor and the recipient organism. The 'r' determinant could be carrying genes to several antimicrobials, hence simultaneous transfer of many antimicrobials can occur (Fig. 1.5.5).

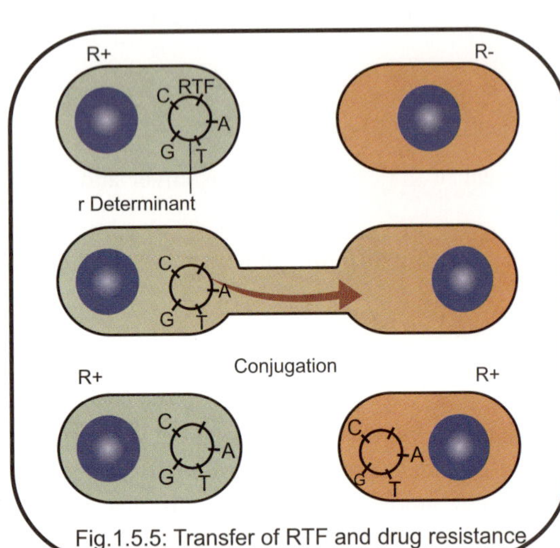

Fig.1.5.5: Transfer of RTF and drug resistance

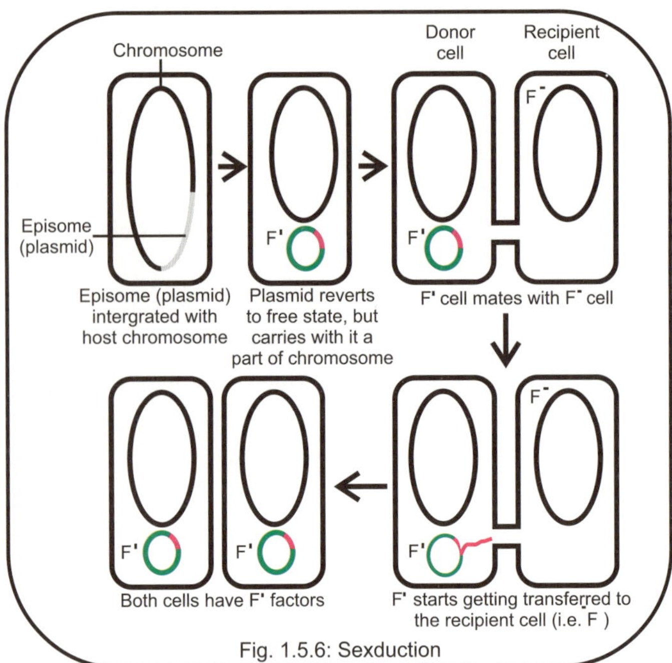

Fig. 1.5.6: Sexduction

Classic example of plasmid mediated drug resistance:

Chloramphenicol was the drug of choice for S. Typhi (enteric fever) for many decades till an outbreak of multidrug resistant (due to plasmid) S. Typhi started in 1989 and peaked in India in 1992-93. This resulted in the change of drug of choice of enteric fever in these areas, from chloramphenicol to ciprofloxacin.

How to halt spread of plasmid mediated drug resistance:

Essentially antimicrobial stewardship programme

1. Proper antibiotic policy: Frequent use of inappropriate antimicrobial can result in increased selection of resistant strains. Hence, it is vital to identify the antimicrobial by susceptibility testing to which the organism is most sensitive, before starting an antimicrobial to treat an illness.
2. Restricted usage of antibiotics: The transfer of plasmids is rapid in the intestines of patients on antimicrobials due to the selection pressure provided by the drug.
3. Prohibit antibiotics in animal feed, as it has been demonstrated that plasmids can spread from animal to human strain.

NB: If RTF dissociates from 'r' determinants in some organism, then resistance can't transfer into another organism, although the concerned organism remains resistant to antimicrobials in healthy individuals.

Describe conjugation with special reference to 'F' plasmid.

A.7 (c) **CONJUGATION**

This process was discovered by Joshua Lederberg in 1946 in *E. coli*. He found that two selective strains of *E. coli,* which couldn't synthesize certain (mutually exclusive) substances (i.e., couldn't be cultivated on a medium that lacked those nutrients) were able to grow on a medium, which lacked all these nutrients, after mixing of these two strains and inoculated onto deficient medium. It indicated, the exchange of DNA between the two strains, leading to complementation of the deficiencies of the two strains.

It refers to a process in which close cellular contact between two bacteria (namely a donor and recipient), leads to a transfer of a large quantity of DNA from the donor to the recipient bacteria. As the process requires cell to cell contact, it is also called *mating*. The process requires that the donor bacterium (also called as male cell) has a plasmid which governs this process rather than the bacterial chromosome. The *donor* (male) cell is able to form sex pili which makes contact with the specific receptor sites on the surface of the *recipient* (female) cell. This adherence between the two cells is important, as a cytoplasmic bridge formed between the two cells is required for the transfer of DNA to be initiated. The DNA transfer is believed to occur through the sex pili, which is a hollow tube.

*occasionally whole chromosome

The process of transfer of DNA gets initiated, when the enzymes associated with the cytoplasmic (mating) bridge makes a single stranded nick in the plasmid at the position of the transfer origin (ori T). One strand of the plasmid starts getting passed on to the cytoplasm of the recipient cell until the entire single stranded copy of the plasmid is in the recipient. As this process is occurring, one strand of the plasmid gets duplicated in the donor cell by the DNA polymerase and a copy of the incoming strand in the recipient cell gets duplicated by the DNA polymerase of the recipient cell. All these functions are performed by a cluster of genes called *transfer (tra) genes*. The recipient cell, which lacks the fertility plasmid (F^-), after conjugating with the donor (F^+) cell; also becomes F^+. The recipient that has become F^+ can now conjugate with other F^- cells and can convert them to F^+.

The F plasmid can integrate into the bacterial chromosome (as a prophage gets integrated) at many possible sites. This process isn't random and specific sites in the chromosome are preferred. Such a strain, where the F plasmid is integrated with the bacterial chromosome is called *HFr strain*, as it can induce highly increased number of recombinations, when the F′ plasmid reverts to free state in comparison to the conventional F^+ and F′ conjugations. When the F' plasmid reverts to the free state, it may carry with it only a part of the F' plasmid with some* additional chromosomal genes.

*In this way an average of ten to twenty percent of the chromosome is transferred, but with this process the entire chromosome may be mapped using a number of different HFrs, whose transferred segments overlap.

Prime (F′) plasmid: The process of integration of the fertility plasmid with the bacterial chromosome can be reversible, i.e., when the F plasmid reverts to the free state, it may again become a 'F' plasmid. However, if the separation is imprecise and it carries with it some chromosomal genes, then the plasmid is referred to as *F′ (F prime) plasmid*. The cells with fertility factor integrated with host chromosome, can transfer chromosomal DNA to recipient cell with high frequency, so also termed as *HFr cells*.

When a cell containing F' plasmid conjugates with a F^- cell, it transfers to the recipient cell, along with the F plasmid (some part) part of the chromosomal genes a process referred to as *sexduction* (Fig. 1.5.6).

A comparison of the selected conjugations is depicted in table 1.5.2.

Table 1.5.2: Outcome in conjugations

Donor	Recipient	Nucleic acid transferred	Outcome
F^+	F^-	F plasmid	F^+ cell
F′	F^-	F′ plasmid with part of chromosomal DNA	F′ cell (sexduction)

NB: Conjugation has also been observed in gram-positive organisms.

Mobilizable transmid: It is a plasmid that has the ability to replicate itself, but lacks the genes to create a cytoplasmic (mating) bridge for the transfer of the genetic material. Hence it requires the presence of the self-transmissible plasmid in the cell which can form the cytoplasmic (mating) bridge between the donor and recipient cell, through which it can transfer the plasmid strand.

Describe transduction (phage).

A.8 TRANSDUCTION:

The phenomenon was discovered in Salmonella in 1952 by J. Lederberg and N. Zinder.

The term is derived from 'trans' which means 'across' and 'ductio' which means 'to pull'.

It is defined as a bacteriophage (virus) mediated transfer of (genetic material) nucleic acid/genes from a donor to a recipient bacterial cell.

Prophage: The integrated form of the phage DNA is called the prophage.

Lysogen: The bacterial cell that harbors a latent prophage (which has the capability of producing phage) is said to be a lysogen.

Lysogeny: The condition of the bacterium harbouring a prophage is termed lysogeny (details A4, p. 389)

Details of bacteriophage, see virology p. 388-390

Highlight the need of control of gene expression and describe the process.

A.9 CONTROL OF GENE EXPRESSION

Bacteria are more versatile than higher organisms in their ability to synthesize most of the organic compound; as carbohydrates, lipids, amino acids and nucleotides. The biosynthetic pathways need to be shut off, when these compounds are readily available in the environment, as less energy would be required to absorb these compounds than to synthesize them. So the concerned enzyme production needs to be turned off. However; when these compounds have to be synthesized, these enzymes need to be turned on. So the bacterium must have the ability to turn on and off in accordance with their needs. Energy, molecules and space are too valuable to be wasted by an bacterium. Bacteria also need to have the ability to adapt to sudden changes in the environment, for which they again have to modulate the gene expression. For instance, bacteria inside a ice cream need survive all changes in environment, when this food is consumed by a human. The bacterium has to survive freezing temperature outside the body but acid hostile environment in the stomach to the varying environment in the small and larger intestines, before their exit to the outside environment.

Operon: It refers to a set of genes that are linked together and transcribed as a single unit, e.g., lac operon

Different mechanisms are available to control gene expression. Generally there are many mechanisms that involve control of gene transcription into mRNA than those that involve control of translation of the mRNA into polypeptide. Two of the mechanisms that have been extensively studied in prokaryotes are *feedback inhibition* and *enzyme induction*. In feedback inhibition as the name indicates, the presence of an end product; as tryptophan (significant level) would inhibit the further synthesis of this amino acid.

The classic example to elucidate of the principle of enzyme induction is the '*operon model*' of French scientists, Francis Jacob and Jacques Monod, who proposed it in 1961 and were awarded the nobel prize for their work in 1965. This concept applies to several operons, but to illustrate the example, we take the case of lac (lactose) operon. This is illustrated in Fig. 1.5.7.

E. coli synthesizes enzymes for lactose metabolism, only if it is present in the artificial medium or in the environment. This phenomenon is called enzyme induction, as the nutrient (here lactose) serves as an inducer of the enzyme production. For the synthesis of enzymes to metabolize lactose, the RNA polymerase must be able to travel from the promoter region to the operator region of the lac operon. The operator region is controlled by a regulator gene, which works in conjunction

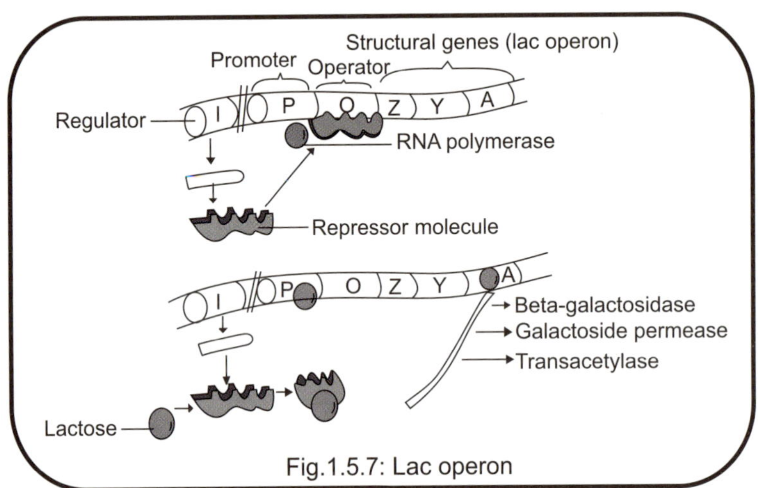

Fig.1.5.7: Lac operon

with the operon, but may be located some distance from it. This gene produces a repressor protein, which when lactose is absent, binds to a specific site on the DNA of the operator site, which is upstream from the promoter region and prevents the RNA polymerase from binding and so preventing the transcription of the operon genes. However, if lactose is present, it binds to the repressor protein, thus preventing the repressor from binding to the operator region, and allowing the transcription of the operon genes to occur. There are three genes in the operon; namely **Z, Y** and **A,** which are transcribed as a single long strand of mRNA. The single mRNA associated with ribosome leads to the production of three enzymes namely β-*galactosidase*, *permease* and *transacetylase;* associated with the **Z, Y** and **A** genes, respectively. The enzyme permease facilitates lactose entry into cells, the β-galactosidase breaks down lactose into galactose and glucose and the function of enzyme transacetylase isn't clear.

NB: The regulator gene is an example of constitutive gene, which is continuously getting transcribed to produce the repressor protein.

Bacterial Growth and Metabolism

- *'What's great about bacteria is you have a surprise every day waiting for you, because they are so fast, they grow overnight.*
- *I think the easiest application to help people understand what quorum sensing is and why it's important to study is to tell them, that if we could make the bacteria either dead or mute, we could create new antibiotics.* — **Bonnie Bassier**

French wine makers in the nineteenth century were losing business, as the wine they were producing was acquiring a sour flavour and was losing its appeal. So they hired Louis Pasteur to solve this problem.

Louis Pasteur concluded after studies that this was occurring due to fruit juice instead of getting primarily converted to ethyl alcohol, was getting converted to acetic acid; which was responsible for the sour flavour. The latter reaction occurred because of the contamination of fruit juice with bacteria. This problem was solved by pasteurization or mild heating of the fruit juice, which killed the contaminating bacteria. This step was followed by inoculation of the juice with the yeast culture. This incident highlights the importance of study of bacterial growth and microbial metabolism. Let's study this aspect in detail.

Describe the process of bacterial division.

A.1 Most of the bacteria undergo cell division by binary fission (unlike eukaryotes where mitosis/meiosis occurs) and in few the cell division occurs by budding (yeasts also undergo cell division by budding). DNA synthesis occurs continuously (unlike eukaryotes, which have cell specific periods of DNA synthesis) and the two strands of the circular double stranded DNA synthesize new complementary strands. The chromosome remains attached to the cell membrane. The dividing cell and the nucleoid appears elongated. A transverse septum grows across the cell membrane and when it is complete separates the organisms into two. The nuclear division precedes the cell division. Incomplete separation of the organism can produce patterns; as short chain, tetrads, sarcinae (groups of eight) or large clusters (as in staphylococci).

Define generation time and explain its importance.

A.2 *Generation time* is defined as the time required for organism to divide into two cells under optimum conditions. The bacteria divide by binary fission. It is a remarkable feat than many organisms; as *E. coli* has a generation time as low as 20 minutes, when cultivated at 37°C in a rich medium. If the division by geometrical progression occurs in this fashion and nutrition is not a limiting factor, a single bacterium can produce 10^{21} bacteria in 24 hours.

One of the *implication* of this fact is that bacteria with longer generation time have to be incubated longer for isolation. For instance; *M. tuberculosis* which has a generation time of 20 hours has to be incubated for weeks to produce colonies in contrast to *E. coli* which can produce visible colonies on solid media in 18-24 hours. One of the bacteria with the longest generation time is *M. leprae,* for which this time is 20 days.

What are the two major components of cellular metabolism?

A.3 Anabolic and catabolic reaction of the cell. *Catabolism* refers to the degradation processes of the food, which result in generation of energy, which can be used for various processes; as organism motility. *Anabolism* refers to the biosynthetic processes, which results in synthesis of molecules; as proteins, DNA and RNA.

Do such bacteria exist in nature that are dependent on their survival on killing of other bacteria?

A.4 Yes, bacterial predators; as bdellovibrios exist.

Classify bacteria on the mode of acquistion of nutrition.

A.5 Basically there are two groups

- *Autotrophs* (use inorganic form; as CO_2 for carbon source)
  - Photoautotrophs – If can synthesize their own food from inorganic substances utilizing light as a source of energy, e.g., cyanobacteria
  - Chemoautotrophs– cannot use light as source of energy but oxidize inorganic compounds for energy production. So use energy and carbon dioxide to synthesize substances; as nitrate, nitrite and sulphate.

    e.g., some Archaebacteria, nitrifying bacteria

- *Heterotrophs* (use organic compounds; as glucose for carbon source)
  - Chemoheterotrophs – cannot use light as source of energy, but use organic compounds for source of energy. e.g., most bacteria, protozoans, helminthes fungi and animals.

Why does one need to study the environmental (physical) factors that can affect growth of bacteria?

A.6 One needs to provide conditions similar to the organisms that they require in their native state, so that they can be cultivated in the lab. Most of the organisms have broad physical range of parameters in which they can survive and proliferate, although the optimal growth may occur under in a small range of conditions. This fact can be appreciated from the fact that microorganisms can inhabit almost all diverse and harsh environments of environment; from Arctic to hot springs. However; there is a group of organisms called *extremophiles,* which as the name indicates can grow only under harsh conditions and do not grow, when cultivated under mild conditions in which most organisms grow. Such organisms have been found in the dead sea, which has a high salt concentration of 30% and at the Yellow stone national park in U.S.A. with temperature as high as 90°C.

What are the environmental/physical factors that can affect the growth of bacteria? Discuss their role.

A.7 (i) *Moisture:* All actively metabolizing organisms require moisture. This is obvious as approximately 80% of bacterial mass consists of water.

Bacteria vary in their capacity of surviving in dry environment. This aspect has an epidemiological importance. Bacteria like *N. gonorrhoeae,* and *T. pallidum* die quickly in dry conditions, whereas *S. aureus* and *M. tuberculosis* can survive for weeks to months in dry conditions.

This factor is employed in *lyophilization* (freeze drying), a technique for preserving bacterial and fungal cultures. Basically in this technique, the organisms in a vial are rapidly frozen, dried (i.e., all water of organism is removed) and sealed under vacuum. This technique is also used in dispensing of certain instant coffee brands, where it helps to maintain the natural flavour of coffee

(ii) *Oxygen requirement*/oxidation – reduction (redox) potential of the culture medium (Eh)

Based on the oxygen requirement of bacteria, they can be categorized into strict (obligate) aerobe, microaerophile, strict (obligate) anaerobe, aerotolerant anaerobe, and facultative anaerobes. This oxygen requirement is related to the *oxidation reduction potential* of the culture media, which is usually about +0.2 volts for media in contact with air in contrast to anaerobic media, which should have an reduced Eh of usually about -0.2 volts. The more oxidized a system, the more positive value it has. Oxidizing potential of a system is measure of its tendency to donate electrons. The redox potential can be measured by the fact that when an unattacked electrode is immersed into solution, an electrode potential difference is set up between the electrode and solution, depending on the state of the oxidation or reduction of the system.

- *Strict (obligate) aerobes* – Grow (preferentially and profusely) in the presence of (normal) oxygen

  N. meningitidis (some), *V. cholerae,* Acinetobacter spp, Alcaligenes spp, *P. aeruginosa,* Pseudomonas spp. (some), *Flavobacterium meningosepticum,*
- *Microaerophiles* – grow only in the presence of low oxygen concentration, e.g., *H. pylori*

  One of the apparatus to create anaerobic conditions is termed McIntosh and Filde's anaerobic jar (Fig. 1.6.1(a) and (b)).
- *Strict (obligate) anaerobe*–grow only in the absence of oxygen.
- *Facultative anaerobes*–Normally grow aerobically (i.e., can make ATP by aerobic respiration); if oxygen is present, but are capable of growing anaerobically; if oxygen is absent (i.e., metabolism switched to fermentative or anaerobic.
- *Aerotolerant anaerobe* cannot use oxygen for metabolism, but tolerate its presence e.g., *C. histolyticum*

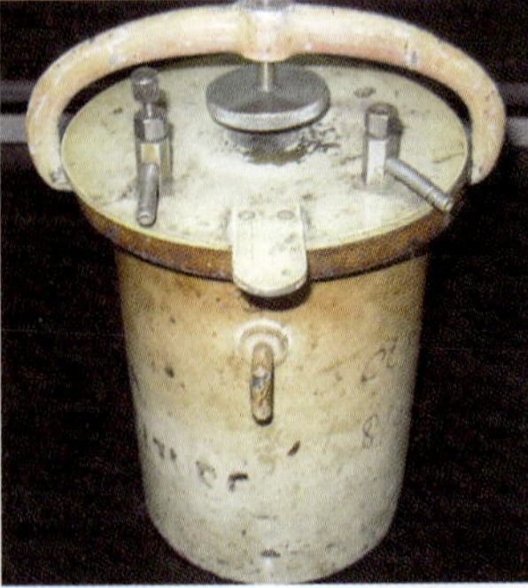

Fig. 1.6.1(a): Mc Intosh Filde's Anaerobic jar

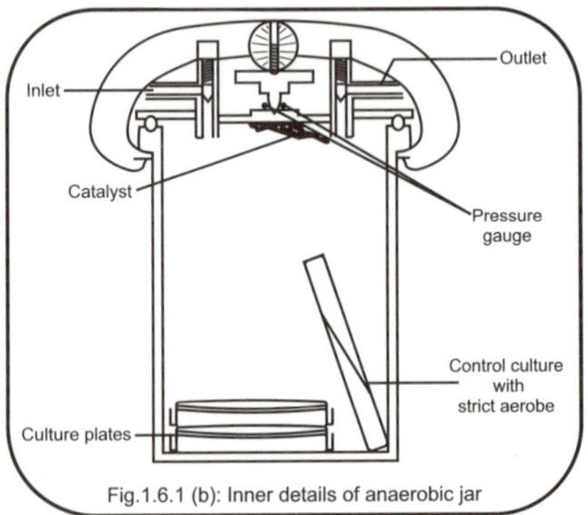

Fig.1.6.1 (b): Inner details of anaerobic jar

(iii) *Carbon dioxide:* All microbes require some CO_2 for their metabolism, which is usually obtained from the carbon dioxide present in the environment. However, some bacteria require an environment with higher carbon dioxide levels in the range of 3-10%, such organisms are called capnophiles, e.g.,

- *S. pneumoniae, N. meningitidis, N. gonorrhoeae, B. anthracis* (for capsulation),
  Brucella abortus (most strains), *B. melitensis* (some strains), Haemophilus spp. (as aphrophilus, paraphrophilus), *M. tuberculosis,* Actinomyces spp., *Gardnerella vaginalis, Erysipelothrix rhusiopathiae* and *Listeria monocytogenes*

The increased carbon dioxide levels are achieved by incubating the inoculated plates in *candle jar or a capnoeic incubator.

*A burning candle is put in a closed small incubator. The lit candle consumes oxygen and increases the carbon dioxide concentration. Such an apparatus is called candle jar (Fig. 1.6.2).

(iv) *Temperature:* Most bacteria have a range of temperature in which they can grow. Within this range, there is an upper and lower limit, at which the organisms do not grow optimally. There is a temperature within this range called optimal temperature; at which the organisms divide most rapidly, i.e., have the shortest generation time.

Bacteria are divided into three major groups depending on their optimal growth requirements, namely mesophiles, psychrophiles and thermophiles.

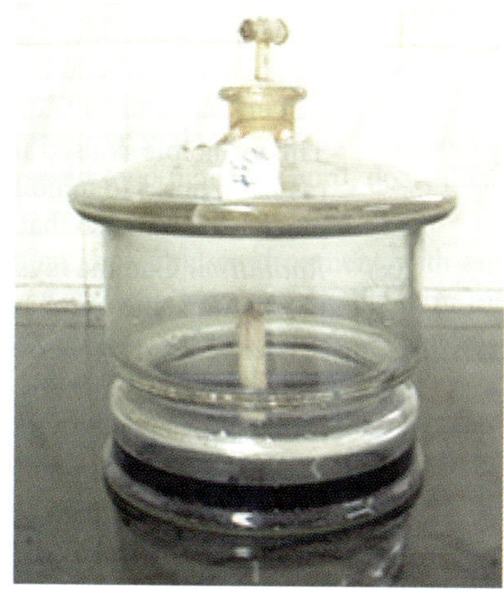

Fig. 1.6.2: Candle jar

Most of the bacteria have moderate temperature requirements in the range of 25°-40°C and are designated *mesophiles*. Most of the human pathogens belong to this category and grow optimally at 37°C, which is the normal human body temperature. The organisms which are cold loving and grow in a temperature range of below 20°C are called *psychrophiles*. Those organisms are rarely pathogenic to man and are mostly found in soil and water including snow bound areas; as Himalayas. The organisms which are heat loving and grow in the temperature range of 45°-80°C are called *thermophiles*. An example; of it is *Geobacillus stearothermophilus,* which grow optimally at approximately 70°C. Another group called extreme thermophiles also exists, in which the organisms have an optimal growth temperature of above 80°C. These organisms are usually isolated from hot springs and erupting volcanos and are often members of Archaebacteria.

The concept has found application in food preservation. As most of the microbes that cause food spoilage are mesophiles, the food items are kept in refrigerators that maintain 4°C. To overcome the problem that psychrophiles can cause at times, food items are also frozen, i.e., kept at temperatures below freezing point.

This concept has also role in the pathogenicity of *M. leprae*, which grows optimally at low temperature, preferentially involves the coolest parts of the body; as feet, finger and ears. Similarly *T. pallidum* affects more the male genitalia (regulated at 32°C), lips and tongue. This principle was also used therapeutically to treat syphilis in the past, where such patients were deliberately infected with malarial parasite. An odd application of the role of temperature on microbes, is few people in Japan put their jeans in freezer and do not wash them, which kills the bacteria and does not make the jeans smell anymore!

(v) *pH:* Most pathogenic bacteria require a pH of 7.2-7.6 for their optimal growth. At pH of 7.0, the number of acidic ions (H+) is the same as the number of basic ions (OH^-, hydroxyl). Most microbes do not grow at a pH more than 1 pH unit above or below their optimum pH. Some organisms can grow within a very narrow range of pH. For instance *Legionella pneumophila* grows well at a pH of 6.85-7.0 and beyond these values is easily killed. To maintain this pH range, media with special buffers are essential.

According to their tolerance for acidic or basic ions, the organisms can be classified into acidophiles, neutrophiles, and alkaliphiles. *Acidophiles* grow best at low (acidic) pH, e.g., lactobacilli, *Helicobacter pylori* and many yeasts and molds.

Most organisms that cause human disease are *neutrophiles*, i.e., grow best at neutral pH (which is neither too acidic nor too basic). *Alkaliphile* grow best at alkaline pH, for example *Vibrio cholerae* and *Alcaligenes faecalis*.

(vi) *Light:* Surprising though it may sound, most bacteria grow well in dark (except phototrophic bacteria). Atypical mycobacteria belonging to the photochromogen category need light for pigment production.

(vii) *Hydrostatic pressure:* It may appear surprising but it is true that certain bacteria can only live at high hydrostatic pressure (e.g., in depth of lake or ocean and die, if kept in the laboratory for few hours at standard atmospheric

7 Culture Media

"Our food should be our medicine and our medicine should be our food (man to provide food in the lab for microbes with the same spirit)."

— Hippocrates

Man must be able to study the role of microbes in disease and other conditions. To achieve this goal, three things must be achieved namely, *I*-cultivation (growth) of the organisms, *II*-isolation (culture) of the organisms (chapter 8) and finally *III*-identification of the organisms (chapter 9).

What is one attempting to do, while cultivating bacteria?

A.1 Basically, one is attempting to simulate the 'in vivo' conditions of the organism in the laboratory, so that the organism can easily be cultivated. This actually does not really occur totally in the laboratory but one attempts to approximate the in 'vivo' conditions of the organism. Since the exact simulation may not many times be possible, so many organisms never get cultivated.

Can the metabolism of an organism be a limit on its cultivation and isolation in the laboratory? Provide a landmark example.

A.2 Yes. Initially it was concluded that *E. coli* was the predominant species of colon, as the cultures were incubated only aerobically. Later it was realized that the colon environment would be anoxic and would have anaerobes. This happened to be true, when the colonic contents were incubated on media, which was heated to expel oxygen and incubated anaerobically. This led to the discovery of Bacteriodes and Peptostreptococci. Bacteriodes spp. happens to be the most predominant organism in the colon,

Are most microorganisms cultivable?

A.3 Surprising it may appear, but most organisms are not cultivable in the laboratory. This fact emphasizes the need of providing appropriate media and environmental conditions in an attempt to cultivate the organisms.

What do you understand by medium (plural-media)?

A.4 They are specific nutrients (liquid or solid form) that can support growth of a group or a subgroup of microorganisms; as bacteria (or fungi)

Broadly what are the physical categories into which the media can be categorized?

A.5
- Liquid media
- Solid media
- Semisolid

What do you understand by 'culture methods or techniques'?

A.6 These are methods used for growing (cultivating) microbes.

What is the key ingredient added to liquid medium to make it solid? How does solid media helps to obtain pure cultures?

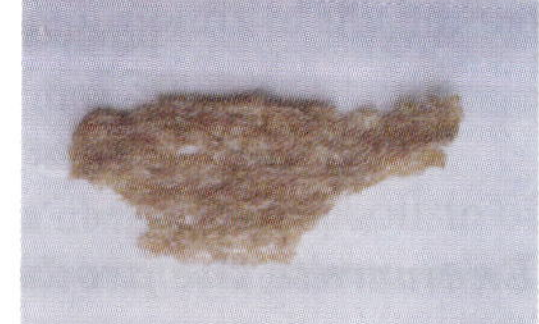

Fig. 1.7.1: Agar shreds

A.7 Agar is added to the liquid medium to make it solid. It is synthesized from agar shreds (Fig. 1.7.1). This agent was suggested to Robert Koch by Angelina Hesse, wife of one of Koch's associates. She used it to harden jelly, while making various recipes in her kitchen.

The inocula (sample) is diluted on the surface of solid media by spreading and thus getting diluted to eventually result in isolated colonies on the surface of solid medium. Previous to agar, gelatin was used to solidify media but it had the disadvantage of liquefying around room temperature.

What are the properties of agar that resulted in it being universally accepted as an ingredient for solid media?

A.8
- It can be sterilized easily by heating and does not get denatured

- It remains stable at high temperature (unlike gelatin, which melts at around room temperature).
- Once melted, it remains liquid until cooled to about 40°C. At a temperature of about 45°C, heat sensitive nutrients and living organisms can be added to the medium without fear of the medium getting solidified (it does not melt below 95°C) but once melted it solidifies around 40°C.
- Very few bacteria can degrade it.

Why does one need to study the nutritional factors that can affect the growth of microorganisms?

A.9 Different organisms have varying nutritional requirements and one needs to cultivate the various microbes in the lab. Broadly the number of nutrient requirement of an organism is determined by the type and number of enzymes it has. Basically, the organisms with many enzymes have simpler nutritional requirements, as they can synthesize most of the substances they require. The organisms with fewer enzymes have complex nutritional requirements, as they are unable to synthesize many substances eg. lactic acid synthesizing bacteria.

What are the nutritional factors that need to be provided for growth of microorganisms?

A.10 *Water* is the most essential requirement, as it is a primary constituent of the organism accounting for about 80% of its total weight. It is a source of hydrogen and oxygen.

Next in importance is a substance acting; as a *carbon* source. This is used as a source of energy and as carbon containing building block for synthesis of cell components. The source of it varies; depending on whether the bacteria is a autotroph (Lithotroph), which uses inorganic chemicals; as CO_2 or a heterotroph (organotroph), if it uses organic carbon sources. Substances acting as nitrogen source are also important, as these are required in the synthesis of enzymes, proteins and nucleic acid. *Sulfur* requirement in the organism is obtained from inorganic sulphate salts and sulfur containing amino acids. *Phosphorus* requirement of the organism is obtained from inorganic phosphate ions ($PO4^{3-}$). Phosphorus is used in the synthesis of ATP, phospholipids and nucleic acids. The above nutrients are categorized as *macronutrients*, as they are required in relatively large amounts and play a key role in cell structure and metabolism.

The nutrients that are required in minute quantities but essential for the functioning of organism; often as part of key enzymes are called *micronutrients*. All organisms require some sodium and chloride. The variety of trace elements that are often required include iron, zinc, copper and cobalt. Certain organism require some other organic factor; as X and V factors required by *H. influenzae*.

What are the key components of culture media?

A.11
- Water
- Electrolytes (often NaCl etc.)
- Peptone–it is a complex mixture of partially digested proteins. They can be of animal or plant (vegetable) source, obtained by enzyme digestion. The latter are preferred by some groups, as there is no fear of infectious agents such as those, which cause Bovine spongiform encephalopathy.

  The preparation contains proteoses, polypeptides, amino acids, inorganic salts (as phosphates), minerals (as K, Mg) and accessory growth factor (as riboflavin).
- Meat extract–it is commercially available as 'Lab lemco'
- Agar (if medium has to be solid or semisolid)
- Other factors (as blood, yeast extract etc. depending on type of medium).

What are the ways in which media can be classified? Explain how do these classifications help the microbiologist and clinician in achieving their mandate.

A.12 I. On the basis of physical state of the medium. It is categorized as

- Liquid • Semisolid (floppy) and • Solid

II. On the presence/absence of molecular oxygen and reducing substances in the media

(i) Aerobic media (ii) Anaerobic media

If from the clinical sample, anaerobic bacteria are expected, then anaerobic media must be inoculated for successful isolation of anaerobes. One has to be very careful in this regard, as even common medium; as blood agar plate, if it not stored in reducing environment, may not support anaerobes. Prolonged exposure of the medium to environmental oxygen may make such medium ineffective for anaerobic work. Ideally PRAS.

III. *Bacterial/fungal*: If the clinical picture suggests a fungal lesion; as dermatophytes or dimorphic fungi, dermatophyte media/Sabourauds dextrose agar should be used additionally to routine media for fungal isolation.

IV. *Synthetic (defined)/complex/undefined*

Most of the media in usage are in the complex category because often what is present as a component in a accurately weighed ground meat, milk or plants is not exactly known. The composition of the medium also varies with the digestion protocol followed, while preparing it with the various enzymes, e.g., nutrient broth, beef extract. It is difficult to know the exact nutrient requirements of a suspected pathogen in a clinical sample and create such an medium. For this reason, clinical microbiology labs often use this complex medium in the primary isolation of an organism.

In the synthetic media (defined), as the name indicates, the composition of the medium is accurately known as only defined and weighed components are added to the medium, e.g., Dubo's medium with Tween 80.

V. *Transport media/plating media*: *Transport media* are those, which are used by the clinician or the patient to transport the specimen to the microbiology laboratory, where the sample processing is to be performed. The composition of these media is to be such that the pathogens present in the sample do not proliferate but remain viable till they reach the laboratory. They usually contain buffers and salts and lack carbon and nitrogen source.

Plating media are those media in which the clinical sample is inoculated in the laboratory. Rarely this medium can also be used to inoculate CSF samples at the bedside and transport to the laboratory.

VI. *Enrichment media/selective media*: Enrichment media; as the name indicates, enrich the desired organisms, from a mixture or organisms present in the specimen, e.g., tetrathionate broth and selenite broth used in allowing preferential growth of typhoid bacilli. These are liquid media, which allow small number of pathogens to outgrow inhibited (commensal) organisms, before subculture on to culture plates. So the indication of using them, is when you want to select out few pathogenic bacterial present in a mixture of unwanted organisms. This medium should not be confused with the enriched media, which is a similar sounding term. Enrichment media are always liquid media and enhance the isolation of desired organism by apparently shortening the lag phase of the desired organisms. This makes these organisms reach earlier the log phase, thus they become relatively predominant in comparison to other commensal bacteria in the earlier period of the growth curve. So to take advantage of this dynamics, sample after 6-8 hours of inoculation into a enrichment medium, must be subcultured onto a selective medium, or the commensal bacteria would also enter log phase, making lose the advantage that may have occurred.

Selective media, as the name indicates, select out the desired organisms from a mixture of organisms by enhancing the growth of the desired organisms and possibly inhibiting the other organisms. These media are always solid. In Deoxycholate citrate agar (DCA), sodium deoxycholate inhibits the growth of gram positive cocci and makes the medium selective for gram negative bacilli. In MacConkey agar, sodium taurocholate inhibits the gram positive cocci making the medium selective for gram negative bacilli. More examples see Table 1.7.1.

VII. *Simple (basal)/Enriched media*: The *simple basal media* are, as the name indicates are the simple and routinely employed diagnostic media. It can be both in liquid or solid forms, e.g., nutrient broth, which contains peptone, meat extract (1%), sodium chloride and water. Addition of 2% agar to nutrient broth makes it *nutrient agar*. Sugar media often used in fermentation tests also belong to this category. It contains 1% sugar (glucose/lactose/sucrose/mannitol) in peptone water along with indicator (often, andrades) and sometimes an inverted tube called Durham's tube (to see gas production).

Enriched media as the name indicates are enriched with blood, serum, ascitic fluid or egg. These are obviously expensive than simple media and are used; if fastidious organisms are expected in a clinical sample or fastidious organisms are to be cultivated.

NB: Many media can also be of multiple types eg differential and indicator. e.g., Blood agar, is both an enriched and indicator medium, L.J. medium is both an enriched and selective medium.

VIII. *Other categories*: *Indicator media* (differential) as the name indicates, provide an indication to the type of growth on the medium. E.g., MacConkey's medium can differentiate between lactose fermenters, and non-fermenters. However, it is also a selective medium, as the sodium taurocholate in it inhibits gram positive cocci. Another example of this would be blood agar, where small pin-point β haemolytic colonies would indicate the organism to be β haemolytic Streptococci. However this plate is also an enriched medium. So this classification for media is not absolute and some media can be categorized into numerous categories.

The commonly used media are categorized in table 1.7.1.

Table 1.7.1: Common media and their characteristics

Media for Transporting Samples		Type	Name & Essentials Components	Role of the Components	Functions of Media
		Pike' s medium	• Blood agar • Crystal violet (1 in 1,000,000) • Sodium azide	• Enriched base • *S. pyogenes*, resistant to it • Preservative	Transport of specimen likely to contain *S. pyogenes*
		Buffered glycerol saline	• Glycerol • Saline • Phenol red	• Prevents dessication • Preserves structures • Indicator (if medium turns yellow, it indicates growth of contaminants)	Transport of stool specimens likely to contain organisms, as Shigella
		Stuart's transport medium	• Soft agar (non nutrient) • Charcoal • Sodium thioglycollate • Sodium glycerophosphate • Calcium chloride • Methylene blue	• To provide solidity • Neutralize bacterial inhibitors • Reducing agent • Buffer • Buffer • Indicator	Transport of fastidious organisms including anaerobes (ensures survival but not proliferation of organisms)
		Cary Blair medium	• Sodium thioglycollate (pH 8.4) • Disodium phosphate • NaCl • Alkaline pH	• Provides low oxidation-reduction potential • Buffers medium • Osmotic equilibrium [non-nutritive] • Minimizes bacterial destruction due to acid production	Transport medium for Shigella, Salmonella and Vibrio
For Fungi	Solid	Sabouraud dextrose agar (Fig. 1.7.2)		• Lower pH favour growth of fungi over bacteria • High sugar concentration also favours growth of fungi	Isolation of fungi
		Sabouraud dextrose agar with antibiotics		• Cycloheximide inhibits molds and yeasts • Chloramphenicol inhibits bacterial gowth	Isolation of fungi from contaminated samples
		Dermatophyte test medium agar	• Nutrient base with glucose • Phenol red • Tetracycline, Gentamicin • Cycloheximide	• Indicator • Inhibits Contaminants	Isolation of Dermatophytes
		Brain heart infusion agar (BHIA)	• Calf brain infusion • Beef heart infusion • Salts and buffers		Growth of Dimorphic fungi
		Cornmeal agar	• Corn meal infusion • Agar	• Stimulate chlamydospore formation	To identify *C. albicans* (formation of chlamydospore, blastoconidia & pseudohyphae, occur in 48 hrs
Aerobic Bacteria					
	Semi-solid	Cragie's tube	• Have 0. 2 - 0. 5% agar		Motility studies
		Oxidation_Fermentation (OF) medium	• Casein enzymic hydrolysate • Carbohydrate • Dipotassium phophate • Bromothymol blue • Agar (low concentration)	• Nutrition. • One to be tested • Buffer • Indicator • Permits motility and diffusion of acidity	Determine oxidative or fermentative metabolism of carbohydrates by GNB
	LIQUID				
	Basal	Peptone water pH 7. 4 (Fig. 1.7.3)	• Peptone - 1% • NaCl - 0. 5%		• Routine culture • As basal medium for carbohydrate Fermentation medium
		Nutrient broth (has variants like Digest broth)	• Peptone water • Meat extract		• Routine culture

Contd.

Contd.

	Enriched	Glucose broth	• Nutrient broth • Glucose - 0. 5%	• Also acts as a reducing agent	• Luxuriant growth of many organism
		Todd Hewitt (meat infusion) broth	• Glucose - 0. 2% • Infusion		• Luxuriant growth of organism's; as Streptococci
		Serum peptone broth	• Serum	• For growth	• For carbohydrate fermentation tests with fastidious organism such as Streptococci, *C.diphtheriae*
		Brain heart infusion broth			• Recovery of bacteria and fungi
		Mueller Hinton broth (Fig. 1.7.4)			• Bacterial susceptibility test medium
		Trypticase soy broth			Cultivation of fastidious organisms; as Brucella
		PPLO broth (medium be free of toxins)	• Bovine heart infusion broth • Horse serum (20%) • Yeast extract (fresh) • Glucose • Phenol red	• For growth • For growth • Indicator	Isolation of mycoplasma
		Middlebrook's 7H10			• For isolation of tuberculosis group of organisms
	Enrichment				
		Bile broth			
		Selenite F broth	• Peptone water • Sodium selenite	• Inhibits most enterobacteriaceae	Enrichment medium for Salmonella & Shigella
		Tetrathionate broth	• Nutrient broth/Peptone base broth • Sodium thiosulphate • Bile salts • Calcium carbonate • Iodine solution	• Inhibits grams positive organism • Neutralizes toxic metabolites • Inhibits enterobacteriaceae	Enrichment medium for Salmonella & Shigella
		Alkaline peptone water	• High pH	• Optimal for vibrio multiplication	Enrichment medium for Vibrio
	SOLID				
	Basal (majority have 2% agar as solidifying agent)	Nutrient agar (Fig. 1.7.5)	• Nutrient broth • Agar (2%)		Routine medium
	Enriched				
		Blood agar (Fig. 1.7.6)	• Nutrient agar • 5 -10% sheep / horse / human blood		For isolating organisms as Group A streptococci, Haemophiius (fastidious organisms)
		Blood agar with *S. aureus* streak	• *S. aureus* streak	*S. aureus* provides V factor	For isolating Haemophilus organisms
		Blood agar with X and V discs	X disc V disc	• Provides hemin • Provides NAD	For isolating Haemophilus organisms
		Chocolate agar (blood agar slowly heated to 80°C) (Fig. 1.7.7)		Heating blood, releases nutrients	For isolation of fastidious organisms as *H. influenzae*, *N. gonoroheae* & *N. meningitidis*, *Gardnerella vaginalis*
		Loeffler's serum slope (has no agar)	• Nutrient broth • Serum (Horse/sheep) • Glucose		For rapid growth of *C. diphtheriae*
		Egg yolk agar	• Proteose peptone • Hemin • Salts • Egg yolk	• Nutrient • Enhance anaerobic growth • Buffer • Lipase (produced by microbes), break down fat into fatty acid, provide iridescence	For Clostridia isolation and other anaerobes

Contd.

Contd.

		Dorset's egg	• Nutrient broth • Hen's egg		For isolation of Mycobacteria & other fastidious organisms
		PPLO agar	PPLO broth • Antibiotics as Penicillin, ampicillin, polymyxin B	• Inhibits contaminant bacteria and Fungi	For isolation of Mycobacteria
		Bordet gengou medium	• Blood • Potato • Glycerol It has methicillin (final conc. 2. 5 µg/ml)	Nutrition	For isolation of Bordetella
		Legionella medium	• Mueller Hinton medium supplemented with ferric salts, L-cysteine etc	• Provides reducing condition (L-cysteine)	For cultivation of Legionella spp.
		Francis blood dextrose cystine agar	• Blood, dextrose • Cystine		For isolation of *Francisella tularensis*
		BHI agar			
	Selective				
		MacConkey	• Peptone • Lactose • Agar • Neutral red • Taurocholate (sodium)	• Indicator substrate • Indicator, dye • Inhibits gram positive cocci	• Routine medium • Differential medium for the demonstration of lactose fermentation by gram negative rods
		Salmonella & Shigella medium	• Bile salts (higher concentration) • Sodium citrate • Ferric citrate	• Inhibits GPCs and coliforms • Blackening occurs due to formation of ferrous sulfide	
			• Lactose • Neutral red	• Indicator substrate • Indicator dye	
		Bile salt agar (alkaline) pH 8.2	• Sodium taurocholate (0. 5%)	Inhibits most gram negative organism	Selective plating media for Vibrios
		Thiosulfate citrate bile salt agar (TCBS)	• Peptone base agar • Yeast extract • Bile salts • Citrate • Sucrose • Ferric citrate • Sodium thiosulphate • Bromothymol blue • pH-alkaline	• Inhibits GPCs • Inhibits most GNBs • Indicator substrate • Allows H_2S detection • Sulfur source • Indicator • Helps recovery of vibrio	Selective plating media for Vibrios (recovery of vibrios)
		Monsur's gelatin taurocholate trypticase tellurite agar	• Gelatin • Sodium taurocholate • Tellurite	• Vibrios can hydrolyze gelatin & produce halo around colonies • Inhibits gram positive cocci • Reduction of it imparts black color to colonies	For isolation and identification of *Vibrio cholerae*
		Vibrio media containing 8% NaCl		Halophilic vibrio can tolerate 8% NaCl but not 10%	Differentiation of halophilic vibrios from *V. cholerae*
		Deoxycholate citrate agar (DCA)	• Nutrient agar • Sodium deoxycholate • Lactose • Sodium citrate • Neutral red	• Nutrition • Inhibits gram positive bacteria • Indicator substrate • Inhibits gram-positive bacteria and intestinal commensals • Color indicator	Selective medium for Salmonella & Shigella
		XLD agar (Xylose Lysine deoxycholate) medium	Details beyond undergraduate level		Selective/Indicator medium for Enterobacteriaceae, especially for Salmonella and Shigella
		Wilson&Blair bismuth sulfite medium	• Bismuth ammonium citrate • Sodium sulfite • Salts	Formation of H_2S renders black color to colonies	Selective medium for S. Typhi

Contd.

Contd.

		Campy Blood agar	• Brucella agar base with sheep blood with Antibiotics as • Trimethoprim • Cephalothin • Polymyxin B • Vancomycin • Amphotericin B	• Inhibits Proteus spp. (contaminants) • Inhibits gram positive organism • Inhibits most gram negative organisms • Inhibits gram positive organisms • Inhibits yeasts	
		Lowenstein Jensen medium (Fig. 1.7.8)	• Eggs • Mineral salts • Asparagine • Glycerol, Malachite green	• Nutrition, solidifying agent • Inhibits organisms other than mycobacteria and provides contrast to buff colored colonies	Selective for mycobacteria
		Dorset medium	Egg based		For isolation of Mycobacteria
		Middlebrook 7H11	Agar based		For isolation of Mycobacteria
		Bile esculin agar	• Nutrient agar base • Esculin • Ferric citrate react with above	Hydrolysis of esculin by Group D streptococci, provide blackening	Differential isolation & presumptive isolation of enterococci
		Crystal violet blood agar	• Blood agar • Crystal violet	In concentration of 1 in 1,000,000 inhibits *Staphylococcus aureus*	Selective isolation of *Streptococcus pyogenes*
		Buffered charcoal yeast extract agar (BCYE)	• Agar • Yeast extract • Salts supplements with ketoglutarate, L-cysteine		Selective for Legionella sps
		Skirrow agar	• Peptone & soy protein base agar • lysed horse blood • Vancomycin • Polymyxin B • Trimethoprim	• Inhibits gram positive organisms • Inhibits most gram negative organisms	Selective for campylobacter & Helicobacter
		Cycloserine-cefoxitin fructose agar	• Egg yolk base Fructose • Neutral red • Cefoxitin • Cycloserine	• Indicator dye • Inhibits gram negative rods • Inhibits faecal flora	Selective for *Clostridum difficile*
		Cystine-tellurite blood agar	• Agar base with 5% sheep blood • Potassium tellurite	Reduction of potassium tellurite produces black colonies	Selective isolation of *C. diphtheriae*
		Thayer Martin agar (variant of choclate agar)	• Blood agar base enriched with haemoglobin and supplement B • Colistin • Nystatin • Vancomycin • Trimethoprim	• Inhibits gram negative contaminants • Inhibits yeast • Inhibits gram positive organism • Inhibits gram negative contaminants	Selective for *N. meningitidis* and *N. gonorrhoeae*
		Mannitol salt agar	• Peptone base • Mannitol • Salt concentration of 7.5% • Phenol red	• Acts as indicator substrate • Inhibits growth of most bacteria • Indicator	Selective for *Staphylococcus aureus*
	Miscellaneous	Cystine Lactose electrolyte deficient agar	• Peptone base agar • Lactose • L. cysteine • Bromothymol blue	• Inhibits swarming of Proteus • Indicator substrate • Indicator dye	isolation & quantification of bacteria
		Modified Kelley's medium (BSK)			Cultivation of *Borrelia burgdorferi*
		EMJH (Ellinghausen, Mc Cullough, Johnson Harris)			Cultivation of *Leptospira interrogans*

Contd.

Contd.

		Castaneda's medium (biphasic medium)	Trypticase soy broth and agar		Cultivation and isolation of Brucella
For Anaerobic bacteria	Liquid	Robertson cooked meat medium (Fig. 1.7.9)	• Meat broth • Solid meat particles • Liquid parraffin	• As nutrient • Lower oxidation reduction potential • Block environmental oxygen	Cultivation of anaerobes support growth of anaerobes, aerobes, microaerophilic & fastidious Organisms
		Thioglycollate broth	• Pancreatic digest of casein • Soy broth & glucose • Thioglycollate • Agar • L cysteine & vitamin	• Lower Eh (reduction potential/ redox) • Act as reducing agent	Cultivation of anaerobes including Actinomycetes
	Solid enriched				
		Blood agar (plain) _PRAS	Pre-reduced anaerobically sterilized medium prepared & packaged in oxygen free environment		Cultivation of anaerobes
		Blood agar (with additives) _PRAS	Yeast extract, haemin, Vitamin K, Neomycin	Support isolation of anaerobes	Cultivation of anaerobes
		Serum/egg yolk agar (6%)	Peptic digest of blood 20% human serum or 5% egg yolk	6% agar Inhibits swarming	To demonstrate Nagler reaction by *C. perfringens*
	Selective				
		Colistin_ Nalidixic acid Blood agar		Antimicrobials make medium selective	Supports selective growth of anaerobic & facultative anaerobes (mostly gram positive, inhibits most gram negative)
		Kanamycin_ Vancomycin Blood agar (*laked blood agar*)	• Kanamycin • Vancomycin • Blood		Selective isolation of anaerobes
		Phenylethyl alcohol sheep blood agar	• Phenylethyl alcohol • Blood		Supports growth of most gram positive & gram negative bacilli
		Bacteriodes bile esculin agar	• Trypticase soy agar base • Hemin • Ferric ammonium citrate • Bile salts, Gentamicin, phenylethyl alcohol	Enriches Gentamicin - inhibits most aerobic gram negative contaminants including Proteus spp.	supports selective growth of Bacteriodes sps, other bacteria can also grow supports growth of most gram positive and negative anaerobes (inhibits facultative, gram negative, bacilli)
Animate media!	Tissue culture (cell lines)	McCoy cells (rendered non-replicating by irradiation or treatment with antimetabolites as cycloheximide)		Organism cannot grow on inanimate media	Isolation of Chlamydia
		HeLa cells (treated with DEAE dextran)			Isolation of Chlamydia
	Chick embryo (6-8 day old)	Yolk sac			For isolation of Chlamydia, Rickettsiae (not suitable for primary isolation)
		Chorioallantoic membrane			For cultivation of *Borrelia recurrentis*, *Leptospira interrogans*
	Laboratory animals	Mice (various routes)	Foot pad of mice		Cultivation of *M. leprae*
			Intranasal		For isolation of Chlamydia
			Intracerebral Intraperitoneal		• Isolation of Rickettsia, *Spirillum minus*, • *Leptospira interrogans*
		Rabbit testes			Cultivation of *T. pallidum, T. pertenue*
		Rabbit kidney (Noguchi's medium)	• Rabbit kidney, • Ascitic fluid		Cultivation of *Borrelia recurrentis*
		Armadillo (*Dasypus novemcintus*)			Cultivation of *M. leprae*

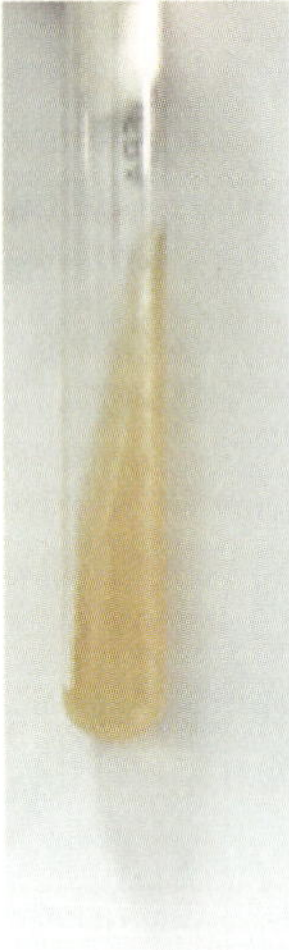

Fig. 1.7.2 Sabouraud`s dextrose agar

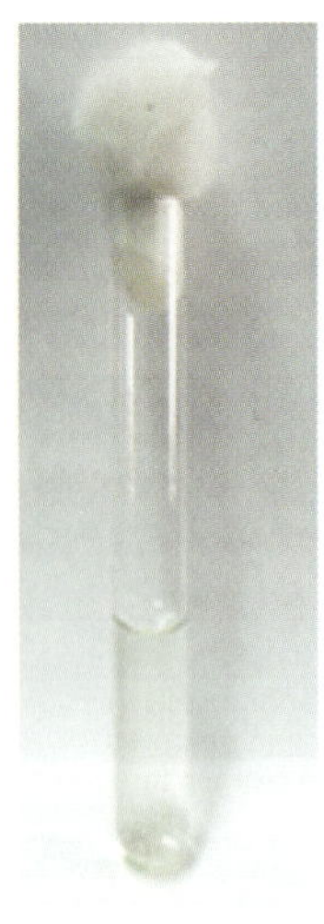

1.7.3: Mueller Hinton broth

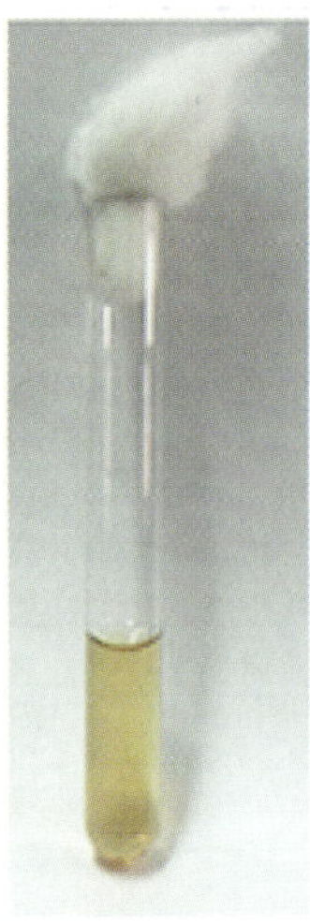

Fig.1.7.4: Peptone water

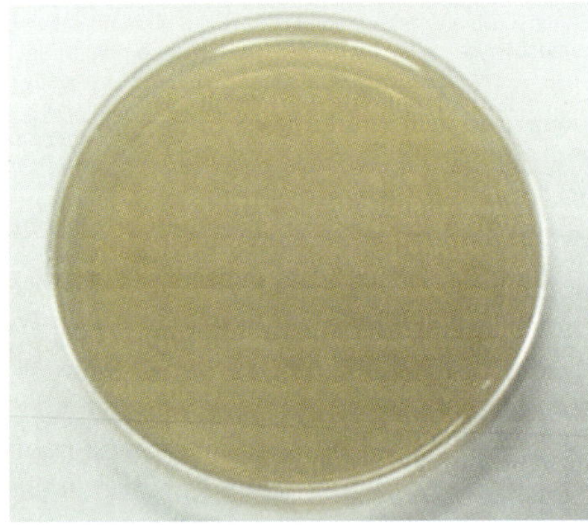

Fig.1.7.5: Nutrient agar plate

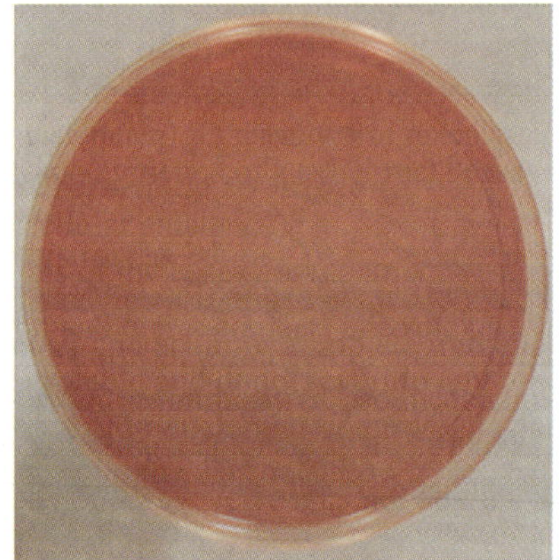

Fig.1.7.6: Blood agar plate

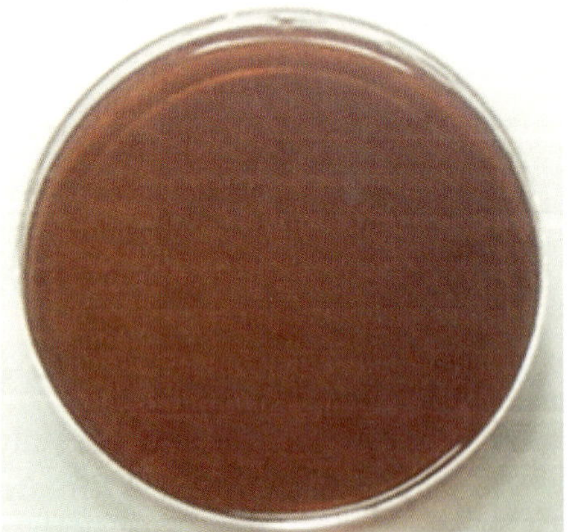

Fig.1.7.7: Choclate agar plate

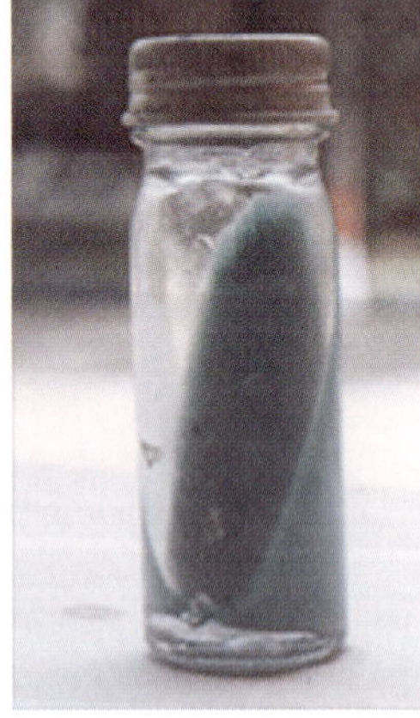

Fig.1.7.8: Lowenstein Jensen edium

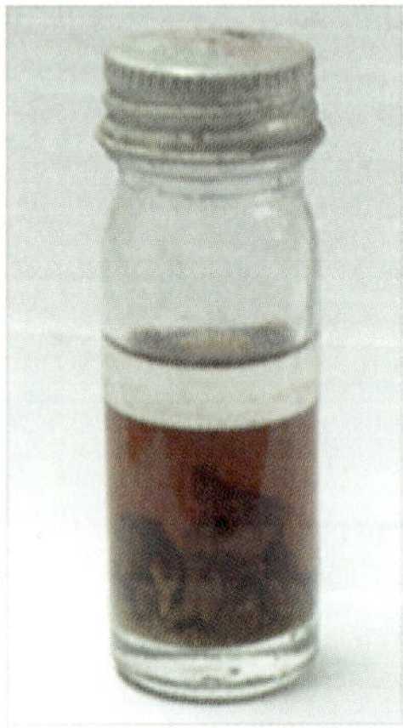

Fig.1.7.9: Robertson cooked medium

Culture Techniques and Growth Curve

The second thing required to study the role of microbes (bacteria) in health and disease is isolation of the microbe.

Let's study the culture techniques, which achieve this goal.

What do you understand by culture?

A.1 It refers to a population of bacterial cells.

What do you understand by pure culture?

A.2 It is a population of genetically homogenous organisms (derived by multiplication from single organism)

What are the uses (indication) of culturing bacteria?

A.3 (i) To isolate bacteria in pure cultures; for instance from the clinical specimens and environmental samples

(ii) To study the various properties of bacteria (in pure cultures); as biochemical characteristics, antigenic characteristics, genotypic characteristics.

(iii) To study the epidemiological and other characteristics of bacteria; as bacteriophage typing, bacteriocin typing and antibiotic susceptibility testing

(iv) To estimate viable counts; as required in diagnosis of urinary tract infections

(v) To main stock cultures; which would help in later study of the organisms.

What do you understand by 'inoculation of culture media?

A.4 It implies introduction (delivery) of material containing suspected or known organism into culture media. This is achieved by using inoculation straight wire/loop or Pasteur pipette (Figs. 1.8.1 and 1.8.2) (for details see practical aspects).

What are the equipment required to obtain liquid cultures?

A.5 Inoculating equipment (see A.4), Test tubes, bottles (as universal containers, McCartney bottles) and flasks (round/conical).

What are the indications of performing liquid cultures?

A.6 (i) When large yields of organisms are required; as for antigen preparation. This is feasible, as the liquid medium can be subject to processes; as agitation aeration, replenishment of nutrients and removal of unwanted metabolites.

(ii) When the bacteria in the inoculum is expected to be low; as performing blood cultures or testing material for sterility.

(iii) When specimens contain substances, which are inhibitory to the cultivation of bacteria, are to be cultured, e.g., antibiotics. The effect of antibiotic gets minimized by dilution.

What is the major disadvantage of liquid cultures?

A.7 Pure culture cannot be obtained from specimen containing multiple organisms.

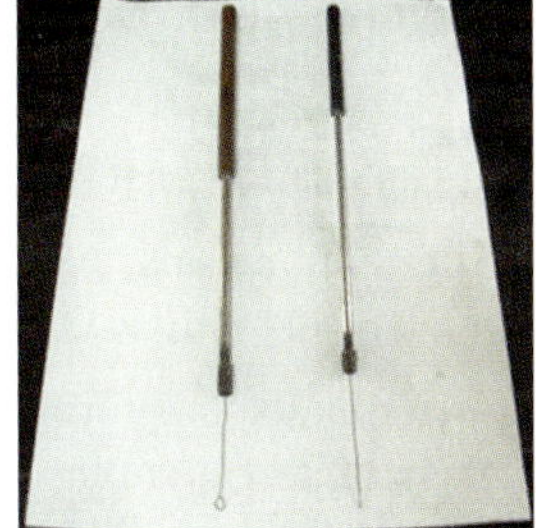

Fig. 1.8.1: Conventional straight wire and loop

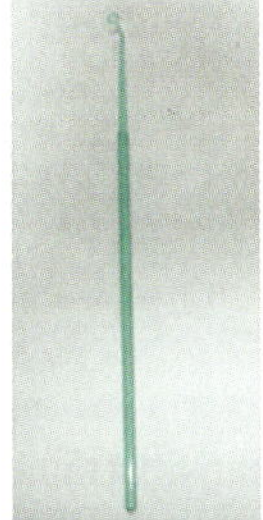

Fig. 1.8.2: Plastic loop

What has been the role of solid media cultures in the development of Microbiology?

A.8 The isolation techniques used to obtain pure cultures in solid media, made it possible for the 'Golden age' of bacteriology to be possible.

What are the techniques available to culture bacteria on solid media?

A.9 (i) *Stroke cultures:* Performed on tubes containing media in the form of a slant. This type of culture is performed, while performing various biochemical tests and to obtain pure growth for performing various slide agglutination and other tests.

(ii) *Stab cultures:* In this, the inoculum is penetrated (stabbed) deep inside the agar medium with the help of a straight wire. This technique is used to study oxygen requirements of bacteria and to stock (preserve) cultures for later study.

(iii) *Streak plate method* (see practical book for technique):

This is a widely used technique to obtain isolated colonies (pure growth) (Fig. 1.8.3).

(iv) *Lawn (carpet culture):* As the name indicates, by various techniques a uniform complete growth is obtained on the surface of the solid medium. This technique is used to perform the antibiotic susceptibility tests (as Stoke's method) or perform the bacteriophage studies (as in *S. aureus*). This principle is also used commercially to obtain large amount of growth, for instance; when the bacterial antigen are to be extracted.

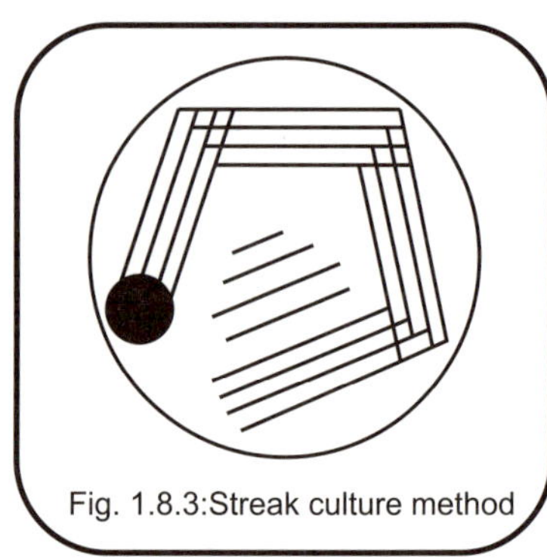

Fig. 1.8.3:Streak culture method

(v) *Pour plate method:* The name of the technique indicates, the medium of the plate (culture) here is poured with the inoculum. The inoculum is diluted in a series of dilutions, so that the final dilution containing about a thousand organisms (this is so done, so that the colonies in the plate finally remain countable). A known amount of the final dilution say 1 ml is mixed with 15 ml of molten agar kept at 45-50°C and mixed well. The contents are poured into a sterile petri dish and allowed to set. After adequate incubation period (usually 18-24 hours) at optimal temperature (usually throughout 37°C), the colonies that form throughout the medium (not just the surface of the medium) are counted using colony counter. This technique is favourable for the growth of microaerophiles which cannot tolerate a concentration of oxygen in the air at the surface of the medium.

How does one separate mixtures of different bacteria contained in a clinical specimen?

A.10 (i) *Surface plating* is the usual method employed in clinical microbiology, however it has limitations, as the study of the subsequent techniques would demonstrate.

(ii) *Enrichment media* are required for specimen containing few bacteria of interest in a sample with predominant other bacteria, e.g., isolation of shigella or salmonella from a stool specimen (here the stool specimen will have few pathogens in contrast to the predominant *E. coli* organisms in the stool specimen).

However subculture from the enrichment medium (after few hours) to the selective medium is necessary.

(iii) *Indicator media*

(iv) Samples containing organisms with varying oxygen requirements would have to be incubated in parallel with *varying environmental* conditions. For instance a sample with both aerobic and anaerobic organisms would have to be incubated both aerobically and anaerobically. The anaerobic concept has been developed in two clinical problems in the Anaerobic infections chapter in the Clinical Microbiology section Pg. 584-585.

(v) Samples containing organisms with temperature requirements can be purified, isolated and separated by incubating *at different temperatures*. For instance a sample containing *N. meningitidis* and *M. catarrahalis* can be purified by incubating at 22°C, where only the latter grows.

(vi) *Pre-treatment* of specimens, with bactericidal substances that can destroy or minimize the unwanted organisms.

e.g., Petroff's method concentration for *M. tuberculosis*. The commensals in the sputum sample are usually susceptible to laboratory protocol involving exposure to extreme of pH unlike *M. tuberculosis*.

(vii) Vegetative bacteria are usually susceptible to *prolonged heat* unlike spore forming bacteria. This technique is useful in the purification of many anaerobic spore forming bacteria; as *C. tetani*.

(viii) *Cragie's tube* technique can help in separation of motile and non-motile organisms and in studying phase variation of salmonella or definitive identification of salmonella.

(ix) In the past *animal pathogenicity tests* used to be performed to proliferate an organisms of interest, e.g., *M. tuberculosis* or *B. anthracis* in guinea pig.

(x) Modern techniques immunological techniques (including *FACS*), can help in separating organisms of interest.

Describe the concept of growth curve.

A.11 *Concept:* If a pure culture of bacteria is introduced into a fresh nutrient rich liquid medium (plural – 'media' – that which supports the bacteria), the rate of increase of bacterial number follows a predictable phases, which characterize the typical standard bacterial growth curve. The regulation of the different phases is accompanied by control of gene expression, which affects the enzyme activity.

- *Why do you need to study it?*
  (i) It is a fundamental process of bacteriology that needs to be studied.
  (ii) Morphological characteristics vary with the phase of the growth curve. This concept should be known, otherwise diagnostic fallacies may occur; as involution forms occur in stationary phase and gram variability may be seen.
  (iii) The concept of growth phases is also seen in the colonies growing on solid medium. A colony is formed, as a result of organism, dividing, exponentially. The growth of colony is more rapid at the edge than at the center, as lesser nutrients and greater toxic substances are found in the center of the colony than at the periphery.
  (iv) Secretion of substances; as exotoxins and antibiotics occur in the stationary phase. This fact should be known, and is exploited in commercial ventures.
  (v) For industrial purposes, it should be known how to minimize the lag period, how to maintain the culture in exponential phase for prolonged period.
- *What are the phases of growth curve?*

Broadly there are four phases (depicted in Fig. 1.8.4).

1st phase: Lag phase

As the name indicates, it is a period in which organism number does not increase significantly. However it should not be conceived that the organism is not metabolically active. The organism is active, adapting to the new environment and incorporating various molecular components from the medium to enlarge in size.

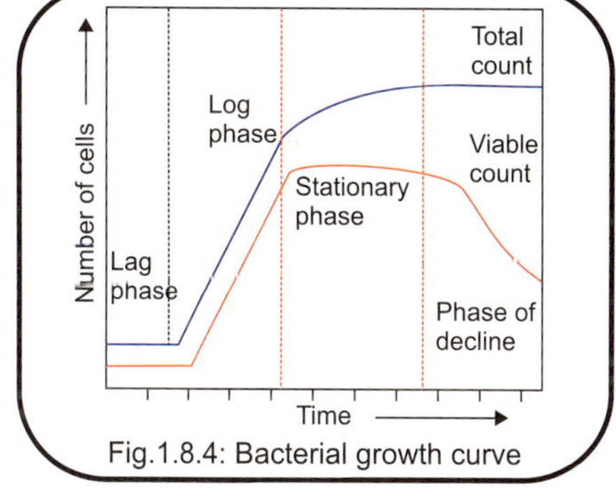

Fig.1.8.4: Bacterial growth curve

The lag period may last a few hours. The length of the period is determined by the genetic characteristic of the organism, the medium characteristics from which the organism is taken and the one into which it is introduced and other growth conditions. The cell acquires maximum cell size towards end of this phase.

2nd phase: exponential phase (logarithmic phase)

The phase starts after the organisms have adapted to the new medium. As the name of the phase indicates, the organism divide at a very rapid rate (called generation time) and population growth occurs at an exponential or logarithmic rate. But this period of constant maximal growth rate occurs, after a brief period of accelerating growth. The logarithm of the viable organisms, when plotted against time gives a steep straight line. This represents a regular increase in number of organisms. The average duration of this phase is a few hours (8 hours).

To maintain the culture in this phase, instruments; as chemostat and *turbidostat are available, which basically infuses fresh medium and takes away (or exchanges) the used medium. This process results in continuous culture of the organism. The process has applications in the research and industrial fronts.

3rd phase (stationary phase)

The steep growth curve slowly starts levelling off (called decelerating phase). This starts occurring due to nutrient depletion, metabolic waste accumulation and loss of other entities; as oxygen for aerobic organisms. Gradually a stage is reached, where the rate at which the organisms divide, becomes the same at which cells die. Then the culture comes

* Basically, as the name indicates, it operates on the principle of turbidity, i.e., when the turbidity in the vessel reaches a certain threshold, an exchange of the used broth with the fresh broth occurs. The chemostat works on the principle of continuous addition of fresh medium, with the total volume of the device remaining constant, with an overflow tube.

in the stationary phase, which is represented by the horizontal straight line. The duration of this phase varies from few hours to few days. Most of the organisms in this phase are not dead, as when inoculated into fresh medium, enter into exponential growth; after a lag phase.

This stage has an industrial application, as some metabolites; as exotoxins and antibiotics get produced during this phase. Morphologically; organisms appear atypical during this phase due to reaction being gram variable, staining irregularly due to formation of intracellular storage granules and formation of endospores.

4th phase

Decline/Death phase: This phase occurs; as a result of the rate of the bacterial division being slower than the rate of death. This is seen as a steep (declining) line in the Figure 1.8.4, which occurs as cell viability is lost by exponential kinetics. This stage results due to the autolysis of the organisms, besides the continued exhaustion of nutrients and accumulation of toxic products. There is decline of both the viable organisms count and the total organism count. Many cells undergo involution during this phase and may assume unusual shapes making them difficult to identify.

How is bacterial growth monitored?

A.12 (i) *Turbidity:* One of the commonest and simplest techniques to monitor bacterial growth is based on degree of turbidity in a transparent (glass) culture tube. The basic principle is that greater is the organism (cell) density in the tube, greater is the turbidity. However, the limitation of the technique is that samples with very high densities must be diluted to ensure accurate readings. Also samples with fewer than 1 million organisms per millilitre may display little or no turbidity, so if subcultures of bottles is based only on turbidity, false negative reporting can occur. It may also be remembered that turbidity can also be produced by dead cells in a culture. The turbidity of samples may be estimated roughly by comparing manually with control tubes as $^{\Delta}$McFarland tubes. Accurate estimation of the turbidity is done using photoelectric devices; as colorimeter or spectrophotometer.

Δ Are reference tubes to adjust turbidity of bacterial suspension, prepared mixing barium chloride and sulfuric acid, which forms barium sulfate precipitate.

(ii) *Serial dilution and standard plate counts:* In this the sample is so diluted that, when transferred to the molten agar medium would give no more than 300 colonies in the plate, after adequate incubation.

This number is so chosen, as more colonies than this would be difficult to count even with a colony counter.

(iii) *Direct microscopic counts:* This technique basically employs different counting chambers; such as Petroff-Hausser, in which the sample is inoculated and later the organism count is done. The limitation of this technique is that it cannot accurately measure samples that have small cell/organisms numbers and one cannot distinguish between living and dead organisms.

(iv) *Filter paper technique:* This technique is based on filtering a known amount of sample (fluid or air) through a filter paper with pores sufficiently small not to allow passage of organisms. The organisms retained on the filter paper are plated on a solid medium and incubated in appropriate environment. The colony count is performed (one colony represent one organism) of the filter paper.

(v) *Most probable number:* In this the number of organisms in the sample is estimated from a most probable number table, which is based on statistical probabilities.

Identification of Bacteria

The third thing to study the role of bacteria in health and disease, after isolation of the bacterium; is the identification of bacteria. Once an organism has been isolated in culture, it must be identified. Let's study the techniques, which can achieve this aspect

What are the advantages of identifying a bacterial isolate?

A.1 (i) helps in the characterization of the isolate, i.e., whether it is a pathogen or a contaminant.

(ii) Identification helps in deciding strategy for infection control in the hospital ward and community, depending on its potential to spread.

(iii) Depending on the isolate, presumptive treatment can be initiated. Susceptibilty data of the local isolates help in deciding empiric treatment (when sample not sent to the laboratory and General Physician dealing with uncomplicated infection.)

(iv) Antibiotic susceptibility test can be performed to further guide treatment. If the report indicates that the administered drug turns is susceptible in the test, then the treatment can continue, otherwise the drug can be changed; depending on the report.

(v) Special tests can be performed to detect drug resistance genes in the organism (sometimes the drug resistance genes do not get expressed during the antibiotic susceptibility test but display clinical resistance 'in vivo'.

What are the two broad categories, into which the tests to identify the bacteria can be categorized into?

A.2 The system to identify the microbes can be categorized into two groups, namely (I) classic phenotypic (conventional procedures) and (II) phenotype–independent methods (essentially nucleic acid based).

Describe the role of the classic phenotypic techniques to identify bacteria and describe them.

A.3 The classic phenotypic techniques are carried out in many of the laboratories, as they are traditional and economical. However they have the disadvantage of being time consuming and lacking specificity. The limitation of time consuming aspect has been to some extent been compensated by automation of tests and improvisation in techniques. The phenotype–independent techniques have the advantage of being specific and often being completed in limited time but have the disadvantage of requiring expensive infrastructure, training and not being available for many pathogens.

The *classic phenotypic techniques* can be categorized into:

1. *Colony morphology on solid medium:* It is a baseline parameter in the study of an organism. This characteristic essentially helps in characterize a colony and give a provisional diagnosis. (in some typical colonies) and differentiate from other organisms. Once a colony is characterized, then further tests can be performed.

   Following are some of the characteristics studied in a colony.

   - Size
   - Surface—smooth/rough/granular
   - Edge (Fig. 1.9.1c)
   - Colour of colony (pigment)
   - Shape (Fig. 1.9.1a)
   - Elevation (Fig. 1.9.1b)
   - Opacity—opaque/translucent/transparent
   - Consistency—mucoid/friable/firm/butyrous

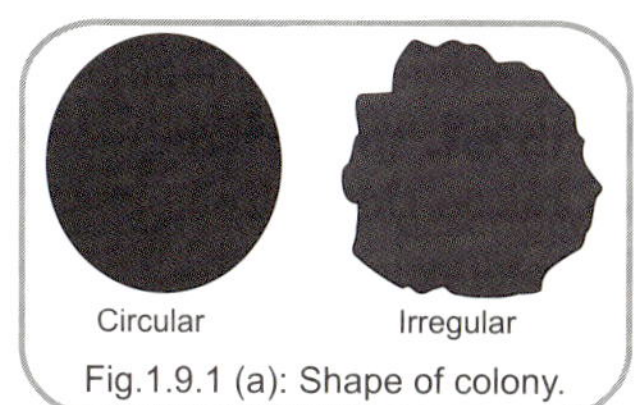

Fig.1.9.1 (a): Shape of colony.

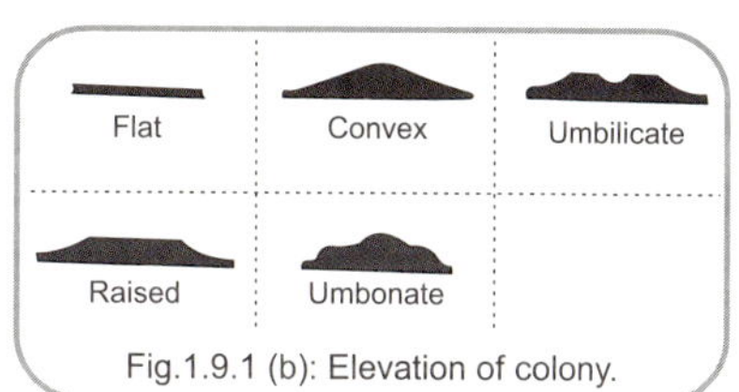

Fig.1.9.1 (b): Elevation of colony.

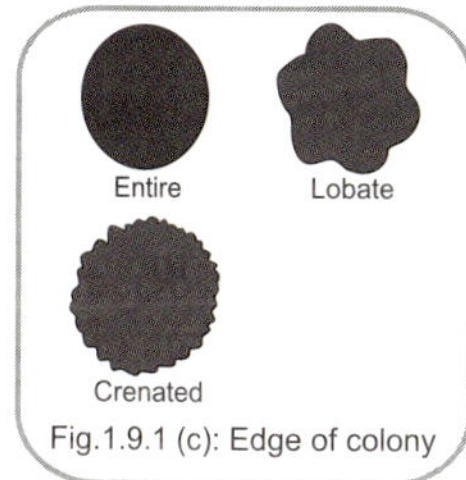

Fig.1.9.1 (c): Edge of colony

Table 1.9.1: Biochemical Tests

Text	Principle	Medium/reagent/constituents	Procedure outline	Colour of uninoculated medium/-ve reaction	Incubation duration	End result/ Colour of +ve reaction	Significance
1. Carbohydrate Fermentation test (sugar fermentation) (Fig. 1.9.2)	Acid production (Carbohydrate fermentation or utilization) is detected by change of colour of medium and gas production by small inverted tube (Dursham's tube)	• Peptone water fermentation medium • 0.5% carbohydrate (to be tested, e.g., Lactose) • 1% peptone • Andrade's indicator	Inoculate growth into medium and incubate	Yellow	18-24 hrs.	Pink (Durham's tube can show gas formation	Specific patterns for various bacteria
2. Nitrate Reduction test (Fig. 1.9.3)	Determines ability of an organism to reduce nitrate to nitrites or free nitrogen gas	• Nitrate broth • 0.1% potassium nitrate	• Inoculate growth and at the end of incubation, add 10 drops of mixture of • 8% sulphanilic acid (in 5N acetic acid) • 5% alpha-napthylamine (in 5N acetic acid)	Yellow	1-2 days	Red	In identification of Enterobacteriaceae
3. Indole formation test (Fig. 1.9.4)	Determines the ability of organism to convert tryptophan to indole, which is then detected with Kovac's reagent	Peptone water (rich in tryptophan) 1% peptone	• Inoculate growth and at the end of the incubation add 5 drops of following mixture of • P-dimethyl aminobenzaldehyde (Kovac's reagent) • Iso-amyl alcohol • Conc.-HCL	Yellow and clear	24 hrs/48 hrs	Pink in alcohol layer	To differentiate *E. coli* from Klebsiella and Edwardsiella from Salmonella
4. Citrate utilization test (Fig. 1.9.5)	Determines the ability of an organism to utilize citrate (of citric acid cycle) as a sole carbon and energy source for growth	(Simmon's citrate) • Sodium citrate (inorganic source) • Ammonium dihydro phosphate • Bromothymol blue [indicator (pH 6.0-7.6)]	Inoculate growth lightly on to the slant and incubate	Green	1-2 days	Blue with growth	In differentiating Salmonella from Edwardsiella Others
5. Urease production (Fig. 1.9.6)	Determines the ability of organism (which have urease) to reduce urea to ammonia	• Christensen's urease medium • 2% urea • 0.1% glucose • Phenol red • [Indicator (pH-6.8-8.4)]	Inoculate heavily on the surface and incubate	Buff coloured	4-24 hrs	Pink	In differentiating *E. coli* and Klebsiella and *P. mirabilis* and vulgaris
6. Methyl red	Detects between strains that produce and maintain a high concentration of hydrogen ions (pH<4.5) and those in which reversion of pH occurs	• Glucose phosphate broth • 0.5% glucose • 0.5% di-potassium hydrogen phosphate	Inoculate growth and at the end of incubation, add 5 drops of 0.1% methyl red	Yellow	2-5 days	Bright red	In identifying various members of Enterobacteriaceae
7. Voges Proskauer test	Detects the ability of organisms to produce acetyl methyl carbinol or it's reduction product (butylene glycol)	do	Inoculate growth at the end of incubation, add 1 ml O'Meara's reagent (40% KOH and 3% creatinine) OR 2.5 ml of Barrit's reagent (1 ml 40% KOH and 3 ml of 5% alpha napthol in alcohol)	Yellow	2 days	Eosin pink (in O'Meara's) or Bright red (in Barrit's)	do
8. Phenylalanine deaminase test (Fig. 1.9.7)	Determines the ability of organism to deaminate phenylalanine with production of phenylpyruvic acid, which will react with ferric salts to give green colour	• PPA Broth • 0.2% Phenylalanine • yeast extract • Others	Inoculate growth and at the end of incubation, add 4-5 drops of acidic ferric chloride	Yellow	18-24 hrs	Deep green	Is characteristic of Proteus, Morganella and Providencia genera

Contd.

Contd.

9. Amino acid decarboxylase test (Lysine/ Ornithine/ Arginine)	To determine the ability of an organism to decarboxylate an amino acid to form an amine with resulting alkalinity	Moller's decarboxylase base • 1% (Lysine/arginine/ornithine) • Glucose • Peptone • Pyridoxal • Bromocresol purple (pH 5.2-6.8)/Cresol red (pH 7.2-8.3)	*Control tube* without an aminoacid should be incubated with each panel of amino acids under investigation. All tubes are overlaid with 2 to 3 ml of sterile paraffin. Prolonged incubation beyond 10 days may be required to demonstrate weak reaction	Yellow colour (only glucose fermentated)	1-5 days	Turbid purple (tinge of yellow may be present)	In identifyng various bacterial groups
10. Oxidation – Fermentation test (Fig. 1.9.8)	To determine the oxidative or fermentative metabolism of a carbohydrate or its non-utilization	Hugh and Leifson's OF basal medium pH 7.1 - Bromothymol blue (indicator) ([pH6 (yellow)-7.6(deep prussian blue)]	*Two tube test*-for each carbohydrate to be tested, inoculate a pair of OF tubes, one open and other sealed with liquid paraffin. Also inoculate a control with no carbohydrate.	Green colour	2-4 days	• Fermentative-yellow in both tubes • Oxidative-yellow in open tube and green in sealed tube • Non utilization blue/ Green in both tubes	• Useful in identifying • Enterobacteriaceae • Micrococci group
11. Oxidase test (Fig. 1.9.9)	To determine the presence of component cytochrome oxidase enzyme, which catalyzes the oxidation of the reduced cytochrome and the reduction of the dye to purple colour	Filter strip coated with Kovac's reagent (Tetramethyl-p-phenylenediamine dihydrochloride)	Incubate a loopful of the colony on to reagent impregnated paper	–	Few seconds	Purplish colour	In identifying Neisseria species and differentiating Pseudomonadaceae from Enterobacteriaceae
12. Catalase test (Fig. 1.9.10)	To determine the presence of enzyme catalase, which splits hydrogen peroxide into oxygen	30% Hydrogen peroxide (stored in dark bottle)	Bacterial colony placed on a slide and then add a drop of Hydrogen peroxide	–	Few seconds	Immediate bubbling	To differentiate Streptococcus from Micrococcus and Staphylococcus group
13. Coagulase test (Fig. 3.2.2, pg. 175)	To determine the ability of an organism to clot plasma by the action of the enzyme coagulase	Plasma human/rabbit	*Slide test:* emulsify the colony in a drop of saline and add a loopful of fresh plasma. Mix. Set up positive and negative controls	–	Few seconds	Formation of white clumps	To differentiate *S. aureus* from other Staphylococcus species
14. Tride sugar Iron agar test	Determines ability of organism to ferment sugars to produce acid with or without acid/H_2S	• Three sugars; glucose sucrose and lactose (1:10:1) • Phenol red ferric salt	Colony is inoculated in butt as stab culture and then streaked on slope	Red color	18-24 hours	• K/A, Glucose fermented • A/A, G and L termented with/without sucrose • K/K, No sugar fermented	Useful in Enterobacteriaceae

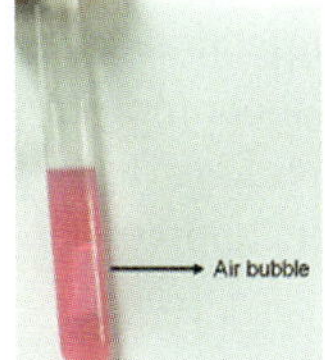

Fig.1.9.2: Carbohydrate fermentation test

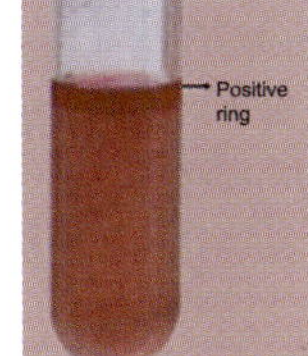

Fig.1.9.4: Indole test

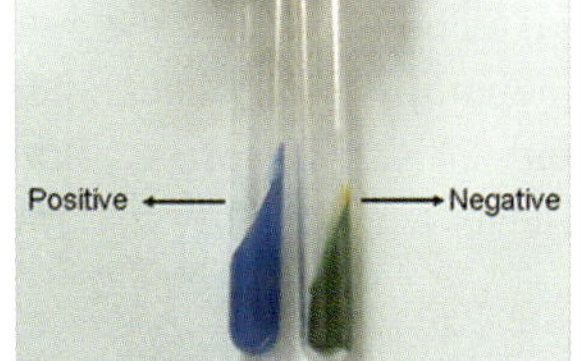

Fig.1.9.5: Citrate test

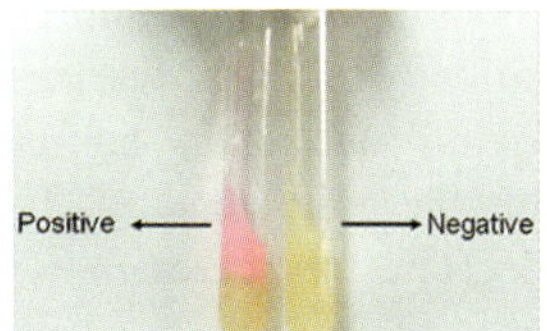

Fig.1.9.6: Urease test

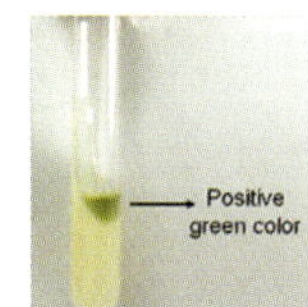

Fig.1.9.7: Phenyl pyruvic alanine test(PPA) test

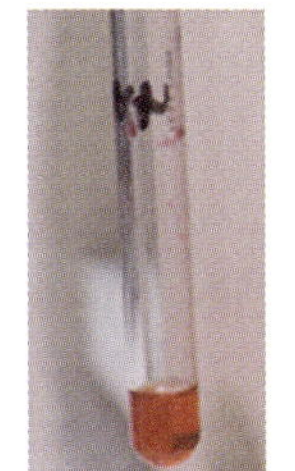
Fig.1.9.3: Nitrate test

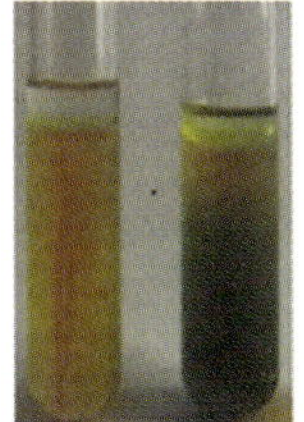
Fig.1.9.8: Oxidation fermentation test

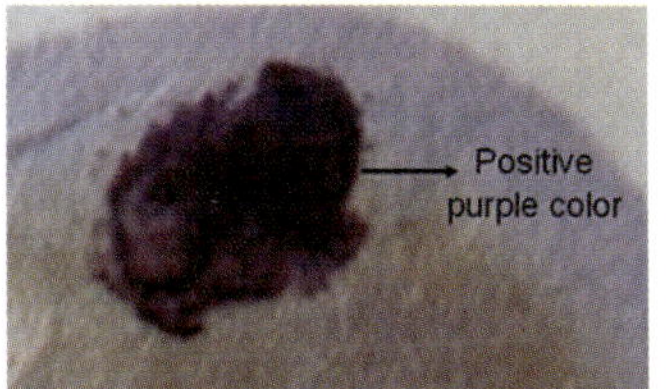

Fig.1.9.9: Oxidase test

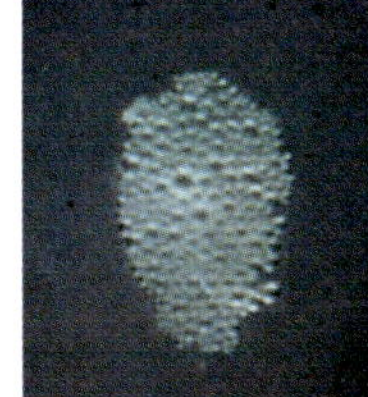
Fig.1.9.10: Catalase test

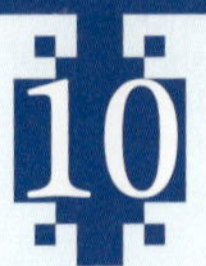

10 Detection of Microbes Based on Molecular Biology Techniques

A phenomenal change has occurred in the technology of detecting (identifying) microbes during the last few decades. The number of these tests and type of these tests keep increasing. Molecular based tests have become increasedly available. Let's study this trend.

What are the reasons that have led to the in changed scenario that is described above?

A.1 The sequencing of many human pathogens and identification of many of their genes have transformed our understanding of pathogenesis of infectious diseases. The availability of the sequence of human genome; following the completion of the human genome project and subsequently the identification of some of the human genes has changed our concepts of pathogenesis of disease. The emergence of *molecular pathology,* which analyzes nucleic acids to diagnose disease also helps to evaluate susceptibility to disease, guide treatment and predict the prognosis of disease. The ability to identify gene expressions helps us to delineate clinically diseases that mayn't have been possible on morphological or other clinical cum laboratory data.

What advantage do the tests based on traditional techniques may have over those based on molecular technology?

A.2 The molecular biology tests used to diagnose infectious agents have many advantages over the traditional microbiological techniques, however they should be seen to overall complement these tests, as a total dependence on them; can at times present an aberrated picture of the disease and miss some benefit that the traditional tests may be providing at times. One of the distinct advantages of culturing a bacterium or a fungus is that, one can provide an antimicrobial susceptibility pattern of the isolate, which isn't exactly possible, after identification of them by tests based on molecular detection.

What are the indications of performing diagnostic tests based on molecular biology?

A.3 Following are some of the applications of tests, based on molecular methods for microbial identification and characterization:

(a) *Detection of:*

(i) slow growing organisms; as *M. tuberculosis*

(ii) uncultivable pathogens; as *T. whipplei.*

(iii) Fastidious organisms: Culture-based techniques were the gold standard for diagnosis of infectious diseases. But currently for many diseases, as hepatitis C, HSV encephalitis, CMV infection (in immunocompromised), enteroviral meningitis, pertusis and *C. trachomatis* (genital infections), molecular biology tests have become the gold standard. These tests are not only are more sensitive but also faster, and can predict prognosis in some cases.

(iv) Identification of bacteria and fungi from culture isolates at genus or species level by DNA sequence of the 16S rRNA gene, which is a stable genotypic characteristic of an organism.

(b) *Guide to treatment*, for instance detection of antibiotic resistance genes in a microbe, e.g., mec A gene for detecting MRSAs. Drug resistance in HIV-1 RT gene, indicate less than optimal response to antiretroviral drugs.

(c) *Prognostication,* e.g., subtyping of respiratory syncytial virus provides information on outcome of infants infected with it, e.g., genotype of HCV can predict response to therapy in a case with chronic HCV infection.

(d) *Monitoring treatment,* e.g., monitoring HIV-1 RNA level is a standard practice in initiating, monitoring and changing antiretroviral therapy.

(e) *Epidemiology*

Classify the molecular biology based detection techniques.

A.4 Classification of techniques:

1. *Nucleic acid probes*
2. *Amplified nucleic acid techniques*
   - Target amplification
   - Probe amplification
   - Signal amplification

   [Details of classification see chapter 9, A4, p 65 (Section 1) and details of technique A6, 7, 8 of this chapter.]
3. *DNA microarray technology*
4. *DNA sequencing*

Describe the nucleic acid probes (non amplified techniques).

A.5 Nucleic acid probes:

This technique is used for direct detection of pathogens from clinical samples; as group A streptococci from throat swab and identification of culture isolates. The obvious limitation of the technique is that it lacks sensitivity and requires approximately 10^4/ml copies of nucleic acid/ml for reliable detection. To overcome this limitation one may use DNA probe, which targets bacterial ribosomal RNA, of which there may be 10,000 copies per cell.

The single-stranded nucleic acid utilized in these assays may be either DNA or RNA, so that DNA-DNA, DNA-RNA and least commonly even RNA-RNA duplexes may form, depending on the type of *hybridization assay*. These techniques are based on the principle that, if two nucleic acid strands sequences are complementary (i.e., are homologous), then they will specifically bind with each other and form a stable double-stranded molecule. Whether such binding has actually occurred, is determined by the test nucleic acid strand that is added in the assay; has a reporter molecule, which can be detected using an appropriate substrate. The reporter molecules can be radioactive (with ^{32}P or ^{125}I), non-radioactive labelled (e.g., biotin, alkaline phosphatse or chemiluminescent based (e.g., acridium). The presence of radioactive reporter molecule in a test sample is detected by autoradiography, in which usually positive hybridization is indicated by black spots on X-ray film, as a result of radioactivity. The nonradioactive reporter molecules are usually detected by colorimetric principles, in which color change is detected visually or using a spectrophotometer. Presence of chemiluminescent reporter molecules are detected using a luminometer, which can detect emitted light.

The commonly used formats include liquid phase (GenProbe) and solid phase. In the *liquid (solution) format*, the probe and target (from clinical sample) nucleotide strands are placed as a liquid reaction mixture, in which reaction occurs faster, when solid formats are used.

In *solid formats*; filter paper hybridizations, nitrocellulose membrane (as in southern blot) and 'in situ' hybridization approaches are often used. *'In situ' hybridization* is a technique often used by pathologists to detect the nucleic acid of pathogen in the pathologic tissue sample, which is used as a solid support phase. This test is sometimes available in 'fluorescent in situ hybridization' (*FISH*) format, wherein the probe is labelled with a fluorescent dye, which is detected by a fluorescent microscope. This technology is also used in 'Southern blot' and 'Northern' blot assay. The probes are available for numerous bacterial, parasitic and viral pathogens.

Describe unique aspects of the amplified nucleic acid techniques.

A.6 (a) Amplified nucleic acid techniques:

These techniques have some unique aspects besides those discussed in the general aspects of molecular biology techniques. *One* is the extreme sensitivity to detect nucleic acids from the clinical sample. This aspect is a distinct advantage but it can become problematic in the interpretation of results. For instance, PCR technique can detect nucleic acid from non-viable microbe, the importance of such a report could be of doubtful importance. Also detection of organisms, which are present in the body in minimal numbers, as a result of their being a part of normal transient flora or as an agent of latent infection. *Secondly*, these techniques can detect previously unknown agents in clinical samples by using broad range primers, which target a region of DNA that is conserved amongst a broad group of organisms; for instance bacteria.

Enumerate the amplified nucleic acid techniques based on target amplification and their characteristics.

A.6 (b) Amplified nucleic acid techniques based on target amplification:

As the name indicates in these techniques, a particular target of DNA or RNA is amplified. Most of these techniques involve two oligonucleotide primers, which bind to complementary sequences on opposite strands of the double-stranded nucleic acid. These techniques are extremely sensitive and can produce billions of copies of the targeted sequence in a few hours. Due to this characteristic, the technique is sensitive to contamination at specimen preparation level and has real cross-contamination problem (i.e., positive amplicon of one test contaminating a subsequent test being performed). These tests are extremely popular because of adaptation of these methods to commercial kits. A summary of the techniques based on this principle is given in table 1.10.1.

Table 1.10.1: Amplified nucleic acid techniques based on target amplification

Technique	Temperature requirement	Target	Enzymes used
PCR	Thermal cycler required	DNA, RNA	DNA polymerase
NASBA	Isothermal	RNA (DNA)	RT, RNAase H, RNA polymerase
Transcription mediated amplification (TMA)	Isothermal	RNA (DNA)	RT, RNAase H, RNA polymerase
Strand displacement amplification (SDA)	Isothermal	DNA, RNA	Restriction endonucleases, DNA polymerase

Describe in detail the PCR technique.

A.6 (c) Polymerase chain reaction:

The idea for this revolutionary technique to make unlimited copies of the specific nucleic acid sequence (of defined length and sequence) theoretically, even from a single copy of it; without cloning (i.e., using a technique involving living cell) came to Kary Mullis, when he was driving his car at night time in the mountains of northern California. The technique was developed by him during 1983-85, while he worked at Cetus Corporation, California, USA. For the almost unlimited applications, the technique has in the scientific world, he was awarded the Nobel prize in 1993 for his commendable work.

The fundamental basis of diagnostic techniques based on nucleic acid is that, every living being in its genome has unique nucleotide sequences in its DNA or RNA, which can be used for its identification (Fig. 1.10.1). Certain features have helped in the development of this technology. *One*, is the ^*de*naturation of the two DNA strands at high temperature like 95°C and their *re*naturation, when exposed to lower temperatures.

^The elevated thermal energy breaks the hydrogen bonds between the complementary deoxyribonucleotides on the two strands of DNA.

Second, is the ability of DNA polymerase to synthesize a complementary strand of DNA, if a specific *primer is available, which can bind to a part of the nucleic acid. *Third* is the ability of old and the newly synthesized nucleic acid strands to be available for further cycles of nucleic acid amplification of the desired region. These features can result in a single molecule of DNA molecule, giving rise to greater than one billion molecules in an hour; in PCR reaction conducted in a thermocycler.

The unique component that is specific for the various PCR protocols. for the different infectious agents; is the pair of primers. The pair of primers have to be so designed, that they are complementary to the opposite strand and chosen to flank the end region of the DNA that is to be amplified. The newly synthesized strands of DNA begin at each primer and extend beyond the position of the primer of the opposite strand. This pattern results in generation of new primer binding sites in both of the newly synthesized DNA.

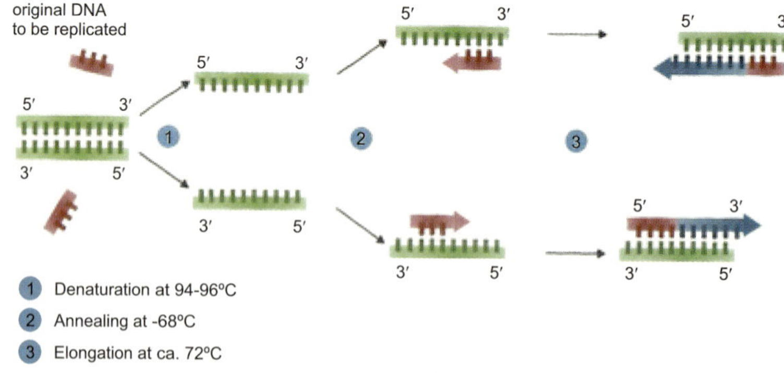

Fig. 1.10.1: Depiction of the three stages of conventional PCR

* Primer is a small sequence of oligonucleotides (usually less than 100), which is complementary to opposite parts of the strand of nucleic acid and can serve as a starting point. Automated synthesizing equipment exist currently, which can make oligonucleotide (oligos, means few) primers of desired sequence and length in less than 24 hours.

Requirements:

- *Thermocycler* (a specially designed machine, which can carry out numerous cycles, in each of which the temperature is changed thrice for the three steps; as required in the protocol. Has a block to hold multiple small vials).
- Deoxyribonucleotide triphosphate mixture (eqimolar mixture of *dNTPs*: dATP, dCTP, dGTP and dTTP).
- *Two oligonucleotide primers* (specific for each protocol, a molar excess of it is provided, so that the targeted DNA anneals preferentially to the primers than to each other).
- *Thermophilus aquaticus* enzyme (Taq) (thermo- 'heat', philus – 'love', aquaticus – from water).

  This enzyme has been derived from the hot springs of Yellowstone, National Park of U.S.A.

  [The discovery of the thermostable DNA polymerase enzyme allowed the cycling of the reaction in a small vial without the requirement of adding new enzyme, after each thermal nucleic acid denaturation step, which is to be performed at a temperature close to the boiling point]
- Buffers as Tris-HCl.
- Electrophoresis machine (to analyze the amplified product).
- Ethidium bromide (a dye that stains DNA).
- Nucleic acid to be amplified (could be in a clinical sample)

NB: If the concerned gene is not in the sample, no amplified product results. The chromosomal DNA exists but at an extremely low level that it can't be demonstrated on a stained gel.

Procedure:

In the PCR machine (thermocycler), numerous cycles of the three step cycle are performed. On an average about 25 cycles can be performed within an hour, depending on the time of each of the three steps. The PCR usually involves 30-50 repetitive cycles.

1st step (Denaturation): In this step, the reaction mixture including the clinical sample is heated at a high temperature approximately 95°C for few seconds, so that the complementary strands of the DNA denature to separate.

2nd step (Annealing): This step is carried at a temperature of less than 60°C. Here, the two primers anneal to the two denatured DNA strands. The exact temperature used in this step varies with the composition of the primers being used and should be less than the melting temperature of the primers being used (Tm).

3rd step (Synthesis): This step is usually carried out at 72°C. In this step, the nucleotides are added along with the primers and DNA polymerase enzyme, resulting in two pairs of nucleic acid at the end of this stage.

The above three steps are repeated number of times, which depends on a protocol being followed.

Uses:

1. The technology helps in rapid diagnosis of infections. For instance, tuberculosis culture may require up to 12 weeks for isolation, but with this technology, the result can be available in few hours.
2. Detection of an infectious agent, which may be present in extremely small amount in a clinical sample or a food product. For instance, demonstration of *S. Typhimurium* in an ice-cream or an egg product.
3. Taxonomic classification of prokaryotes and eukaryotes (16SrRNA and 18SrRNA)
4. Forensic medicine: For instance, PCR and DNA analyses of the semen sample can be done to free the innocent or convict the guilty.
5. Detect genetic diseases: Using allele specific oligonucleotide probes.

Describe the modification of the PCR technique used to study the syndromic approach to diseases.

A.6 (d) Multiplex PCR:

It is an alternative technique to broad based PCR for detecting multiple pathogens. Here instead of one pair of broad-range primer, multiple pairs of primers are used, which are designed for multiple targets. So, in this approach technically, multiple amplicons may be produced in a situation, if co-infections are present. The technique is complicated and is less sensitive than classic PCR assay, as the primers have to be so designed that they have similar annealing temperatures and lack complementarity. Such as approach helps in implementing the *syndromic approach* to diseases. Such approach has been used detecting the various bacterial/viral causes of meningitis, detecting common respiratory viruses and detecting wide variety of adenovirus subtypes or serotypes that cause human infection.

Describe the other modifications of PCR.

A.6 (e) Several modifications of the classic PCR format have been made, which have resulted in the expansion of the use of this test. Some of the modifications are given below:

RT-PCR (Reverse transcriptase):

In this technique, amplification is performed of the RNA rather than of the DNA, which is performed in the traditional PCR. This process is accomplished by the reverse transcriptase enzyme, which can produce a cDNA copy from the RNA. The cDNA produced is then amplified with the traditional technique. Currently a single thermostable DNA polymerase is used in the protocol, which also has significant RT (reverse transcriptase) activity.

This technique is useful for detecting RNA viruses; as viruses causing meningitis and detecting other organisms targeting their ribosomal RNA. The technique can also be useful in studying the genetic expression of microbes and eukaryotes, if the mRNA is detected. Quantitative RT-PCR assays for HCV and HIV help to determine the amount of viruses in the patient's blood, i.e., the 'viral load' and are helpful in monitoring the response of the individual patient to therapy.

Broad-range PCR:

As the name indicates, here a pair of broad-range PCR primers are used, which focus on a larger group of characteristics. For instance; primer for gram positive bacteria, primer for mycobacteria as a group, primer for common bacteria as a group, primer for common bacteria causing bacterial meningitis or endocarditis. One can choose any group of related microbes or other characteristics. When one chooses genes that encode for bacterial, fungal or parasitic ribosomal DNA, one can gather a lot of information on their taxonomy. Once a positive result has been obtained with this technique, one can assess by multiple techniques the particular organism that can be present in the group. This approach can be time saving and help in the discovery of new pathogens. By this technique *T. whipplei* and *B. henselae* were discovered.

Nested PCR:

It is a modification of the PCR with the aim of increasing the sensitivity and specificity of the PCR assay. It utilizes two pairs of primers. The products of the first round of amplification are subjected to a second round of amplification with the second set of primers, which anneal to the sequences of the first round products. The disadvantage of this technique is the high rates of contamination, as the process requires open manipulations, after the first round of amplification. This approach is useful in detecting microorganism, which may be in low quantity in the blood, CSF or tissues; for example Rickettsia, herpes viruses and enteroviruses.

Real time PCR:

The name 'real time' is used in this type of PCR, as the evidence of amplification occurs during the PCR reaction in 'real-time'. In this type of PCR, the target amplification and detection occurs simultaneously in the same tube. Here fluorogenic molecules are used for the detection of the amplified products, which are present in the same reaction vessel that is used for amplification. A special type of thermocycler is required here, which has precision optics that can determine fluorescence emission from the sample wells. The computer software supporting the thermal cycler monitors the data at every cycle and maintains an amplification plot for the process.

The fluorogenic molecules used for detection of amplified nucleic acids may be of nonspecific or specific category. An example of the former category is the SYBR green, which detects any amplified nucleic acid. An example of the specific probes is the TaqMan or hydrolysis probes.

This technique has several advantages; as quantitation of the nucleic acid in the clinical sample and minimal amplicon contamination, as the reaction vessel doesn't have to be opened to analyze the amplicon. It also gives rapid results, as reaction proceeds rapidly, uses smaller reaction volumes and obviously no post PCR processing is required.

Describe transcription mediated amplified techniques.

A.6 (f) **Nucleic acid sequence-based amplification (NASBA)** and **transcription mediated amplification (TMA)** technique -are examples of transcription-mediated amplification method. These techniques have the greatest strength in the amplification of ssRNA rather than DNA. These techniques have several advantages. *Firstly*; as these are single tube assays and the end product is RNA which is labile, so the risk of contamination is low. *Secondly*, it involves rapid kinetics and doesn't require a thermal cycler, as no denaturation step is required, which is partly responsible for changing the temperature of incubation. The limitation of this technique is that it gives poor performance with DNA targets.

The *procedure* involved here is, first the synthesis of cDNA (complementary) from the target RNA. This step is possible using one type of primer that has T7 RNA polymerase binding sequence on the 5' end of the molecule and the reverse transcriptase enzyme. In the next step, the RNase H enzyme degrades the strand of RNA in the cDNA/target RNA hybrid, leaving the single-stranded cDNA. In the next step, a second (type) primer binds to the cDNA strand and converts to a double stranded DNA. Currently both strands of DNA are flanked by T7 RNA polymerase promoter regions. Consequently, using RNA polymerase, several copies of RNA can be transcribed.

The NASBA based kits are used for detection and quantification of HIV-1 RNA and CMV-RNA. TheTMA based kits are available for detection of *M. tuberculosis* and *C. trachomatis*.

Describe the amplified nucleic acid techniques based on probe amplification.

A.7 Amplified nucleic acid technique based on probe amplification:

The techniques involve geometric multiplication of the number of probes in comparison to the target amplification techniques, in which geometric accumulation of the target site occurs. One of the techniques in this category is the **ligase chain reaction,** which requires thermal cycler, in which the target can be either DNA or RNA. Two sets of primers hybridize adjacent to each other on each of the denatured DNA strands with a small gap between the two. The thermostable DNA ligase 'ligates' (joins) the two set of primers. Amplification of the probes (ligated products) occurs exponentialy in fashion similar to PCR, in which the amplification of the target site occurs. This method is not used these days.

Describe the signal amplification techniques.

A.8 Amplified nucleic acid techniques based on signal amplification:

A detailed description of these techniques is beyond the undergraduate curriculum, however a summary of the techniques and their features is depicted in table 1.10.2

Table 1.10.2: Signal amplification techniques

Technique	Temperature requirement	Target	Amplification system
Branched DNA assay (bDNA)	*Isothermal	DNA, RNA	bDNA probe
Hybrid capture assay	Isothermal	DNA, RNA	Anti DNA-RNA hybrid antibody

* Require no changes in temperature of incubation, so no requirement of thermal cycler unlike PCR technique.

Signal amplification techniques:

These techniques are based on increasing the concentration of labelled molecule/reporter molecules to the target or by increasing the intensity of the signal from the probe. The concentration of probe or target site doesn't occur with these techniques. These techniques are generally considered less sensitive than amplification techniques based on probe or target amplification. However they have many other advantages. These techniques are less likely to produce false-positive results, as there is reduced risk of contamination in comparison to other amplification techniques. These tests are more amenable to the development of quantitative assays, as number of target molecules isn't altered and the amount of signal is directly proportional to the amount of target sequence in the clinical sample. These techniques aren't affected by the presence of enzymatic inhibitors in clinical samples, as signal amplification process isn't dependent on enzymatic processes.

Describe the microarray technique.

A.9 Microarray ('Gene chips'):

The term *microarray* literally means arrangement at microscopic level. The arrangement is of the thousands of hybridization sites, each of which is an olgonucleotide, to which labelled amplification product is hybridized. The signals generated may be fluorescent or electrical. The device can detect multiple signals simultaneously, which can help in detecting DNA differences or differences in expression of mRNA. These features make this system expensive and dependent on software packages for extensive data analysis. The microarray analysis can be useful in discovery of new infectious agents, discovering new drugs, detecting genetic determinants of resistance and to study host response to infection (study gene expression).

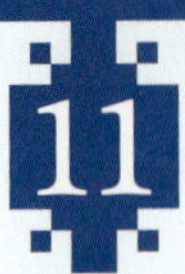

Bacterial Taxonomy

– *God's Registrar (Referring to Carolus Linnaeus, who is also known as 'Father of Taxonomy'*

– *Think of the earth as a living organism that co-exists with billions of different species. Thus the need to classify them.*

Pneumocystis jirovecii **was first described in 1909 and thought to be a protozoan having 'trophozoite' and 'cyst' stages. There was not much interest in this organism until the AIDS emerged in the 1980s, when it became a common opportunistic pathogen in these cases. The population of immunocompromised individuals also increased recently due to increased usage of immunosuppressants in organ transplant cases. This organism was an eukaryotic microbe of uncertain taxonomy with many workers concluding it to be a protozoan on the basis of morphological, ultrastructural findings and its susceptibility to common antiprotozoal drugs; as pentamidine and Trimethoprim-sulfamethoxazole. The controversy about its classification continued for a long time till a study in 1988 strongly indicated it to be a fungus on the basis of phylogenetic analysis of the organism's 16S like rRNA sequence alignments showing close similarity with *Saccharomyces cerevisiae*. Further epidemiologic studies on its transmission have also supported its fungal lineage. Currently the organism is the prize possession of the mycologists, having been snatched from the protozoologists (parasitologists). Let's study the interesting topic of bacterial taxonomy.**

What do you understand by taxonomy?

A.1 It is an art of biological classification, which provides for an orderly basis for the naming of bacteria and placing them into a category or taxon (pleural taxa). The future taxonomic studies would have to depend on DNA chip technology to cope with the challenge of intraspecies classification.

What is the need of bacterial taxonomy?

A.2 The types of bacteria in this universe would be probably millions. If the same organism is studied with a different name in different regions of the world, the progress in bacteriology would be slow, as the scientists may be repeating the work that had already been done and won't be able to share the information they are gathering.

Depict evolution of life on earth.

A.3 Earth is about 4.5 billion years old. It has passed through various phases, as initially its surface was very hot and subsequently had volcanic activity and had other adverse conditions. The life that the planet supported at that time correlated with its physical conditions. Currently we are aware of few organisms that can survive adverse conditions, e.g., *Thermophilus aquaticus* can survive boiling. *Dienococcus radiodurans*, a bacterium can survive 300 times greater radiation than what man can tolerate.

What is the criticism of the science of bacterial taxonomy?

A.4 It is said that taxonomy is written by taxonomists for taxonomists and is of no relevance for non-taxonomists. It is a subjective branch and in many ways is an art than a science.

What would be the characteristics of the taxonomical techniques that would make them ideal?

A.5 The system should be stable (not affected significantly by genetic variation), objective (be able to be verifiable by any observer), predictive and should be based on non-expensive and simple technology. It would group organisms that are related through evolution and separate the unrelated ones.

What are the benefits for classifying microorganisms?

A.6 (i) It provides information on evolution of organisms.

(ii) It arranges related organisms into groups.

(iii) It establishes criteria for identifying microorganisms. Identification relies on comparing the characters of an unknown organism with fully identified organisms in order to name appropriately.

Who is the father of Taxonomy? Describe his key contributions.

A.7 Carolus Linnaeus, the Swedish botanist (eighteenth-century) is considered to be the father of taxonomy. He is credited with introducing the binomial nomenclature, a system which is still being used. In the binomial or 'two name' system, the first name designates the genus (plural 'genera') of an organism and the second name stands for species. The first letter of the genus is capitalized. The species name is not capitalized. Both words are italicized in print but underlined, when handwritten. The International code of nomenclature of bacteria provides rule for naming bacteria at different taxonomic ranks (this 'namkaran' ceremony in humans is performed by pundits/priests). The goal of the nomenclature is to provide the organism with an exclusive name that carries valuable information, e.g., Salmonella Typhi.

What are some of the problems that occur during microbial classification?

A.8 (i) It is difficult to decide what constitutes a kingdom.

(ii) It is difficult to decide what constitutes a species. In higher organisms, characteristic of successful mating to produce fertile offspring helps in identifying species. In bacteria; such criteria cannot be applied and there is a limited feature of lateral gene transfer (gene transfer between two numbers). The fossil records are also incomplete. It is difficult to decide, how different two organisms must be in order to be classified as separate species. One of the important criteria for species definition is approximately 70% or greater DNA relatedness with a Tm of 5°C or less (thermal stability of duplex), besides phenotypic agreement (greater the complementary strands fit together, more are the two strands resistant to dissociation by heating).

(iii) Evolution occurs continuously and rapldly in microbes, which requires continuous updating.

Which would be the best classification scheme to group organisms?

A.9 One that would group organisms that are related through evolution and separate that are unrelated.

Which is the most accepted classification system? Mention about the five kingdom classification system.

A.10 No single classification system is totally accepted by all biologists.

The five kingdom classification system is one of the most accepted classification systems. One of the advantages of this system is that it effectively deals with all microorganisms. The five kingdoms in it are Monera (prokaryotae), Protista, Fungi, Plantae and Animalia. All monerans are unicellular, which consists of all prokaryotes, which includes eubacteria cynaobacteria and the archaebacteria. The eubacteria are of most important in medical microbiology. The cyancobacteria were formerly known as blue-green algae, are photosynthetic, non-invasive and don't pose any significant health threat to humans. Rarely, they are responsible for algal blooms, in which a thick layer of algae growth forms on the surface of water. These blooms can release toxic substances that can make the water malodorous and can harm the life dependent on that water. The Archaeobacteria as the name indicates are primitive prokaryotes adapted to extreme environments, e.g., halophiles, thermoacidophiles and the methanogens (which reduce carbon containing compound to methane gas).

What are the ranks (categories) in a microbial classification system)? Give an example for a bacterium.

A.11 At the lowest level we have the strain. Several similar strains are grouped into a species. Several similar species are grouped into a genus and many similar genera are included into a family. Many families are grouped into orders and many orders characterize class and several such classes constitute a division. Many related divisions constitute a kingdom, e.g., for *E. coli* strain K12 (Fig. 1.11.1).

'Escherichia' is derived from *Theodor Escherich*, who described it and 'coli' from colon, from where it is frequently isolated.

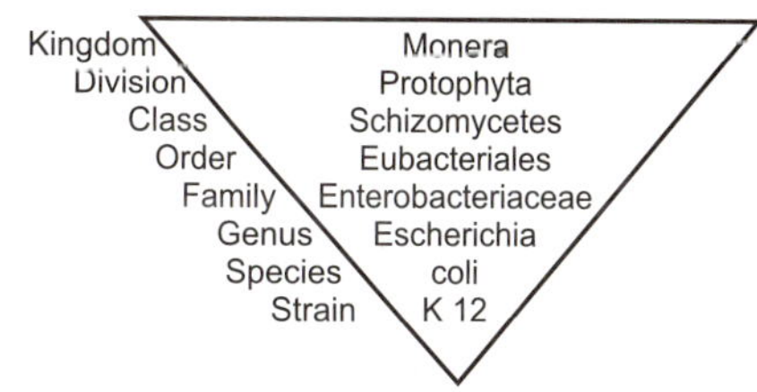

Fig. 1.11.1: Bacterial classification *E.coli*

What is the importance of culture collection. Give an example.

A.12 For many research procedures, genetical identical microbes have to be used, so that work carried out in different parts of the world can be correlated. For commercial products; as wine and cheese to have almost identical end product with same flavour, genetical identical microbes have be used. Two types of culture collections are available, namely National Type Culture Collection (NTCC) and American type culture collection (ATCC). Anybody can purchase the various microbial cultures available at a nominal cost and these are delivered by surface mail.

Mention about Bergey's manual.

A.13 There is no internationally accepted phylogenetic system and bacterial classification scheme. Bergey's manual is one of the most accepted references for identification of bacteria.

When can you presume that a new organism has been isolated?

A.14 When the properties of the newly isolated organism don't tally with any of the descriptions in Bergey's manual, then one can presume to have isolated a new organism.

Enumerate the key classification approaches for organism classification and describe them.

A.15 (i) Adansonian/numerical

(ii) Genetic/phylogenetic

(iii) Intraspecies classification (strain typing)

Describe Adansonian classification.

A.16 The Adansonian classification is named after Michael Adanson, who introduced it in the 18th century. It is based on the principle that increasing the number of study characteristics, would increase the accuracy of grouping of organisms. Hence; it also called as the numerical (phenetic) classification. It makes no phylogenetic assumption and gives equal importance to all characters. Each characteristic is given a value of '1' if present and '0' if not present. A computer program helps to prepare a similarity coefficient for a pair of organisms. If two organisms have more than 90% similarity coefficient, they are presumed to belong to same species.

Describe Phylogenetic classification.

A.17 This classification is based on the principle that phylogenic (natural) groups exist in nature for the organisms. The differentiation is based on certain characteristics that may vary in importance in their classification. Several ranks as kingdom, division, class, order, family, genus and species (serotype) are designated.

A key technology that helps in studying these phylogenetic relationships are the rRNA homology, studies. rRNA is a probabe target, as it is present in all bacteria, functionally constant and composed of highly conserved as well as variable domains. Currently these techniques have been replaced by studies on 16S or 23S rRNA, which yield the dendrograms, which provide the critical information for bacterial taxonomy.

– The sequence of 16S rRNA component is critical in studying evolutionary relationships for several reasons. One of the key reasons is that the ribosomes have evolved slowly, as the probability of nucleotide sequence to change but allow the ribosome to function is limited. The role of ribosomes in protein synthesis is indispensable. The other reasons for using rRNA as target, is that it is present in all bacteria and is composed of highly conserved as well as variable domains. 16S rRNA has approximately 1,500 nucleotides. Their sequence can be determined by direct rRNA sequencing techniques or recently by newer techniques that rely on PCR technology. Every organism has unique base consequences, designated signature sequences. If the nucleotide sequences of 16S rRNA molecules of two organisms is similar then the two are likely to close evolutionarily. However, these techniques are expensive, difficult to perform and available only in few research laboratories.

– DNA base composition

G + C value

It varies between 24 and 76% for the bacteria. The range observed within a genus should not be more than 10% and within a species should not be more than 3%. This value is a classical genotypic characteristic and is part of the routine description of bacterial taxa.

The DNA base composition of an organism is unique, as the number of molecules of adenine A equals that of thymine (T) and the number of molecules of guanine (G) equals that of cytosine (C). However some different organisms may have nearly identical G + C content, as vastly different humans and *B. subtilis* both have nearly identical GC content in their DNA. The GC content is expressed as:

$$\frac{\text{moles G} + \text{moles C}}{(\text{moles G} + \text{moles C} + \text{moles A} + \text{moles T})} \times 100$$

Describe the classification methods for performing intraspecies classification of bacteria.

A.18 The methods can be categorized into phenotypic and genotypic (includes phylogenetic details). Currently great emphasis is given on the genotypic methods.

Phenotypic methods - (all that don't focus on DNA or RNA) – Morphology, staining characteristics, cultural characteristic, antigenic characteristics, biochemical characteristics, phage typing, Whole cell proteins profile (by sodium dodecyl sulphate polyacrylamide gel electrophoresis)*, aminoacid sequencing, serology.

* SDS; act as detergent, dissolves the proteins of the lysed protein.

Genotypic method: see section 17, p.. 621-623

What are the uses of studying intraspecies classification?

A.19 Most often these techniques are used in the outbreak of infectious diseases, where they can help in tracing the source and path of the disease transmission. This is of vital importance, as this can lead to immediate control measures and help in preventing such outbreaks in future.

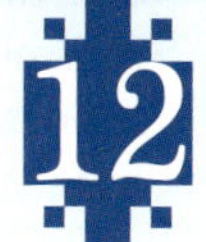

Epidemiology of Infectious Diseases

- *Infections are most often transmitted from patient to patient by the hands of healthcare workers.* — *Dr William Jarvis*
- *Epidemiology is like a bikini: what is revealed is interesting; what is concealed may be crucial.* — *Peter Duesbergh*

After the mysterious outbreak of pneumonia (Legionnaire's disease) in 1976 in a hotel in Philadelphia, *Legionella pneumophila* became recognized as a common cause of nosocomial pneumonia. However the source of this organism and methods of control of this disease remained unknown for some time. The crucial work in this area was done by two teams (Best *et al.* and Johnson *et al.*) who applied Evan's modification of Koch's postulates and found potable water in the water distribution to be a key source of this organism. They found that decrease in the number of this organism in the water supply led to decrease in nosocomial pneumonia cases.

One of the achievements of the last century has been the marked increased in life expectancy. One of the key contributors to this has been the reduced morbidity and mortality from infectious diseases. This has been possible because of the correct application of the science of epidemiology of infectious diseases. Let's study this aspect.

Selected Epidemiologic Terms

Common source:	The etiologic agent responsible for an epidemic or outbreak originates from a single source or reservoir
Etiological agent:	A microorganism responsible for causing infection or infectious disease
Mode of transmission:	Means by which etiologic agents are brought in contact with the human host (e.g., infected blood, contaminated water, insect bite)
Nosocomial infection:	Infection in which etiologic agent was acquired in a hospital
Outbreak:	A larger than normal number of diseased or infected individuals that occurs over a relatively short period
Pandemic:	An epidemic that spans the world
Reservoir:	Origin of the etiologic agent or location from which they disseminate (e.g., water, food, insects, animals, humans)
Strain typing:	Laboratory-based characterization of etiologic agents designed to establish their relatedness to one another during a particular outbreak or epidemic
Surveillance:	Any type of epidemiologic investigation that involves data collection for characterizing circumstances surrounding the incidence or prevalence of particular disease or infection
Vector:	A living entity (animal, insect, or plant) that transmits the etiologic agent
Vehicle:	A nonliving entity that is contaminated with the etiologic agent and as such is the mode of transmission for that agent

How is epidemiology defined? Mention one of its earliest successful applications.

A.1 Epidemiology is defined as the study of occurrence of health related conditions/disease, its distribution and factors associated with it and its control/prevention in populations. One of the earliest successful applications of it was the John Snow's application, which led to the correct investigation of the 'Broad street' pump outbreak of cholera in London in 1851. This led to a legislation mandating all water companies to filter their water. One of the most recent applications has been the description of the AIDS syndrome in 1981, hypothesis of an infectious aetiology, identification of the HIV virus and the subsequent control and preventive measures.

What is the role of the microbiologist and clinician in the application of epidemiology?

A.2 Epidemiological analysis has several goals. Some of these, which directly involve the microbiologist include identifying outbreaks or unusual rates of disease occurrence or detecting new/rare diseases, provide laboratory based efforts to identify the infectious agents, help in understanding of disease pathogenesis, characterize factors that contribute to disease transmission and develop/evaluate primary, secondary and tertiary control/prevention measures.

Every clinician should be aware of regional patterns of infection for effective diagnosis, treatment and prevention of them. This requires the study of incidence rate and prevalence rate of infections. For acute infections lasting a few days/weeks, the incidence rate may be high in comparison to the prevalence rate that may be low. In contrast, for chronic infections lasting months/years, the prevalence rate may be very high in comparison to the incidence rate. Early diagnosis of numerous outbreaks of infection, e.g., methicillin resistant *S. aureus* that occur in the nurseries and ICUs, before they can create havoc, depend on an efficient hospital infection team including microbiologist.

What are the forms in which infectious disease in a geographical place can present as?

A.3 (a) **Outbreak:** A cluster of cases in a single household/locality or small area. A local source is indicated, which has to be identified before further transmission can be stopped.

It is defined as an unusual or unexpected increase of cases to a known microbe or emergence of cases of a new infection.

Endemic: Infections that have a stable incidence within the population or are constantly present in the population.

e.g., Sexually transmitted diseases (STDs) in hilly regions of Himachal Pradesh

Hyperendemic: If infection within a population has very high incidence.

e.g., Trachoma in a large rural district

Sporadic: Cases which are often unconnected, i.e., scattered (from the aspect of source of infection).

Epidemic: An increase in infectious cases of one infection over a large area; for instance a country over a prolonged period of time. e.g., 'Swine flu' in 2009

Prosodemic: epidemic that is smoldering and chiefly transmitted by contact (person to person)

Pandemic: An epidemic that involves a larger area in a short period; for instance several countries or continents, e.g., the classic 1918-19 pandemic of influenza (killed 20 million people).

What are the three components of transmission of infection, whose knowledge should be existing in order to control the infection in the community?

A.3 (b) These are namely

(i) Reservoir of the infection

(ii) Modes of transmission and

(iii) Susceptible host

The relationship of infection to these is depicted below in a figure.

I	II	III
Reservoir of infection→	Modes of transmission→	Susceptible host

Describe the role of first component, i.e., 'reservoir of infection' in the transmission of the infection.

A.4 *Reservoir of the infection:* It is defined as living beings (man, animal or plants) or other material as soil, in which the infectious agent can survive, live or multiply.

A term related to it is the source of infection, which implies the various living beings or other material, from which the infectious agent can transmit to the host. The reservoir and source of the infection are usually same for most of the infections but sometimes can be different in some diseases.

The *source of infection* may be endogenous or exogenous. The *endogenous* source refers to the individuals own normal flora present in the body becoming infections, e.g., the *E. coli* present as perineal flora can ascend the urinary tract of the (same) person and cause urinary tract infection. Another example would be the normal 'viridians', streptococci present in the oral flora of an individual entering blood during a dental procedure; as tooth extraction (not performed under cover of antibiotics) causing bacteremia and/or bacterial endocarditis.

The *exogenous* source indicates infectious agents from outside the body of the individual (host) causing infections. These include: (a) Human cases (here in a different context) are acting as sources of infection for other individuals than themselves) (b) Human carriers, (c) Animals, (d) Insects, (e) Soil, (f) Water and (g) Food

(a) The **human case** usually becomes a source of the infection in the prodromal period (i.e., before signs and symptoms manifest) to many weeks after it (in some cases, the person may remain infectious for his life as TB, toxoplasma, HIV infected individuals).

(b) **Human carrier:** A carrier is defined as a person who harbours the infectious agent, who can infect others (including oneself) but causes no morbidity (ill health/signs or symptoms) in the individual itself.

The carriers can be categorized into:

(i) *Convalescent carrier:* It is the probably the group that has the largest number of any type of carrier. It is defined as the individual who continues to harbour the infectious agent despite or after having recovered from the disease.

(ii) *Healthy carrier:* It is the individual, who harbours the infectious agent but has never succumbed to it, i.e., has suffered because of it.

(iii) *Temporary carrier:* It is the individual, who harbours the infectious agent up to 6 months after having recovered from that disease.

(iv) *Chronic carrier:* It is the individual, who carries the infectious agent for years, after having recovered from that disease, e.g., 'typhoid Mary' see. p. 269

e.g., Herpes simplex oral infection case

e.g., Infectious mononucleosis case

(v) *Contact carrier:* It is the individual, who acquires the infectious agent from (another) patient.

(vi) *Paradoxical carrier* is the individual, who acquires the infectious agent from another carrier!

(c) **Animals:** Some diseases of animals can also be transmitted to man, so these infectious agents in symptomatic and asymptomatic animals can act as reservoir of infection. Details see chapter 2, section 17 p. 597-598

(d) **Insects:** Numerous insects can act as source of infection. These are the ones in which the infectious agent develops and multiplies as part of its life cycle, before being transmitted to man, e.g., plague bacillus and malarial parasite in rat-flea and mosquito, respectively.

(e) **Soil:** it can act as source for many bacterial pathogens as Nocardia, spores of *C. tetani* and *C. perfringens*, fungal pathogens; as blastomyces, histoplasma, Cryptococcus, mycetoma agents and helminthic agents; as filariform larvae of *Strongyloides stercoralis* and *Ancylostoma duodenale*.

(f) **Water:** It acts as a source of many bacterial, viral and parasitic infectious agents. This could be due to the presence of agents (see chapter, vehicle and vectors, p. 595).

Agent – Bacterial – *V. cholerae*

Viral –Hepatitis A, Hepatitis E

Vectors – *Dracunculus medinensis* in Guinea worm

(g) **Food:** It acts as a source of infection for many diseases; as eggs and meat for S. Typhimurium, sweets for *S. aureus* food poisoning and rice for *B. cereus* infection.

Describe the role of second component i.e., 'modes of transmission' in the transmission of infection.

A.5 Infectious agents can transmit from source (environment) or from one host to another by mechanisms, which can be classified as either **direct** or **indirect**. The different modes in the former include

(i) Close contact; as in touching, kissing, or sexual activity, e.g., in primary syphilis, gonorrhoea

(ii) Droplet spread (include large drops/particles greater than 100 μm) that does not spread beyond a distance of about 1 mt from infected individuals onto the conjunctiva or to the nose/mouth of an individual.

(iii) Susceptible tissue coming in contact of a bite of an infected animals or material; as soil containing infectious agent, e.g., rabies following dog bite

(iv) Vertical (congenital), this occurs when the infectious agent can travel from mother to fetus 'in utero' transplacentally, e.g., congenital syphilis and TORCH* infections. The latter infections are called teratogenic, as these are often associated with congenital malformations in the fetus.

*TORCH is acronym for Toxoplasma, Rubella, CMV and Herpes.

INDIRECT modes of transmission indicate that the infectious agent gets transmitted to the infected host indirectly.

(a) *Vehicle borne:* this occurs, when any substance serves as an intermediate means of introducing the infectious agent into the susceptible host. These substances include:

(i) Water (details see chapter 2 section 17, p. 595)

(ii) Food (refer chapter 7, section 6, p. 271-272)

(iii) Fomites (application, see A8a, p. 265)

(iv) Infected instruments (iatrogenic)

E.g., Hepatitis B and HIV

(b) *Vector borne* (details see chapter 2 section 17, p. 599-600

The vectors can serve as a means of transmitting infectious agents by mechanical means or biologically. The example of the former is soiled (contaminated) feet of housefly transmitting dysentery or vibrio organisms to the food that it comes in contact with. The biological mode occurs; when the infectious agent needs to develop, multiply or undergo cyclopropagative (both development and multiplication) before it can transmit the infectious agent to the man.

(c) *Airborne* (inhalation): this occurs by airborne route and involves spread with aerosols (with infectious agents) with particles in the range of 1-5 µm. These particles can spread great distance, as remain suspended in air for long periods (unlike droplets and large particles) and cause outbreaks of measles and anthrax.

Applied importance: see chapter 1, section 17, p. 596-597

Describe the role of the third component, i.e., 'Susceptible host' in the transmission of the infection.

A.6 The characteristics of the individual play a vital role in eventual outcome of the host-parasite (infectious agent) interaction. The host factors can be classified into two categories as depicted below:

I. *Factors that determine exposure*

(i) Sex

(ii) Age (as child may be attending a childcare facility, whereas a young adult might be staying in military barracks)

(iii) Socio-economic status could determine good diet, hygiene and life-style diseases

(iv) Behavioural factors; as using alcohol or I/V drugs or risk behaviour

(v) Sex habits: homoxsexual/heterosexual, number of partners

(vi) Occupation

(vii) Travel to endemic areas

(viii) Vector exposure

II. *Factors that determine occurrence of infection and its severity*

(i) Genetic constitution of the individual: A large number of human genes have been found to be associated with altered susceptibility to infectious agents. It is likely that a significant functional variation in the human genome has evolved to facilitate human defense against the infectious agents.

(ii) Immunity status of the individual including vaccination status. The inflammatory response of the host is critical for initiating the infection or resolving the infectious process. Bacterial infection initiates a triple series of host responses involving the complement, kinin and coagulation pathways. C3a, C5a and other components are inflammatory and cause inflammatory cells to migrate from the luminal side of the vessel to the site of infection.

(iii) Quantum and virulence of the infectious organisms; as antibiotic resistance.

(iv) Duration of exposure and route of entry of the infectious agent

(v) Coexisting infections

(vi) Vaccination

The outcome of the infection would depend on the interaction between factors which influence microbial pathogenicity and the various host factors mentioned including its immune status (see section of immunology, p. 138 and 145).

Note:
- Many factors that determine exposure would also influence the occurrence and severity of infection
- Identification of many clinical syndromes; as haemolytic-uremic syndrome required extensive microbiological testing. For instance, the former syndrome required isolation of the organism (*E. coli*) from the sample, testing with specific antisera and pulse field gel electrophoresis of the isolate (to comment on the identity of strains involved at source level in the outbreak).

Microbial Pathogenicity

- *You can find bacteria everywhere. They are invisible to us. I have never seen a bacterium except under a microscope. They are so small, we do not see them, but they are everywhere.* — *Bonnie Bassier*

Let's study how microbes cause pathogenicity with three integrated clinical based studies

Integrated Clinical Case Based Study 1

Three months back Shefali, a twenty three years old female was treated for a lower urinary tract infection with ampicillin to which she had responded well. Currently, she has again presented with similar complaints and urine culture has revealed *E. coli* count of >10^5 CFU/ml. The antimicrobial susceptibility report of this isolate has revealed it to be resistant to ampicillin.

What is the likely reservoir of organism for causing UTIs in this case?

A.1 (a) They are likely to have acquired from the organisms present in the patient's GIT, which have colonized the perineal area. Most of the UTIs are endogenous in origin.

Describe the terms saprophyte, opportunistic pathogen, pathogen, pathogenicity, virulence and parasite.

A.1 (b)

- *Saprophyte:* These are free living organism, who don't need a host (living being) to survive, but can survive on decaying and dead organic matter. These organism cannot invade a host, but under circumstances of lowered resistance of the host may cause infection, e.g., *B. subtilis*.
- *Opportunistic pathogen:* Some microorganisms (saprophytes or commensals) can cause damage under certain conditioning; as Micrococci/coagulase negative staphylococci in immunocompromised individuals or an organism getting introduced into a normally sterile site; as Proteus spp. in blood.
- *Pathogen:* These are microorganism that regularly causes disease or are capable of causing disease in some proportion of apparently immunocompetent host.
- *Pathogenicity:* It refers to the ability of microorganisms to cause disease.
- *Virulence:* It refers to degree to which a given microorganisms is pathogenic. It is measured by *ID50* (I= infectious and D=dose) and *LD50* (L=lethal, and D=dose). The former is defined as the number of organisms required to cause infection in fifty percent of those exposed to the pathogen, whereas the latter is defined as the number of organisms required to kill fifty percent of test animals exposed to the pathogen. However it should be clear that the virulence of the organism must be viewed in the perspective of the host. For instance; whether Hepatitis B infection causes asymptomatic infection or fulminant hepatitis depends on the genetic constitution of the host and the immune mediated mechanisms, besides varying virulence of HBV.
- *Parasite:* This term needs clarification because one often talks of host-parasite relationship in general microbiology and immunology. Truly speaking in latter context, parasite refers to any organisms (as bacteria, viruses etc.) which are dependent on other organisms (host) for their sustenance but in medical terminology, it classically refers to a protozoan or helminth.

Distinguish between commensalism and parasitism.

A.1 (c) *Commensalism* is a relationshp between two organisms in which one benefits and the other (host) is not harmed whereas *parasitism* is a relationship in which one organism benefts and the host gets harmed.

Depict in a figure; the relationship between contaminants, infection and disease.

A.1 (d)

Constant interaction of billions of microorganisms with host result in →	Some microorganisms **contaminate** the host →	The microorganism remain present on the host for prolonged time, results in **colonization** of the host but does not elicit an immune response or multiplication, can lead to →	**Infection** (microorganism start multiplying on or within host) can lead to→	→**Disease** →*Cure* →*Carrier state*
A related term that one should known is *syndrome,* which is defined as a disease, characterized by certain combination (complex) of signs and symptoms.				

What is the most common relation between the prokaryotes and the human body?

A.1 (e) The body of man carries billions of prokaryotes, the number of which is many times the total number of cells (eukaryotic) the human body has. The current study of microbial pathogenicity at molecular level has revealed that most! infections are beneficial to both the microbe and the host, for instance the microbial colonization and infection provides protective flora to the host and stimulates the immune system. The central question that arises is what makes the microorganism pathogenic? The answer is not simple, as the process starting with contamination/colonization to disease involves many processes and depends on several factors.

When is disease is said to have occurred?

A.1 (f) Disease is said to have occurred, when the multiplying infectious agent cause injury to host tissues and as a result sign and symptoms are produced in the host.

What are the microbial determinants of virulence?

A.1 (g) (i) *Infectious dose*: Infectious dose is defined as the minimum number of organisms that can initiate an infection. The ID varies from one organism in Q fever, to about 10 in rabies and tuberculosis, 100 in Shigella and 1000 in enteric fever.

(ii) *Route of infection*: It should be noted that many organisms can cause disease or are infective, only when they enter the host by an optimal route, e.g., *Vibrio cholerae* causes diarrhoea only, when it enters orally. However some organisms can cause infection by multiple routes, e.g., *S. aureus.*

(iii) *Expression of microbial virulence factors*

- Adhesins (help in colonization) Table 1.13.1(p. 84)
- Enzymes (help in tissue invasion)
- Siderophore (seen in many pathogens (including *Entamoeba histolytica*) is a substance that can steal iron from the host's iron carrying proteins. Optimal iron concentration is required for pathogen growth and multiplication)
- Antiphagocytic factors
- Toxins – exotoxins, endotoxins
- Miscellaneous – Vi-antigen

Others: as Vi antigen of S. Typhi (promotes virulence of typhoid bacillus) and K antigen of *E. coli* help to resist phagocytosis and lytic action of complement. Haemolysin and leukocidins are cytotoxic and damage RBC and WBC, respectively.

(iv) *Host factors:* Numerous factors including cytokines IL-1, IL-6 and TNF produced by the host in response are responsible for numerous manifestation; as fever, muscle proteolysis etc.

(v) *Regulation of pathogenicity:* A successful parasite should be able to continuously sense its local environment and be able to distinguish those that favour rapid growth from those that are inhospitable and require adaptation. It should also be able to make drastic transitions required, when the pathogen changes host during it's life cycle, e.g., *Y. pestis* has to shift from rat flea (arthropod vector) to human. The pathogen must be able to express differentially their genome to survive in all situations.

Describe the type of infection the lady in the above case is having.

A.2 (a) The lady is having an acute, localized reinfection.

Categorize the various types of infection.

A.2 (b) (i) According to degree (region) of infection

- *Localized* – confined to a small area or an organ, e.g., amoebic liver abscess.

- Generalized – spread to many regions, e.g., meningococcemia with petechial rash

(ii) According to chronology (sequence of infection)

- *Primary:* Initial infection with a pathogen, e.g., colitis due to *Shigella flexneri.*
- *Reinfection:* Subsequent infection with the same pathogen in the same host, e.g., second attack of *E. coli* UTI.
- *Secondary:* Invasion by a (different) pathogen subsequent to primary infection, e.g., chicken pox lesions (primary infection) on skin getting infected by *S. aureus* following child scratching the itchy lesions, e.g., bacterial (*H. influenzae*) pneumonia following viral (Influenza) lung infection.

(iii) According to duration

- *Acute:* Rapid onset (hours) and brief duration (days)

  e.g., staphylococcal food poisoning
- *Chronic:* prolonged duration (weeks)

  e.g., TB of lung

(iv) According to presentation

- *Subclinical (asymptomatic):* When clinical signs and symptoms are not manifest (detectable)

  e.g., most common state for most infections, indicates a desirable state for both the host and the pathogen, as it is not detrimental for either.
- *Persistent:* It is one in which organism (virus) remains continuously (usually at low level) present over a prolonged time after the acute infection has ended; as chronic active hepatitis (Hepatitis B)
- *Latent:* The pathogen remains remains viable but does not proliferate till the conditions appear favourable for its multiplication.

  It is usually differentiated from a persistent infection by the pathogen not being demonstrated continuously.

  E.g., Herpetic infection of ganglia, TB infection of lymph node
- *Opportunistic:* Opportunistic pathogen (see A.1b) p 81
- *Fulminant:* Infection that occurs suddenly and intensely.

  e.g., Cholera (diarrhoea), Gas gangrene of gut
- *Cross:* When a patient already suffering from a disease, acquires new infection.
- *Mixed:* Two or more pathogens infecting same tissue eg gas gangrene, wound infections, human bite infection, dental caries.

  HIV and tuberculosis in an individual is better termed as co-infection
- *Iatrogenic:* It is an infection, which results as a result of patient's therapeutic or investigative procedure, e.g., UTI following urinary catheterization in an admitted case
- *Nosocomial:* These are infections acquired following admission in a hospital. Traditionally; defined as occurying after 48 hours of admission in hospital to differentiate from community acquired infections.

How has this individual likely acquire the UTI?

A.3 **(a)** The individual has likely acquired the infection by an ascending route i.e. the bacteria in the perineal region colonized the urethra and ascended to the urinary tract resulting in UTI.

Describe the role of adhesins in microbial pathogenicity.

A.3 **(b)** They explain the process of how the microbes attach to living surface. The first step a pathogen has to undergo before it can colonize/infect a host, is that it must adhere/attach to the surface of the human host. For this to occur the pathogen usually have adhesins, which adhere to receptors on the host cell. The list of such adhesins is depicted in table 1.13.1. The adhesins prevent the pathogen from being removed from the host by various physiological processes; as persistalsis in the gut, coughing in the respiratory tract or flushing in the genitourinary tract. Some examples are polysaccharide slime in *Staphylococcus epidermidis* and alginate in *P. aeruginosa.* The proximity of the pathogen to the host; as a result of adhesins, help in toxin action and invasion of the host.

Knowledge of adhesins can be used in the prevention of disease, as antibody to the adhesins may prevent the first step of host parasite relationship to occur. This approach has been to certain extent successfully utilized in prospective vaccines for gonorrhoea.

Table 1.13.1: Adhesins of common human pathogens

Pathogen	Adhesin	Adhesion mechanism/host receptor
S. aureus	Lipoteichoic acid	Receptor unknown
Staphylococcus sps	Slime	Receptor unknown
Group A Streptococcus	Lipoteichoic acid and M. protein (LTA-M)	Receptor unknown, anchor to epithelium
Group B Streptococcus	Protein	N-acetyl glucosamine
Streptococcus mutans ('viridans')	Dextran slime layer	Tooth surface (caries)
N. meningitidis	Fimbriae	Attach to mucosa of pharynx
N. gonorrhoeae	Fimbriae	Attach to cells of genitalia, N-acetyl glucosamine
C. diphtheriae	Surface protein	Pharyngeal mucosa
E. coli	-Type I fimbriae -Colonization factor antigen 1 fimbriae (well developed K antigen capsule)	D-mannose GM ganglioside
E. coli (fimbrial)	p fimbriae	Uroepithelium
Shigella	Type 1 fimbriae	D-mannose
Vibrio spp.	Glycocalyx	Intestinal epithelium
T. pallidum	P1P2P3	Fibronectin
Pseudomonas aeruginosa	Fimbriae and slime layer	-
M. pneumoniae	Protein P1	Sialic acid
Chlamydia spp.	Lectin	N. acetyl glucosamine
Human immunodeficiency virus	gp 120	CD4 antigen
Influenza virus	Viral spikes	on epithelium
Polio virus	Capsid protein	on mucosa
Entamoeba histolytica	Galactose-binding lectin	galactose

Describe the role of enzymes in host invasion by a pathogen.

A.3 (c) **Invasiveness** is defined as the ability of the organism to enter host cells, penetrate mucosal surfaces (including tissue destruction) and spread within the host after colonization. This is facilitated by numerous enzymes; which include:

(i) Protease (ii) Nuclease – breakdown (depolymerise) nucleic acid (iii) Lipase

(iv) Mucinase – breakdown mucin protective coating on mucous membrane (e.g., by *V. cholerae*, *E. histolytica*)

(v) Keratinase: digest keratin chief component of hair and skin, e.g., most dermatophytic fungi

(vi) Collagenase: digests principal fibre of connective tissue e.g. Clostridium species

(vii) Hyaluronidase: Breaks down hyaluronic acid, a polysaccharide present in connective tissue that helps to cement animal cells. So; this enzyme helps in spreading of pathogen, is also called 'spreading factor:', e.g., by staphylococcus, streptococci, pneumococci, clostridia, other anaerobes

(viii) Lecithinase: breakdown lecithin, e.g., by Clostridia

(ix) Streptokinase (fibrinolysin) breakdown fibrin e.g., Streptococci spp.

This enzyme is life saving in treatment of myocardial infarction, as can dissolve the fibrin clots in coronary arteries

(x) Coagulase: This converts fibrinogen into fibrin and form a wall around bacteria in infected area, thus preventing the bacteria from phagocytosis

(xi) IgA1 protease: This splits the key mucosal antibody and facilitates infection, e.g., by *Neisseria gonorrhoeae*

(xii) ß lactamases: These inactivate the beta lactam ring of antibiotics, hence make them ineffective. Thus the pathogens can survive the hostile environment containing β-lactam antibiotics

What in this case's history may explain the resistance of E. coli to ampicillin?

A.4 Presence of antimicrobials in the gut can accelerate the mobilization of plasmids resistant to ampicillin and other antimicrobials to transfer to other previously susceptible organisms, in this case to *E. coli*. This may explain the current *E. coli* isolate causing UTI to be resistant to ampicillin.

Integrated Clinical Case Based Study 2

Understanding pathogenicity of disease is crucial and complex. However, one of the well understood concepts in pathogenicity, is of toxin, which is a soluble product secreted outside the bacteria. The bacteria that cause the disease by this mechanism need not even invade the body, just colonization is enough. Modifying this toxin has made the public health team, control many dreaded disease.

What is the name of this toxin?

A.1 Exotoxin

What are the human diseases attributed to exotoxin? Mention the part of the bacterial genome carrying the gene for the toxin.

A.2 MAJOR CLINICAL AND SYNDROME/DISEASE IN WHICH EXOTOXIN IMPLICATED

Table 1.13.2: Part of the Implicated Genome

	Toxins	**Part of implicated genome**
Food poisoning (*S. aureus*)	Enterotoxin (types A-E)	Plasmid
Diarrhoea (*E. coli*, enterotoxigenic)	LT and ST (labile and stable toxins)	Plasmid
Haemorrhagic colitis syndrome (EHEC, Enterohaemorrhagic *E. Coli*)	Shiga like toxin (SLT)	Phage (lysogenized or transformed genome)
Diarrhoea (*V. cholerae*)	Choleragen	Chromosomal genes
Pseudomembranous colitis (*Clostridium difficile*)	Toxin A and B	Chromosomal genes
Tetanus (spastic paralysis) (*C. tetani*)	Tetanospasmin	Phage (lysogenized bacterium)
Diphtheria (*C. diphtheriae*)	Diphtheria toxin	Phage (lysogenized bacterium)
Pertusis (*B. pertusis*)	Pertusis toxin	PT operon
Scalded skin syndrome (*S. aureus*)	Exfolative toxin	Phage
Toxic shock syndrome (*S. aureus*)	Enterotoxin	-
Scarlet fever (*S. pyogenes*)	Erythrogenic toxin	Phage T12 has role

Other pathogens which have partly their pathogenicity dependent on exotoxins: *B anthracis, B cereus, K. pneumoniae, S. flexneri, S. Typhimurium, Y pestis Y. enterocolitica and Aeromonas hydrophila.*

Compare and contrast the characteristics of exotoxin with endotoxin.

A.3 **(a)** Exotoxins are proteinaceous in nature. So the exotoxins has all its properties as mentioned in table 1.13.3. They are one of the most poisonous substances, as it has been estimated that a few pounds of botulinum toxin can wipe out the entire human population.

Table 1.13.3: Characteristics of Exotoxin and Endotoxin

	Exotoxins	**Endotoxins**
Structure	Protein in nature	Lipopolysaccharide in nature
Components	Most are composed of two subunits, fragment B is the binding fragment and fragment A is the active one, having enzymatic activity	See A3b, p. 87
Action	Enzymic	Non enzymic
Source	Some gram negative, mostly gram positive bacteria	Gram negative bacteria
Effects on body	Specific to tissue, e.g., tetanus toxin on nerve endings	Non-specific (generalized)
Functional types	Three namely: Enterotoxin, Neurotoxin and Cytotoxin	Non-specific
Production	By secretion	By lysis of organism
Genetics	Often encoded on plasmid (e.g., LT and ST toxins of EPEC), also on lysogenic phage, e.g., *C. diphtheriae*	Chromosomal Origin is from cell wall
Characteristics	Highly potent (few microgram of can kill man)	Weakly potent
	Highly antigenic (stimulates antitoxin production)	Weakly antigenic (doesn't stimulate antitoxin production)
	Can be toxoided	Cannot be toxoided
	Heat labile (at ≥60°C)	Heat stable (withstands 100°C for 1 hour)
	Can be neutralized by antibody	Cannot be neutralized, pyrogenic (sepsis shock occur)
	Non-pyrogenic	Pyrogenic

Contd.

Contd.

Identification	– Immunoassay (antisera helpful) – Ileal loop assay (classical test) – Cell culture (e.g., effect on vero cells	• Immunoassay (recently developed) • Limulus amebocyte lysate test (ability of endotoxin to clot lysate of amoebocyte cells from horseshoe crab, rabbit pyrogenicity
Vaccine	Antitoxin (specific antibodies available for some toxins, as toxoids)	None

Tabulate the effects of exotoxins produced by different pathogens.

A.3 (b) Effects of exotoxins

Table 1.13.4

Bacterium	Name of toxin or disease	Action of toxin	Host symptoms
• *Bacillus anthracis*	• Anthrax (cytotoxin)	• Increases vascular permeability	• Hemorrhage and pulmonary edema
• *Bacillus cereus*	• Enterotoxin	• Causes excessive loss of water and electrolytes	• Diarrhoea
• *Clostridium botulinum*	• Botulism (eight serological types, neurotoxins)	• Blocks release of acetylcholine at nerve endings	• Respiratory paralysis, double vision
• *Clostridium perfringens*	• Gas gangrene (alpha toxin, a hemolysin)	• Breaks down lecithin in cell membranes	• Cell and tissue destruction
	• Food poisoning (enterotoxin)	• Causes excessive loss of water and electrolytes	• Diarrhoea
• *Clostridium tetani*	• Tetanus (lockjaw) (neurotoxin)	• Inhibits antagonists of motor neurons of brain	• Violent skeletal musclular spasms, respiratory failure
• *Clostridium botulinum*	• Progenitor toxin	• Blocking release of acetylcholine at synapses and n/m junction	• Botulism (foodborne, infant and wound)
• *Corynebacterium diphtheriae*	• Diphtheria, (produced by virus infected (cytotoxin) bacteria)	• Inhibits protein synthesis	• Heart damage can cause death weeks after apparent recovery
• *Escherichia coli*	• Traveller's diarrhoea (enterotoxin)	• Causes excessive loss of water and electrolytes	• Diarrhoea
• *Escherichia coli* (0157. H7)	• Hemolytic uremic syndrome	• Destroys intestinal lining and causes haemorrhages in kidney	• Bleeding and kidney failure
• *Pseudomonas aeruginosa*	• Various infections (exotoxin A)	• Inhibits protein synthesis	• Lethal, necrotizing lesion
• *Shigella dysenteriae*	• Bacillary dysentery (enterotoxin)	• Cytotoxic effects	• Diarrhoea
• *Staphylococcus aureus*	• Food poisoning (enterotoxin)	• Stimulates brain center that causes vomiting	• Vomiting
	• Scalded skin syndrome (exfoliatin)	• Causes intradermal separation of cells	• Redness and sloughing of skin
• *Streptococcus pyogenes*	• Scarlet fever (erythrogenic, or red-producing toxin)	• Causes vasodilation	• Maculopapular (slightly raised, discoloured) lesions
• *Vibrio cholerae*	• Cholera (enterotoxin)	• Causes excessive loss of water (up to 30 liters/day) and electrolytes	• Diarrhoea; can kill individual within hours

Enumerate the common vaccines based on modification of exotoxin.

A.4 Diphtheria and Tetanus are the classic diseases in which toxoid based vaccines are used. Toxoid based vaccines have been used for anthrax and botulism. For cholera, toxoid based vaccines have not been successful. Toxoids are modified toxins that have lost toxigenicity but retained antigenicity. Formalin is often used to convert toxin into toxoid.

Integrated Clinical Case Based Study-3

In the popular 'Man vs. wild' series on discovery channel of TV, a prominent trekker in the forest of South America is rescued by the emergency team. On examination he was found to have fever, hypotension, hyperventilation and several infected wounds, which resulted from his frequent falls on the ground, while trying to escape from the jungle.

What is the provisional clinical diagnosis of the trekker?

A.1 Septic shock

What class of microbes are likely to be responsible for the clinical entity?

A.2 Gram negative bacteria such as *E. coli*, Klebsiella spp, Pseudomonas spp. and Bacteriodes spp. are more likely to be responsible for causation of septic shock than gram-positive bacteria.

What toxin is responsible for his condition?

A.3 (a) Endotoxin

What is the structure of this toxin?

A.3 (b) It is a heat stable lipopolysaccharides as depicted in table 1.13.3. They are integral part of outer membrane of gram negative bacteria and get released into circulation following lysis of some bacteria. Lipopolysaccharide (LPS) consists of polysaccharide O (somatic antigen), a core polysaccharide and lipid A that faces the cell interior.

On hospitalization, besides administration of fluids, the case is also administered antimicrobial agents. His condition was found to have deteriorated (instead of improvement)!

What may be the likely cause of his deterioration?

A.4 The destruction of numerous gram negative bacteria by the antimicrobial administration can cause a massive release of endotoxin, which may be responsible for the clinical worsening.

Depict diagrammatically the pathogenesis of endotoxic shock.

A.5 Endotoxins cause activation of complement, coagulation system and macrophages. The activation of the latter results in release of numerous cytokines, which play a key part in the pathogenesis.

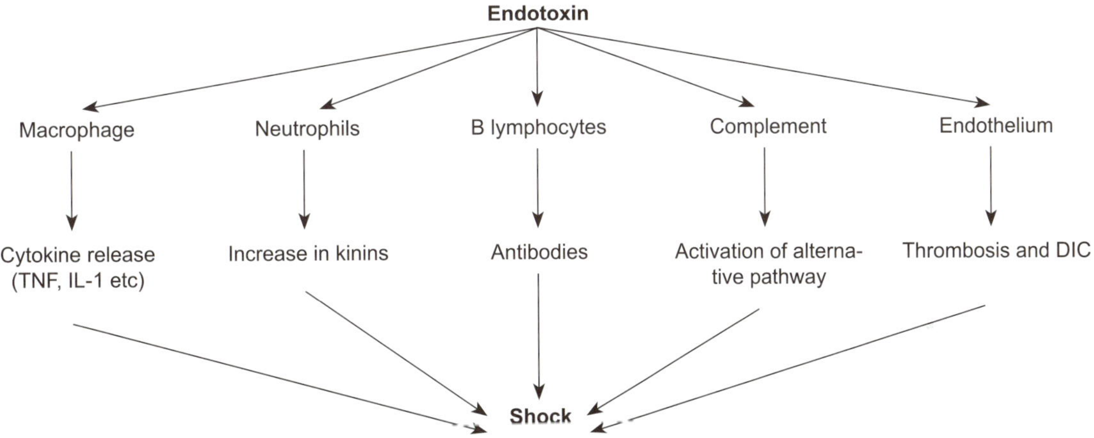

Fig. 1.13.1: Pathogenesis of endotoxic shock

Depending on the amount present in the circulation, it's effect may include fever, cardiovascular shock (in large amounts) and thrombosis, the condition known as endotoxic shock. Death can result from multiple organ failure. Such condition commonly occurs following blood infection by *E. coli*, Salmonella spp. and *N. meningitidis*.

The hospital perfusion team (including nurses) should realize that fever occurring shortly after starting i.v. drip, may be due to contamination of the fluid with gram negative bacteria. In such an event, the incriminated fluid should be replaced with a new lot and the contaminated lot should be sent for testing of endotoxin. Autoclaving is unlikely to inactivate the endotoxin, as it is heat resistant.

Describe the strategies deployed by the pathogen to outwit the phagocyte.

A.6 Phagocytes form an important component of the host to counter the advancement of the pathogen. The pathogen, if it has to succeed must form strategies to avoid the phagocyte. These strategies are numerous and are designated antitiphagocytic. *First* amongst this is the elaboration of toxins; as leucocidins (leuco=white, cidin=destroy), which destroy the white cells, e.g., by Staphylococcus and *Entamoeba histolytica*. *Secondly*, some pathogens secrete a capsule or slimy layer (extra cellular surface layer) that prevents the interaction of the pathogen and the macrophage, e.g., *S. pneumoniae*, *N. meningitidis*, *Y. pestis* and *Cryptococcus neoformans*.

Thirdly certain pathogens; as *M. tuberculosis*, Chlamydia spp. and Toxoplasma spp. prevent the fusion of phagosome and lysosome (containing the destructive chemicals) in the macrophage, thus these pathogens can survive intracellularly and escape the host immune response. *Lastly* some pathogens as Rickettsia, Leishmania and *Trypanosoma cruzi* produce some substance that let them escape from the phagosome of the macrophage into the cytoplasm of the host cell, before the phagosome fuses with the lysosome in the macrophages.

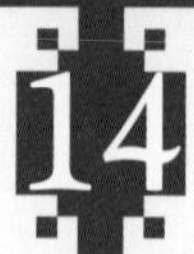

Chemotherapy of Bacterial Diseases

- ***Antibiotics are truly miracle drugs that have saved countless lives.*** — ***Betsy Bauman***
- ***If at the first sign of infection, you jump in with antibiotics, you do not give the immune system a chance to grow stronger.*** — ***Andrew Weil***

The term chemotherapy was coined by the German Nobel laureate, Paul Ehrlich; who believed that chemical substances could selectively kill pathogenic organisms; without injuring the host. It was his firm conviction, that his 606th attempt led him to launch a compound called 'Salvarsan', which had some clinical value for syphilis and was used for a few years. This was an arsenic based drug that was toxic to both *Treponema pallidum* and unfortunately also to humans. It was because of the lack of selective toxicity, that the drug got discontinued. In the present scenario, this drug would have been categorized as one with low therapeutic ratio. The term chemotherapeutic drug is used for any chemical that is used in the treatment or prophylaxis of disease. Let's study these agents.

Describe the discovery and marketing of penicillin.

A.1 Penicillin discovery in 1929 in the London laboratory of Alexander Fleming is well known. A plate of *Staphylococcus aureus* became contaminated with the mold (fungus) *Penicillium notatum* and inhibited the growth of the bacterium around it. It was inferred that some compound may be secreted by the fungus that inhibits the bacterium. A compound called penicillium was extracted from the fungus, which had antibacterial activity. However this great discovery had to wait almost a decade before Howard Florey and Ernest Chain realized the potential of the discovery and went in for industrial production of penicillin in UK. The clinical trials of the drug occurred in 1941 and proved its effectiveness (and high *therapeutic ratio). However gross misuse of it led to decline of its efficacy, as the drug resistance rate went high.

Highlight the importance of antimicrobial drugs.

A.2 The importance of antimicrobial agents can be gauged from the fact that currently more than 250 such agents are in use worldwide and their production is exceeding 100,000 tons/year (including veterinary, agricultural and medical fields). These have reduced the incidence of many diseases and have increased the life span of man.

What is the limitation of the antimicrobial usage in the control of infectious diseases?

A.3 Because of its excellent effectivity in many diseases, one should not go with the misconception that they may lead to eradication of some diseases in the future. Such a scenario may never come. Only an integrated approach can help achieve such a goal, as has occurred in small pox.

What is the basis on which antimicrobials are chosen for clinical use.

A.4 Ideally a large difference should exist between the antimicrobial level that is inhibitory to the microorganism and the concentration that is toxic to the host cells. The principle on which antimicrobial agents are chosen in their selective toxicity towards the microbe rather than the host. The selectivity of these drugs towards microbes is not absolute, as some harm to host does occur with some antimicrobial agents; as amphotericin B.

Describe the evolution of the term 'antimicrobial agents'.

A.5 Initially the compounds acting on microbes were mainly *antibiotics*, i.e., chemical substances that were produced by metabolism of microorganisms that had the capability of inhibiting or destroying microbes. Later on came the category of semi-synthetic drug and synthetic drugs. The *synthetic drugs* are those that are totally synthesized in the laboratory, e.g., Trimethoprim and the *semi-synthetic drugs* are those that are partly made by the microorganism and partly by the laboratory synthesis, e.g., cephalosporins. Currently the distinction between antibiotics and synthetic drug is of little relevance, as many antibiotics; as chloramphenicol and aztreonam are produced synthetically. Currently the term *antimicrobial agents* is often used. It also avoids the confusion the term chemotherapeutic drug can cause, as drugs used against malignancies are also known by this term.

* Therapeutic ratio may be defined as the highest dose a patient can tolerate without side (toxic) effect, divided by the dose required to control a microbial infection.

What is the basis of categorizing antimicrobial agents into bacteriostatic and bactericidal categories?

A.6 One way of classifying antimicrobial drugs is by categorizing into bacteriostatic and bactericidal drugs. *Bacteriostatic*; as the name indicates are drug that inhibit the activity of microbes, but do not destroy/kill them. It is important to use these drugs, where the human defence mechanisms are intact. The suppression of the metabolic activity may be a reversible inhibition one, i.e., once the levels become suboptimal the microbe may resume their metabolic activity. The *bactericidal* (cidal means destroy) *drugs;* as the name indicates are drug agents that can destroy the microbes, if used in optimal concentration. It must be remembered that MIC assays can be run for both type of drugs, but MBC assays can be run for only bactericidal drugs.

What is the basis of characterizing the antimicrobial drugs on the basis of the spectrum of activity?

A.7 Antimicrobial drugs are also classified on the basis of the spectrum of activity. The two categories are namely, *narrow-spectrum agents* and the broad-spectrum agents. The former as the name indicates act on a small number of infectious agents, e.g., Benzyl Penicillin acts primarily against gram positive and negative cocci with little activity against enterobacteriaceae (enteric gram negative bacilli). *Broad-spectrum agents;* as the name indicates have an activity against wide range of gram positive and gram negative bacteria including certain obligate intracellular agents. These are basically indicated, when pathogen is unknown, e.g., septicaemia and when multiple pathogens are possible, e.g., perforated colon. Ideally; as far as possible, narrow spectrum agents should be used in therapy of infections, as then the chances of super infection, drug resistance and adverse reactions are minimized. However, if the clinical condition is such that the aetiological agent is not known or infection with multiple microbes is suspected, then broad spectrum agents should be considered.

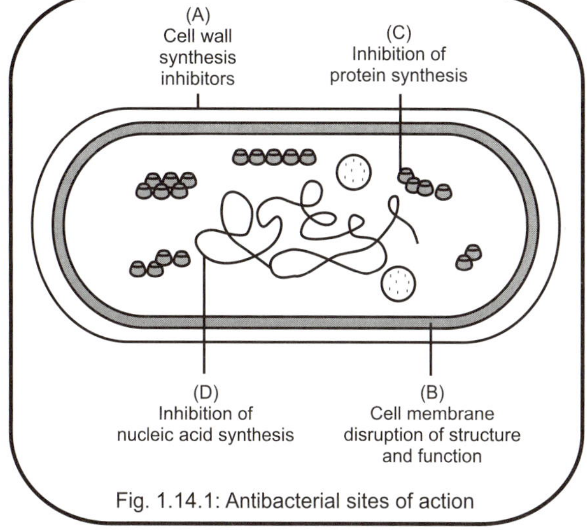

Fig. 1.14.1: Antibacterial sites of action

What is the basis of characterizing the antimicrobial drugs on the basis of the site of action in the microbe?

A.8 The classification of the antimicrobial agents on the basis of site of action in the microbe is depicted in table 1.14.1 and Fig. 1.14.1.

Table 1.14.1: Classification of antimicrobial drugs on the basis of site of action in the microbe

I. Cell Wall Synthesis Inhibitors	II. Action On Cell Membrane	III. Inhibition of Protein Sythesis	IV. Inhibition of Nucleic Acid Synthesis
Beta lactams; as Penincillin, Cephalosporins, Methicillin, Carbenicillin	Polymyxins	Tetracycline	Quinolones; as Nalidixic acid Ciprofloxacin Norfloxacin
Bacitracin (polypeptide)	Colistin (Polymyxin E)	Amino glycosides (as Streptomycin, Gentamicin)	Nitrofurantoin, (Nitrfurans)
Cycloserine	Gramicidin (eye drops)	Chloramphenicol	Nitroimidazoles; as Metronidazole Tinidazole
	Amphotericin B	Macrolides; as Azithromycin, Roxithromycin, Clindamycin Lincomycin	Rifamycins; as Rifampicin Rifabutin
Carbapenems; as Imipenem, Meropenem	Nystatin (Mycostatin)	Oxazolidinones as Linezolid	Sulphanilamide, Dapsone, PAS
Monobactams; as Aztreonam		Streptogramins	Trimethoprim, Trimethoprim-Sulfamethoxazole
Glycopeptides; as Vancomycin, Teicoplanin, Daptomycin			

This categorization would be followed in this text-book, while studying treatment aspects.

15 Assessment/Examination Questions

Chapter 1

1. Describe the contributions of Anton van Leeuwenhoek. Table 1.1.1., p. 2
2. Describe the contributions of Robert Koch. A 6, 7., p. 4,5
4. Describe the contributions of Louis Pasteur. A 5,6., p. 3
5. Describe the contributions of Paul Ehrlich. A 9., p. 5

Chapter 2

1. Discuss the role of staining and microscopy in study of microbes. p. 7-11
2. Describe the principle and types of stains. A 2-10., p. 7,8
3. Describe Gram's staining. A 9-17., p. 8,9
4. Describe Z.N. (acid fast) staining. A 18-20., p. 9
5. Describe Dark ground microscopy. A 30-35., p. 10
6. Describe Fluorescent microscopy. A. 37, 38 ., p. 11
7. Describe Electron microscopy. A 39-42., p. 11

Chapter 3

1. Enumerate the differences between prokaryotes and eukaryotes. A 5., p. 17-18
2. Draw Labelled diagram of bacterial cell. Fig. 1.3.1., p. 12 and Fig. 1.3.12., p. 17
3. Describe Bacterial capsule. Table 1.3.1., p. 13 and Fig. 1.3.2., p. 18
4. Describe Bacterial cell wall. Table 1.3.1., p. 13, Table 1.3.2., p. 18 and Figs 1.3.3, 1.3.4., p. 18, 19
5. Enumerate Differences between cell wall of cell wall of gram positive and negative bacteria. Table 1.3.1., p. 13.
6. Describe Cytoplasmic cell membrane. Table 1.3.1., p. 13.14 and Fig. 1.3.5., p. 19
7. Describe Bacterial flagella. Table 1.3.1., p. 14-15 and Fig. 1.3.6. and 1.3.7., p. 19
8. Describe Bacterial fimbriae. Table 1.3.1., p. 14 and Fig. 1.3.1., p. 11
9. Enumerate the differences between common and sex fimbriae. Table 1.3.1. , p. 14
10. Describe differences between flagella and fimbriae. Table 1.3.1., p. 15
11. Describe Bacterial spore. Table 1.3.1., p. 16 and Figs. 1.3.8, 1.3.9., p. 19
12. Describe Intracytoplasmic inclusions in bacteria. Table 1.3.1., p. 16
13. Describe L forms of bacteria. Table 1.3.1., p. 13 and A4d., p. 347

Chapter 4

1. Define sterilization and mention differences from disinfection. Classify sterilization agents. A1 (a-d)., p. 20
2. Discuss the Role of sterilization and disinfection in a healthcare setting including Tyndallization and Inspissation A1e, A3, A4d., p. 21-22
3. Classification of critical and semicritical agents according to Spaulding. A3., p. 23
4. Describe the principle, functioning of autoclaves including monitoring of its efficacy (role of moist heat in sterilization). A5, 6, 3., p. 21-22
5. Describe Hot air oven. A4c., p.21
6. Describe Plasma sterilization. A14., p. 26
7. Describe Sterilization by filtration. A1-6., p. 26
8. Describe Sterilization of heat sensitive agents. A9a,b and A4-6., p. 26-27
9. Describe Disinfection techniques used in hospitals, their principle and use. A7-11., p. 24-25
10. Describe Disinfection of skin. Table 1.4.1., p. 27

11. Describe Vapour phase disinfectants (gaseous sterilization agents). A13a,b., p. 25,26
12. Describe Sterilization controls. A3, A4c., p. 21, A13., p.26
13. Describe Sterilization by radiation including 'Hot sterilization systems and Cold' sterilization agents. A8-10., p. 27
14. Describe Chemical agents as sterilization agents including alcohols, aldehydes, dyes, halogens, phenols, surface active agents and metallic salts. A 10., p. 24-25
15. Describe methods of testing disinfectants including Rideal Walker test, Chick Martin test and 'In –Use test'. A11, p.25
16. Mention about Household water purification systems. clinical based study 3., p. 26

Chapter 5

1. Discuss the terms Phenotype and genotype. A 1, 2 ., p. 34-35
2. Describe Methods of gene transfer among microbes resulting in variability in microbes. A3., p. 34
3. Describe Structure of bacterial DNA and method of its replication. A4., p. 30, 31
4. Describe Structure and function of RNA. A5., p. 31
5. Define gene and related terms. A6., p. 31-32
6. Describe Transcription and Translation. A9., p 33-34
7. Define mutation, describe types including tests to detect mutation. A4., p. 35-38
8. Describe Transformation including types and importance. A5., p-38-39
9. Describe Transposition (Transposons). A6., p. 39-40
10. Describe Plasmids including definition types, role, laboratory detection. A 7 a,b., p. 40-42
11. Describe 'R' plasmids. A7b., p. 41-42
12. Describe Conjugation. A7c., p 42-43
13. Describe Transduction (Bacteriophage its structure, types, life cycle and typing). A 8., p. 43
14. Describe Lysogenic conversion. A4., p. 389
15. Describe control of gene expression including lac operon. A9., p. 43

Chapter 6

1. Discuss Generation time and give its classic examples. A2., p. 45
2. Describe Autotrophs and Heterotrophs (and their types). A5., p. 45-46
3. Describe Fermentation (including the historical aspect). Vignette., p. 45, A 8-10., p. 48
4. Mention applications of fermentation A 13-15., p. 49
5. Describe Physical factors affecting growth of bacteria A7ii., 46-48
6. Enumerate metabolism categories in microbes and discuss them (aerotolerant, aerobic, facultative anaerobic and anaerobic). A7 ii., p-46
7. Describe capnophiles, micraerophiles, extremophiles. A7 ii, iii, iv, v, vii-ix., p 46-48
8. Describe Redox potential. A7ii., p. 46

Chapter 7

1. How can role of microbes be studied in health and disease? Mention the goal tried to achieved, while cultivating bacteria. Vignette and A1., p 50
2. What do you understand by medium (plural media)? A4., p. 50
3. Classify culture media and discuss them. A5, A7-A12., p. 50-52
4. Describe the following categories of media including enriched, enrichment, selective, indicator, differential, sugar, transport and anaerobic. Table 1.7.1., p. 53-58
5. Describe the following types of media namely blood agar, chocolate agar, Sabouraud dextrose agar and Lowenstein–Jensen media. Table 1.7.1., p. 54, 56

Chapter 8

1. What do you understand by 'culture' and 'pure culture'? A1, 2., p. 59
2. What are the uses/indications of culturing bacteria? A6., p. 59
3. Describe briefly the aerobic culture techniques. A 9., p. 60
4. What is the major limitation of the liquid culture technique? A7., p. 59
5. What are the techniques to culture media on solid media (including streak culture, lawn culture, pour plate method)? A 9, 10., p. 60

6. How does one separate mixtures of different bacteria contained in a clinical sample? (incld cragie's method) A 10 ii
7. Describe the anaerobic culture techniques. A3a., p. 586
8. Describe principle and use of Mc Intosh and Filde's anaerobic jar. A3a., p. 586 and Fig. 1.6.1 a,b., p. 46
9. Describe briefly the Gaspak system. A 3a., p. 586
10. Describe briefly the RCM medium. Table 1.7.1., p. 57
11. Describe the concept and phases of the growth curve with the help of a figure and mention its industrial application. A. 11., p 61-62
12. Describe the techniques to monitor bacterial growth. A. 12., p. 62

Chapter 9

1. What are the advantages in identifying an isolate in culture? A1., p. 63
2. What are the two broad ategories of tests to identify the microbes? A2., p. 63
3. What is the role of the classic phenotype based tests in the identification of the microbes? A. 3., p. 63-64
4. Describe the following phenotype based tests; namely IMViC (indole, methyl red, Voges Proskaeur, Citrate utilization, catalase test, Phenylalanine deaminase test, decarboxylase test and TSI test. Table 1.9.1., p. 66-67
5. Enumerate the two categories of the nucleic acid tests (phenotype independent) and their sub categories and their examples. A4., p. 651

Chapter 10

1. Describe the technique of detection of microbes by nucleic acid probes A5., p. 69
2. Describe the principle, steps and limitations of the classical PCR test. A6c., p. 70-71
3. Describe the types of PCR tests and their applications. A 6d., p-71-72
4. Describe the technique Trancription mediated amplification (TMA) and Ligase chain reaction (LCR) A6f., p 72-73

Chapter 11

1. What would be the characteristics of an ideal microbial taxonomical science? A5., p. 74
2. Describe bacterial taxonomy. A4-A 19., p. 74-76
3. Describe the Adansonian (numerical) and Phylogenetic classification methods. A 16, 17., p. 72

Chapter 12

1. Describe a recent disease, in which epidemiological work up of it, led to control of the outbreak. Vignette., p. 73
2. Define the terms endemic, hyperendemic, sporadic, epidemic, prosodemic and pandemic. Table., p. 73
3. Enumerate various modes of transmission of diseases and give examples. A5., p 79-80
4. Describe the role of vehicles and vectors in the transmission of the microbial agents. A5a,b., p 79-80

Chapter 13

1. Describe briefly the following terms: saprophyte, opportunistic pathogen, pathogen, pathogenicity, virulence and parasite. A 1b., p. 82
2. Diagrammatical depict the relationship between contaminant, infection and disease. A.1d., p. 81-82
3. Describe the key microbial determinants of virulence. A1g., p. 82
4. Describe the role of adhesins in microbial pathogenicity. A3b., p. 83-84
5. Describe the role of enzymes in invasion of the host by a pathogen A 3 c., p. 84
6. Categorize the types of infection, according to degree of infection, and chronology sequence of infection, A2 bi, ii., p. 83.
7. Enumerate the human diseases, in which exotoxin is implicated and mention the part of microbial genome responsible for it. A2., p. 89
8. Compare and contrast the characteristics of exotoxin and endotoxin. A 3a., p. 85-86
9. Enumerate the common vaccines in human usage based on modification of exotoxin. A 4., p. 86

Chapter 14

1. Classify the antimicrobial drugs on the basis of their action and give examples. A8., p. 89
2. Write briefly on beta lactam antibiotics, cepalosporins, carbapenems, macrolides and quinolones. Table 1.14.1., p. 89

Section II: Immunology

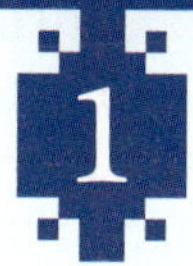

Introduction to Immunology

An immune system of enormous complexity is present in all vertebrate animals. When we place a population of lymphocytes from such an animal in appropriate tissue culture fluid, and when we add an antigen, the lymphocytes will produce specific antibody molecules, in the absence of any nerve cells. I find it astonishing that the immune system embodies a degree of complexity, which suggests some more or less superficial though striking analogies with human language, and that this cognitive system has evolved and functions without assistance of the brain.

— Niels K. Jerne

Let's make a beginning of the study of this interesting subject.

What makes the study of Immunology very exciting?

A.1 (a) The word 'immunity' is derived from Latin 'immunitas' which means 'freedom from'. Immunology helps us to understand the ^pathogenesis at molecular level of the inflammatory, infective, autoimmune, immunodeficient and neoplastic (some) disorders. It also helps in the treatment of the various infective, immunodeficient and autoimmune disorders by specific immunoglobulins, immunomodulators and cytokines. The highest form of preventive medicine may lie in immunological interventions including vaccines.

^innate and adaptive immunity response critical to understanding

Immunology was practiced even before the immune system could be delineated and the microbes were characterized. Give an example of a viral infection for which vaccination was available, even before the implicated virus could be identified, isolated and cultivated?

A.1 (b) Small pox.

Who introduced the small pox vaccination initially? Mention the principle used in this vaccination (hint-cross-reactivity) and the route used to administer this vaccine.

A.1 (c) Edward Jenner. The origin of immunology in the modern medicine could be attributed to Edward Jenner, who in 1796 discovered that cowpox or vaccinia infection; induced protection against human small pox. He described this procedure as vaccination, a term that is still used.

The principle of cross reactivity was used in this procedure. The cow pox virus has some similarity in the structure with the small pox virus and immune response (protective) against cow pox also helped against small pox.

The parenteral (intradermal) route was used for administration of this vaccine.

The kings in the olden times used to raise a special human population, by which they could eliminate their enemies. What was this class of individuals named?

A.2 (a) 'Vishkanya' (Vish = poison, kanya = girl) (Fig. 2.1.1)

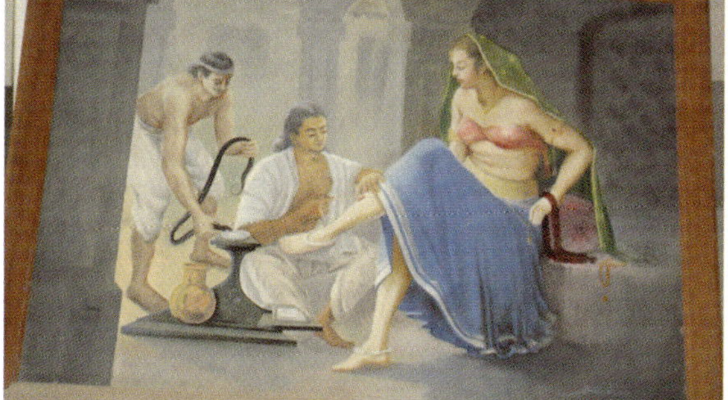

Fig.2.1.1: Vishkanya (being exposed to snake bite)

What was the principle and procedure used to raise this class of individuals?

A.2 (b) The idea was to eliminate the enemies, when they would physically come in contact with the 'Vishkanyas', raised by the kings.

The girls were given parenterally increasing graded doses of snake venom over periods that lasted many months. The idea was that these girls would become immune to the snake toxin themselves but the level of toxin in their secretions, as saliva would be lethal to their enemies, when introduced.

Why did some of these individuals (girls) die in the process of their raising?

A.2 (c) The science of immunology was crudely practiced. Many girls would succumb to this 'vaccination' method but those that survived had snake toxin in their secretions, that was lethal, when introduced into others (as by salivary secretion exposure), but had no effect on self.

Depict the key historical developments in Immunology/Molecular biology.

A.3 (a)

1796	• Edward Jenner an English surgeon introduces vaccination for small pox
1869	• A Swiss pathologist, Johann Miescher, discovers the presence of complex acids (termed DNA, RNA) in the cell nucleus
1883	• Elie Metchnikoff, a Russian biologist, discovers phagocytic cells and proposes the concept of cellular immunity
1885	• Louis Pasteur develops vaccines for rabies (neural), anthrax and fowl cholera (a disease in which cholera like disease occurs in fowl)
1888	• Roux and Yersin discover mechanism of diphtheria toxin
1889	• Charrin and Roger discover agglutination of bacteria by immune serum • Kitasato discover that *Clostridium tetani* produces tetanus toxin
1890	• Emil Von Behring, a German and Shibasaburo Kitasato, elicit the presence of antibodies in serum that neutralize the toxins of diphtheria and tetanus
1894	• Pfeiffer discover the property of immune serum to cause bacteriolysis (destruction of bacteria)
1894	• Jules Bordet, a Belgian biochemist, discovers complement and describe its properties as haemolysis.
1896	• Widal and Grunbaum, developed an serum agglutination test for diagnosis of typhoid fever
1897	• Kraus discovery of precipitins • (Paul) Ehrlich proposes side chain theory of antibody formation
1901	• Bordet and Gengou develop complement fixation text
1902	• Portier and Charles Richet (French) demonstrated the phenomenon of anaphylaxis and showed its clinical importance
1903	• James Wright, an American pathologist, with his team demonstrate the presence of antibodies in the blood of immunized animals
1906	• August Wasserman, a German bacteriologist with his colleagues develop the first serologic test for syphilis
1914	• Tetanus vaccine available
1920	• TB vaccine become available
1930	• Diphtheria and Yellow fever vaccine become available)
1940	• Medawar and his colleagues proposed the concept of immunological surveillance.
1944	• Oswald Avery, Colin MacLeod and McCarty demonstrate that DNA is the genetic material • Joshua Lederberg and El Tatum demonstrate conjugation in bacteria
1953	• James Watson, Francis Crick, Rosalind Franklin and Maurice Wilkins determine the structure of DNA
1959-1960	• Gerald Edelman and Rodney Porter determine the structure of antibody
1967	• Burnet propose the concept of immunological surveillance and clonal selection theory
1972	• Paul Berg develops first recombinant DNA in a test tube
1973	• Herb Bayer and Stanley Cohen clone first DNA using plasmid.

Mention the key vaccines available currently and their introduction years.

A.3 (b) Vaccines

1796	Small-pox (Edward Jenner)
1885	– ^Fowl cholera (*Louis Pasteur) – Anthrax – Rabies
1890-1904	Test vaccines for Diphtheria and Tetanus (Von Behring and Kitasato)
1914	Tetanus vaccine available
1920	T.B. vaccine
1930	Diphtheria and yellow fever vaccine
1954	Japanese encephalitis (killed mouse brain)
1955-60	Salk and Sabin vaccines
1960	Measles and Rubella vaccine *Rabies (HDCV, tissue culture vaccine)
1970	*N. meningitidis* and chickenpox vaccine
1980	Hepatitis B and MMR combination vaccine
1990	*Haemophilus influenzae* vaccine
Currently	Typhoid vaccine (Ty21a), work in progress for HIV vaccine

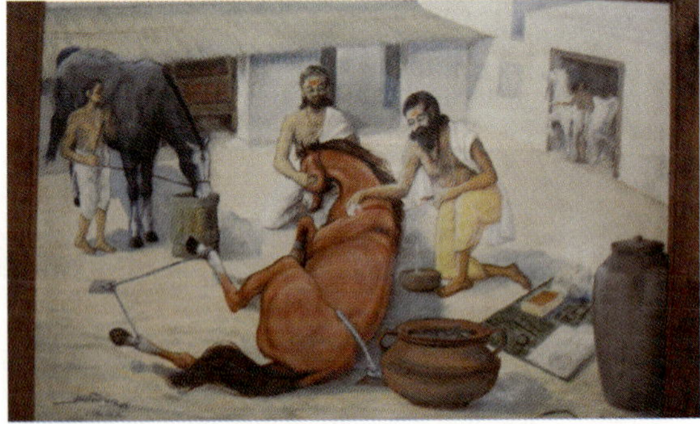

Fig. 2.1.2: Horse (traditionally used for antisera production)

* Almost a century after Jenner's vaccine, Louis Pasteur used his ingenuity to create the ^fowl cholera, anthrax and the rabies vaccines. The last vaccine was first received by Joseph Meister a boy of nine years, who was severely bitten by a rabid dog. He was saved from the deadly disease and subsequently because the custodian of the famous Pasteur Institute in Paris. During the 2nd world war about fifty five year later, when the Nazis occupied Paris, he sacrificed his life rather than hand over the keys of the institute to the Nazis.

^cholera like disease in fowl

Enumerate key scientists who were awarded Nobel prizes for contribution in immunology in twentieth century.

A.4 Nobel prizes for contribution in immunology

Year	Recipient	Country	Contribution
1901	Emil von Behring	Germany	Serum antitoxins in Diphtheria (Fig. 2.1.2)
1905	Robert Koch	Germany	Cell-mediated immunity in tuberculosis
1908	Elie Metchnikoff Paul Ehrlich	Russia Germany	– Phagocytosis – Antitoxins in immunity
1913	Charles Richet	France	Anaphylaxis
1919	Jules Bordet	Belgium	Complement-mediated bacteriolysis
1930	Karl Landsteiner	USA	Human blood groups discovery
1951	Max Theiler	South Africa	Yellow fever vaccine
1957	Daniel Bovet	Switzerland	Antihistamines
1960	F. Macfarlane Burnet Peter Medawar	Australia U.K.	Discovery of acquired immunological tolerance
1972	Rodney R. Porter Gerald M. Edelman	U.K. U.S.A.	Antibody structure
1977	Rosalyn R. Yalow	U.S.A.	Radioimmunoassay test development
1980	George Snell Jean Dausset Baruj Benacerraf	U.S.A. France U.S.A.	Major histocompatibility complex
1984	Cesar Milstein Georges E. Kohler Niels K. Jerne	U.K. Germany Denmark	Development of monoclonal antibody Immune regulatory theories
1987	Susumu Tonegawa	Japan	Gene rearrangement in antibody to explain its diversity
1991	E. Donnall Thomas Joseph Murray	U.S.A. U.S.A.	Advances in transplantation immunology
1996	Peter C. Doherty Rolf M. Zinkernagel	Australia Switzerland	Role in M.H.C. in antigen recognition by T cells
2002	Sydney Brenner H. Robert Horvitz J.E. Sulston	S. Africa USA UK	Apoptosis (genetic regulation of cell development)

Mention the various periods in development of Immunology till date.

A.5 The period of 1890-1950 is referred as the *'age of serology'*, where contributions were made in the serological identification of bacteria, application of sera and vaccines to pathogenic diseases and in aspects of antibody diversity and specificity. Allergy clinics also came up in this period. Contributions were made mainly by German and French scientists.

Critical observations and analysis have contributed in a big way in the development of immunology. The period of 1950s was one of *'cellular immunology'* and the selection theories (as clonal selection). It is possible that one of the key events leading to the modern theories of immune cell origin was the atomic bomb attacks on the two Japanese cities of Hiroshima and Nagasaki. The animal experiments conducted later could explain the cause of human deaths that resulted in these attacks from intense radiation exposure. The whole body radiation exposure killed the generative blood forming and lymphoid organ cells. As a result these people died of haemorrhage and infections. This condition, as we know now currently can be treated with bone-marrow transplantation.

The period of 1980s to the present (A4) is one of *molecular immunology*, T cell receptor studies, transplantation and AIDs. It was again a meticulous epidemiological and virological work on the group of patients in 1981, who presented with opportunistic infections and reduced CD4 cell counts that a new syndrome; as AIDS and HIV virus could be identified. The HIV virus infects the very immune cells, which are to defend human body.

Mention the key lymphocyte subsets in man on basic of antigenic determinants

A.3 **(d) Table 2.2.1(b)**

Table 2.2.1(b)

Cell type	Marker
B cell	CD 19
Pan T marker (Present on all T cells)	CD3, CD2
T_H/T_{DTH}	CD4
T cytotoxic/suppressor	CD8

Outline the T cells subsets on basis of function

A.3 **(3)**

Regulatory T Cell	• T-helper (CD4) • T-suppressor (CD8)
Effector T cell	• Tc-Cytotoxic T cells • T_{DTH}–Delayed type hypersenstivity

Which cells are involved in innate immunity? Describe them.

A.4 **(a)** List see A2c)

Neutrophils (Fig. 2.2.1): They are the first cells to arrive at the site of infection from blood. They play a key role in the innate defense against bacteria and fungi. This is evident in the 'chronic granulomatous disease' patients, who have increased susceptibility to bacterial and fungal infection and whose neutrophils NADPH phagosome oxidase is unable to generate oxidizing species as depicted below:

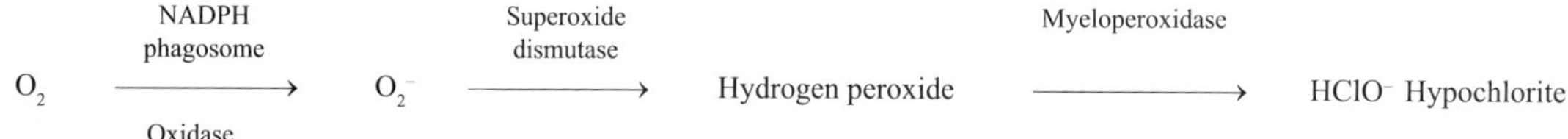

Neutrophils have Fc receptors for IgG (CD16), which facilitate the phagocytosis of opsonized bacteria. They also have receptors for activated complement components; as C3b', Toll-like receptors on them; as TLR2 and TLR4 which facilitate the detection of gram positive and gram negative bacteria (by detecting peptidoglycan and lipopolysaccharies, respectively).

The neutrophils have azurophilic granules containing lysozyme, myeloperoxidase and other granules (containing lysozyme, lactoferrin, elastase and others) besides the superoxide radicals, which are responsible for their antibacterial//antifungal activity, besides also damaging the host tissue at times.

Human antimicrobial peptide defensins kill a wide variety of bacteria. One of their rich sources is neutrophil. They kill microbes rapidly within minutes, usually by disrupting microbial membranes. The mechanism of their discriminating between microbial and host membranes is not known. These are not in clinical use, for it is feared that the bacteria might rapidly acquire resistance to these agents.

Eosinophils (Fig. 2.2.5a): Like neutrophils, they are also present in many forms of inflammation and act as amplifier and effector of the innate immune response; especially for parasitic infections. They express Fc receptors for IgG (CD32) and are powerful cytotoxic effector cells in numerous parasitic infections. They contain in the cytoplasm; major basic protein, and cationic proteins, which may damage the host tissue and may play a part in the hypereosinophilic syndrome. The eosinophil also contains anti-inflammatory enzymes; as phospholipase and histaminase, which may downregulate the inflammatory process.

Macrophages (Fig. 2.2.2): They arise from the blood monocytes, after they have migrated out of the circulation into the extravascular pool or tissues. They are found in the liver (Kupffer cell), spleen, lymph nodes peritoneal/pleural/synovial cavities, lung, bone (osteoclast) and CNS (microglia). They are the first line of defense in the innate immunity by carrying out non-specific phagocytosis. They also play the later role of clearing the 'mess' created by the infection and inflammation. They also mediate elimination of antibody-coated bacteria, malignant cells and even normal blood cells in certain types of autoimmune blood disorders. Transferrin an serum beta globulin in them competes with bacteria for iron and removes it.

They play a major role in the recruitment of the acquired immune response by presenting the foreign antigens to the lymphocytes. However; they are not the major antigen presenting cells and now dendritic cells are known to be the most effective APCs for the organism. The macrophages also secrete numerous biological compounds including cytokines that play a part in the inflammation and the recruitment of the acquired immune response.

Dendritic cells (Fig. 2.2.3): These cells acquired its name, from its long membranous extensions resembling dendrites of nerve cell. They are more important APCs than the macrophages. They are distinct from the macrophages and are derived from both lymphoid and myeloid lineages. They lack the standard T, B, NK and monocyte cell markers but express CD83 molecule that helps in its identification, besides it's dendritic morphology with multiple fine membrane projections. The two classes of it namely lymphoid dendritic cells and myeloid dendritic cells (further divided into follicular and langerhans) provide an important role in the communication between innate and acquired immune systems. They vary in their display of the class I and II MHC molecules (required as stimuli for T lymphocyte) and co-stimulatory molecules; as CD80 and CD86. On their maturation, the dendritic cells shift from their residency in the peripheral tissues to the lymphatic organs (where T cells reside) through the lymphatic and/or blood circulation. The binding of the infectious agents products to the TLRs of dendritic cells produces cytokines, that activate the cells of the innate immune system and recruit T and B cells of the acquired immune system.

Natural killer cells (Fig. 2.2.4)

These innate lymphoid cell, have been named so, because of their non-specific cytotoxicity, Their activity is non-immune (i.e. without the effector cell having come in contact with the target) and without any MHC restriction.

Their *discovery* occurred accidentally, when the scientists were measuring the ability of certain tumor specific cells to be lysed by certain constituent of the mice with tumor. Surprinsingly, the control mice (negative controls) with no related tumor had also this ability to significantly lyse the tumor cells.

The *characterization* of these cells revealed them to belong to the population of large granular lymphocytes, which constitute 5-10% of the circulating lymphocyte population. These cells play an important *part in* the killing of viral infected cells, malignant cells and transplanted foreign cells. These cells can also mediate antibody dependent cellular cytotoxicity (ADCC). The NK cells can be stimulated to become **lymphokine activated killer cells (LAK)** on exposure to high concentration of IL-2, which kill tumor cells more efficiently. Almost all NK cells express CD16 (a receptor for the Fc region of IgG) and CD56. These molecules have diagnostic significance and a cell preparation treated with anti-CD16 will have no NK cell activity.

These cells do not develop exclusively in the thymus unlike the T-lymphocytes. They kill the cells by a process similar to the cytotoxic T-lymphocytes (CTL). The large activated granules of the NK cell (unlike CTL which have to be activated) degranulate, after adhering to the target cell and releases the perforins and granzymes at the junction between interacting cells (similar to apoptosis).

The *mechanism* by which the NK cells recognize altered self cells is unique, as the NK cells do not express antigen-specific receptors (a mechanism by which other lymphocytes recognize unique antigens). It has two type of receptors, namely lectin like and killer-cell immunoglobulin like (KIR). Both have inhibitory and activating receptors. The current theory of the opposing signals model explain the recognition of the normal/altered cells by a balance between the two types of signals (activating and inhibitory). Another observation is that the ability of the NK cells to kill target cells is in inverse relation to the target cell expression of the MHC class I molecules, i.e., NK cells kill target cells with low or no levels of MHC class I molecules.

NK/T cells: This cell has a hybrid quality, as it has characteristics of both NK cell and CTL. NK/T cells are NK cells that also express CD3 and oligoclonal forms of T-cell receptor. The TCR on these cells cannot recognize MHC-bound peptides but instead lipid molecules of certain intracellular organism;s as *Listeria monocytogenes* and *M. tuberculosis*. They probably play an important part in defending the body from them, but their exact role is not clear.

(The following is **not** a cell, but an alteration in its structure and function, can affect the innate and acquired responses.)

T cell receptor – (TCR, Fig. 2.2.5b) As the name indicates it is the receptor that is present on the T cell that interacts with the combination of antigen plus MHC combination on the antigen presenting cell. Unlike the B-cell receptor, it can not bind directly the antigen (Fig. 2.5.2b). It is important to study it, as it is believed that some alteration on it could be a factor in the pathogenesis of infectious diseases, which result from alteration in cell mediated response.

It is a *transmembrane protein,* which is a heterodimer of alpha-beta (95%) or gamma-delta chains (5%). The rearrangement of the α and β genes during the T cell development is responsible for the milions of combination of TCRs. Each chain contains 4 separately encoded regions of V (variable), D (diversity), J (joining) and C (constant) regions analogous to regions of antibody. The TCR functions in combination with the CD3 complex, which consists of three pairs of dimers, namely delta-epsilon ($\delta\varepsilon$), gamma-epsilon ($\gamma\varepsilon$) and zeta-homodimer (Fig. 2.2.5b). After the binding the antigen MHC complex to TCR, the generated signal gets transmitted through the CD3 complex, activating the T cell.

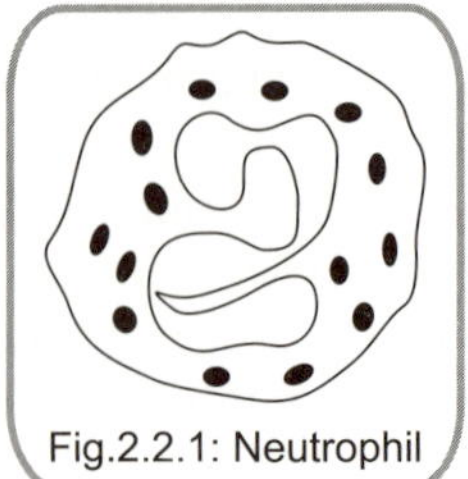
Fig.2.2.1: Neutrophil

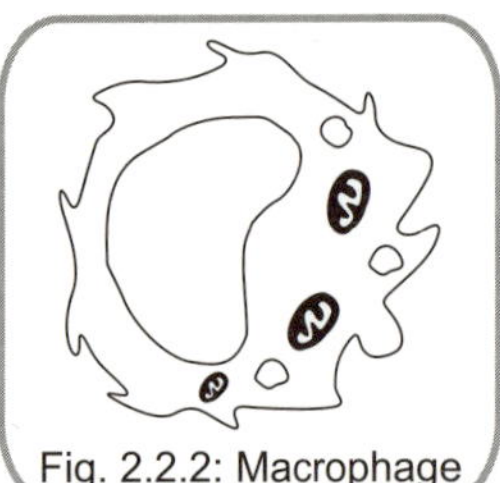
Fig. 2.2.2: Macrophage

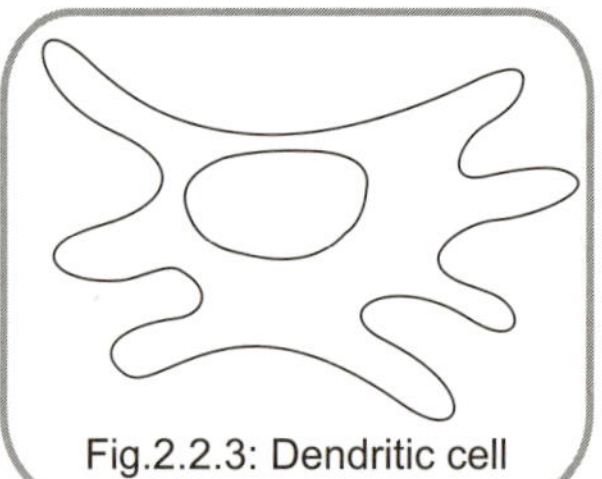
Fig.2.2.3: Dendritic cell

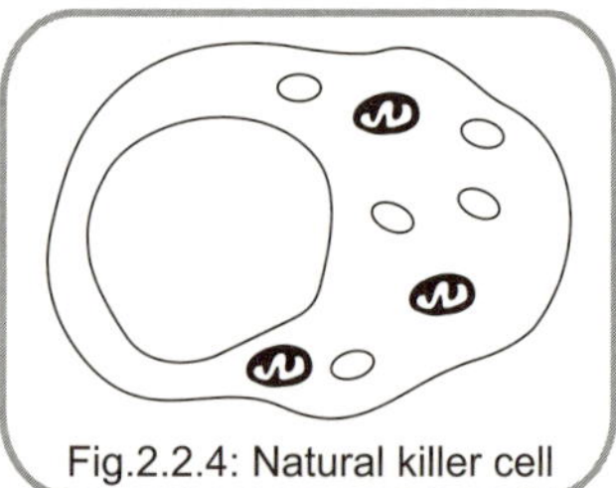
Fig.2.2.4: Natural killer cell

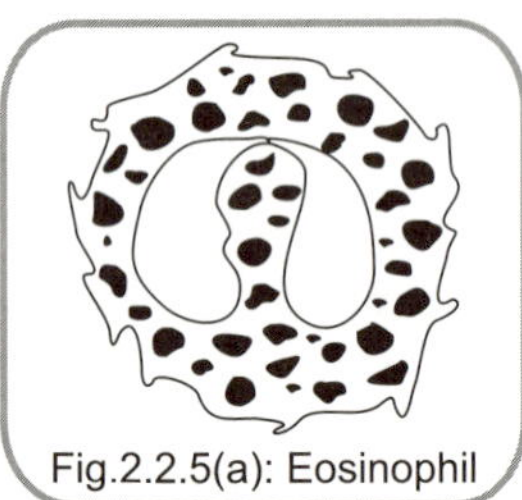
Fig.2.2.5(a): Eosinophil

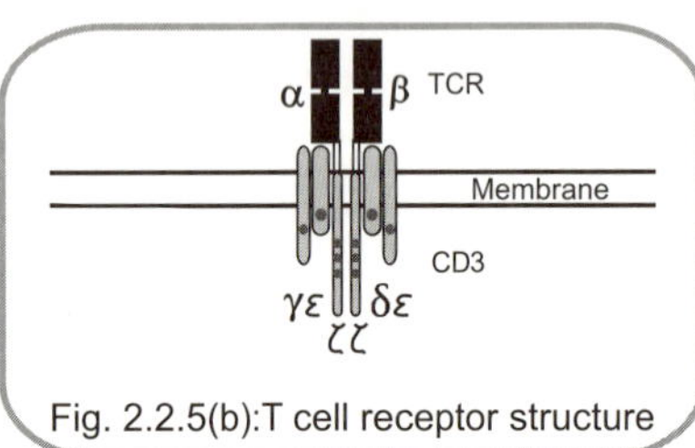

Fig. 2.2.5(b):T cell receptor structure

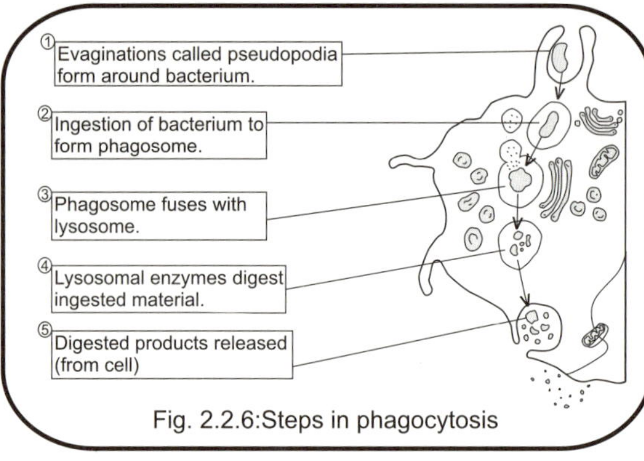

Fig. 2.2.6:Steps in phagocytosis

Diagrammatically depict the steps of phagocytosis.

A.4 **(b)** See Fig. 2.2.6

What is acute phase response? Explain how C-reactive protein (CRP) help in providing innate immunity.

A.5 During the acute phase of disease, changes in the serum protein concentration occur (increase and decrease), which is called **acute phase response.** The biological significance of some of these proteins is understood, which are chiefly synthesized in the liver, after it receives signals through the blood from sites of the injury or infection. The major signals inducing this response are the proinflammatory cytokines, Tumor necrosis factor-alpha and interleukins (one and six).

C-reactive protein is an acute phase response protein. It belongs to the group of pentameric proteins called pentraxins. The ligands it can bind include polysaccharide on *Streptoccus pneumoniae* and phosphorylcholine on many other pathogens. This binding facilitates the uptake of these pathogens by the phagocyte and the activation of the complement cascade. *Mannose-binding lectin* (MBL) is another acute phase protein that triggers the complement attack on the pathogens, to which it binds.

Discuss the role of pattern recognition receptors (PRRs) and pathogen-associated molecular patterns (PAMPs) in providing innate immunity.

A.6 Once a pathogen breeches the anatomical, physiological and some of the biological substance barriers,the infectious agent can elicit a complex cascade of events known as the *inflammatory response*. Many times the acute inflammatory response that occurs, can combat the infection successfully. However; sometimes the chronic inflammatory response sets in with damage to the host and is unable to eradicate the infectious agent.

The innate defense system must be able to detect the microbial invader and mount an elaborate response to attack the invader. Once the pathogen is recognized by the molecular sensor, different components of the immunity may come into play; as complement and opsonins. During the invasion, infectious agent interacts with the soluble/membrane bound molecules of the immune system capable of differentiating between the self and the infectious agent. These molecular sensors are able to detect broad structural motifs of microbes and are called **pattern recognition receptors** (PRR). The corresponding patterns, when found on infectious agents are called **pathogen associated molecular patterns** (PAMP) (Table 2.2.2).

The receptors (*pattern recognition receptors*) that exist on the innate immune system, which recognize the components of the pathogen (PAMPs) are important. Amongst these the Toll-like receptors are the most important. These are related to the Toll, which is a transmembrane signal receptor protein. Eleven TLRs have been discovered in humans, out of which functions for nine have been determined. Their activation results in promotion of expression of gene with effects in leucocyte activity, antigen presentation and intercellular signaling. Other common receptors include CRP, MBL and others (Table 2.2.2).

Table 2.2.2: Major pattern recognition receptors (PRR) of the innate immune system

Receptor	Sites of expression	Ligand (PAMP)	Effect of recognition
Toll like receptors (belong to family of Leucine rich protein)	Dendritic cells, macrophages and others	Lipopolysaccharide (LPS)	Cytokines produced required for innate and adaptive immunity
C-reactive proteins (belong to family of pentraxins)	Plasma protein (blood and tissue fluids)	Phosphatidyl choline	- Opsonization - Complement activation
Mannose binding Lectin (MBL)	Plasma proteins	Mannose microbial carbohydrates	- Complement activation - Opsonization
Macrophage scavenger receptors	Macrophage	Bacterial cell wall	Phagocytosis of bacteria
Complement	Plasma proteins	Microbial cell wall	- Complement activation - Lysis - Other effects
LPS binding protein	Plasma protein	LPS	Binding LPS and transferring it to CD14

What is signal conduction pathway?

A.7 After the cellular receptor (of the immune system) is occupied by a pathogen associated molecular pattern of a microbe, a signal must be transmitted inside the cell for an action to be generated. This pathway for the signal transduction is called the **signal conduction pathway**, which is constituted of the *'signal → cellular receptor → signal transduction → effector process'*, e.g., a bacterial product (signal) on a leucocyte PRR generating a signal transduction, resulting in the destruction of the bacterium (effector). The different pathways and their description is beyond the undergraduate curriculum.

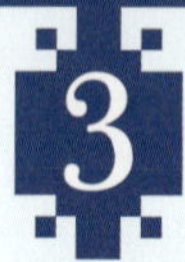

Acquired/Adaptive/Specific Immunity

Vertebrates have been evolving for millions of years. In this period they have acquired a process of specific (adaptive) immune response, which has given them an edge in their fight with microbes. This immunity has been given many names as acquired/adaptive/specific; which indicate the characteristics of this immunity. The term 'acquired' means that it is not present at birth time but it is acquired later on exposure to the antigens. The term 'adaptive' indicates that it is an response which is tailor made for a pathogen, so it is very specific. As this process is seen only in vertebrates, it is a character which has been acquired late in the evolution and gives the organism advantages in their survival. In the battle of supremacy between the microbe and the host, this process gives the latter a new dimension in protection from the ingenious microbe, which can always come up with strategies to defeat the host.

Let's study it.

How can immune response be best defined as? Discuss it's various characteristics.

A.1 It is very difficult to define it, as it is still being understood (studied) and has countless processes, for many of which the understanding is lacking. For understanding sake, it can **defined** as an altered reactivity to specific molecular configuration (i.e., antigen), which follows contact with it and is mediated by antibody and/or sensitized lymphocytes (T_H, Tc and their products) interacting with the other cells of the innate immune system.

Let us analyze this process. The word *'altered'* indicates that second time the organism interacts with the same antigen, the response is different. A classic example of this could be a second exposure of human-being to chicken pox infection, in which case the person would become immune to the disease.

The organism retains this information, which is explained as the body having *'immunological memory'*. The term 'specific' configuration indicates that the characteristic of *'altered reactivity'* is only towards the antigen to which the organism has been previously exposed. So; in the above example the human being won't show the protection to measles infection to which the body had no exposure.

Another characteristic of this response besides the specificity is the *diversity* of the response. What it implies, is that this response can be tailor-made for billions of different antigens.

One more characteristic that is often seen in this response is that the immune response, differentiates between the *'self'* and the *'non self'*, i.e., it mounts a response only to the foreign molecular configurations and not to the host cells (antigens). However, many times the immune response occurs significantly against the host resulting in autoimmune diseases. Damage to the organism can also occur, if there is excessive immune reactivity to innocuous substance resulting in hypersensitivity diseases. A final point that needs to be understood is that the organism is often protected from a second attack by the same microbe, because of an increased (heightened) state of immune reactivity.

Introduce the concept of immunological tolerance.

A.2 (a) Can sometimes, a decreased reactivity occur, following second time exposure to the same antigen in an organism? Yes! It can and this phenomenon is called immunological tolerance, which we shall be discussing later. It can be described as *specific *hyporesponsiveness* to specific molecular configuration, which follows contact with it and is mediated by antibody and/or T lymphocyte and its products.

*i.e., the body's immune response against other antigens is not decreased; remains maintained.

Describe a non-immunological tolerance process observed in human body?

A.2 (b) The immunological tolerance should be differentiated from other types of tolerance seen in the human body, **not** mediated by B and/or T cells and their products. One of the classic example is the tolerance to foetus by the pregnant woman. The fetus carries paternal MHC antigens different from the mother and mother becomes sensitized to them during the course of pregnancy, as is evident by presence of anti-HLA antibodies and cytotoxic T cells against paternal histocompatibility antigens. What are the mechanisms, which prevent the foetus from potential immunological attack? A number of hypotheses has been put forward to explain this. One of them is that placenta, which is a fetal derived tissue shields the immunological attack. The placenta lacks class I and class II MHC antigens, thus these cells lose much of their antigenicity.

Another hypothesis to explain this is the immunosuppressive environment in the fetus. This is likely to be due to the presence of high levels of ∝ fetoprotein in fetal blood, which is a fetal form of albumin, functioning as a immunosuppressive molecule. This would impede the immune response from occurring against the antigens.

Give classic examples in the body, in which tolerance is observed.

A.2 (c) Tolerance to infectious agents; as rubella and CMV virus is seen in congenital rubella syndrome and* congenital CMV infection. This can be explained on the basis that, since these infectious agents got introduced in the fetal period, they are treated as self by the immune system and hence no immune response is mounted against it.

*In this the viruses multiply in fetus causing viraemia in body, which persists after birth and there is minimal or no antibody or cell mediated response against these infectious agents.

Depict diagrammatically the key cells (players) involved in the immune response namely APC, T_H (helper T cell). Tc cell (Cytotoxic T Cell)

A.3 (a) Fig. 2.3.1 (Antigen presenting cell), Fig. 2.3.2 (T_H cell) and Fig. 2.3.3 (T_C- cytotoxic cell).

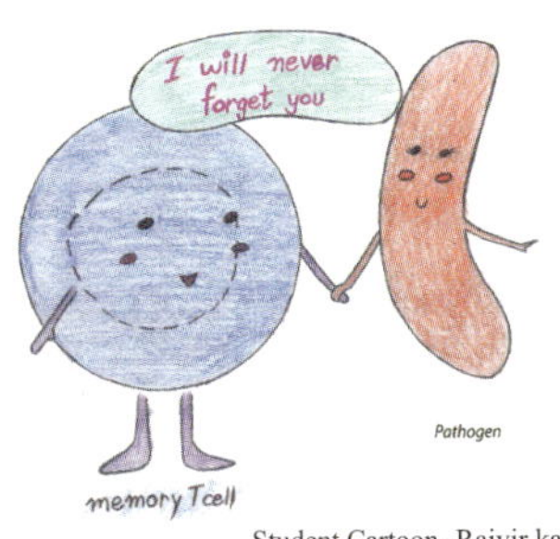

Student Cartoon -Rajvir kaur

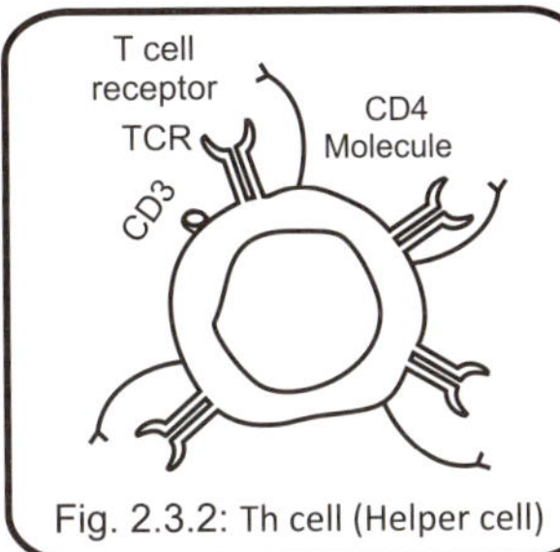

Fig. 2.3.2: Th cell (Helper cell)

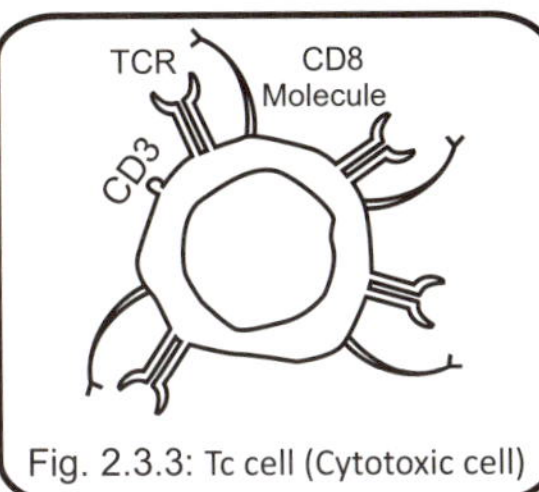

Fig. 2.3.3: Tc cell (Cytotoxic cell)

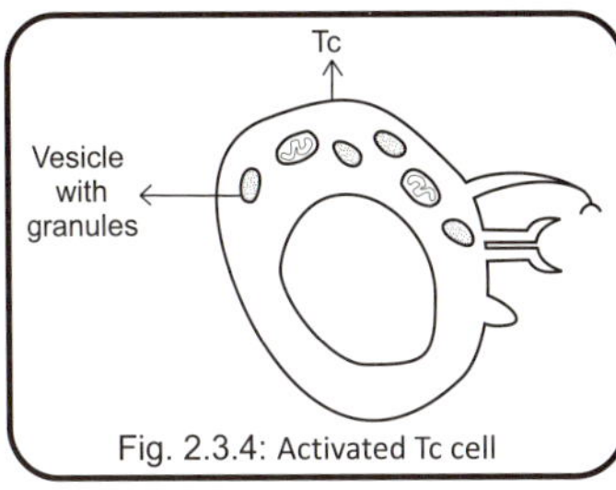

Fig. 2.3.4: Activated Tc cell

Illustrate diagrammatically the process of immune response.

A.3 (b) The steps involved in the immune response are

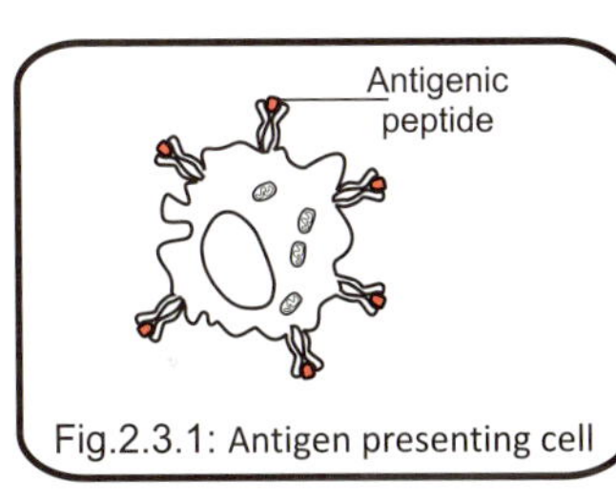

Fig.2.3.1: Antigen presenting cell

Invasion by (infection/vaccination) microbe
↓
Neutrophils joins (1st immune cells)
↓
Complement joins (alternate pathway)
↓
Presentation of antigen by APCs
↓ ↓

For intracellular microbe
↓
Formation of peptide- class I MHC complex and
↓
Interaction with Tc [CD8+ TCR)
↓ IL-2 induced
Expansion of Tc clone
↓
Interaction with infected cells leading to their destruction (of microbe) because of perforin and cytokine release
↓
Suppressor T cells send signals to stop immune response
↓
memory T and B cells remains

For other proteins

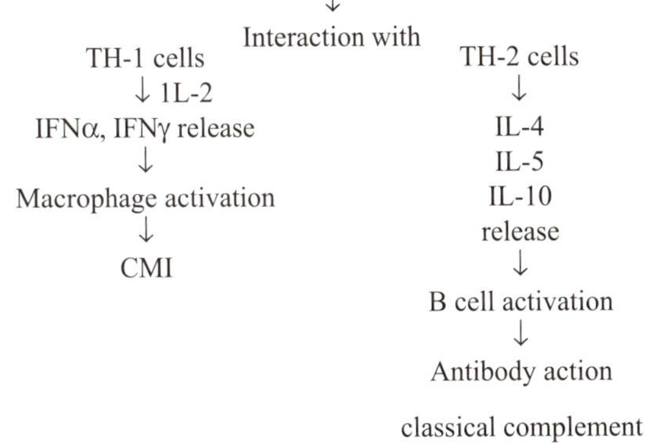

Depict the spectrum of the processes that are associated with the immune reactivity.

A.4 The immune response can be active/passive,protective/harmful and increased/decreased resulting in different states as depicted in Fig. 2.3.5 and Table 2.3.1.

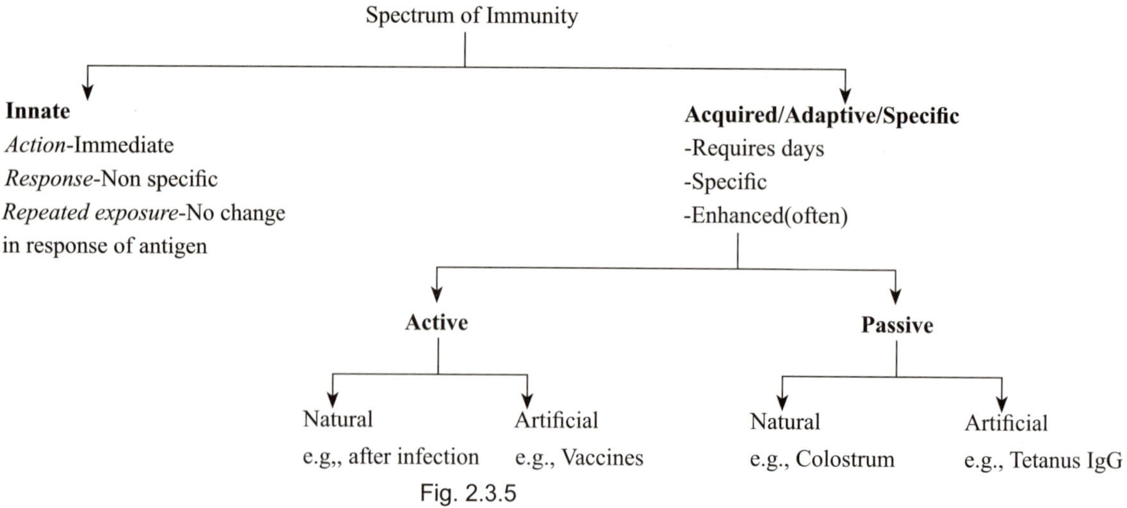

Fig. 2.3.5

Table 2.3.1: Spectrum of Immune reactivity, according to activity characteristics

Heightened ↑↑ (increased) Immune reactivity	*Helpful To organism*	Eliminates (controls) Pathogens & altered cells	• Mediated primarily by antibody (A.M.I.) • Mediated primarily by T cells (C.M.I.)
	Causing damage To organism	- Inappropriate (besides increased)	• Hypersensitivity Disorders
		- Targeting self antigens	• Autoimmune Disorders
		Targeting grafted Organs	• Rejection of transplant
Decreased ↓↓ Immune reactivity	*Beneficial to organism*	Targeting graft	• Acceptance of transplant
	Detrimental to organism	Targeting various molecules	• Tolerance phenomenon (as some persistent infections)

Tabulate the differences between innate, active and passive immunity.

A.5 Types of Immunity

Characteristic	Innate	Active	Passive
Source	Anatomical structure, Physiological processes and Chemical substances	Immune response (including cytokines) to antigens	Ready made Antibodies
Constitutents	Physical barrier, Chemical agents, Cells	Antibodies/activated lymphocytes (cytokines) Interacting with other cells	Plasma/from mother
Elicitment	Normal Genetic expression	By disease/vaccination	By colostrum, transport across placenta, Immune sera
Kinetics	- Slways present - No lag period - No negative phase	- Appear a week after antigen introduction - Lag period present - May be present (negative phase)	- Immediately - None - None
Limitation	- May not be able to deal severe infection	- Can deal with severe Infections but not applicable to immunodeficient states	- Valid for limited infections
Duration	- Life long	Months to years	Days to weeks

What is herd immunity? Discuss its possible role in outbreak causation.

A.6 Herd immunity:

It refers to the overall level of immunity in a community. This concept is very important in the disease eradication programmes. Many disease eradication/control programme aim at achieving a certain definable prevalence of immunity in a population, so that the concerned pathogen cannot circulate freely amongst the susceptible population. This leads to indirect protection of susceptible population. This indirect protection of the unvaccinated persons is called the herd immunity effect. This concept is important, as most vaccines are not 100% effective and in any vaccination programme, certain population would remain deprived of the vaccination due to different reasons. So the implementing agency must know that for a certain disease control, what percentage of population must be vaccinated?

This level of vaccination coverage varies for different pathogens. Infectious agent; as measles have higher transmission rates than *S. pneumoniae*, so require higher level of vaccination coverage for the disease control to occur.

This concept also explains the numerous outbreaks and epidemics that occurred in different parts of the world due to complacency in the immunization programmes. One classic example is the diphtheria epidemic in mid 1990s in several parts of the former Soviet-Union due to decreased vaccination rate after the breakup of the Soviet Union. So when the herd immunity is low in a region due to any reason, probability of epidemics in that region may increase.

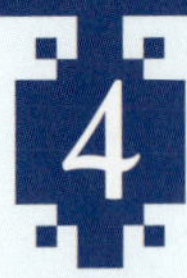

Antigen

A biomedical engineer, along with an orthopaedician; Dr Alok Sood are devising an unique knee prosthesis with features; as very low weight and non antigenicity. What should be the characteristics of this material in reference to the antigenic properties? Let's study this aspect.

Define antigen and mention its importance in immune response.

A.1 Broadly, it can be *defined* as a substance that when introduced into an organism with a functioning immune system elicits a specific immune response and reacts specifically with antibody and/or T cells.

Antigen is the key cornerstone in the organisms immune response against the numerous infectious diseases and even the malignancies. It's study provides the insight in these processes, which are often studied 'in-vitro' and then applied efficaciously 'in-vivo', for instance the various grades of intradermal administration of antigens with the aim of controlling allergy to them.

What are the two key properties of antigen? Describe with special reference to haptene.

A.2 Properties of antigen:

(i) *Immunogenicity:* It is the ability to induce a humoral and/or cell mediated immune response. Another term for antigen is the immunogen.

(ii) *Antigenicity:* It is the ability of the antigen to react specifically with the antibody (it produces) and/or with the receptors of the T cell.

Most molecules that possess immunogenicity also have antigenicity but the reverse may not be true; as in the case of haptens.

Karl Landsteiner did pioneering work in the 1920s in the area of epitopes and gained information into the specificity of the antigen-antibody reactions. *Haptens* are partial antigens that possess antigenicity but not immunogenicity, e.g., Dinitrophenol (DNP) and penicillin. They can not cause the production of antibodies or activate lymphocytes however can react with them. To make them acquire the characteristic of immunogenicity, they have to be coupled to large carrier molecules; as albumins or globulins. When such hapten-carrier is injected into an organism, three types of antibodies may be formed as depicted below:

Injection of guinea-pig with	Response
• DNP (hapten)	• No antibodies
• BSA (protein carrier)	• Anti-BSA antibodies
• DNP-BSA conjugate	• Anti-DNP antibodies (major) • Anti-BSA antibodies • Anti-DNP/BSA (combined) antibodies

An application of this phenomenon is that many peptide and steroid hormones, which are haptens can be bound to carrier proteins to produce antibodies against them, which can be then used in their detection or measurement from clinical samples.

What is the basis on which antigen gets classified?

A.3 Classification of antigens

On chemical composition	• Proteins/polypeptides • Glycoproteins • Polysaccharides • Others; as glycolipids

Contd.

Contd.

Completeness	• Complete - have both key characteristics • Incomplete - has only one characteristic
Type of response elicited	• Increased/heightened- (called *immunogen*) • Decreased - (called *tolerogen*)
Recruitment of MHC molecules for their presentation	• Certain antigens do not need MHC • Most antigens require to be presented with MHC molecules for them to be effectively presented.
Source of antigen	- *Endogenous* antigens (another term is intracellular pathogen/cytosolic pathogen) Viruses are degraded endogenously in the cytosol by proteasomes, assembled with class I MHC molecules in the endoplasmic reticulum system and exported to the cell membrane by golgi apparatus (to interact with CD8+ T- cells) - *Exogenous:* Antigens/protein; as some extracellular pathogens are taken inside the cell by endocytosis (or internalized), degraded within the acidic endocytic compartment and subsequently combine with MHC II molecules to present in a combined form on the cell membrane to CD4+ T_H cells.
T_H cell help	• *Thymus dependent* (require presentation to T cells for antibody production) • *Thymus independent* (do not require presentation to T cells, have large repetitive structures; as flagellin and Lipopolysaccharide.
Site of antigen	• *Sequestered:* Antigens are in a site in the body, where it doesn't come in contact with antibody producing cell, e.g., cornea (non-vascularized), brain (no lymphatics) • *Exposed* (non-sequestered)

What are the factors that affect antigenicity?

A.4 1. *Foreignness:* The antigen must be foreign to organism to which it is being administered to be immunogenic; for example bovine serum albumin, which is a normal component of the cow serum, is strongly immunogenic in rabbit but not in cows. When an antigen is introduced into an organism, the degree of immunogenicity depends on the degree of foreignness. Generally, the greater the phylogenetic disparity between the organisms, the greater is the structural disparity between their constituent molecules. The grading can be understood in the context of grafting.

(a) *Autologous* antigens: are found within the same individual, e.g., a skin graft from an individuals back to his arm is an autograft.

(b) *Syngeneic* antigens: are found between identical twins or in individuals of an inbred strain (extensive inbreeding, that the loci have become identical), e.g., graft between members of an inbred strain is an isograft or a syngeneic graft.

(c) *Allogeneic* (homologous) antigens: are found within the same species but different individuals, e.g., two individuals of different nationalities have B blood group.

(d) *Xenogeneic* (heterologous) antigens: are found across species limits, e.g., transplant of a baboon heart to human would be a xenograft.

2. *Chemical composition:* This is an important factor in determining the ability of a molecule to be immunogenic, besides its size and foreignness. The majority of the immunogens are proteins because they have the biggest array of building blocks (namely amino acids). Lipoproteins are components of many cell membranes and also act as antigens.

Most polysaccharides are incomplete immunogens or haptens and lack the degree of chemical diversity seen in proteins. The polysaccharides are usually degraded rapidly limiting their contact with the immune system to elicit an immune response. However some polysaccharides are utilized as successful immunogens; as pneumococcal capsule polysaccharide vaccine.

Blood group antigens A and B are example of glycoproteins. Nucleic acids are usually non-immunogenic, however nucleoproteins can elicit an immune response; as is seen in SLE cases. Lipids are also non-immunogenic, however glycolipid can act as antigens as seen in the cell mediated immune response in *M. tuberculosis* infection.

3. *Macromolecular size:* Generally substances with a molecular mass less than 10,000 Da (Dalton) are weakly antigenic or non-antigenic. Larger molecular mass (as > 100,000 Da) are usually strong immunogens; as they would have greater number of epitopes and would have to phagocytosed, increasing their interaction with the immune system.

4. *Susceptibility to antigen processing and presentation:* The macromolecules must be able to be degraded and presented with MHC molecules for T-cell-mediated and some antibody mediated (thymus dependent) immune

responses; for instance polymers of D-amino acids are poor immunogens, as the degradative enzymes within the APCs can degrade only proteins with L-amino acids.

5. *Dose:* Generally speaking, below a certain threshold dose, most proteins do not elicit a primary immune response. Above the threshold level, there is a gradual increase in the response, followed by a decrease response at very high level (Fig. 2.4.1).

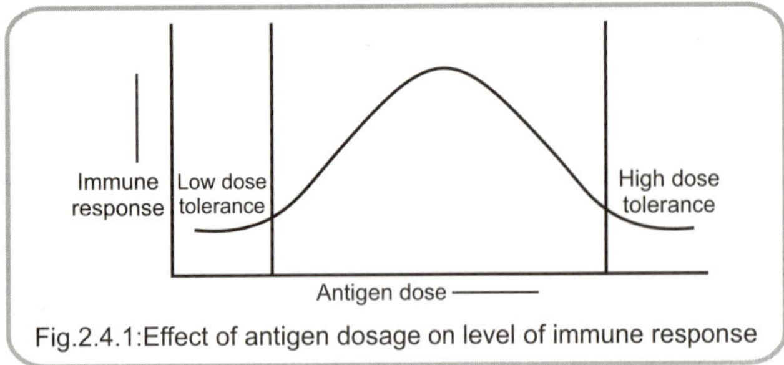

Fig.2.4.1:Effect of antigen dosage on level of immune response

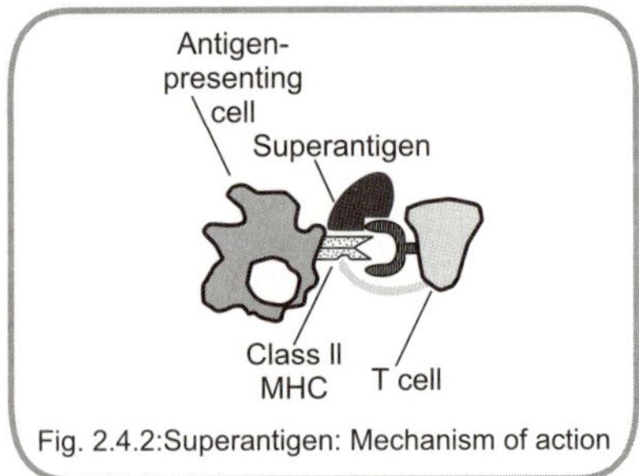

Fig. 2.4.2:Superantigen: Mechanism of action

An antibody response may be measured by determining the level of antibodies in the serum of the immunized vertebrate animal. The T-cell responses are difficult to evaluate but may be measured by observing the increase in T-cell receptors that recognize the antigen. An inadequate dose won't activate enough lymphocytes to induce an immune response. The inhibition of the response at very high levels may be important in maintaining tolerance to abundant self proteins; as plasma proteins.

6. *Route of antigen administration:* Generally the subcutaneous route is the most effective in generating strongest immune response. It is followed by intraperitoneal, intravenous and the intragastric routes in a decreasing order.

   The principle of an antigen, e.g., food producing least immune response, if administered intragastrically is used in preventing some allergies. Some antigens; if administered intragastrically with a view of controlling their allergic responses results in poor systemic immune response, when subsequently administered by other routes.

7. *Form of antigen:* Generally speaking, antigens that are particulate and denatured are more immunogenic than soluble and native antigens.

8. *Genotype of the recipient:* It is important for a species to survive that the immune response should vary amongst it, so that the response to a pathogen is not constant or all of it may be eliminated in response to a new pathogen. This is exactly so in the humans, who have the extremely polymorphic MHC genes, whose products play an important role in the presentation of the processed antigen to the T cells. Variability in the immune response is also provided by the difference in the genes that encode B, T cell receptors and are involved in the immune regulation.

9. *Malnutrition:* Protein and/or carbohydrate deficiency inhibits the immune response.

10. *Multiple antigens:* The administration of multiple antigens to an organism can result in variable results. The response may be enhanced by taking optimal amounts of the antigen; as is done for the triple vaccine of DPT.

11. *Role of adjuvant:* The word adjuvant is derived from the Latin 'adjuvare' which means 'to help'. So these are substances that when combined with the antigen and administered, enhance their immunogenicity. These have a role in the research and the therapeutics, where it can be used with vaccines to increase their efficacy. However a distinction may be made from the protein carriers, which form stable linkages with the immunogen; for instance the protein carrier (as tetanus toxoid) used to carry the polysaccharide vaccine of *H influenzae*.

    Historically the first adjuvant was introduced by Jules Freund and is known as *Freund's complete* adjuvant and consists of a water-in-oil emulsion, which means that the aqueous solution of antigen with killed *M. tuberculosis* antigen is dispersed in the oil. This acts by delayed release of antigen, enhanced uptake by APCs and induction of co-stimulators in macrophages. This is not used in human, as it can induce granulomas locally and in the draining lymph nodes. Modification of the Freund's complete adjuvant include a preparation, in which muramyl dipeptide (a component of mycobacterial cell wall) is added. *Freund's incomplete* adjuvant consists of antigen in aqueous solution with a mineral oil and emulsifying agent. This also acts by delayed release of antigens and enhanced uptake by APCs.

    A number of other agents can act as adjuvants, which include silica particles, bentonite and ISCOMs (immune stimulatory complexes). Aluminium potassium sulphate (alum) is the only chemical approved by the FDA for human use. It prolongs the persistence of antigen. ISCOMs are immune stimulatory complexes of antigens held within a lipid matrix that enhance the immunogenicity of the antigen by enabling it to be taken up into the cytoplasm, after fusion with the lipid in the plasma membrane. These carriers have minimal toxicity.

12. Heterophile specificity:
    - *Definition*: Heterophile antigens are same or closely related antigens that are present in different species.
    - *Example*: *Forssman antigen* is a lipoprotein-polysaccharide complex found in widely diverse species; as man, animals, plants, birds and bacteria.
    - *Implication*: Antibodies formed against antigen of one species may react with another species and vice versa.
    - *Utility (application)*: For many infectious agents, antigen preparation of them can be challenging due to different reasons; as the agent may be difficult to cultivate. In such circumstances, heterophile antigen can be utilized to devise a serological diagnostic test.

      Weil Felix reaction (pg 348-349, A3b, Chapter 5, Section 10)

      Cold agglutination test (pg 347, A3c, Chapter 4, Section 10)

      Paul Bunnel test (pg 418-419, A8c Chapter 7, Section 12)

What is the basis of antigenicity?

A.5 Entire antigenic molecules do not react with the antibody or the T-cell receptors. Instead distinct antigenic determinants on the antigen called *epitopes* participate in the binding. The basis of the specificity between the epitope and the antibody/T cell receptor is stercochemical, i.e., depends on the chemical composition and the spatial arrangement of the chemical groups. The precise area of the antibody that binds with the epitope is called *paratope*.

The surface of an antigen may present a large number of potential antigenic sites. The valence of the antigen will be equal to the total number of epitopes the antigen possesses. However, in an organism the number of epitopes that the immune system recognizes is usually less than the potential antigenic profile. Certain epitopes induce a more pronounced immune response than others and are called *immunodominant*.

Generally the *epitope* is composed of 4-5 amino-acid or monosaccharides. The epitope may be composed of a linear sequence of amino-acids or a non-sequential/conformational one, in which the elements are brought together by the folded conformation of the antigen. The size of the epitope is generally 25-30°A. B cell epitopes are generally accessible and hydrophilic in comparison to the T cell epitopes, which may be internal and brought to the surface by antigenic processing and presentation. The antigen molecules can be altered by adding or taking away epitopes, e.g., some epitopes may be lost on heating the antigen.

How many structures exist in the environment that can be immunogenic (antigenic)?

A.6 Probably the number is *infinite*. In other words, any molecular configuration, when presented appropriately to the immune system can be antigenic. But does that mean that there are also almost infinite antibodies or T cell receptors; as the reaction between the two entities is specific. There are actually billions of antibodies and T cell receptors according to estimates, so at times cross-reactions occur between similar molecules.

What is the importance of studying antigenic presentation?

A.7 The ultimate that can be practiced in the infectious disease, is the prevention of the diseases, as by vaccines. For many diseases that we do not have an efficacious vaccine; as for TB. In such a scenario, it may be possible to have a TB vaccine in the future, if *M. tuberculosis* antigens could be effectively presented to the immune cells. Similarly, for AIDS vaccine development, study of the HIV antigen presentation is of paramount importance.

Where does antigen localize in the body after its introduction into it? Mention the sequelae.

A.8 The localization of the antigen in the body, depends on the route by which it is introduced, as illustrated below:

Route by which antigen introduced	Primary site where it localizes
Subcutaneous	Draining lymph nodes
Upper respiratory tract	MALT (Mucosal associated lymphoid tissue)
GIT (orally)	MALT
Intravenously	Spleen/liver

The antigen is usually degraded by the mononuclear phagocytic system within a few days, if it is a protein and may take a few weeks, if it is a polysaccharide.

Antibodies to the antigen that are formed later accelerate the elimination of both the particulate (insoluble) and soluble antigen, which form antigen-antibody complexes. The soluble antigen when administered intravenously undergoes three phases namely (a) the brief equilibrium phase characterized by rapid outflow of antigen into the extravascular space (b) slow metabolic delay (c) rapid immune elimination because of the formation of antigen–antibody complex clearance by the macrophages.

Antigen that induce humoral response interact directly with the B lymphocytes (B. cell receptor) however the antigens that induce cell-mediated response must be processed by the APCs and presented with the MHC molecules to the T lymphocyte (T cell receptor).

How does one separate (purify) antigen (protein) for 'in-vitro' studies.

A.9 Different techniques exist to separate the protein fractions; as sodium dodecyl sulphate-polyacrylamide gel electrophoresis (SDS-PAGE) and isoelectric focusing. The latter technique consists of an electrophoretic technique in which proteins migrate in a pH gradient until they reach the place in the gradient, at which their net charge is neutral, their isoelectric point.

How does one detect antigen 'in vitro'?

A.10 Different antigen-antibody techniques exist for their detection. These are discussed in Chapter 6, p124-134.

What are antigen presenting cells?

A.11 Antigens of pathogens need to be processed and presented by specific cells, so that they can interact with the immune cells and elicit an immune response. Native antigens mostly can't elicit the immune response. The cells of the body that can perform the job of antigen presentation on the surface of cell are called *antigen presenting cells* (Fig. 2.3.1). All cells can be designated such but strictly speaking the cells that display peptides associated with class II MHC to CD4+ T_H cell are called APCs and cells that display peptides associated with class I MHC molecules to CD8+ cells are referred to as *target cells*. Initially it was believed that macrophages are the key APCs but now it is realized that dendritic cells are the key APCs, with this function being possible to be performed by almost any type of cell.

The APCs can be broadly categorized into two categories as depicted in Table 2.4.1.

Table 2.4.1: Categories of Antigen Presenting Cells (APCs)

Professional (constitutively or easily activated to express class II MHC/costimulatory signal)	• Dendritic cell • Macrophage • B cells
Non-professional (need to be induced to express class II MHC or costimulatory signal and can function for short periods)	• Fibroblasts (skin) • Vascular endothelial cell • Glial (brain) cells • Thymic epithelial cell • Thyroid epithelial cell • Pancreatic beta cells

How does antigen processing occur in the cell?

A.12 It would depend on type of antigen (see A.3). Major histocompatibility complex (MHC) would play a key role in the response (see Chapter 11, Sec. 2).

What is superantigen?

A.13 These are designated; such as they can cause significantly increased nonspecific activation of T cells, resulting in massive release of cytokines that can result in pathology (application, see Staphylococcus problem pg. 181. These antigens cause such pathophysiology, as they can bind directly to the T cell receptor and class II MHC molecules, without the need of binding to the peptide cleft (Fig. 2.4.2).

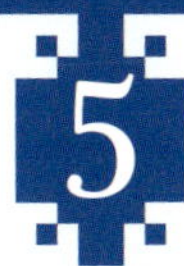

Immunoglobulin (Antibody)

The innate immune defense can deal effectively with the numerous pathogens that the vertebrate organism encounters. But often the pathogen acquires a character that can outwit the defense of the organism. Then what can the organism do? Let's take the example of rough colony type of *Streptococcus pneumoniae*, which when introduced into a mouse, gets quickly killed by the mouse macrophages. But when the smooth (having capsule) colony type of *S. pneumoniae* is introduced, the mouse succumbs to the infection. This occurs because the capsule of this organism, prevents the effective interaction of the macrophages and the neutrophils with the pathogenic organism.

How must the organism overcome this situation? The organism must generate specific entities to overcome this disability. It has been seen that people who survive a pneumococcal type 3 pneumonia attack, are protected (immune) from an attack by this specific organism but not from the other numerous serotypes of same pathogen. From many studies, it was demonstrated that the serum of these individual acquire a specific entity (antipneumococcal antibody), which is of protective nature.

Let's study this aspect in detail.

Describe an animal experiment to demonstrate the specificity aspect of antibody.

A.1 (a) There are more than 90 serotypes of virulent pneumococci in existence. If any of them is injected in big numbers into a mouse, it succumbs to the infection. However, if a specific type of pneumococcus, let's say type 4 is mixed with a drop or two of serum taken from a man, who has recovered from type 4 pneumococcus and then injected to mouse, the animal survives. This protection entails from the fact that serum has specific antipneumococcal antibodies (to type 4 pneumococcus). So if mouse is injected with pneumococcus of type 4 with few drops of antiserum taken from a man, who has recovered from type 5 pneumococcus, the mouse succumbs to the infection.

What should be the structure of the antibody that can perform the function of adaptive immunity?

A.1 (b) The antibody molecule should have two ends, one end should be antigenic, i.e., should be able to identify the antigen and the other end should have the biological properties; as stimulation of phagocytes, functional capacity and other activation properties, as for complement.

What is the actual structure (broadly) of the immunoglobulin?

A.2 The immunoglobulin structure is seen to have an similar structure and function, as postulated above. Later studies confirmed these postulates.

In which fraction of the electrophoresed serum proteins, do the antibodies belong to? Elucidate this aspect in an experimental set up.

A.3 (a) In the gamma fraction of the gamma globulins.

Arne Tiselius and EA Kabat (1939) resolved the serum proteins in electrophoresis into three non-albumin fractions, namely *alpha, beta and gamma* and demonstrated that most serum antibodies were found in the gamma fraction. A simple experiment in the laboratory demonstrated this. An electrophoresis of an rabbit serum sample (who has been immunized with killed type 3 *S. pneumoniae)* performed in a standard buffer at pH 8.6 is depicted in Fig. 2.5.1. Serum albumin which is most negatively charged, migrates most rapidly to the anode.

Precipitation reaction of the purified polysaccharide of pneumococcus (i.e., antigen) would occur only with the gamma-globulin fraction of this serum and not with the others. Later studies have found some antibodies to be also present in the alpha and beta globulins.

A serum that contains a specific set of antibodies is called *antiserum*.

What is the composition of the antibody?

A.3 (b) Antibody can be described; as glycoproteins present chiefly in serum (and other biological fluids) globulins, produced chiefly by plasma cells (also by lymphocytes) in response to exposure to an antigen.

Chemically the antibodies are *globulins*. Serum globulins can be separated into water soluble *pseudoglobulins* and water insoluble *euglobulins*. Most antibodies belong to the latter category.

The heavy chains of some classes (γ, α and δ) contain an extended peptide sequence between the CH_1 and CH_2 domain, which is not homologous with any other known domain. This is called the *hinge region*. The extended polypeptide conformation is created by the large number of proline residues, which makes it more exposed, hence becomes the site of enzymatic action of pepsin and papain (on either site, disulphide bonds). The increased flexibility that this area provides, as the name 'hinge' suggest permits the Fab fragments to change their angle to accommodate nearby epitope sites that may vary slightly in distance and position.

Table 2.5.2: Properties of Human immunoglobulin classes

	IgG	IgA	IgM	IgD	IgE
Molecular weight	150,000	160,000	900,00- to 1,000,000	180,000	190,000
Usual forms	Monomer	Monomer/Dimer	Pentamer/Hexamer	Monomer	Monomer
Sedimentation coefficient	7	7	19	7	8
Heavy chains	Gamma (1 – 4)	Alpha1, Alpha2	Mu	Delta	Epsilon
Light chain	K or L	K or L	K or L	K or L	K or L
Other Chains	–	J or SC	J	–	–
Synthesis rate mg/kg/per day	33	65	7	0.4	0.016
Antibody Valence	2	2, 4	10, 12	2	2
Classical Complement pathway activation	+	–	++	–	–
Alternate complement pathway activation	–	+	–	–	–
Present in Milk	+	+	–	–	–
Serum Concentration (mg/ml)	12	2	1.2	0.03	0.0003
Binding cells via Fc on	Macrophage, Neutrophil, Large granular Lymphocyte (LGL)	Lymphocyte	Lymphocyte	–	Basophil, B cell
Biological properties	Placental transport, Secondary antibody response	Mucosal transport (Secretory)	Primary Antibody response	–	Allergy, Anaphylaxis
Heat stability (56°C)	+	+	+	+	–

Can antibody act as an antigen?

A.4 (c) Yes, antibodies are proteins and when injected in another animal; for which they are foreign, will result in the formation of 'anti-antibodies'. Thus antibodies can act as antigens.

Describe the major types of immunoglobulin antigenic determinants; namely isotypic, allotypic and idiotypic.

A.5 The antigenic determinants or the diversity of antibodies that can be produced (or exist), can be categorized into isotypic, allotypic and idiotypic.

Isotypic *(Iso = same)* – These are antigenic determinants that are shared by all members of a species. Thus; if anti-isotypic antibody is to be produced, the antibody must be injected into another species, which will recognize it as foreign. The isotypic determinants are constant region determinants that define each heavy-chain class, subclass and each light-chain type and subtype within a species. In a specific species, each individual would express all isotypes in the serum. These arise because of the different constant regions inherited and expressed as different isotypes. As an example; if human immunoglobulins are injected into guinea-pig, antibodies would form against the human immunoglobulin. The guinea-pig antiserum on electrophoresis analysis would be found not so have a single component but isotypes of IgG, IgM and IgA antibodies. Isotypes IgD and IgE would require more sensitive assays to be detected, as their concentration is very low.

Allotypic *(allo=other)*: These are antigenic determinants that exist in different individuals of the same species. To generate anti-allotypic antibody, the immunoglobulin can be raised in the same species, if the recipient and donor's immunoglobulin have different allotypes. For a rough analogy, example could be taken of injecting RBCs of blood group A of one human into another human of blood group B and generating anti-A antibodies. The allotypic determinants are present on the constant regions of the heavy and light chains. These differences arise because of multiple alleles existing for some of the genes of isotypes. These alleles encode subtle amino-acid differences called *allotypes*. In humans, allotypes have been described for all four IgG subclasses, one IgA subclass and for one kappa light chain. Markers on γ chains are designated *Gm*, markers on α chains are designated *Am* and markers on κ are designated *Km*.

Idiotypic:

These are unique antigenic determinants (see Fig. 2.5.2b, 2.5.3a) in the V_H and V_L domains of the immunoglobulin that may be associated with the antigenic binding capability of the immunoglobulin. To raise anti-idiotypic antibodies (antisera), an animal of the same species have to be chosen that have identical (or minimal variation) allotypes. Alternatively Fab fragment has to be chosen for raising antisera or extensive absorptions would have to be carried out the remove anti-isotypic and anti-allotypic antibodies, before injecting for raising anti-idiotypic antibodies.

There are many antigenic determinants on the variable region of the immunoglobulin called *idiotopes*. These stimulate production of anti-idiotypic antibodies. On the variable region of the immunoglobulin, some of the idiotopes are the actual antigen binding sites whereas some comprise variable-region on sequences outside of binding site. The sum of the individual idiotopes of an immunoglobulin would be it's *idiotype*.

What are the mechanisms that lead to immunoglobulin acquiring the phenomenal diversity?

A.6 One of the unique properties of the antibody is the ability to bind specifically to the almost infinite type antigen structures. So the immunoglobulin must be able to exist in millions of structures to match the antigen variability. What mechanisms does the immune system utilize to produce these diverse antibodies? Two theories have existed to explain this process, namely the **germline** and the somatic-variation theory. According to the former theory, the cell has dedicated a substantial portion of the genome to code for antibody variability, hence no other mechanism is necessary to produce the diverse antibodies. The **somatic variation** theory is based on the mutation and the recombination processes; yielding the diverse antibodies. Both the theories could not explain the characteristic of the antibody molecule having tremendous variability in the variable region, while having few structural variations in the constant region. To overcome this limitation, W. Dreyer and J Bennett (1965) suggested the model of two separate genes encoding a single Ig heavy or light chain, one gene for the V region and the other gene coding the constant region. They suggested that these two genes must be integrated at a later stage and translated into a single immunoglobulin (heavy or light) chain. Theoretically the assembly of two or more genes into a single polypeptide is possible by two other mechanisms, namely genes being transcribed separately but the resulting RNA being joined and the other mechanism being the genes being transcribed and translated separately but the linkage occurying at the polypeptide level. Subsequently *S. Tonegawa and N. Hozumi* in 1976 confirmed experimentally the theoretical model of Dreyer and Bennet, which postulated the DNA of two genes joining and then being transcribed and translated together (Fig. 2.5.6). This was a revolutionary concept in immunogenetics, for which Susumu Tonegawa was awarded the Nobel prize in 1987. So the plasma cell (mature B cell) chromosomal DNA is not identical to its germ cell. So, *genomic rearrangement* is a characteristic feature of B cell development, which questions the stable genetic blue print character of the genomic DNA.

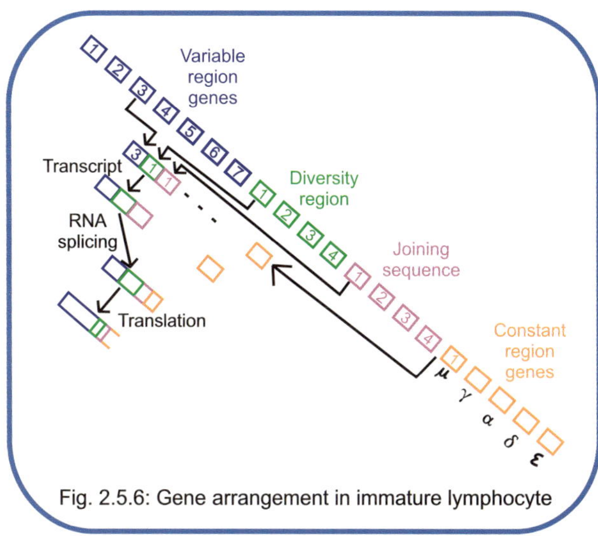

Fig. 2.5.6: Gene arrangement in immature lymphocyte

The current concept of the immunoglobulin genetics is of *multigene organization*. The genes for the λ light chain, K light chain and heavy chain occur on the 22nd, 2nd and 14th human chromosome, respectively.

The κ and λ light chain families contain the V, J (joining) and C gene segments. There are separate sets of genetic building blocks for the light chains, which rearrange to form the VJ segment which then associates with the constant region C gene segment. The heavy chain have additionally the D (Diversity) segment, so in it, VDJ rearranged segments combine with the C gene segment to form the heavy Ig. The subsequent assembly of the light and heavy harms and the formation of the intrachain and interchain disulphide bonds and the addition of the carbohydrate occur in the rough endoplasmic reticulum. The assembled immunoglobulin is finally transported to the golgi apparatus; where it gets bound in secretory vesicles, to be finally integrated with the cell membrane. So the diversity of the Ig arise from the different ways the multiple V-(D)-J-C germ-line gene segments combines, besides the combinational association of the light and heavy chains. The hundred-thousand fold higher mutation rate in the V-D-J segments called *somatic hypermutation*, also contributes to the diversity in the immunoglobulin. The other processes; as P and N nucleotide region addition and junctional flexibility, also contribute to the diversity, but are beyond the undergraduate level discussion.

Illustrate the mechanisms by which immunoglobulins act in the body.

A.7 Mechanism of action:

1. *Neutralize:* toxins (Fig. 2.5.7)
2. *Prevent entry* and spread: by binding pathogen on surface, e.g., by sI_gA

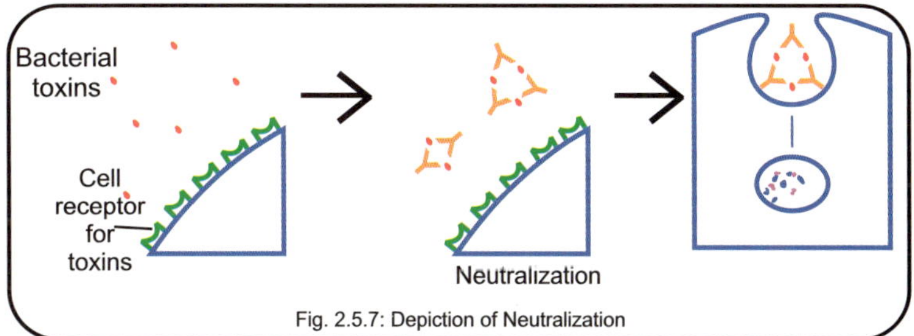

Fig. 2.5.7: Depiction of Neutralization

3. *Opsonization:* Coating pathogen by Fc end of antibody, facilitates recognition by Fc receptor on cells; as macrophages, results in enhanced phagocytosis (Fig. 2.5.8).
4. Antibody dependent cellular cytotoxicity (*ADCC*) (Fig. 2.5.9): This mechanism is utilized by cells; as natural killer cells, eosinophils and neutrophil.
5. Activating classical complement pathway: initiated by binding of complement fixing antibody on surface of pathogen results in recruitment of inflammatory cells and generation of membrane attack complex (MAC).

Enumerate disease conditions in which abnormal immunoglobulins are formed in body.

A.8 Multiple myeloma, cryoglobulinemia and Heavy chain disease.

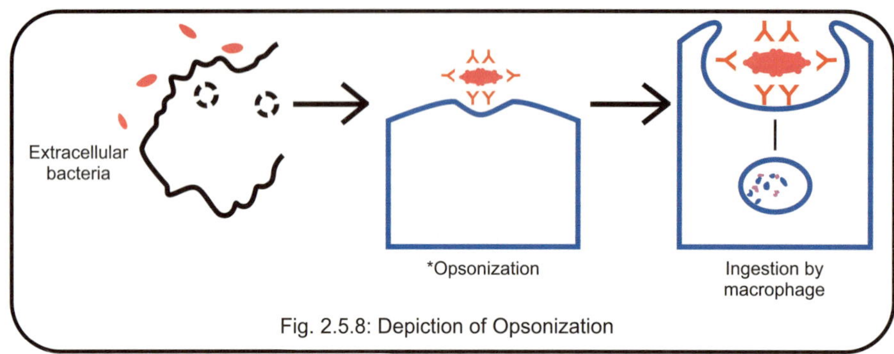

Fig. 2.5.8: Depiction of Opsonization

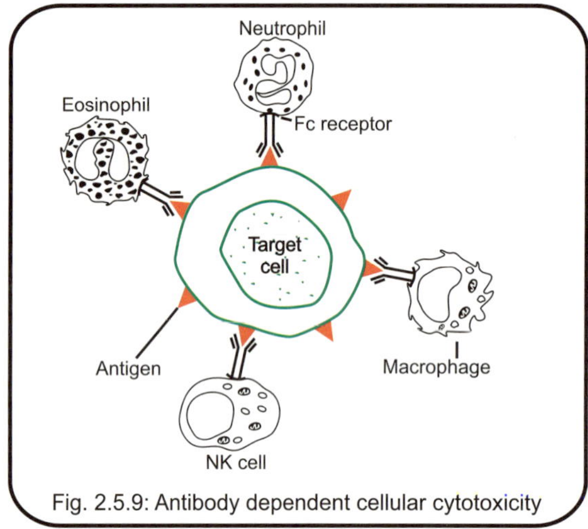

Fig. 2.5.9: Antibody dependent cellular cytotoxicity

“**B cell**
Born as a warrior
But
I am also canny
A loyal subject to my host
Protecting her from all odds
But seem harmless and idle
But I recognize the enemy at a glance
Recruit my fellow generals
And send my loyal troops—
IgA, IgM, IgA, IgD and IgE
Go further marching !
PROTECTING !”

–Deborah (4th semester student)

Monoclonal Antibody

A four month old male infant, Shahid is admitted in a paediatric ICU with severe respiratory infection due to respiratory syncytial virus. To therapy being instituted, Palivizumab is added, which happens to be life saving.

What class of drug does Palivizumab belong to?

A.1 The suffix *'mab'* in the drug indicates it to be a monoclonal antibody and the affixing of *'u'* to mab indicates it to be a humanized monoclonal antibody.

What is the mechanism by which Palivizumab acts?

A.2 The drug is used in the treatment of respiratory syncytial virus infection, where it results in reduction of the morbidity. It is directed to an epitope in the 'A' antigenic site of the F protein of the virus.

Compare and contrast the terms monoclonal antibody and polyclonal antiserum (antibodies) and mention the difficulties in producing monoclonal antibody.

A.3 (a) The term *monoclonal* antibody indicates single clone of antibody from a single B cell lineage. This term contrasts with the term *polyclonal* antiserum (antibody), which means that the serum has antibodies with multiple specificities derived from several clones having different B cell lineages. For medical, diagnostic and therapeutic purposes, monoclonal antibodies are required but these are not often available. The commonly available antiserum has multiple antibodies due to heterogeneous antibody responses. The reason for it is that, when an antigen is introduced into an organism, several clone of B cells proliferate, producing different antibodies, as an antigen has multiple epitopes.

The history of monoclonal antibody dates with the discovery of (tumor) multiple myeloma in mice, which consisted of genetically identical plasma cells and produced pure antibodies of single specificity indefinitely.

Who are the two scientists credited with the discovery of monoclonal antibodies, for which they were awarded the Nobel prize?

A.3 (b) The technological breakthrough to produce monoclonal antibodies was achieved by *G. Kohler* and *C. Milstein* in 1975, using the hybridoma technology for which they were awarded the Nobel prize in physiology/medicine in 1984. Hybridoma technology is based on the principle that when two cell types are mixed in culture in the presence of chemical (as polyethyelene glycol), it is possible to fuse two different cells.

Describe the principle and procedure of synthesis of monoclonal antibodies. Diagramatically illustrate the procedure of synthesis of monoclonal antibodies.

A.4 It is extremely difficult to stimulate a specific clone of lymphocytes in 'vivo' and to collect the resulting antibodies. In lab it, would be possible to isolate a single specific B cell, stimulate it and collect the antibodies, however the antibody production would be short lasting.

Immuni--zation
Antigen
Mouse myeloma cells (tissue culture)
Spleen cells
Cells mixed to fuse, to make hybridomas
Fusion
Hybridoma cells are grown in tissue culture.
Limiting dilution
Cloning
Microwell plate
Clonal expansion
Monocl--onals
MONOCLONAL ANTIBODIES
MONOCLONAL ANTIBODIES

Fig.2.6.1:Schematic representation of technique of monoclonal antibody production

Kohler & Milstein developed the ingenious technique (for monoclonal antibody production) in which they used the growth potential of myeloma cell and fused with the specific antibody secreting B cells of the spleen (Fig. 2.6.1). The rate of successful hybrid formation is very low, hence in the technique, the need to develop a strategy to select the rare successful fusions. The myeloma cells that are used, lack the capacity to synthesize hypoxanthine-guanine-phosphoribosyl-transferase (HGPRT) enzyme (this enzyme enable the cell to synthesize nucleotides, using hypoxanthine as a precursor in the 'salvage pathway'). Such cells cannot survive in a basal medium containing HAT (hypoxanthine, aminopterin and thymidine), as the cells cannot use the 'denovo' pathway for nucleotide synthesis, as the aminopterin binds competitively to the dihydrofolate reductase enzyme to block tetrahydrofolate synthesis (which is essential for purine and pyrimidine synthesis. Thus only those hybrid cells can survive indefinitely that have taken the HGPRT enzyme from the B cells and the growth potential from the tumor cell (depicted in flow diagram below).

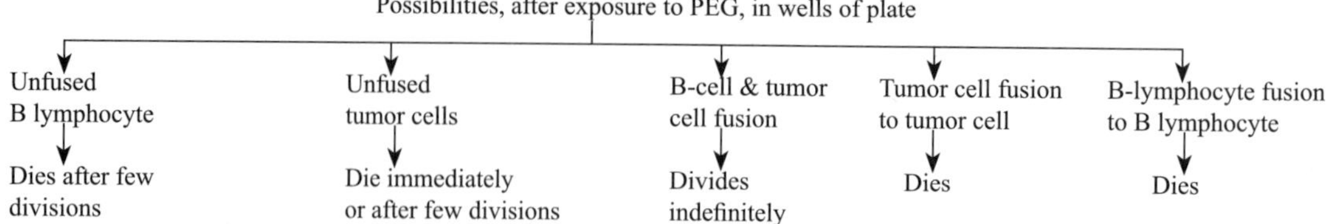

Procedure:

1. Antigen of interest injected into experimental animal; usually a mouse following a certain protocol
2. After adequate period, splenic lymphocytes (B) are harvested
3. The spleen lymphocytes are incubated with mouse myeloma cells (HPRT enzyme deficient) grown in culture (tissue culture bottle) with polyethylene glycol, so that fusion of cells can occur.
4. The resulting cells are diluted, such that each microwell has one (fused) cell. The basal culture contains HAT.
5. The microwells are tested for (hybrid) clones (by looking for products)
6. The clone that makes appropriate antibody is selected out, using an appropriate assay. The process uptil this step may take many months to years to standardize.
7. The isolated clone can be grown in large culture vessels to obtain significant amount of antibody. The clone (*hybridoma*) can also be cultivated (propagated) in mice to obtain greater amount of antibodies.

What are the clinical limitations of the monoclonal antibodies raised in mouse?

A.5 (a) Until recently, only mouse monoclonal antibodies were available. These had the limitation in therapeutic use, when used in human of evoking a human antimouse antibody response, that resulted in an (obtained with mouse myeloma cell line) accelerated clearance of the monoclonal antibodies from the blood stream and lowering the effectiveness of the administered antibodies.

How can these limitations be overcome?

A.5 (b) One technique to overcome this limitation is to synthesize human monoclonal antibodies by *genetic-engineering techniques* for clinical use. However due to technical problems, generation of hybridomas secreting human antibodies is difficult. To overcome these limitations, genetic engineering including recombinant technology has been employed. This has resulted in the creation of *human-mouse chimeric* monoclonal antibodies, which as the name indicates are chimeras (molecular hybrids of human and mouse antibody). Another variant available in the market for clinical use is called the *humanized monoclonal antibody*, in which the antibody is such engineered, such that all of the antibody is human except for the complementarity determining regions in the variable portion of the light and heavy chain.

In the product Inflixbimab, what does 'imab' indicate?

A.6 It indicates that it is a chimeric monoclonal antibody

Mention the uses of monoclonal antibodies and name the key drugs based on monoclonal antibodies available for clinical usage?

A.7 One of the common applications of monoclonals is in the diagnostics and imaging. This occurs, as monoclonal antibodies are standardized and would give same results, when used anywhere in the world, due to standardized technique in their raising. One of the such kits commercially available in the market, is the pregnancy kit, which can detect the HCG hormone in the serum in just 10 days after conception. Other available kits based on this technology are useful in rapid diagnosis of many infections; as Hepatitis, Herpes and Chlamydia.

Radiolabelled monoclonal antibodies are useful in imaging of some primary and metastatic tumors in patients, which would go undetected by some other lesser sensitive scanning techniques, for instance some monoclonal antibodies labeled with Iodine-131, when introduced into blood, permit earlier detection of spread of breast tumor into regional lymph nodes.

Monoclonal antibodies have great potential in treatment of human disease but are limited by the fact that most monoclonal antibodies are of mouse origin and many humans are hypersensitive to them. Many methods are under development which would use appropriate drug or radioactive substance to be attached to a monoclonal antibody to be delivered exactly at the cells bearing the appropriate antigen. Currently a wide range of drugs are available for use in transplantation, viral chronic diseases and malignancies. Some examples are depicted in table 2.6.1.

Monoclonal antibodies are also used in other diverse applications as measuring blood levels of various drugs, enumerating human lymphocyte subpopulations, matching histocompatibility antigens and detecting specific tumor antigen.

Table 2.6.1: Some monoclonal antibodies in common clinical usage

Monoclonal antibody	Nature of antibody	Target	Treatment for
Muromonab CD3□	Mouse mAb	T cells	Acute rejection of liver and kidney transplants
Infliximab	Human-mouse chimeric	TNFα (tumor necrosis factor α)	Rheumatoid arthritis and Crohn's disease
Palivizumab*	Humanized mAb	Respiratory syncytial virus (on F protein)	RSV infection
Rituximab$^{\Delta}$	Human mouse chimeric	B cell	Relapsed or refractory non-hodgkin lymphoma

NB: Abzymes-This term is derived from antibody (ab) and enzymes, indicating monoclonal antibodies to be having enzymatic activity, which can be clinically utilized.

Δ Suffix *'imab'* indicates chimeric antibody.

□ Suffix *'monab'* indicates mouse monoclonal antibody.

* Suffix *'umab'* indicates humanized monoclonal antibody.

Complement

An eight year child, Aakrosh, presented with history of repeated bacterial infections. An analysis of the immunoglobulin levels revealed them to be within normal range.

What immune deficiency is likely to explain his clinical profile?

A.1 (a) C3 'component' of the complement

Mention the origin of the term 'complement' and the history of development of this concept.

A.1 (b) The term 'complement' is derived from the ability of the non-specific proteins in the normal human serum to complement (i.e., initiate) some innate and humoral immune defense mechanisms.

The concept of these proteins was first put forth by Jules Bordet in 1890, when he was working at Pasteur Institute at Paris. He demonstrated that sheep antiserum to vibrio could lyse this bacterium, but if the antiserum was heated, it lost the bactericidal activity, which was regained, if fresh serum was added (which contained no antibodies against the bacterium). So; it was inferred that serum contained something, which was responsible for this activity.

Initially it was believed that a single substance complements the immunological reactions, but now we know that the complement system is composed of more than 20 large regulatory proteins.

What is the normal serum complement level of C3?

A.2 (a) 1.3 mg/ml

What is the technique by which complement levels are measured using RBC lysis?

A.2 (b) Classically complement activity is measured by CH_{50}, which is *defined* as the highest dilution of the serum, which lyses 50% of the sheep RBC coated with amboceptor (anti sheep RBC antibodies raised in rabbit).

What are the usual commercial techniques available to measure complement levels?

A.2 (c) For clinical usage in laboratories, technique of radial immunodiffusion in agarose is often used to estimate the levels of complement components in serum. Other techniques are also available.

What is the complement component at which key regulation of complement occurs and tremendous (hundred fold) amplification occurs?

A.3 C3 is a central (point) component at which key regulation occurs (Fig. 2.7.2). This is due to numerous reasons, which are:

(i) It has the highest concentration in the serum (1.3 mg/ml).

(ii) It is the step at which tremendous amplification occurs (hundred fold amplification, not on one to one basis).

(iii) C3 stands at intersection of three pathways namely classical, alternate and mannose binding lectin (MBL) (Fig. 2.7.1b).

Describe the nomenclature of complement.

A.4 (a) The complement components are designated by numerals, namely 1-9. These are designated in the sequence in which they were discovered. This occurred before the cascade sequence was deciphered. For this reason, the cascade sequence is not sequential (apparently). Many components exist by cleavage into two components, namely 'a' and 'b'. The smaller is usually designated 'a' and larger as 'b' (excepting 2a which is larger). These are designated by lower case letters; as C3b. Of the two components, one component sticks to cell surface and contribute to the cascade, while the other component goes to the fluid.

The components which are activated or those with enzymatic activity are depicted with a horizontal bar over as $\overline{C5b67}$.

Where do the complement components get synthesized?

A.4 (b) They are synthesized mainly by liver hepatocytes. The synthesis also occurs in blood monocytes, tissue macrophages and epithelial cells of gastrointestinal tract and genitourinary tract.

Amount: It constitutes 5% of serum globulins. These proteins account for approximately 10% (by weight) of all plasma proteins.

NB: The source of complement for laboratory work is guinea pig serum

What are the key functions of the complement?

A.5 Many of the protective activities system mediated by the humoral limb of the immune system are in reality implemented by the complement system. The functions are:

1. *Immune adherence and opsonization:* The C3b component attaches to some cells; as bacteria. These attach readily to C3b receptors; as CR3 found on cells; as macrophages, neutrophils and eosinophils, promoting their destruction.

   The C3b coated cells tend to aggregate, a process called *immune adherence,* which may promote phagocytosis.
2. *Inflammatory function:* Certain components result in stimulation of inflammatory response, e.g.,

   C3a and C5a act as anaphylatoxins.

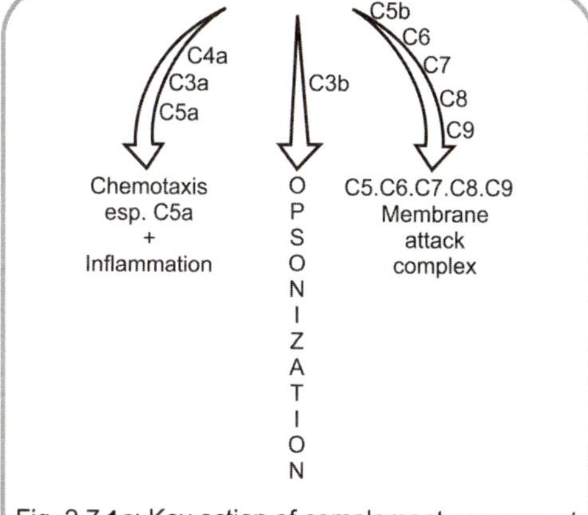

Fig. 2.7.1a: Key action of complement components

3. *Neutralization of virus infectivity:* Some viruses as the retroviruses, Epstein-Barr virus can activate the complement pathways and mediate virus neutralization by a number of mechanisms (this function is different than opsonization).
4. *Cytolysis/cytotoxic:* In the final stage of complement cascade, C5-9 attaches to membranes of target cells, as bacteria, tumor cells and RBC and cause their lysis (death).
5. *Basis of complement fixation test:* As some antibodies require/fix complement, which is tested by lysis of (antigenic) target cell.
6. Role in *pathogenesis* of:
   (a) Certain type II hypersensitivity diseases; as incompatible blood transfusion and type III hypersensitivity diseases; as serum sickness.
   (b) Endotoxin: can activate alternate pathway
      – Excessive C3 activation leads to tissue damage by DIC
      – In dengue with septicaemia, C3b sticks on platelet by immune adherence, causing lysis of platelets with release of inflammatory mediators
   (c) One paradox function is in clearance of immune complexes in autoimmune disease; as in Systemic lupus erythematosus, where individuals also have cellular pathology because of complement mediated type II and III hypersensitivity reactions.

What are the general characteristics of the complement?

A-6 (a)
- Most complement components circulate in an inactive form.
- The activated components become inactive, unless it reacts with the next component.
- The next activated molecules can bind through hydrophobic and/or covalent interactions to each other.
- All C factors need to be activated except C5-C9.
- The complement cascade/pathway can be initiated/activated by specific substances; as antibody, however its effects are non specific.
- They are heat labile substances that get inactivated by heating the serum at 56°C for 30 minutes. The importance is this fact, is that in serological tests especially complement fixation test, serum needs to be heat inactivated before the start of the test.
- Activation of each member in complement pathway occurs, as a result of proteolytic cleavage of molecule (transient exposure of sites). This confers proteolytic activity on the molecule (i.e., acts as an enzyme) to act on the subsequent molecule and activate it.
- Many molecules instead of one molecule may act as a substrate of a prior component and in turn activate many subsequent ones.

The cascade reaction is characterized by a set of reactions that amplify some effect, i.e., greater product is formed in the second reaction than in the first, still greater is formed in the third than in the second, and so on. In cascade, different components; are activated in a fixed sequence with the first substance activating the next, which activates the next and so on. For example; a complement path getting initiated with one IgM molecule, generates hundreds/ thousands of various molecules in the complete complement pathway.

What are the pathways by which complement gets activated? Illustrate them.

A.6 (b) The sequential activation of complement, in a cascading manner occurs via three pathways; alternate, classical and lectin (Mannose-binding lectin).

Generally (for understanding sake) the complement cascade can be divided into three stages, namely; *initiation*, *amplification* and the *membrane attack* stage. The final steps in the membrane attack stage, is common in all the three pathways.

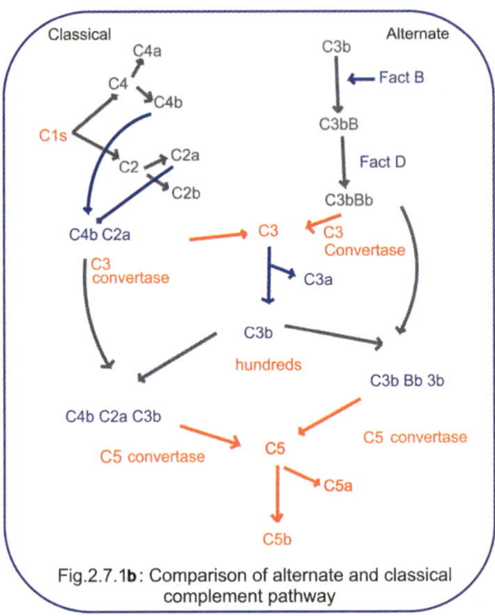

Fig.2.7.1**b**: Comparison of alternate and classical complement pathway

Alternate pathway (Fig. 2.7.1b): It is a more primitive system than the classical pathway. It does not require antibody (except IgG, IgA, IgE in complexes), so it is a component of the innate immune system. It is of special importance in early response to infection, when classical pathway cannot participate due to time required for specific antibody to form.

It *differs* from classical pathway in (i) being less efficient in cell lysis (ii) requiring different initiators (iii) not requiring antigen-antibody complexes for activation and not dependent on antibody (iv) not involving early complement components as C1, C4 and C2.

The *initiators/activators* of this pathway can be categorized into those of *pathogen origin* and non pathogen origin. In the former category are included lipopolysaccharides from gram negative bacilli, teichoic acid from gram positive cocci, fungal and yeast walls (zymosan), some viruses and parasites; as trypanosomes. In the *non pathogen* category are included human IgG, IgA and IgE in complexes, cobra venom factor and anionic polymers; as dextran sulfate.

The initial recognition event for this pathway is the presence of C3; specifically C3b, which is most probably being produced in minimal amounts in the circulation. The composition of C3 convertase in this pathway is different from that in the classical pathway and requires factor B factor D and properdin for its generation and activity (see Fig. 2.7.1b).

Lectin pathway (MBL): This is a recently discovered pathway, which can be considered to be a part of the innate immune defense mechanism. However, unlike the alternate pathway, which it resembles in it's primitiveness, it starts with activation of C4, unlike alternate pathway which starts at C3/C3b.

This pathway gets initiated, when mannose-binding lectin (MBL) bind to mannose residues on surface of microorganisms. This results in the secretion of two MBL-associated serine proteases; namely MASP-1 and MASP-2, which act like C1r and C1s and activate C4 and C2. The rest of the pathway is like classical pathway. However it does not require specific antibody for the pathway activation.

Classical pathway (Fig. 2.7.2): It is *initiated* commonly by the soluble antigen-antibody complexes or with the binding of complement fixing antibody on the surface of targets; as bacterial cell. Certain subclasses of IgG (human IgG1-3) and IgM can initiate this pathway.

We are taking here the *model of a bacterium,* on which IgM attaches. The activation of C1 is the first step in this pathway. The C1 is actually a complex consisting of one C1q and two molecules each of C1r and C1s. This IgM binds to the bacterial surface, which then binds to (this process is complex and its detail are beyond the UG level) C1q in the serum, which gets activated and subsequently there is activation of C1r and C1s. The activated C1s (protease) acts first on C4, splitting it into C4a and C4b. The larger of which is C4b, attaches to bacterial surface and the smaller C4a diffuses away. Then C2 gets split by C1s into C2a and C2b. The larger of these namely C2a attaches to bacterial surface along with C4b, while C2b diffuses away. The C4b2a complex is called C3 convertase and rightly so, as it converts hundreds of C3, into C3a and C3b. This step is critical, as *tremendous amplification* is observed here. The larger of the two fragments, namely C3b attaches to the bacterial surface along with C4bC2a and acts as a C5 convertase. The latter converts C5 into C5b and C5a, the latter diffuses away.

The C5b binds to the bacterial surface and serves as locus for the assembly of single molecule, each of C5, C6, C7, C8 and C9; which acts as the membrane attack complex (MAC). This results in the formation of large transmembrane channels, which ultimately leads to formation of pores in the cell membrane and *lysis of the bacterium* (Fig. 2.7.2).

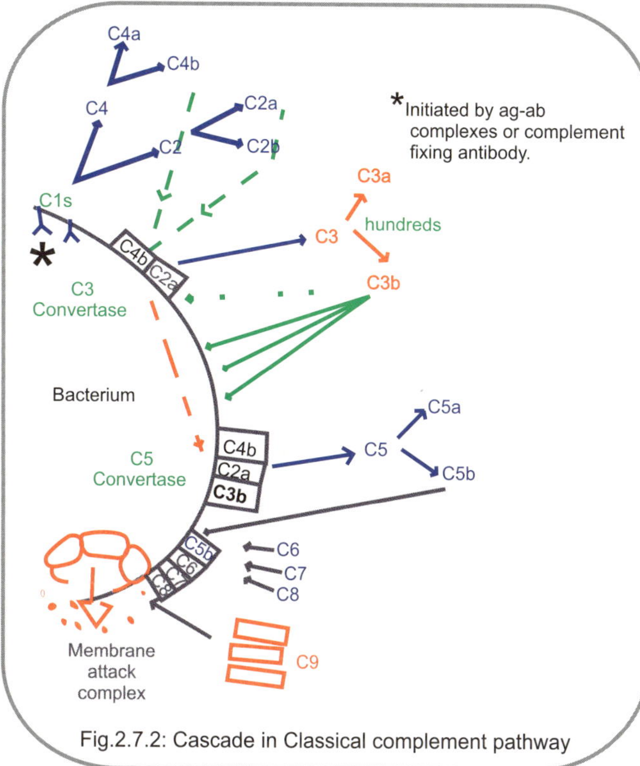

Fig.2.7.2: Cascade in Classical complement pathway

What are the diseases associated with various complement deficiencies?

A.6 (c) The several components of the complement provide many possible sites for the deficiencies to occur. These deficiencies do occur and can be divided into two categories, namely *defects in control proteins* and *defects in complement components*. One of the classical examples of the former category is the *hereditary angioedema*, which is characterized by deficiency of inhibitor of C1. It is an autosomal dominant condition and characterized clinically by oedema in the bowel, which can manifest as abdominal pain and when present in the upper respiratory tract manifests, as airway obstruction, which may be fatal. It's pathogenesis and treatment are beyond the UG level. Another disease associated with defect in complement regulation is *paroxysmal nocturnal hemoglobinuria*.

Deficiencies of early components; as C4 and C2 are associated with immune complex disease, which indicates that one of the function of these components could be to dissolve immune complexes. A high incidence of SLE like syndromes is associated with this deficiency.

As we know C3 plays a key role in the complement pathways, including the formation of MAC, so expectedly a deficiency of it is associated with severe bacterial infections including those caused by *N. meningitidis* and *S. pneumoniae*.

Describe the need and mechanism of complement control.

A.7 The complement system works as a cascade, so it is all the more important to regulate it, otherwise these proteins would be entirely consumed and significant damage to the host (self) could occur. The need to discriminate the self from the nonself becomes more relevant with the alternate pathway, which gets activated non-specifically by many components.

The *passive control* is mainly exerted by the extreme lability of many active components, which lose reactivity; unless they react with subsequent components. Damage by C3b to host is prevented, as this molecule undergoes spontaneously hydrolysis, once about 40 nm away from the C3 convertase.

The initiation of the classical pathway is inhibited by a soluble protein called C1 inhibitor (C1 Inh), which is a serine protease inhibitor. It's deficiency results in hereditary angioedema..

Factor 1 mainly cleaves free C3b in solution, unless bound on cell surface. Factor H blocks formation of C3 convertase by binding C3b.

What are the mechanisms by which microbes can evade complement function?

A.8 Some gram-negative bacteria; as *E. coli* and Salmonella have developed long polysaccharide side chains in the cell wall lipopolysaccharide, which prevents insertion of MAC (membrane attack complex) into bacterial membrane, thus leading to complement resistance.

Most gram-positive bacteria are generally resistant to complement mediated lysis due to presence of thick peptidoglycan, which prevent insertion of the MAC into the (inner) cell membrane.

8 Antigen-Antibody Reactions

The nearer the colloid particle approximates to the normal electrolyte, the nearer its compounds must obviously come to conforming to the law of simple stoichiometric proportions, and the compounds themselves to simple chemical compounds. At this point, it should be recalled that Arrhenius has shown that the quantitative relationship between toxin and antitoxin is very similar to that between acid and base.

— Karl Landsteiner

A follow up case of primary syphilis, Shahid is being clinically examined. As a part of the over-all evaluation, the physician also ordered the VDRL test. The test got reported as non reactive. This discrepancy; expecting a reactive (positive) report was reported to the chief of the Laboratory services, who requisitioned that the VDRL test be repeated after dilution. The test now gets reported as reactive (positive)!!

What type of antigen antibody reaction is the VDRL test?

A.1 (a) It is a type of flocculation (precipitation) reaction (details, see A.7a, pg126 + pg. 301). As the name indicates, they are reactions between antigen and its specific antibody.

What are the two broad categories of antigen–antibody reactions?

A.1 (b) (i) 'In vivo' (in body) reactions-which are basis of immunity, hypersensitivity and autoimmune disorders.

(ii) 'In vitro' (outside body, in laboratory) are called serological reactions. It should be clear that these reactions can be used to detect not only antibodies but also antigens.

What are the factors that can affect the antigen–antibody reactions?

A.2 (a) (i) State of the antigen and the antibody. Soluble antigen lead to precipitation reactions whereas the particulate antigen leads to the agglutination reactions.

(ii) Appropriate pH and solute concentration in the reaction vessel.

(iii) The antigen and antibody reacts in proportions. The antibody is usually bivalent whereas the antigen may have upto hundred binding valencies.

(iv) Optimal temperature: This is usually 37°C.

What are the features of antigen-antibody reactions?

A.2 (b) (i) The reaction is specific with some exceptions

(ii) The reaction occurs at the surface. Hence, generally the surface antigens are important immunologically and antibodies formed against it may be protective.

(iii) Entire molecules react and not just fragments. For this reason, if an antigenic fragment is present on a carrier molecule, the whole unit participates in the reaction with the antibody and is seen in the final reaction, which may be seen; as in haemagglutination.

(iv) The antigen and antibody react in optimal proportions. The antibody is usually bivalent, whereas the antigen has numerous binding valencies. The reaction say precipitation, occurs only in the zone of equivalence, where lattice formation occurs. (Fig. 2.8.1)

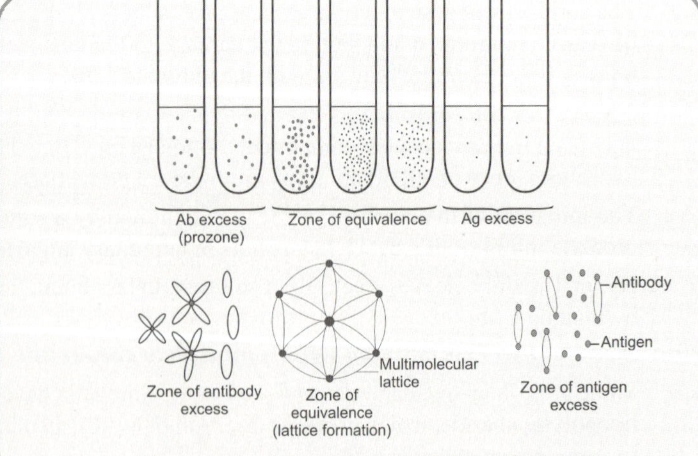

Fig. 2.8.1: Lattice hypothesis to explain proportion and prozone concept

(v) The antigen-antibody reaction is firm but reversible (in primary stage). No denaturation of the antigen or the antibody occurs during the reaction.

How do you explain the VDRL test becoming reactive, after the test was put up after diluting the serum?

A.3 After diluting the serum, the high antibody titer in the serum was reduced, resulting in optimal antigen –antibody reaction. The case had high antibody titre, which resulted in no floculation. The phenomenon of high antibody titer resulting in a false negative test is called *prozone phenomenon*. (Fig. 2.8.1)

What are the uses of the antigen-antibody reactions (in vitro)?

A.4 (i) Detection and quantification of specific antigens and antibodies.

(ii) Detection of non–infectious agents; as the enzymes.

(iii) Diagnosis of infectious and non infectious diseases.

(iv) Useful in epidemiological studies.

(v) Prognosis and monitoring treatment of diseases. A change in titer can be a useful parameter.

What are the characteristics that an antigen-antibody test being developed should possess?

A.5 (i) *Minimal cross reactivity*

The reaction between an antigen (epitope) and its antibody (paratope) is highly specific, however cross reactions may occur.

(ii) *High sensitivity:* It means that the test detects high percentage of true positive cases, i.e., identify those who have actually have the disease.

(iii) *High specificity:* It means the test detects high percentage of true negative cases, i.e., who do not have the disease.

(iv) *Optimal affinity:* A very high affinity may lead to increased false positivity (cross reactivity) in the test.

Affinity may be described as intensity of attraction between an antigenic determinant and antibody combining site.

(v) *Optimal avidity:* Less avid antibodies may be specific but too weak to be of any clinical use.

Avidity refers to the strength of the bond between antigen and antibody, after their combination. It may depend on the multiple antigenic determinants and multivalent antibodies.

Aspects related to case theme/examination evaluation

What are the common measures used to detect (quantitate) antigen and antibody?

A.6 **(a)** The measure may be in terms of mass or more commonly; as units or titer.

Titer is a common unit used to measure the antigen or antibody. *Titer* is defined as the reciprocal of highest dilution of a solution that gives positive result/test.

What are the stages of interaction in antigen-antibody reactions?

A.6 **(b)** (i) *Primary stage:* It is the initial interaction between an antigen and antibody; without any noticeable effect. This reaction is reversible and is initiated by weaker intermolecular forces; as ionic bonds, hydrogen bonds, Vanderwaal forces and hydrophobic bonds. Examples: ELISA test, IFAT.

(ii) *Secondary test:* In some of the reactions, the initial stage is followed by this stage, in which some demonstrable effect; as precipitation, agglutination, or fixation of the complement is seen. e.g., VDRL test, CFT. This reaction is initiated by strong intermolecular force of covalent binding between antigen and antibodies.

(iii) *Tertiary stage:* In few reactions, the antigen-antibody reaction occurying 'in vivo', initiate reactions; as chemotaxis, neutralization of toxin, phagocytosis or tissue damage.

How do you classify the antigen–antibody reaction on the basis of the stage of the stage of reaction?

A.6 **(c)** The example of tests in the category of primary stage are ELISA, Immunofluorescence and Chemiluminescence. These tests have the highest sensitivity and can detect the analyte in the range of pg/ml

The tests belonging to the secondary stage include precipitation, agglutination and haemagglutination reactions. These tests have intermediate sensitivity and can detect the analyte in the range of ng/ml to µg/ml. The tests belonging to the tertiary stage have the least sensitivity

Define precipitation reaction and mention its mechanism.

A.7 (a) When a soluble antigen reacts with its homologous antibody in the presence of appropriate electrolytes (as NaCl) at an optimal temperature and pH, the antigen-antibody complex; forms an insoluble precipitate, the reaction is called *precipitation*. For mechanism, see A.2b(iv), p. 124. When the precipitate remain suspended instead of sedimenting, the reaction is termed, as flocculation.

Classify and describe the types of antigen-antibody reactions based on precipitation.

A.7 (b) Types of antigen-antibody reactions based on precipitation reactions

Precipitation in liquid	
Types: 1) *Ring test* Examples: - C-reactive protein determinantion - Streptococcal Grouping (Lancefield method)	Procedure and interpretation: - Antigen is layered over antiserum in a narrow tube. Shortly a precipitate forms at the junction of the two liquids
2) *Flocculation test* Examples: - VDRL test (slide flocculation test) - Kahn test (tube flocculation test) - Standardization of toxins and toxoids	Procedure and interpretation: - Antigen solution and antiserum (patients serum) is allowed to react in a slide or a tube and the reaction of flocculation is looked for (details see A8, p.301)
Precipitation in gel (agarose)	
Antibody and its homologous antigen; when placed in gel, diffuse towards each other and form a band of precipitation at the junction of their diffusion. The precipitation in gel has following advantages over precipitation in solution namely (i) the reaction is distinct, can be stained and preserved (ii) number of different antigens can be observed in the sample (iii) Identity, crossreactions and non identity can be observed	
Types: - *Single diffusion in single dimension* (Oudin procedure)	Procedure and interpretation: - Antibody is incorporated in the gel in the test tube. The antigen solution is layered over it and allowed to diffuse downwards. Wherever it forms an optimal concentration with antibody, an precipitate is formed. The number of lines of precipitation indicate the numbers of antigen and antibodies present. (Fig. 2.8.2)
Type: *Double diffusion in one dimension* (Oakley-Fulthrope procedure)	Procedure and interpretation: - Antibody is incorporated in a gel in a test tube. Above it is placed an column of plain agar, over which is placed the antigen. The antigen and antibody both diffuse toward each other (in one dimension) through the intervening agar and form a band of precipitation at the zone of optimal concentration (Fig. 2.8.3)
Type: - *Single diffusion in double dimension* (Radial immunodiffusion) Example: - Estimation of immunoglobulin classes as IgG etc. in serum (Tripartigen plates) - Screening sera for antibodies; as to Influenza viruses	Procedure and interpretation: - The antibody is incorporated in a gel placed on a petri dish or slide. One well or multiple wells are cut in the gel, depending on the number of samples to be tested. The antigen diffuses from the well radially (i.e., in two dimensions) and forms a ring of precipitate at the zone of optimal concentration. The *larger* the concentration of the antigen, the *farther* it has to diffuse, before it finds an optimal concentration of the antibody. Therefore the diameter of the precipitate provides an estimate of the concentration of the antigen. (Fig. 2.8.4)
Type: - *Double diffusion in two dimensions* (Ouchterlony procedure), determines relatedness of various antigens, partial identity indicates sharing of some epitopes Examples: - In the diagnosis of many microbial diseases including parasitic and fungal - Elek's test for toxigenicity of *C.diphtheriae* (is a variant of above)	Procedure and interpretation: - Using a template, a central and multiple peripheral wells are cut in the gel formed on a slide. The antibody (antiserum) is placed in the central well and the antigens in the peripheral wells and allowed to react. If two adjacent precipitin lines fuse with each other completely, it indicate *complete identity*. If two adjacent precipitin lines form a spur like formation, it indicate *partial identity*. If two adjacent lines cross each other, it indicates *non identity*. (Fig. 2.8.5)
Type: - *Immunoelectrophoresis* (technique combines electrophoresis and immunodiffusion) Examples: - Detection of normal and abnormal proteins as myeloma proteins.	Procedure and interpretation: - On a gel on a slide, well and trough is cut (parallel to the direction in which antigen would be later electrophoresed). First antigen is placed in the well, which is followed by electrophoresis. Subsequently antibody (antiserum) is put into the trough and diffusion is allowed for 18-24 hrs. Precipitin arcs form, wherever antigen and antibody meet in optimal concentration. (Fig. 2.8.6a,b)

Contd.

Contd.

Type: - *C.I.E.P.*	*Procedure and interpretation:* - Counterimmunoelectrophoresis (CIE) is a type of antigen-antibody reaction of the type resembling double diffusion in single dimension, which is accelerated by the electric field. The rate of migration of a charged ion in an electric field depends on the strength of the field, net charge, size and shape of molecule. The ionic strength, viscosity and the temperature of the medium also plays a role. This technique is based on the ability of antigen and antibody to form a precipitate in an agar gel in the equivalence zone. This technique is more sensitive and rapid (result in 10 to 30 minutes) than conventional diffusion in agarose. (Fig. 2.8.7 a,b) This technique can be used to detect both antigen and antibodies from body fluids and microbial cultures. The technique is available for many microbes including *Streptococcus pneumoniae, Neisseria meningitidis, Candida* spp. and others.
- *Rocket electrophoresis* (one dimensional single electroimmunodiffusion) Example: - Quantification of antigens	- The antibody (antiserum) to the antigen that is to be estimated is incorporated in a gel (agarose) on a slide. The antigen is placed in multiple wells (in increasing concentration) in the gel. Electrophoresis is then performed such that the antigens get driven in a perpendicular fashion into the gel. Precipitin bands form in the pattern of 'rockets'. The lengths of the rocket correspond to the concentration of the antigen.
Type: - *Laurell's two dimensional immunoelectrophoresis* Example: - Quantification of several antigens	*Procedure and interpretation:* - It is a variant of 'rocket' electrophoresis. Initially the antigen mixture is electrophoretically separated to be followed by electrophoresis in direction perpendicular to the initial direction.

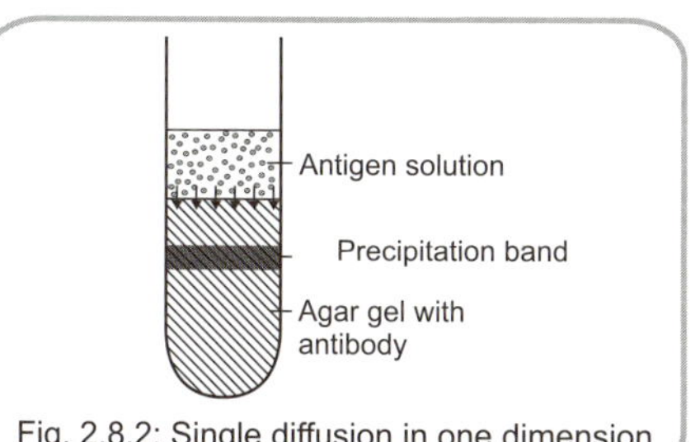

Fig. 2.8.2: Single diffusion in one dimension

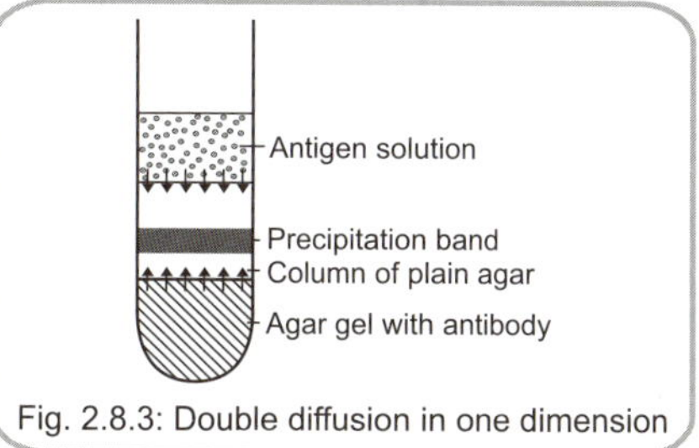

Fig. 2.8.3: Double diffusion in one dimension

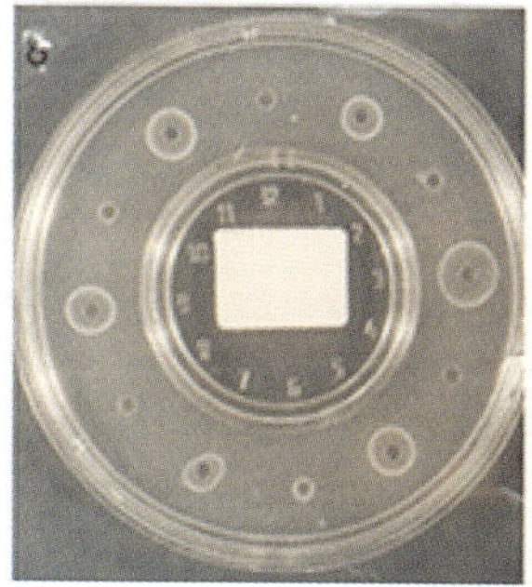
Fig.2.8.4 (a): Tripartigen plate

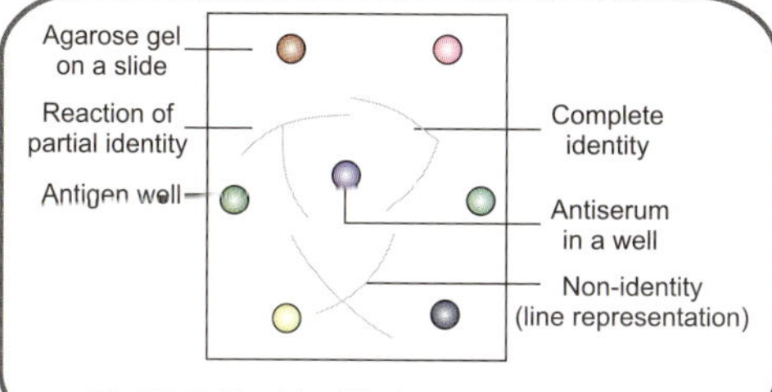

Fig.2.8.5: Double diffusion in two dimensions

Agarose gel with antibody
Antigen in the well
Precipitation band

Fig. 2.8.4(b): Single diffusion in two dimensions

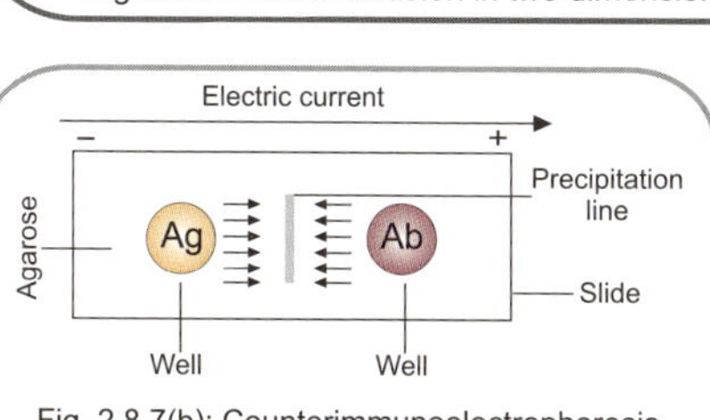

Fig. 2.8.7(b): Counterimmunoelectrophoresis (line diagram)

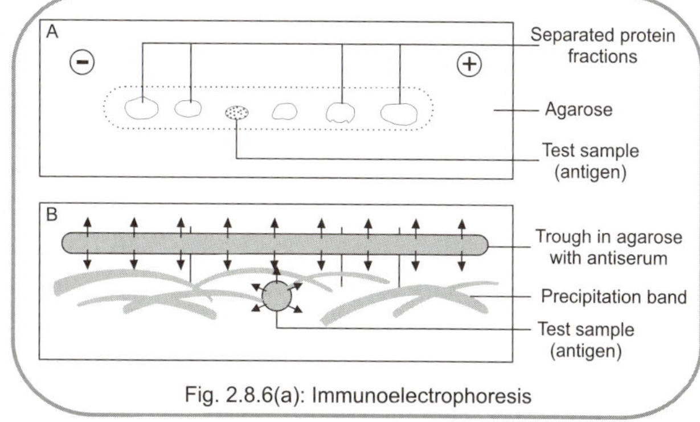

Fig. 2.8.6(a): Immunoelectrophoresis

Fig. 2.8.6 (b): Immunoelectrophoresis

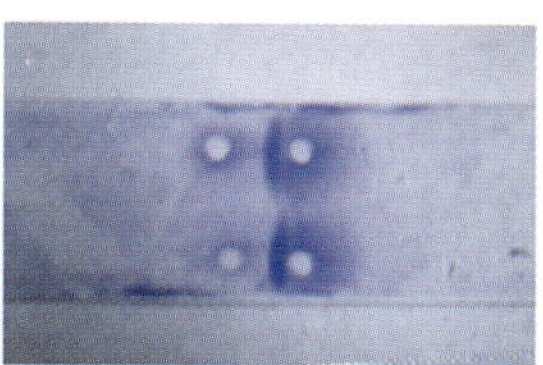
Fig.2.8.7 (a). Counterimmunoelectrophoresis

Describe role of radioimmunoassay in microbiology diagnosis.

A.7 (c) Radioimmunoassay:

- **Historical:** First described by Berson & Yalow in 1960. In 1977, Yalow was awarded the Nobel prize for it.
- **Status:** It is a very sensitive and specific technique, which can measure antigen and antibodies upto picograms amounts. So in the earlier periods it was used to detect drugs, hormones, IgE, and viral antigens, which are present in very low amounts. However due to the risks of radioactivity, requirement of the lab to be certified by BARC for testing and availability of simple tests by other principles with similar sensitivity, this test is not very popular at present.
- **Principle:** This test can be used to detect any substance that is an immunogen (i.e., against which antibody can be raised) and which can be labeled with radioactive isotope as I_{125}. Gamma spectrometer is used to detect the gamma radiation.

  The test involves competitive binding of the radiolabelled antigen and unlabelled antigen (in the clinical sample, whose detection is required) to high affinity antibody. A standard graph (curve) is obtained by adding samples of unlabelled antigen of known concentration in progressively larger amounts.
- **Types:**
  (i) *Classical:* In the past, this was the technique, which was performed and the test was conducted in the solution. The combined antigen complex with the antibody was separated from the unlabelled antigen by various techniques, as using salt or anti-immunoglobulin or other techniques. In the Farr technique, 50% ammonium sulphate is used.
  (ii) *Solid phase RIA:* In this type, as the name indicates the reaction is carried out on the solid phase support, which has the ease of separating the unlabelled antigens from the immune complexes. This technique is currently in vogue (practice).
  (iii) *Variant technique:* Radioallergosorbent test (RAST) is carried out on filter paper to detect specific IgE antibodies.

Describe the tests based on Enzyme Linked Immunosorbent Assay (ELISA) technology.

A.8
- **Status:** An excellent test of tremendous potentiality used in diagnosis of most diseases (antigen and antibodies), some hormones and drugs. It is commonly used to demonstrate HIV antibodies, Rotavirus in stool and hepatitis B markers in serum.
- **Definition:** Enzyme immunoassay for identification of antigen or antibody; by linking antibody to enzyme, in which the immunological (biological) ability of the antibody, antigen and enzyme is retained.
- **Requirements:**
  - Solid phase support, e.g., plastic surface/paper disc for adsorbing antigen or antibody (anti IgG/anti IgM)
  - Pure antigen or antibody (depending on which is to be assayed)
  - Enzyme linked antibody conjugate (commonly alkaline phosphatase or horse-raddish peroxidase)
  - Substrate (paranitrophenyl phosphate for alkaline phosphatase and orthophenyl diamine for horseradish peroxidase). It develops color after enzyme action, as yellow color with the substrate for alkaline phosphatase.
  - Stopping solution (to stop the reaction of enzyme on the substrate)
  - Positive and negative cut off controls (Figs. 2.8.8(a) and 2.8.8(b))
  - Spectrophotometer (to quantify the color change)
  - Micropipettes (to dispense micro amounts), Incubator and buffers.
- Types:
  - Macro ELISA (done in polystyrene tubes) and Micro ELISA (done in polyvinyl microtiter plates
  - Indirect, Competitive, Sandwich, Cylinder/Cassette (Table 2.8.1)

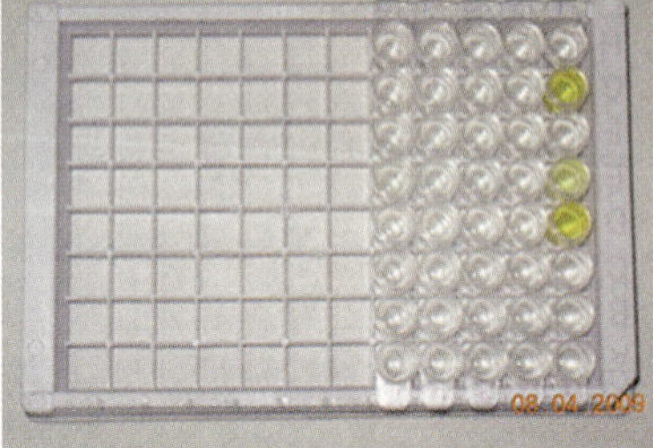

Fig. 2.8.8 (a): ELISA test (depicting +, -ve and cut off controls)

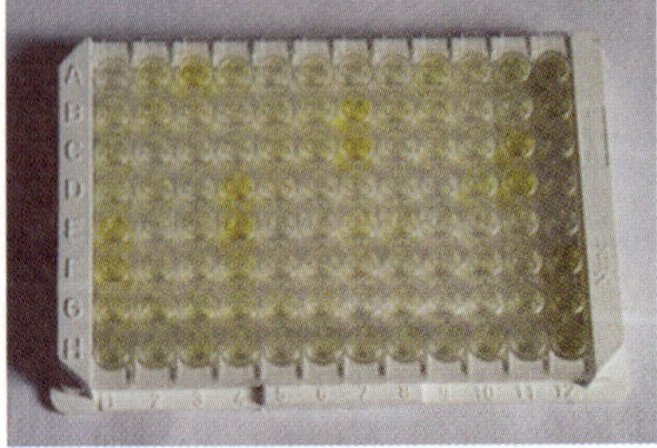
Fig. 2.8.8 (b): ELISA test (all 96 wells used)

Table 2.8.1: Comparison of common types of ELISA

	Indirect ELISA (Fig. 2.8.9)	**Sandwich ELISA** (Fig. 2.8.10)	**Competitive ELISA** (Fig. 2.8.11)
Uses	Detection of antibodies as HIV-1, HIV-2, dengue, Japanese encephalitis etc in serum	Detection of Hepatitis A, Rotavirus, amoebic antigen in stool, *H. influenzae* antigen in CSF	Detection of HIV antibodies in the serum
Procedure	- Wells are coated with antigen	- Wells are coated with specific antibody against the antigen to be detected	- Wells are coated with antigen
	- Serum (sample) added to well	- Specimen as faeces added to well	- Specimen containing suspected antibody and conjugate antibody added
	- Incubate, Wash	- Incubate, Wash	- Incubate, wash
	- Add enzyme linked antibody (conjugate) against antibody to be tested	- Add enzyme antibody linked (antibody conjugated) against above antigen	
	- Incubate	- Incubate	
	- Add specific substrate	- Add specific substrate	- Add specific substrate
	- Incubate	- Incubate	- Incubate
	- Measure color intensity by spectrophotometer (increased color intensity indicates positive reaction, i.e., presence of antibody	- Measure color intensity by spectrophotometer (presence of increased color/intensity indicates presence of antigen)	- Measure color intensity by spectrophotometer (Absence of color/decreased intensity, indicates presence of antibody in the sample). This occurs as conjugated antibody and antibodies in the sample compete for limited antigen sites in the sample.

- *Cylinder/Cassette ELISA:* It is a modification of ELISA, in which results are obtained in a few minutes, in contrast to few hours in classical ELISA, indicated when few samples need to be tested, e.g., for HIV antibody detection.
- *ELISPOT assay:* It is a modification of ELISA, in which cells layered onto bottom of wells, producing specific type of antibodies are detected. Each point of color/light is determined. This technique has been used in quantitation of cytokines.
- **Dot blot test/Dipstick** ELISA (Fig. 2.8.12(a))

  ELISA tests though very popular have some limitations; as requiring trained personnel, specialized instrument; as ELISA readers and being time consuming. These limitations have been overcome in tests called *dot blot*, so named; as these produce well circumscribed color dots on solid surface. These tests have the advantage of being a simple test being completed in a few minutes. It uses specific antibodies on membranes; as nitrocellulose membrane for the detection purpose. The protocol is similar to an EIA. This method, unlike other blot techniques, as Western blot offers no information on size of molecule, as no electrophoresis is performed.
- *Immunochromatographic tests (ICT):* It is one of the most popular one step rapid tests based on lateral flow immunoassay technology. The appeal of the test lies in the simplicity, economy, high sensitivity and specificity. The test is commonly available for detection of HBsAg, HIV antibody etc.

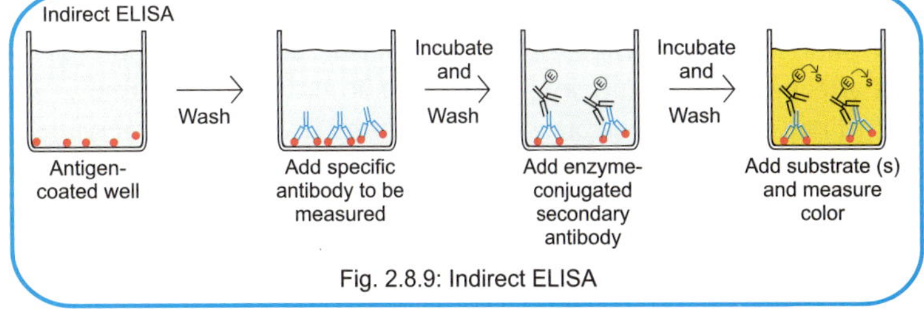

Fig. 2.8.9: Indirect ELISA

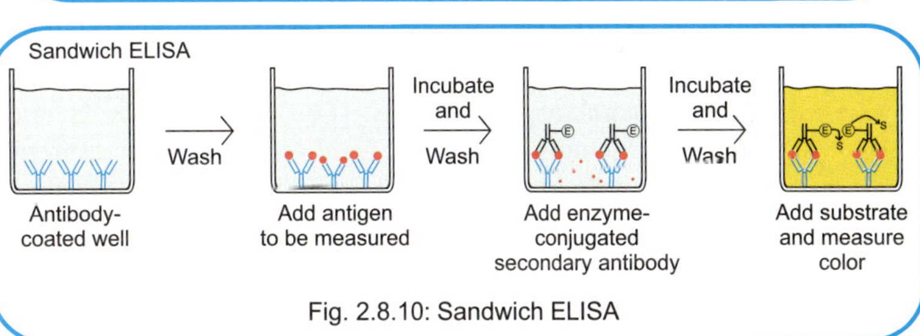

Fig. 2.8.10: Sandwich ELISA

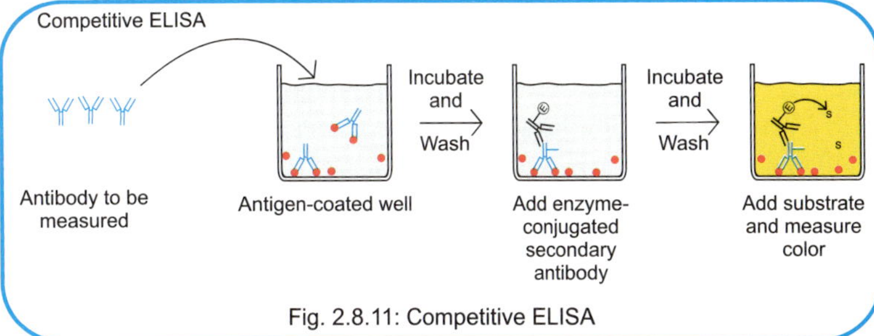

Fig. 2.8.11: Competitive ELISA

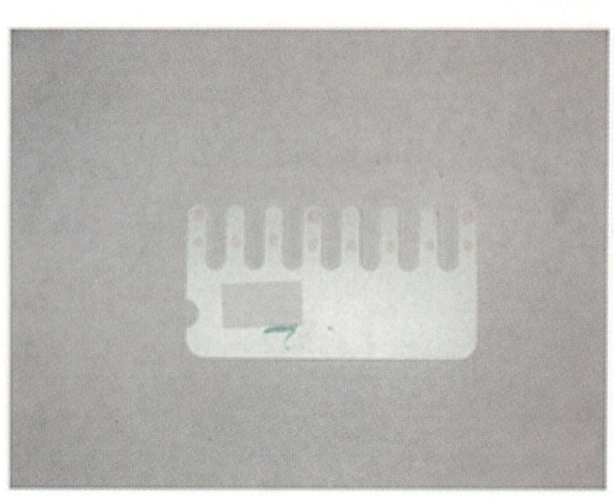

Fig.2.8.12 (a): Dot Blot Test

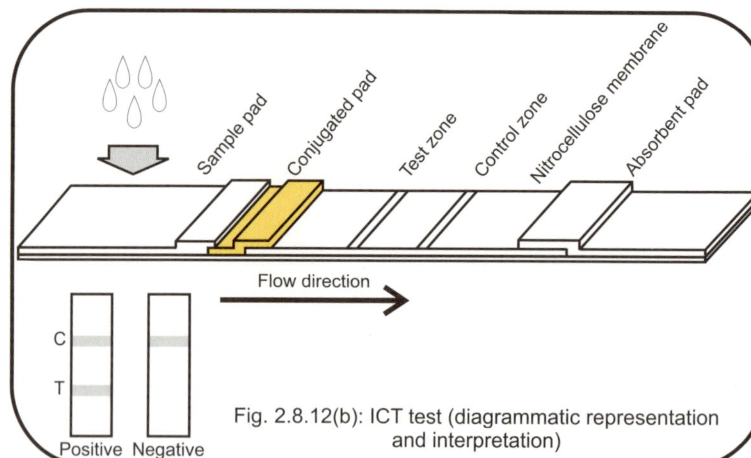

Fig. 2.8.12(b): ICT test (diagrammatic representation and interpretation)

The test strip usually contains three windows. In the *first* window, the test serum is applied, which travels upstream by capillary action. It reaches the *second* window (also called conjugate pad), where it reacts with specific conjugate to produce a specific reaction. A specific reaction (e.g., band) should also be produced in the *third* window, which is an inbuilt control to make the test valid, an absence of reaction in this window, makes the test invalid (Fig. 2.8.12b).

Describe the antigen–antibody tests based on Immunofluoresence technology.

A.9 Coon and his colleagues (1942) demonstrated that antibodies (Fc end) could be conjugated to fluorescent dyes without affecting their specificity. These could be antibodies in tissues. *Fluoresence* is the property of certain dyes to absorb rays of one particular wavelength and emitting rays of different wavelength. *Fluoresent dyes* (as Fluorescein isothiocyanate, FITC) absorb ultraviolet light (lower wavelength, invisible to eye) and convert it to higher wavelength (visible eye), e.g., Fluorescein absorbs 490 nm (blue) and emits (517 nm) yellow green light, Rhodamine absorbs 515 nm (yellow green) and emits 546 nm (red fluorescence). These tests are more sensitive than precipitation reactions and complement fixation tests. These tests can detect tissue antigens, antigens of pathogens and tissue antibodies (including autoantibodies). For it, an fluorescence microscope is required, which can generate UV light (from mercury lamp) instead of normal visible light. As the UV light is injurious to man, a secondary filter near eye piece is placed to protect the observer eye.

- *Direct immunofluorescence test* (Fig. 2.8.13): This technique is used for bacterial and viral antigen detection in a tissue section or a smear fixed on a slide. For example, to detect rabies antigen in a brain smear, specific antibodies to rabies virus conjugated to FITC is used for detection. Apple green fluoresence in the antigen in the slide is indicative of a positive test (see Fig. 2.8.14). A disadvantage of this technique is that specific labeled antibodies to each antigen (pathogen) have to be prepared.
- *Indirect immunofluorescence test* (Fig. 2.8.15): This technique is used for detection of specific antibodies; as in syphilis, malaria, amebiasis and other infections. In this test, the slide is fixed with antigen (known), against which antibodies are to be detected. To the slide fixed with antigen, the test sample containing suspected antibodies is added. If the sample contains the specific antibodies, these attach to the antigen fixed on the slide. These antibodies are detected by a standard (common to all) fluorescent dye labeled antibody to human immunoglobulin, An example of this test is FTA-ABS test in syphilis.

The advantage of this technique is its greater sensitivity, flexibility and saving of time (as single conjugated antiserum is used). Generally immunofluorescence tests have the disadvantage of requiring expensive equipment, trained personnel and a subjectivity in the interpretation of results, which can generate variable results.

Define agglutination reactions.

A.10 (a) It is an antigen–antibody reaction, in which a particulate antigen, when it combines with its homologus antibody in presence of electrolytes, appropriate temperature and pH; results in *clumping/agglutination* of particles.

The same principle (lattice formation hypothesis) governing precipitation also holds true for agglutination. These reactions occur better with IgM antibody than IgG antibody and these reactions are more sensitive than precipitation reaction for the detection of antibodies. (Fig. 2.8.16)

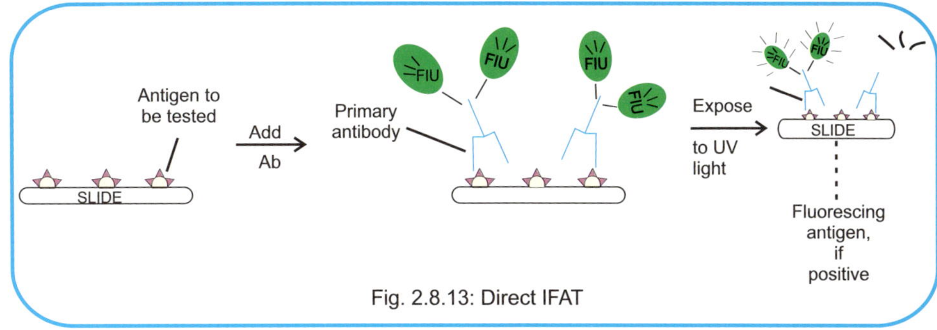

Fig. 2.8.13: Direct IFAT

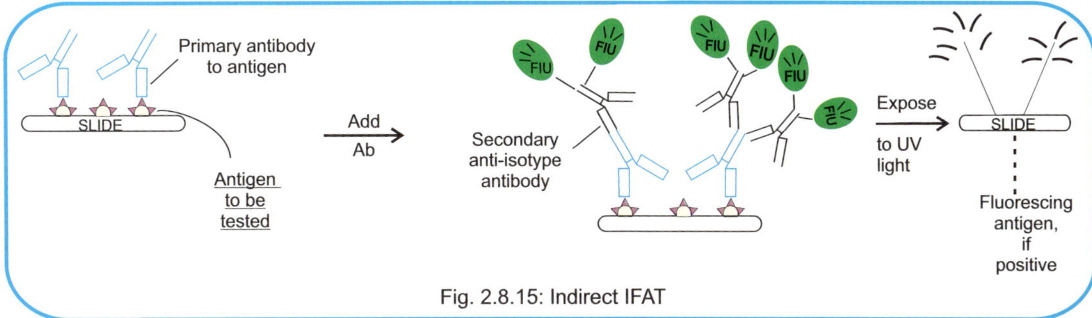

Fig. 2.8.15: Indirect IFAT

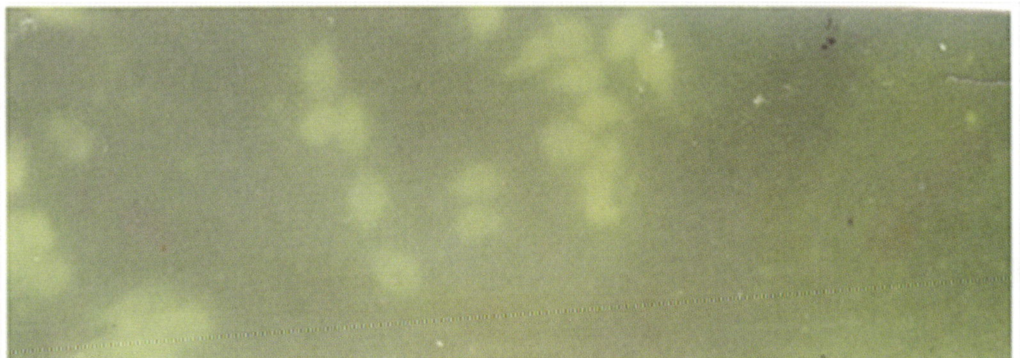

Fig. 2.8.14: Fluorescing trophozoites of *Giardia lamblia*

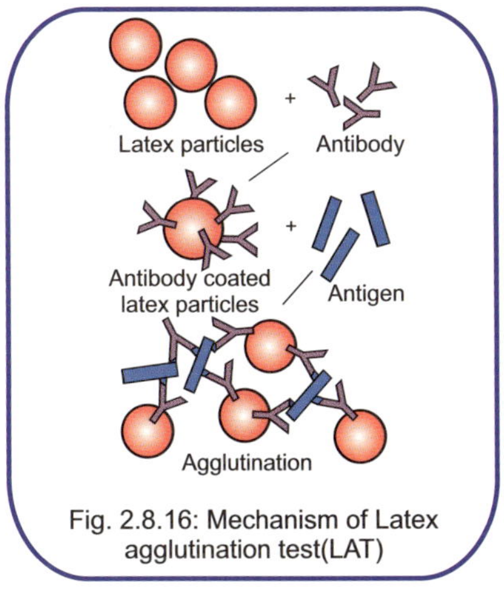

Fig. 2.8.16: Mechanism of Latex agglutination test(LAT)

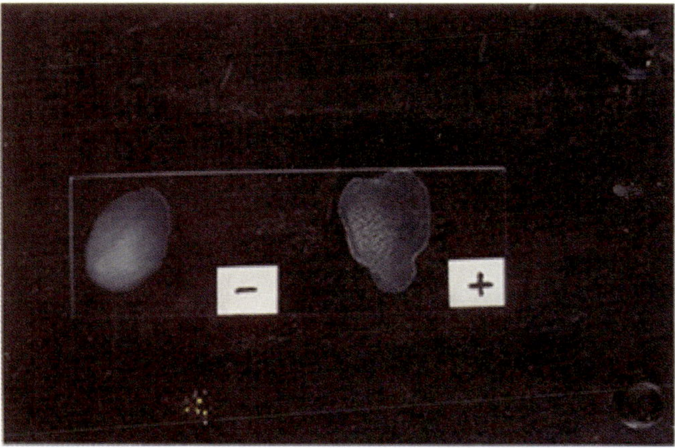

Fig. 2.8.17: LAT test

Classify the antigen-antibody tests based on agglutination principle and describe them.

A.10 (b)

Category/Type	Example	Procedure
Direct (reactions involve naturally occurying particle)/ *Slide agglutination test*	- Identifying bacterial isolates; as Salmonella, Shigella, and Vibrio from culture plates (isolates from clinical samples) - Blood grouping	- The antigen suspension (from culture plate) is made in normal saline and mixed with antiserum. The slide is rocked and clumping within a minute indicates positive reaction. An antigen control (i.e., antigen solution without antiserum) is run with the test to exclude 'autoagglutinable' reaction. (Fig. 2.8.17)
Direct/*Tube agglutination reaction*	- Widal test - Weil –Felix reaction - Paul Bunnel test	- Here the test is carried out in tubes instead of slide. Prozone phenomenon and blocking antibodies can affect the quality of reporting of these tests. The high concentration of antibodies, as in brucellosis can result in false negative result, this problem can be obviated by carrying out the test in multiple dilutions. Blocking (incomplete) antibodies can result in false negative results. To obviate this problem, the test may be carried out in hypertonic saline (5%) or albumin saline or preferably the Coomb's (antiglobulin) test may be carried out. The incomplete antibodies are commonly seen in brucellosis cases and in individuals possessing anti-Rh antibodies.
Direct/*Antiglobulin (Coombs test)*	- This test was originally devised by Coomb and colleagues in 1945 to detect incomplete anti-Rh antibodies. The anti-Rh antibodies coat the Rh +ve RBC, but are unable to agglutinate them for unknown reasons	• *Direct Coomb test* (Fig. 2.8.18): The red cells* to be tested (as of erythroblastosis patients), are mixed with a drop of anti-globulin/Coomb serum (rabbit antiserum against human antiglobulin). Presence of agglutination indicates coating of the RBCs with incomplete antibodies 'in vivo'. *are washed free of unattached protein • *Indirect Coomb test* (Fig. 2.8.19): The test is used to detect the presence of incomplete antibodies present in the serum. So to detect them the normal cells are first allowed to interact with the antibodies (of patients serum), before the antiglobulin is added. So here the sensitization of cells with incomplete antibodies is done 'in vitro', i.e., outside the body.
Passive agglutination	These involve coating soluble antigens onto carrier particles; as latex particles and performing the test. By this process the precipitation tests get converted into agglutination tests and get advantage of increased sensitivity and convenience.	
Passive agglutination/ *Latex agglutination test (Fig. 2.8.17)*	Commonly performed to detect CRP, ASO, RA factor, HCG (pregnancy test), detecting bacterial antigen from CSF	The specific particles of polystyrene latex have a diameter of 0.8-1 µm and can adsorb different types of antigens and immunoglobulins. In one of the modifications (passive agglutination), the antigen is adsorbed to the latex particles. The initial step in the test is the linking together of the latex particles by antibody particles that specifically attach to the antigenic determinants on the surface of these particles. There is formation of large lattices through the cross links. These larger lattices sediment readily due to large size of the clumps and are visible to the unaided eye within a minute.
Passive agglutination/ *Haemagglutination test*	- Indirect haemagglutination test for diagnosis of parasitic diseases; as amoebiasis, toxoplasmosis, syphilis (TPHA)	The RBCs of many species as human, sheep, etc. are used to adsorb the antigen. In the presence of specific antibodies these cells demonstrate haemagglutination (passive haemagglutination test)
	- Haemagglutination inhibition test	- Many viruses as Influenza, Mumps and Measles can agglutinate RBCs, however these are not antigen-antibody reactions. These reactions can be inhibited by specific antibodies against the virus.The viral haemagglutination inhibition test is form of a haemagglutination inhibition test.
	- Rose-Waaler test	- In Rheumatoid arthritis, an autoantibody (RA factor), i.e., antibody to gamma-globulin appears in the serum of cases. This can agglutinate RBCs coated with gamma-globulin (suspension of sheep erythrocytes sensitized with a subagglutinating dose of rabbit erythrocyte antibody, such an preparation is named amboceptor)
Passive agglutination/ *Coagglutination test*	- Used to detect specific bacterial antigens in body fluids; as serum and CSF, e.g., S. Typhi antigen in blood in early phase of disease	- Sensitized Staphylococcal cells, when mixed with homologous (test) antigen leads to agglutination. Sensitization means presence of protein A on the Staphylococcal cells. Such an antigen is usually present on Cowan 1 strain. This protein A has the characteristic of binding IgG molecules, non specifically through Fc region leaving specific Fab sites free to combine with specific antigen.

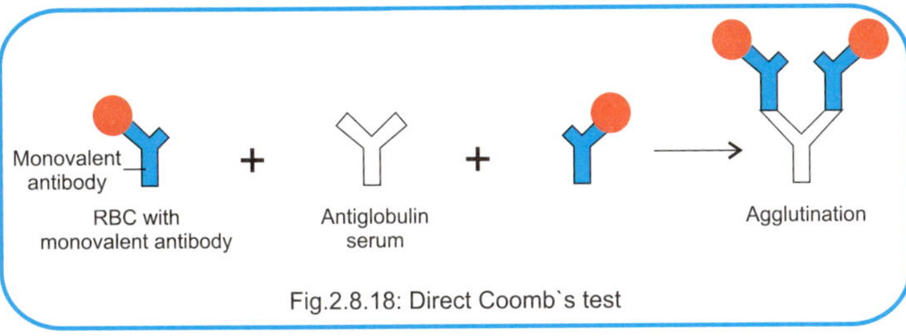

Fig.2.8.18: Direct Coomb`s test

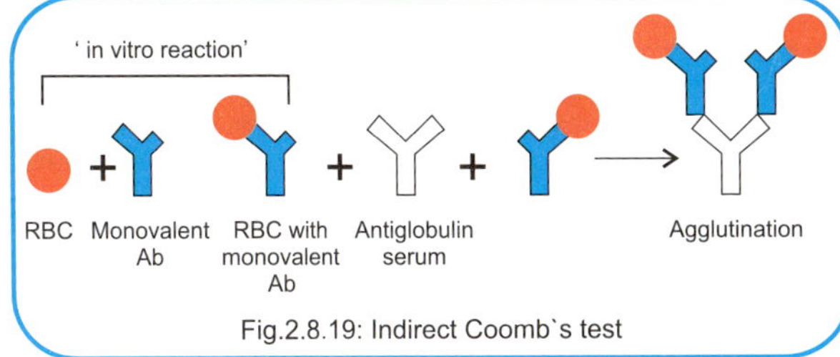

Fig.2.8.19: Indirect Coomb`s test

MISCELLANEOUS TESTS

What is the principle of the complement based tests?

A.11 (a) Complement is a part of the normal serum, which participates in many antigen-antibody reactions. Complement which consists of many proteins has the ability of lysing erythrocytes, killing bacteria, inhibiting motility of organisms and immune adherence. These activities are useful in assay of the complement activity.

What is the source of complement in the classical complement fixation tests? Explain how complement activity is titrated and the reason for taking CH50 (50% lysis point), as a reference in classical complement fixation tests.

A.11 (b) Guinea pig serum is used as the source of complement.

The lysis of antibody coated erythrocytes has been long used as a means of estimating the complement activity of a serum. As more complement is added to the antibody-coated erythrocytes, the proportion of the lysed cells increase. However, as the curve approaches 100% asymptotically, it is difficult to determine the total lytic unit of complement (CH_{100}). It is for this reason, the test is defined by the 50% lysis point (CH_{50}). One *M.H.D.* of complement is defined as the least amount or highest dilution of the guinea-pig serum that lyses one unit volume of washed sheep erythrocytes in the presence of excess of haemolysin amboceptor within a fixed time (usually 30 or 60 minutes) at a fixed temperature 37°C.

Describe the classical complement fixation test.

A.11 (c) *Complement fixation reaction* (Fig. 2.8.20) is a very sensitive technique, as it can measure <1µg of antigen or antibody. This is possible because of the amplifying cascade sequences in complement, a small amount of antigen, – antibody complex will cause massive complement fixation or consumption. In this technique, the patients serum is first heated at 56°C for 30 minutes to inactivate any available free complement. The test involves two distinct reactions. In the *first*, the antigen and antibody (one of which is known and the other unknown) are allowed to react with a fixed amount of pretitrated complement. The *second step* involves testing of the free complement by utilizing an indicator system. This system is usually sheep red blood cells and homologous antibodies (haemolysin) for the red blood cell antigens. Hemolysis of red blood cells indicates presence of free complement and so a negative test. In contrast, absence of hemolysis indicates fixation of the complement by the antigen-antibody complex and so a positive test.

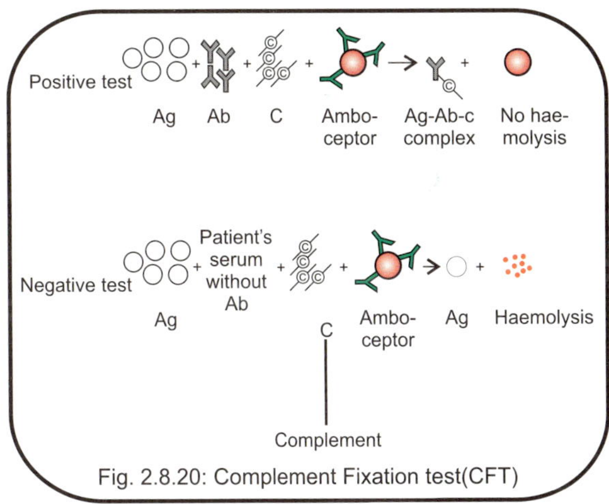

Fig. 2.8.20: Complement Fixation test(CFT)

If either antigen or antibody can inactivate the complements it is unsatisfactory for the test. Anticomplementary antigens or sera can sometimes be removed by heating or dilution. The antigen and antibody controls ensure that they are not anticomplementary. *Cell control* is required to see that the sensitized erythrocytes don't undergo lysis in absence of complement. *Complement control* is required to assess the complement activity.

What is the status of complement based tests? Classify them and give examples.

A.12 Complement based tests have good sensitivity and specificity, however these tests are cumbersome and technically demanding; as require lengthy standardization (Table 2.8.2). Therefore these tests are used in few laboratories, as easier and faster tests are available.

Table 2.8.2: Classification of complement based test

Type	Example
1. Classical complement reaction	- Wasserman complement fixation test for syphilis (more specific than VDRL in diagnosis of primary syphilis) - Available for all complement fixing antigens of the bacterial, fungal and viral categories.
2. Indirect Complement fixation test	- When certain avian (as ducks, parrot) and mammalian (horse, cat) sera, which do not fix guinea pig complement are to be used
3. Conglutinating complement adsorption test	- Used for sera which do not fix guinea pig complement. The test uses horse complement (non haemolytic), so interpretation is reverse of classical CFT.
4. Immobilization test	- *T. pallidum* immobilization test (*T. pallidum* in presence of specific antibody (patients serum) and complement, gets immobilized (inhibition of motility)
5. Cytolytic/Cytocidal test	- Vibriocidal antibody test (*V. cholerae* in presence of specific antibody and complement gets killed)
6. Immune adherence test	- Bacteria; as *V. cholerae* or *T. pallidum* in presence of specific antibody and complement adhere to RBCs or platelets, a process known as *immune adherence*. This process facilitates phagocytosis of organism.

Describe neutralization tests.

A.13 The homologus antibodies can neutralize the biological action of toxin, enzymes and viruses. Such antibodies are called neutralizing antibodies and form the basis of the *neutralization tests*. These can be categorized as:

– *Toxin neutralization* → 'in vitro' -1) Antistreptolysin 'O' test
-2) Nagler reaction in *Clostridium perfringens*
→ 'in vivo' -1) Schick test
-2) Toxigenicity test of *C. diphtheriae* in experimental animal

Virus neutralization test: This can be demonstrated in various systems; as laboratory animals, embryonated eggs* and tissue culture. An example of the latter is inhibition of the plaques of lysis produced by bacteriophage, when specific antiphage serum is incoroporated in medium.

*are growing (viable) eggs and not non-viable eggs used for food.

Describe Chemiluminescence immunoassays.

A.14 Here luxogenic (chemiluminescent) compounds; as luminal dye are used, which generate light on oxidation. These take the place of chromogenic substrate in conventional ELISA. The light (signal) can be amplified and measured and so the concentration of the analyte (antigen or antibody) can be measured. This method has been totally automated and application of this has been the antimicrobial susceptibility testing of *M.tuberculosis.*

Describe Immunoelectronmicroscopic tests.

A.15 In these the antigen-antibody reactions are visualized by electron microscope. These are of two types:

(i) *Immunoelectron microscopy:* This technique is used to detect hepatitis A and viruses causing diarrohoea; as Rotavirus.

In this the viral particles, when mixed with specific antisera, get demonstrated; as clumps of virion particles.

(ii) *Immunoferritin tests:* Ferritin an electron-dense substance is conjugated with antibody and such labeled antibodies are used to detect specific antigens in tissue sections, visualzed under electron microscope.

Describe a test based on Immunoblotting technique.

A.16 *Western blotting* is a technique to identify a specific protein (often antibody) from a mixture. This technique has a greater specificity than ELISA. For this reason, this test is often considered to be a confirmatory test for the serodiagnosis of HIV. Also; with this technique, one can characterize the types of antibodies present against specific antigens of HIV.

To perform this test, initially one has to perform SDS polyacrylamide gel electrophoresis of the protein. It is then followed by blotting (transferring) the electrophoresed proteins to a nitrocellulose membrane strip. This is followed by reacting the test sera with, the strip to be followed often by an enzyme conjugated anti-human immunoglobulin. To detect, if the specific antibodies (of test serum) reacted with the antigen, a suitable substrate is added. Development of specific color, where separated antigen reacts with specific antibody, indicates a positive test. This technique may be considered to be a variation of ELISA.

Describe Opsonization.

A.17 An opsonin can be an antibody or a complement component. *Opsonization* refers to the facilitated phagocytosis process with the aid of opsonins. Phagocytic index refers to the phagocytic activity of the blood, which is the average number of phagocytosed bacteria per polymorphonuclear leucocyte. *Opsonic index* refers to the the ratio of the phagocytic activity of the patients blood to a particular bacterium, to the phagocytic activity of blood from a normal individual.

Antibody Mediated Immunity

A 25 years old young male, Hashmeen was brought to the medical emergency of Medanta hospital in a critical condition, with history of a cobra snake bite. The physician administered immediately a specific injection and the case improved within few hours.

What is the composition of the injection that has been administered?

A.1 (a) Polyvalent anti-snake serum (having antibodies) against snake venom.

What was the first human disease, where such therapeutic approach was used?

A.1 (b) Diphtheria

What is the mechanism of action by which the agent in the administered injection acts?

A.2 The antibodies (against the snake venom) in the antiserum neutralize the snake venom present in the body of patient, making it functionally ineffective.

What is antiserum and in which animal it is often raised?

A.3 (a) A serum that contains a specific set of antibodies is called *antiserum*. It is the serum of an animal or human containing antibodies against specific disease agent. It confers passive immunity to that disease.

It is essentially raised in horses (Fig. 2.1.2). One advantage of this animal, is its large size resulting in raising (production) large amount of antiserum.

What is the procedure utilized to raise the antiserum?

A.3 (b) An immunization protocol is followed, in which many injections (of antigen, here snake venom) are given parenterally to the animal over a period of few weeks. After this period is over, the animal is bled. The serum is separated from the blood and the appropriate fraction containing the specific antibodies is separated and purified. The serum is filter sterilized and stored.

What can be the side-effects of administering antiserum (raised in animal) to man?

A.4 (a) One major side effect of raising antiserum in animal, is the serum sickness (type III hypersensitivity reaction) reaction and anaphylaxis that can occur in the man with heterologous serum therapy.

How can these side-effects be prevented?

A.4 (b) These side effects can be prevented by raising homologous serum, i.e., raising serum in the same species in which it is to be administered, if possible (here man)

In which other human diseases, can passive immunization be life-saving?

A.5 Diphtheria (Horse antitoxin), Tetanus, rabies, hepatitis A&B, gas gangrene and botulism (horse antitoxin).

Aspects related to case theme/examination assessment

What is the spectrum of biological activity, where antibody mediated immunity (AMI) plays a key role?

A.6 Role/Spectrum:

- *In defense against infectious agents*
  - Primarily extracellular (Bacterial) pathogens and toxins
  - Primarily viruses and parasites infecting/entering through the gastrointestinal tract, respiratory tract and urogenital tract.
- *In pathogenesis of*
  - Type I, II and III hypersensitivity reactions
  - In some autoimmune disorders; as Rheumatoid arthritis
  - In allograft rejection

Outline the stages (levels) involved in humoral response.

A.7 Stages (levels) involved in humoral (antibody) immune response:

- *Afferent limb*
  - Antigen entering (routes)
  - B cell dependent tissues
  - Classification of antigen

    Thymus dependent

    Thymus independent
- *Central function*
  - Processing of antigen, by Antigen presenting cells APCs (for most antigens)
  - Antigen complex selects appropriate lymphocyte

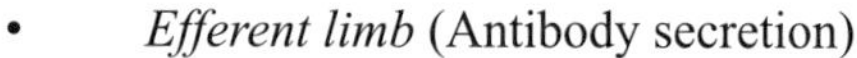

- *Efferent limb* (Antibody secretion)

  Primary humoral response

  Secondary response

  Ontogeny of immune response

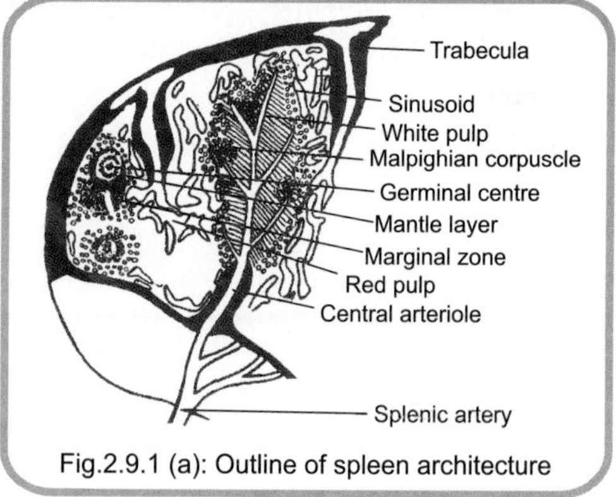

Fig.2.9.1 (a): Outline of spleen architecture

Describe the afferent limb of the immune response.

A.8 Antigen can enter the body from various sites; as oral, respiratory tract or parenteral. The antigen gets deposited at the draining sites.

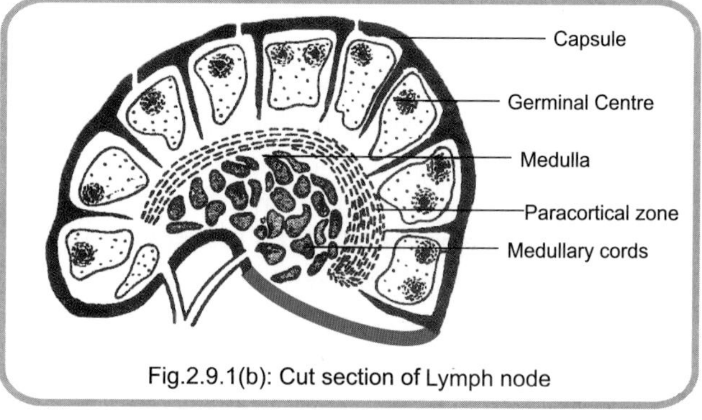

Fig.2.9.1(b): Cut section of Lymph node

There are B cell dependent areas in the peripheral lymphoid organs, where antigen dependent B cell activity (proliferation) occurs. *In lymph node*, such areas are predominantly cortical region (Fig. 2.9.1a). The paracortex region is rich in T cells (Fig. 2.9.1b).

In spleen, the predominantly B cell area is the marginal zone.

The antigen; as far as the antibody mediated immune response is considered can be categorized into thymus independent and thymus dependent antigens.

The term *thymus independent* antigen, indicates that for these antigens, T-cell help is not required to generate immune response. Examples of this category, include lipopolysaccharide, endotoxin, ferritin and flagellin. One of the characteristic of this category of antigens is that, it has naturally repeating epitopes, which can cross-link sufficient number of surface antibody of B cells to activate them into proliferation. An application of this fact is that vaccine target antigens, which are T-cell independent are not desirable, as they cannot generate predominantly IgG1 (opsonizing) antibodies and memory cells. Hence vaccine target antigen should ideally be T-cell dependent type.

Majority of the antigens belong to the category of *thymus dependent*, i.e., these antigen require the help of T cell to generate AMI to these antigens. The common examples belonging to this category are soluble protein antigens; as serum protein. The implication of this is that in humans, in which thymic development is lacking or fails to develop, won't be making functional T cells. Hence not be able to make antibodies to these antigens.

Describe the common theories that explain antibody production.

A.9 There are basically two groups of theories that have been used to explain the antibody production or (AMI). One is the **instructive** group of theory, in which it is believed that the antigen serves as a template for the antibody production, which instructs the synthesis of unique immunoglobulin structure molecules. This theory was found to be incorrect, as it was seen that a denatured antibody could renature in the absence of the antigen, if the physiological conditions were restored. It could not also explain the secondary immune response, which is different from the primary immune response.

The second group of theories are the **selective** theories. The concept to this arose, as a result of a proposal by Paul Ehrlich, who at the beginning of the twentieth century, proposed the existence of immune cells bearing hundreds of different receptors that could bind to the antigen. The current modern *theory of clonal selection* has also contribution from Burnet, Jerne and Talmadge. According to it, an organism; as human carries heterogenous population of lymphocytes, which can specifically bind to antigen (antigen binding cell). The specificity of an antigen-binding cell resides in the structure of receptor molecules present on its surface. Once the antigen interacts with specific receptors on antigen binding cells, they are stimulated to undergo mitosis and develop into a clone of cells, expressing the same receptor specificity. The diversity is introduced by the process of recombination.

Describe the activation of resting B cell and the consequent synthesis of antibody.

A.10 To activate a naïve/resting B cell to go through various phases (as G_1 → S phase → G_2) to proliferate and differentiate into various types of plasma cell, at least two signals, are required; namely signal 1 and signal 2. *Signal 1* is generated, when B cell, acts as an antigen presenting cell, presents to B-Cell membrane; a peptide class-II MHC complex. This leads to expression of co-stimulatory B7 molecules and CD molecules on B cell. These cells having processed antigen along with other molecules, when it enters secondary lymphoid organ, confronts lymphocytes (T_H) bearing a tremendous array of antibody receptors. It selects only that lymphocyte, with which it makes close fit. These interact with CD28 and CD40L (ligand) on T_H cell to generate *signal 2*, which is IL-1. This leads to expression of various cytokine and cytokine receptors; especially IL-2. This leads to B cell activation, proliferation (clonal expansion) and differentiation into various types.

Immunoglobulins are synthesized in the ribosome of plasma cells, where both the chains (heavy and light) are synthesized by different ribosome and released into the cisternae of endoplasmic reticulum for final assembly and release from the cell.

Describe primary and secondary immune response (including ontogeny).

A.11 *Primary humoral response* (Fig. 2.9.2): It is immune response resulting, when man encounters an antigen for the first time. It results from activation of naïve B cells. Some of the B cells that become activated upon interaction with antigen do not differentiate into plasma cells but persist in body for many years without dividing as memory cells.

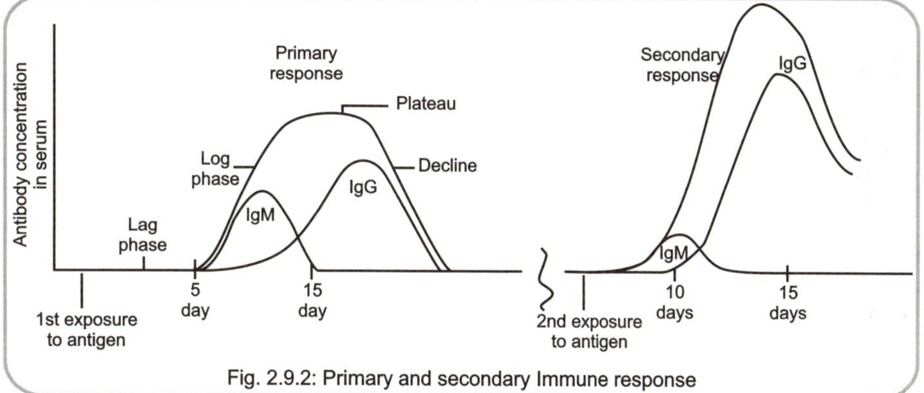

Fig. 2.9.2: Primary and secondary Immune response

Secondary response: It is the immune response resulting, when man encounters a specific antigen (or closely related cross- reactive) for the second time. It results from activation of B cells that had been previously primed to the same antigen.

The primary and secondary humoral response vary in many characteristics for the four phases; namely lag, log, plateau and decline phase; which exist in both the responses.

The *lag phase* is the first phase following antigen stimulation, when antibodies cannot be detected in the circulation. The lag phase lasts approximately 7 days but can be longer depending on the nature of antigen. This fact has many applications. *One*, a clinical sample taken for demonstrating antibodies in this period by a serological test, may yield a non reactive (negative) result; as in a Widal test. *Secondly*; an administration of antimicrobial during this phase can impede or stop the production of antibodies. This stage is followed by the *log phase*, where as the name indicates is characterized by steady rise in titre of antibodies. This is followed by the *plateau phase*, where the antibody titre remains more or less constant as the antibody synthesis and catabolism rates remain in an equilibrium. The decline phase as the name indicates is characterized by fall in antibody titre, as the catabolism rate exceeds the synthesis rate of antibodies.

The primary humoral response to antigen begins with the naïve B cells undergoing selection to be followed by clonal expansion and differentiation into plasma cells.

During the primary humoral response, IgM is secreted initially. This is followed by switching to predominant IgG synthesis, which results from class switching, in which gene rearrangement of same V_H (variable heavy chain) with different C_H (constant heavy chain) occurs.

The other characteristics of this response are depicted in Fig. 2.9.2 and table 2.9.1 of the immune response.

Ontogeny: IgM synthesis occurs in fetus and is the major antibody produced by fetus. However, IgG is the major fetal antibody that is acquired transplacentally.

The *secondary humoral* response results from activation of memory lymphocytes, which are formed as a consequence of the primary response. This response depends on the existence of population of both memory B and T cells. The response characteristics of this differ from those of primary response; as depicted in Fig. 2.9.1 and table 2.9.1. IgG is the predominant response in this, in contrast to IgM isotype, which predominates in the primary response. This aspect is utilized in clinically in differentiating a primary infection from a secondary infection. Obviously a predominant IgG response indicates a secondary (relapse) infection.

Table 2.9.1: A comparison of Primary and Secondary antibody response

	Primary antibody response	**Secondary antibody response**
Responding B cell	*Naïve B cell (virgin)	Memory B cell
Lag period	4-7 days (long	1-3 days (short)
Time of peak response	7-10 days (slow)	3-5 days (fast)
Magnitude of peak response (titre)	Varies depending on antigen (low)	Many times higher than primary (high)
Persistence of response	Shorter	Longer
Isotype produced	IgM predominates initially (to be followed by IgG)	Small IgM response followed by predominant IgG
Antigens	Thymus (T cell) dependent and independent	Thymus dependent
Antibody affinity	Lower	Higher

*Naïve B cell have lower receptor affinity than of memory B cells (due to affinity maturation). In diagnosis of toxoplasmosis, if one is detecting IgG and its avidity happens to be say less than < 0.3, it indicates recent infection.

What are the factors that can affect antibody production?

A.12 1. **Age:** The human embryo is immunologically immature, the antibody production starts at about 3-6 months of gestation. A birth, the infant is not fully immunologically competent and acquires complete immunocompetence by the age of 5-7 year for IgG isotype and 10-15 years for IgA isotype.

2. **Genetic factors:** Different individuals vary in their immune response to same antigen, due to immune response being under control of immune response gene (Ir) gene located on the short arm of the 6th human chromosome. The individuals; who respond to a particular antigen are called *'responder'*, whereas those; who don't respond are termed '*non responder*'. One of the applications of this fact is that some individuals, who are non responder to some vaccine antigen; as hepatitis B may not be able to get benefit from the vaccine.

3. **Nutritional status:** Deficiencies of proteins and some vitamins are known to suppress both the humoral and cell-mediated immune responses.

4. **Route of administration:** The immune response may vary in a host depending on the route of administration of an antigen. For many antigens, parenteral administration of an antigen induces a better immune response than the oral or nasal route administration. IgA isotype production for many antigens is better following oral or nasal administration. Similarly the IgE isotype production response to pollen antigen occurs chiefly after intranasal administration.

5. **Immunogen dosage:** A critical immunogen dosage is required to elicit an optimal immune response. A dose below the optimal dose may fail to elicit the immune response, possibly enough lymphocytes aren't stimulated. Similarly, very high dose of antigen may fail to elicit immune response by inducing tolerance.

6. **Multiple antigens:** When multiple antigens need to be administered simultaneously to man; for instance during vaccination, their nature and relative proportion need to be critically adjusted to have an optimal response to all the antigens, as in DPT vaccination.

7. **Presence of adjuvant:**

   – *Derivation* (of term 'adjuvant'): In Latin 'adjuvare' means to help

   – *Definition:* These are substances, which when mixed with an antigen and administered, enhance the immunogenicity of that antigen.

   – *Uses:* In research setting to boost the immune response of an antigen with low immunogenicity or when low amount of antigen is available.

– In vaccine formulation, to optimize immune response with minimal antigen administration.

Examples:

– Aluminum potassium sulfate (alum) is the only adjuvant approved for human use.

– Freund's incomplete adjuvant is an antigen; as aqueous solution in oil.

– Freund's complete adjuvant incorporates heat killed mycobacteria; as an additional component to the Freund's incomplete adjuvant. This adjuvant attracts lymphocytes and macrophages to the local site of administration, resulting in formation of a granuloma.

– Chemicals; as bentonite and silica particles.

Mechanism of action:

The exact mechanism by which they augment the immune response is not known. In general it has the following effects:

- Antigen persistence is prolonged.
- Local inflammation is increased.
- Co-stimulatory signals are enhanced (some being recognized as ligands) for antigen presenting cells.
- Enhance nonspecific proliferation of lymphocytes.

8. **Usage of immunosuppressive agents:**

These can inhibit the immune response and are useful, when the graft needs to be retained by the host and in some diseases especially of autoimmune nature, where the immune response is required to be selectively inhibited.

Examples:

– X-rays or irradiation.

– Radiomimetic drugs ('mimetic' means-mimics), e.g., cyclophosphamide and nitrogen mustard. They selectively inhibit B cell replication.

– Antimetabolites: Folic acid antagonists; as methotrexate, analogues of purine (azathroprime), cytosine (cytosine arabinoside) and uracil (5-fluorouracil) inhibit DNA and/or RNA synthesis leading to inhibition of cell division and differentiation, which are necessary for both humoral and cellular immune responses.

– Corticosteroids: These are anti-inflammatory drugs, which diminish the responsiveness of both B and T cells. These drugs are often misused by quacks at high doses, but when used in therapeutic doses with clinical indication, have minimal inhibitory effect on immune response.

Antilymphocyte serum: It is a heterogenous serum antiserum raised against T lymphocytes, for use in graft rejection in transplantation surgery. This substance is effective primarily against T lymphocytes and being a foreign protein can cause hypersensitivity reactions. Currently, monoclonal antibodies against specific lymphocyte membrane antigens are available.

How is the humoral immune (antibody) response regulated? Explain giving a clinical example.

A.13 Once the immune response starts, it is very important for the body to modulate it. *Modulation* implies upregulation and downregulation of response, according to need! What is implies, here is that once the function of antibodies is over, its production must stop, otherwise it would result in a waste of energy and can lead to pathological states; as autoimmune disease. Information about these regulatory events to date aren't very well understood. These can allow us to selectively manipulate the desirable responses by upregulating the desirable and downregulating the undesirable ones.

One of the important factors in the regulation of the immune esponse is the *antigen*. Broadly, the presence of the antigen induces the response and its elimination by antibody leads to a decrease in the immune response. It is for this reason that in certain infections, where the body is not able to eliminate the intracellular pathogens, pathological immune state results.

Antibody also plays an important role in the regulation by exerting a negative feedback. This aspect is utilized in the therapeutic administration of anti-D antibody to RhD negative mothers, who have been sensitized by RhD positive red blood cells of the fetus. The IgG anti-D antibodies can combine with any Rh-D positive erythrocytes, which may have entered the maternal blood stream from fetal circulation, before the maternal immune system can react with them, thus preventing maternal sensitization. Another regulator is the *suppressor T cells*, which help to suppress the immune response. Cytokines and idiotypic networks also play and key role.

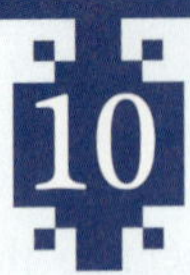

10 Cytokines

Implementation, integration and modulation of the immune response (innate and adaptive) are performed by molecules designated as cytokines. Let's study them.

How are cytokines defined?

A.1 (a) *Cytokines* (cyto-cell, kinein-to move) are low molecular weight soluble proteins, produced by a variety of hematopoietic and non-haematopoietic cell types. They are critical for innate and adaptive immune response. Their expression is altered in inflammatory conditions and in the immune responses associated; with infectious diseases.

How are cytokines differentiated from interleukins and hormones?

A.1 (b) *Cytokines* must be differentiated from *interleukins* (lymphokine and monokine, are old terms) and hormones. Interleukins are some cytokines, which are secreted by leucocytes and act on leucocytes. The differences of cytokines from hormones as depicted in the table below.

	Hormones	Cytokines
Production	– Constitutive	Short lived
Periods	– For long periods	Short periods
Place of action	– Act at long distances	Self act on (autocrine) (Fig. 2.10.1) or at short distance (paracrine)
Site of action	– Act on one/few types	Act on cells of varied types

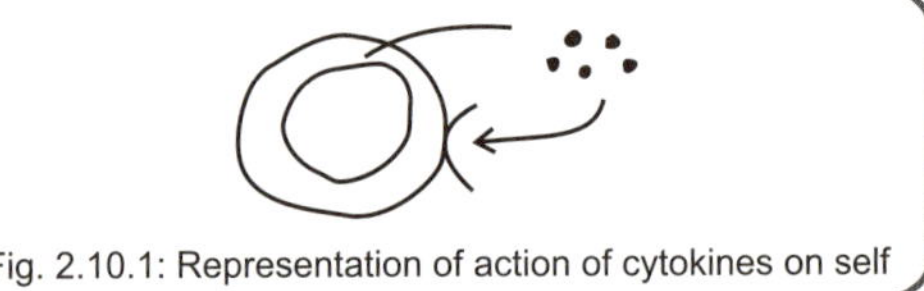
Fig. 2.10.1: Representation of action of cytokines on self

Note: Both hormones and cytokines have action at picomolar concentration.

Why did the cytokine purification work have to wait till the 1980s?

A.2 There are a number of reasons for this:

(i) The concentration of this substance is low in the body.

(ii) Gene cloning was not possible till 1970s, hence these substances would not be synthetized in the laboratory.

(iii) Monoclonal antibodies to these substances could not be synthesized for a long time, hence quantitative assays were not possible.

How are cytokines classified?

A.3 (a) There are classified into four groups:

1. Haematopoietic family
2. Interferon family
   - INF α
   - INF β
3. TNF family
   - TNF α
   - TNF β
4. Chemokine

Cytokines generally have molecular weight of < 30 kDa.

Illustrate diagrammatically the sequential action of cytokines

A.3 (b) (See Fig. 2.10.2)

Enumerate some cytokines involved in adaptive immunity? Mention their key functions.

A.3 (c) Summary of action of selected cytokines

Cytokine	Actions
IL-1	• Enhances activity of NK cells • Attracts neutrophils and macrophages to site of inflammation
IL-2	• Induces proliferation of antigen-primed T cells • Enhances activity of NK cells
IFN-γ	• Enhances activity of macrophages and NK cells • Increases expression of MHC molecules • Enhances production of IgG2a and IgG3
TNF-α	• Cytotoxic effect on tumor cells • Induces cytokine secretion in the inflammatory response

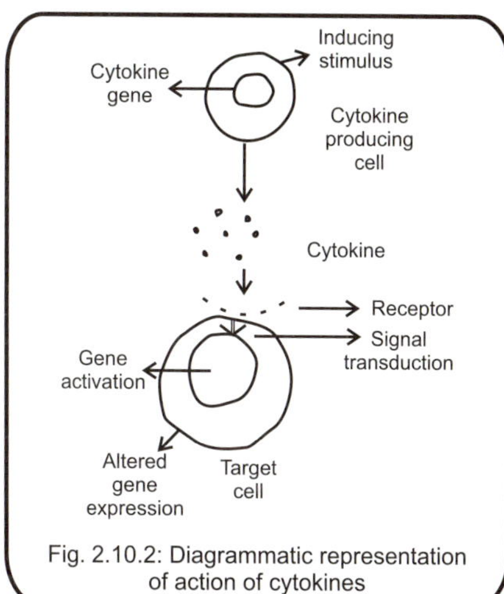

Fig. 2.10.2: Diagrammatic representation of action of cytokines

How are the effects of cytokines studied?

A.3 (d) They are studied by 'in vitro' studies of pure cytokines. These may not be able to predict the 'in vivo' effect, as in the body there is usually an exposure to a mixture of cytokines, who's combined synergistic and antagonistic effects may be different.

What are the key cells involved in cytokine synthesis?

A.4 (a) Dendritic cells, Macrophages, T_H cells and others

What are the key attributes of cytokines?

A.4 (b)
- **Pleiotropy:** It implies same cytokine can have different biological actions on different target cells.
- **Redundancy:** It means two or more cytokines are having similar functions on different cells.
- **Synergy:** New activity induced, e.g., IL-4 and IL-5 → B cell → IgE.
- **Antagonism:** One cytokine blocks action of another cytokine.
- **Cascade effect.**
- **Affect nonspecifically:** Affect any cells in surrounding that bear appropriate receptors.

How are cytokine receptors classified?

A.5 (a) They are categorized into:
1. Ig super family ligands: IL-1 to IL-18
2. Class I cytokine receptors: IL-2 to IL-7, IL-9, 11-18
3. Class II cytokine receptors: IFNα, β and γ
4. TNF receptors
5. Chemokines 1-8

Enumerate examples of cytokine mediated diseases.

A.5 (b)
- Severe combined immunodeficiency disease (SCID)
- Some people who are prone to mycobacterial infection have defect in INF-γ receptor.
- Most individuals with septic shock have increased levels of TNFα and IL-1β. The significance of this is that, neutralizing these cytokines, may have a therapeutic value.
- In Chagas diseases, altered IL-2 receptors have been detected.
- In malignancies as of lymphoid and myeloid lineages, abnormalities in production of cytokines and their receptors have been observered.

Enumerate some diseases in which cytokine therapy has a role.

A.5 (c)
- Monoclonal antibodies against TNFα are in use for rheumatoid arthritis.
- IFNα 2a is useful in hepatitis B infection.
- IFNα 2b is useful in hepatitis C infection.
- Experimentally IL-2 has been tried in AIDs cases, for restoring decreased CD4 counts.

11 Major Histocompatibility Complex (M.H.C.)

The intracellular pathogens can evade the antibody mediated limb of the adaptive immunity by hiding inside the host cells. Alerting the host that some of it's cells have been infected is important. Presenting a part of the intracellular antigen of the pathogen to outside of the cell for specific cell-mediated immune response elicitation is performed by MHC molecules. Let's study them.

Comment on the discovery of MHC molecules.

A.1 These were discovered during allograft rejections experiments in inbred mice performed in the 1930s. The MHC molecules are encoded by a continuous stretch of genes in the human in the 6th chromosome. The major histocompatibility complex, which is responsible for the MHC molecules in man is called the HLA (human leukocyte antigen) system.

Diagramatically illustrate the HLA complex, depicting sequentially the three MHC classes, genes and gene products.

A.2 The three regions of MHC (HLA) are depicted in Fig. 2.11.1.

Their functions are:

Class I: Encode glycoproteins expressed on all nucleated cells and present to CD8 + T cells (presence on all cells ensure, that any altered cell gets eliminated).

Class II: Encode glycoprotein, expressed on all APCs and present to CD4 + cells

Class III: Encode secreted proteins, which include complement components; as C2, C4 and other molecules as TNFα.

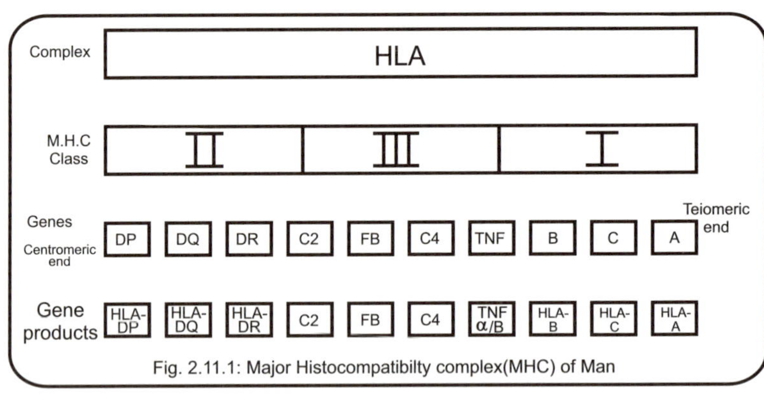

Fig. 2.11.1: Major Histocompatibilty complex(MHC) of Man

Describe the characteristics, transport and evolutionary significance of MHC molecules.

A.3 *Characteristics:* The MHC molecules are transmembrane heterodimer glycoproteins. (Fig. 2.11.2)

The characteristic of the two classes are:

- Class I: molecules are composed of:
  - Alpha chain (43 kDa), organized into α1, α2, α3 and a cytoplasmic chain
  - Beta chain (beta2 microglobulin).

  The antigenic peptide groove of this molecule is formed in the cleft between α1 and α2 domains.
- Class II: molecules are composed of:
  - Alpha – 38 kDa chain
  - Beta – 28 kDa chain

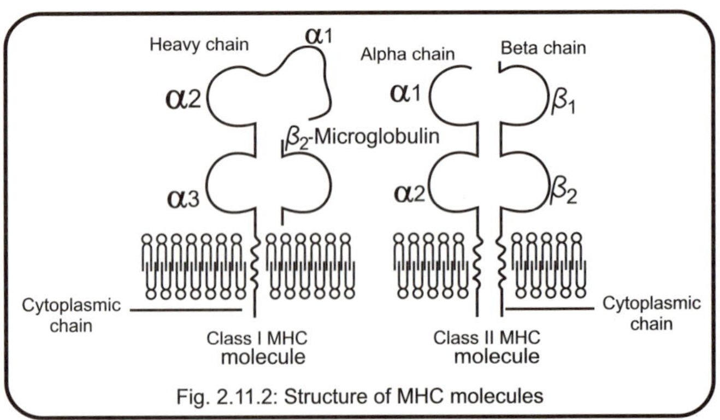

Fig. 2.11.2: Structure of MHC molecules

The antigenic (peptide) groove of this molecule is formed in the cleft between α1 and β1 domains.

These molecules are:

- *Polygenic* – many genes are required to code for one molecule.
- *Polymorphic* – Each gene has many alleles.

These two features combine to extend the range of peptides that can be presented to T cells by individuals.

- *Transport*: The site of synthesis of MHC molecule is endoplasmic reticulum for both MHC I and II molecules. They are transported to cell surface by Golgi apparatus.
- *Evolutionary significance*: MHC molecules help in the presenting the antigens especially of the intracellular organisms, so that the immune response can be made against them. The ubiquitous distribution of MHC I molecules in all cells ensure that any cell may be eliminated by T-cell.

  It could also have a 'energy economy' aspect in the host, as wasteful immune reaction against dead or circulating antigens would be avoided.

  The availability of the extended range of peptides (of MHC) appears to have an evolutionary significance. It provides a tremendous variety of immune reactivity, so that no microbial antigen could be equally pathogenic to every member of species. So, it allows atleast some individuals to survive an exotic outbreak of infection, whenever it may arise.

What is MHC restriction? Describe its relevance.

A.4 It implies that antigen presenting cells, when they present their antigen to T cells, must have the same MHC, as on the T-cell for successful immune response to occur. One of the implication of this is that, if specific sensitized T_H cells to a particular antigen are to transferred to a new host, the transfer of immunity to the new host would only be effective, if the donor and recipient have the same MHC class.

A.5 Precisely the steps that are involved in this process is *not known*, because if these were known, then we would have had a vaccine against dreaded disease of tuberculosis. The first stage in the induction is called *primary CMI response,* in which the specific T-cell receptor (TCR) on a lymphocyte interacts with microbial antigen and a self MHC on the antigen presenting cell. During this phase, APCs move from the infection site to secondary lymphoid organs,where the lymphocytic activation occurs. One of the key cytokine that is produced by the APC in this interaction, is interleukin 1, which activates the T cell (Fig. 2.12.3). The T cell, further secretes an interleukin 2, which acts on self and leads to morphological changes in the lymphocyte, leading to its transformation to blast cell. This differentiates into memory cells and different effector cells as helper T cell (Th), suppressor T cell (Ts), cytotoxic T cell (Tc) and Td (involved in hypersensitivity). Subsequently clonal proliferation of key T cells occurs. This is important, as the body has to deal with numerous (even millions) microbes, which could be present in the host. During this stage the activated T cells and other cells are directed to the site of infection by chemoattractants.

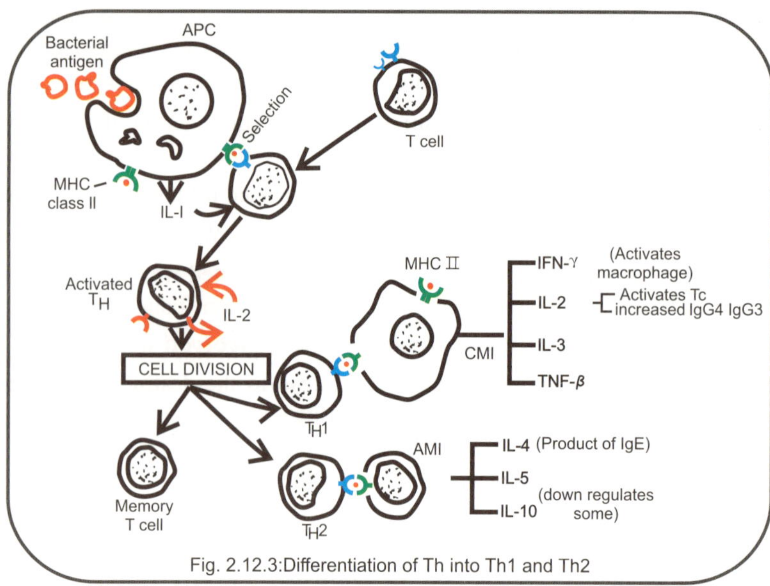

Fig. 2.12.3:Differentiation of Th into Th1 and Th2

On a subsequent exposure of the same antigen, the response is more pronounced and more rapid because of the availability of the memory cells. This is sometimes called the *secondary CMI response* unlike the previous, which is called primary CMI response.

Enumerate and describe the tests to evaluate CMI (delayed hypersensitivity)

A.6 Test to demonstrate CMI (delayed hypersensitivity):

These can be categorized into

'In vitro'	*'In vivo'*
• Leucocyte migration inhibition test (LMIT)/Macrophage migration inhibition test (MMIT)	• CD4/CD8 ratio (n) 1.8 – 2.2 (reversal occurs in AIDS)
• Lymphocyte transformation test	• Delayed hypersensitivity skin testing, e.g., tuberculin testing
• Mixed lymphocyte reaction (MLR)	• Mouse foot pad assay (increase in foot pad thickness in experimental animals)
• Target cell destruction (cell mediated lympholysis) of culture cells by CD8 lymphocytes sensitized against then	
• Measure products as cytokines, e.g., IL-2 by activated T cells	

LMIT/MMIT:

Depending on whether the predominant cells being tested are leucocytes or macrophages, the test is accordingly called as LMIT or MMIT.

This is one of the classic tests used to assess 'in vitro' the cell mediated hypersensitivity (delayed hypersensitivity).

Principle: Macrophages/leucocytes* (actively motile cells), placed in capillary tube (with nutrients) migrate out in a fan like pattern. However, if these are cultured (placed along with) an antigen to which the lymphocytes are sensitized, the migration of macrophages/leucocytes is inhibited. This inhibition occurs, due to production of a lymphokine called macrophage migration inhibition factor, that is released by the sensitized lymphocytes, on contact with the antigen.

*A good source of cells is the peritoneal exudates; containing macrophages and lymphocytes, obtained following injection of the irritant into the peritoneal cavity.

Procedure: Place two capillary tubes with test cells in culture medium. In only one, add the test antigen. In the test tube with antigen, inhibition of the migration of macrophage/leucocytes occurs.

Lymphocyte transformation/proliferation test

This test is based on the principle, that if lymphocytes are placed in culture along with only antigen, some of them will be stimulated to undergo mitosis. This can be measured by providing radiolabelled (tritiated) thymidine (^{3}H-TdR) to the culture medium. This tagged thymidine will be incorporated (by the lymphocyte) during the synthetic phase of the cell cycle. The uptake of the radioactive label can be measured from the lymphocytes, after removing them from the culture medium. The specificity of the proliferative response can be shown by testing the lymphocytes with several different antigens.

Nb: The population of lymphocytes that mediate this response (DTH) to a specific antigen is only small fraction of the total lymphocyte pool of the organism.

Mixed-lymphocyte reaction (MLR) - (See pg 165, A.4c(ii)

Cell-mediated lympholysis (target cell destruction of culture cells by CD8 lymphocytes):

One of the important pathways, by which the cell-mediated immunity acts is by cytotoxic T-lymphocytes (CTLs), so this is an important test. In this assay, suitable target cells (i.e., cells that are target of CTLs) are radiolabeled ion (as; chromium-51) and incubated with activated CTLs for a standard period. After that the amount of radioactive ion released (here; ^{51}Cr) is estimated, which correlates directly with the number of target cells lysed.

- **Measure products as cytokines, e.g., IL2 by activated T cells**-It is an important test as many times the defect lies in the profile of the cytokines secreted by the T cells

CD4/CD8 ratio: Normally this ratio varies between 1.8 - 2.2. However in many diseases, this ratio can vary, so this can act as an indicator of the immune function. In AIDS, this ratio can get reversed. This parameter is assessed in microbiology labs in our country, by fluorescent activated cell sorter (FACS) machine, funded by National Aids Control Organization (NACO) .

Delayed hypersensitivity skin testing: (also see pg. 157-158- A5, A7, A9)

It is a commonly employed test to assess the reaction of the host to numerous antigens that are administered intradermally. The commonest examples of it, are tuberculin and lepromin test.

Mouse foot pad assay:

It is an experimental model system (in laboratory animals; as mice) to assess the response of antigens administered intradermally. This test is based on the principle that increase in foot pad thickness occurs with an effective (positive) antigen as compared to the control food pad of a mouse, that has been only injected with the same amount of saline. However to rule out a false positive reaction, it is advisable to study histologically the tested tissue for strong mononuclear infiltrate.

13 Hypersensitivity Reactions (Diseases)

- *'It is not necessary to react to everything that may interact with self'.* — **VSR**
- *Do not get upset with people and situations, they are powerless without your reactions.* — **Gautama Buddha**
- *Psychoneuroimmunology is defined; as study of interaction of consciousness, central nervous system and body's defence against......* — **Robert Ader**
- *Modulation of delayed type hypersensitivity ('Mantoux' reaction), in the skin by hypnosis is documented.* — **Roitt's Essential Immunology**

A 10 year old girl, Babita gets severe bronchial asthma attacks every year in the month of April. She stays close to Lodhi garden, New Delhi; which has plenty of flowering trees.

What is the likely cause of her respiratory problem?

A.1 It is likely to be an atopic type 1 hypersensitivity disorder.

What are the common allergens to which a person can have type 1 hypersensitivity reactions?

A.2 See table 2.13.1

Describe common localized type 1 hypersensitivity disorders.

A.3 See table 2.13.2

Describe the term hypersensitivity and explain how this concept evolved (including historical aspects).

A.4 The term hypersensitivity implies an excessive or increased response, but the immune response in the hypersensitivity reactions is not always increased, so this condition may better be described as inappropriate response to antigen.

The term *immunopathology* is sometimes used for hypersensitivity, autoimmune and other disorders, where the immune system, instead of protecting the host from pathogens, reacts in a way that is detrimental to the host and thus causes a pathology in the individual. The difference between hypersensitive and autoimmune disorders is that in the former, the reaction is especially often to harmless innocuous substances; whereas in autoimmune disorders, the response is to self tissue antigens. The term atopic allergy implies a genetic predisposition to manifest hypersensitivity disorders; as asthma, rhinitis, urticaria and eczematous dermatitis conditions.

Normal immune based effector mechanisms result in elimination of antigen without excessive tissue injury whereas the inflammatory response results in significant host injury. It must be emphasized that the hypersensitivity reactions clinically manifest only after second exposure to the same antigen. In literature, one would find several anecdotal reports of individuals becoming hypersensitive upon first contact with an allergen, but these would be false. *Priming/sensitizing stage* is necessary before the *shocking stage* can manifest in the individual. In the *sensitizing stage,* the antigen (allergen) leads to priming of the B/T lymphocytes. The problem then is how to explain the anaphylactic reactions occurring on apparent first exposure to the allergen? The common explanation for this could be, that an unknowing contact in the past could have occurred. Other explanations could be contamination of foods consumed with allergens, as penicillins or fetal exposure to allergens from the maternal blood.

The term *allergy* is often used as a synonym for hypersensitivity, but this should be avoided, as many people use it for disorders that aren't immunological reactions to innocuous substance, for instance; toxic reactions to drugs (called *idiosyncratic reaction*) mediated by non-immunological mechanism and digestive disorders from non immunological response.

To understand the pathologic role of the immune system to harmless substances, *an experiment* can convey the message. One milligram of ovalbumin administered to an unprimed guinea pig produces no harmful effect. But the same dose given intravenously to this guinea pig, after 14 days produces severe pathological changes in the animal, which dies in a few minutes. So here the antigen itself was harmless, but an immune response to it on second exposure killed the animal. Like all immune responses, the hypersensitivity reaction displays memory and specificity. The latter aspect implies that if the guinea pig had been injected the second time, to another antigen say, rye grass, the animal would not have succumbed to the administration of the antigen.

These aspects were studied in the early twentieth century, when Prince of Monaco engaged two French scientists, namely Paul Portier and Charles Richet to solve the problem of bathers in Mediterranean sea reacting violently to the sting of jelly fish. In their experiment, they tried the vaccination approach. In it, purified toxin of jelly fish was injected into experimental dogs, but the dogs instead of heaving a reduced (or a protective) effect on second exposure to toxins, died of asphyxia. So; Charles Richet coined the term 'anaphylaxis' from Greek to contrast with the phenomenon of 'prophylaxis'. Charles Richet subsequently received the Nobel prize in physiology/medicine in 1913 for the discovery of anaphylaxis.

Classify hypersensitivity disorders and tabulate the key differences between them.

A.5 Hypersensitivity reactions may develop in the course of either a humoral or a cell mediated immune response. Initially hypersensitivities were defined as either immediate or delayed, depending upon time elapsed between contact with the antigen and onset of clinical symptoms. In actuality, there may a very complex spectrum of reactions. A scheme often followed to aid in delineating the pathogenesis of hypersensitivities was proposed by *Gell and Coomb*. It categories *4 types* of hypersensitivity reactions. Type I, II and III are antibody-mediated and designated as immediate type hypersensitivity reactions; whereas type IV is cell-mediated and is designated as delayed hypersensitivity reaction. However it must be realized that a complicated blend (mix) of antibody and cell-mediated immune responses are often seen in hypersensitivity disorders that can blur the boundaries between the four categories. The important characteristics of the four types of hypersensitivities is depicted in table 2.13.1.

Table 2.13.1: Characteristics of hypersensitivity reactions

Characteristics	Type I hypersensitivity	Type II hypersensitivity	Type III hypersensitivity	Type IV hypersensitivity
Other name	IgE mediated hypersensitivity	IgG/IgM mediated cytotoxic hypersensitivity	Immune complex mediated hypersensitivity	Cell mediated hypersensitivity
Antigen	Soluble/particulate antigen	Cell/matrix associated antigen	Soluble/ particulate antigen	Cell-associated antigen (also soluble)
Cells involved	Mast cells, basophils	Various host cells	Various host cells	Various host cells
Type of antibody Involved	IgE	IgG/IgM	IgG/IgM	No antibody
Effector mechanism	Mast cell activation	Cell destruction via complement activation or ADCC	Complement activation via Ag-Ab complexes induce inflammatory response by infiltration of neutrophils	Sensitized T_H1 cells release cytokines, which activate macrophages, APCs and Tc
Mediators	Histamine, serotonin, SRS etc	Complement	Complement	Cytokines
Transfer of immunity	By serum	By serum	By serum	By T cells (also by transfer factor)
Reaction time	Few seconds to minutes	Few hours to days	Few hours to days	Days
Skin reaction	Wheal and flare	None	None	Induration and erythema
Classic example	Anaphylaxis, Asthma	-Transfusion reaction -Hemolytic disease of newborn	-Serum sickness -Farmer's lung	-Tuberculin reaction -Contact dermatitis

Classify type 1 hypersensitivity disorders.

A.6 The type I hypersensitivity reactions can be classified into two categories as depicted in table 2.13.2. The localized hypersensitivity reactions are limited to a specific target tissue or organ. The tendency to manifest the localized hypersensitivity reaction is inherited and is called *atopy*.

Table 2.13.2: Classification of type 1 hypersensitivity reactions

		Common Allergen/type	Route of entry	Response
Systemic reactions	*Systemic Anaphylaxis*	• Penicillin and other drugs • Venoms (as bees, wasp) • Serum therapy (serum sickness • Also an example of Type III disorder) • *Four cases of sexual intercourse	Parenteral (commonly)	• Anaphylactic Shock • Oedema • Vasodilation • Broncoconstriction • Circulatory collapse
Localized reactions (atopic Disorder)	*Allergic rhinitis (hay fever)*	• Pollens (rye grass, dust, mite)	Inhalation	• Nasal Irritation • Oedema of nasal mucosa, (Manifesting as running nose, sneezing etc)
	Bronchial Asthma (allergic)	• Pollens • Dust • Mite	Inhalation	• Bronchial constriction • Increased mucus production
	Food Allergy	• Milk • Eggs • Nuts,spices • Seafood	Oral	• Vomiting • Diarrhoea
	Atopic Dermatitis (as wheal and flare)	• Insect bite • Allergy testing	– Subcutaneous – Intradermal	• local oedema • Local Vasodilation

Describe pathogenesis and mediators of generalized hypersensitivity reactions.

A.7 Type I hypersensitivity reaction are triggered by certain types of antigens designated as allergens (Table 2.13.2). The response induced by these allergens is similar to a normal humoral response except that antibody secreted by plasma cells is chiefly IgE in response to activation of allergen specific T_{H2} cells. The IgE class of antibody has the characteristic of binding with high affinity Fc receptors present on basophils and mast cells, causing them to degranulate and cause the disease (Fig. 2.13.1). The distribution of the mast cells and basophils in body is of ubiquitous type. Mast cells are present in almost all organs, but particularly high concentration is seen in lungs, gastrointestinal tract, skin and genitourinary tract. Basophils though present in the blood can migrate readily into any tissue.

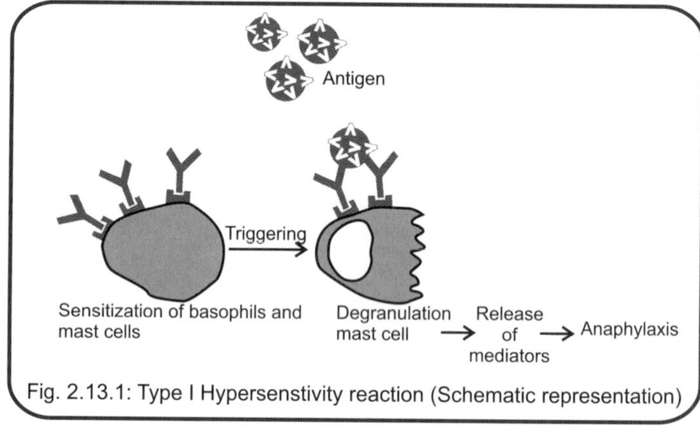

Fig. 2.13.1: Type I Hypersenstivity reaction (Schematic representation)

Physiochemical studies in IgE could not be made initially due to its very low intrinsic levels,but when the discovery of the IgE myeloma was made in 1967, it could be characterized. It has a M.W. 1,90,000 which is higher than IgG, IgD, IgA due to additional constant region CH4, has half life 2-3 days, once bound to mast cell/basophil remains stable for weeks.

The reaction can be seen to be occurring in stages. *In the first stage*, the allergen primes the immune system for a subsequent encounter with the same allergen, but produces no symptoms. Here the allergen enters the body, passes through the tissue fluids, lymphatics and reaches the lymph nodes. It is taken up by the antigen presenting cells (as dendritic cells) and with the help of T-helper cells, activate specific clone of B cells. Uptil here the response is like an usual infection, but for reasons, which are not completely understood, the activated B cells convert to plasma cell and produce IgE antibodies instead of the usual IgM antibodies. The IgE antibodies have specific Fc receptors by which they attach with great affinity to the glycoprotein receptors on the mast cells and basophils.

On the second or subsequent encounter with the same allergen, there is cross-linking of the bound IgE molecules, which leads to a process called degranulation and release of mediators, which mediate the clinical symptoms (Fig. 2.13.1)

Mediators of type I reaction:

Several mediators are released during mast cell or basophil degranulation that mediate allergic reactions in the individual. Many of these mediators have been identified and the differing manifestation in these reactions could be explained by the qualitative and quantitative differences in the profile of the mediators released in an individual. The mediators can be classified as primary or secondary (see table 2.13.3). The *primary mediators* are readymade mediators stored in the granules. The *secondary mediators* are those, which are synthesized after target cell activation or released by the breakdown of membrane phospholipids during the degranulation process.

Their study is important because to manage the type 1 hypersensitive cases, their activity has to be controlled; for instance usage of antihistamines to treat allergic rhinitis.

Schultz Dale phenomenon demonstrates the type 1 hypersenstivity concept experimentally. In it, if an isolated muscle or intestine sensitized to an antigen is placed in ringer lactate, it contracts; when the specific antigen is put in the experimental system.

Table 2.13.3: Key mediators in type 1 hypersensitivity reaction

Primary	*Kinetics*	*Action*
• Histamine	• Most important (profuse and fast acting), obtained by decarboxylation of histidine	• Increases smooth muscle contraction of bronchi and intestine causing difficulty in breathing and increased intestinal motility. But decreases vascular smooth muscle activity and dilates arterioles and venules. This gives rise to wheal and flare phenomenon and symptoms; as pruritus, flushed skin and headache, increased permeability of capillaries
• Eosinophil chemotactic factor (ECF-A)		• Eosinophil chemotaxis
• Neutrophil chemotactic factor (NCF-A)		• Neutrophil chemotaxis
Secondary		
• Leukotrienes (previously known as SRS-A) i.e. slow reacting substance of anaphylaxis	• Appear slowly, but effects are more potent than histamine and effect lasts longer	• Key mediator of bronchoconstriction (effect not inhibited by antihistamines) • Increased vascular permeability and mucus production.
• Prostaglandins	• Also appear slowly and effects are very potent, certain anti-inflammatory drugs act by preventing the synthesis of prostaglandins	• Platelet aggregation, vasodilation, broncho-constriction
• Bradykinin	• are kinin.	• Smooth muscle contraction and increased vascular permeability

It is useful to differentiate the two phages of anaphylaxis, namely the immediate and late phase because it is useful to know some of the clinical manifestations may begin 4-6 hours after the immediate phase and may persist for 1-2 days. Neutrophils and eosinophils play a key role in the late phase reactions.

Describe the clinical aspects of generalized anaphylaxis.

A.8 It is a generalized, severe, acute life threatening reaction that is characterized by its onset within second to minutes, after the introduction of the antigen, usually by parenteral route. Insect bites (as bee), penicillin-injections and vaccines are probably the commonest causes of this reaction. Different animals vary in the clinical profile in the manifestation of this entity. The variation in symptoms probably reflect differences the distribution of mast cells and the biological content of the granules. The animal model for studying systemic anaphylaxis is guinea pig.

In man, it presents as anaphylactic shock, which occurs as a result of loss of fluid from the blood vessels into tissues and due to blood vessel dilation, which result in tremendous fall of blood pressure and occurence of generalized oedema. The acute respiratory distress occurs due to bronchoconstriction, which may include respiratory obstruction and presence of mucus secretions in the respiratory tract.

The anaphylactic reaction must be differentiated from *anaphylactoid reaction* that is caused by some drugs and iodinated contrast media; used in some radiologic procedures. These reactions have no immunological basis (i.e., not IgE mediated and require other pathogenetic mechanisms for their manifestation.

Describe pathogenesis of atopic disorders.

A.9 The importance of the atopic disorders (allergies) can be gauged from the fact that they affect at least 20% of the population in developed countries, which results in work absenteeism and economic loss. These allergens are often of environmental origin and one cannot do almost nothing to avoid them. The list of allergens is endless and keeps growing with the thousands of commercially synthesized chemicals and drugs getting added for usage. The atopic individuals usually have higher levels of circulating IgE (upto 10 µg/ml) in contrast to the normal individuals. This characteristic is linked to multiple genes. One locus is on the chromosome 5, which is linked to a region that encodes numerous cytokines as IL-3, IL-4, IL-5 and IL-9. These individuals also have increased circulating eosinophils. What is the evolutionary benefit of inherting these responses, that cause misery in 20% of the individuals of developed countries (by reacting against harmless antigens and causing localized hypersensitivity reaction)? These IgE responses were meant for defense against parasitic diseases; especially helminthic diseases. It is believed that with a drastic decrease in the helminthic infections, in some individuals these responses get triggered abnormally to benign environmental stimuli. In developing countries, these allergies are uncommon. Most allergens are small, soluble, glycosylated proteins or protein bound substances having a molecular weight varying between 15-40 kDa. Few of the common allergens that have been purified and characterized include rye, grass pollen and ragweed pollen.

Allergic rhinitis (hay fever): It is probably the commonest atopic disorder affecting a significant population. The incriminating agents are often the pollens from trees, which have a seasonal variation. The airborne allergens react with the sensitized mast cells in the conjunctiva and nasal mucosa, initiating the release of mediators from the mast cells causing localized vasodilation and increased capillary permeability, which manifest as watery eyes, sneezing and nasal congestion. This syndrome should be differentiated from *common cold*, which it resembles clinically, caused by viruses and nasal secretions not having the increased number of eosinophils.

Bronchial asthma: It can be of two types, namely *intrinsic* and extrinsic. The former type is caused by non-immunologic means whereas the *extrinsic* type is caused by minute amount of allergen; especially of the inhalant category. So one category of asthma can be considered as another type of immediate (type 1) hypersensitivity disorder. It is characterized by bouts of difficulty in breathing. Here, chiefly the mast cells of the lower respiratory tract are involved, whose degranulation lead to spasms in the bronchial tube causing difficulty in breathing. As mainly leukotrienes and prostaglandins are responsible for bronchospasm and increased mucus production, antihistamines are of no value in treatment of this disorder.

Food allergy: The common agents causing this type of allergy include peanuts, fish, milk, eggs and soya beans. The mode of entry for these disorders is intestinal, but these allergies can also affect the skin and respiratory tract. Here chiefly the mast cells of the gastrointestinal tract are involved, the symptoms can be nausea, diarrhea and abdominal cramp. In case, the allergen after absorption from the intestinal tract, reaches the skin and reacts with the mast cells there, then predominantly cutaneous manifestations occur. In someone with lobster allergy, the key manifestation is urticaria[Δ] (hives).

Atopic dermatitis (allergic eczema): It is an inflammatory disease of the skin, sometimes called eczema and frequently seen in children. Surprisingly, sensitization occurs more through oral and respiratory route than through skin. The lesions are erythematous and if get secondarily infected with bacteria, than get filled with pus. These lesions can progress slowly to dry, scaly and thickened (lichenified) nature. When the allergen enters through skin, it causes the classic wheal and flare reaction, characterized by erythema, swelling and pruritus. These lesions contain T_{H2} cells and increased eosinophils unlike the lesions caused by delayed type hypersensitivity reactions, which are characterized by T_{H1} cells. The common examples are insect bites and skin allergen testing.

Δ Urticaria (hives) an allergic skin reaction characterized by formation of wheals, itchy red swellings (resembling mosquito bite.

Describe the treatment of type 1 Hypersensitivity reaction with special reference to the treatment approach in this case?

A.10 Treating a case of systemic anaphylaxis is a medical emergency, as a delay of few seconds or minutes in the treatment can make the difference between life and death. For this reason, the individuals allergic to some entities; as drug or food items, should carry an identification tag mentioning the allergens to which they are hypersensitive and kit containing tourniquet (to help make veins prominent for parenteral drug administration), syringe and ampoules of epinephrine for administration without delay, if necessary. Corticosteroids can also be life saving.

For treating the symptoms of localized anaphylaxis conditions, there is a whole range of drugs available from decreasing the IgE production from plasma cells to neutralizing the mediator release from mast cells or blocking the mediator from binding to target cells.

Corticosteroids inhibit the production of IgE antibodies from the plasma cells. They also stabilize lysosomal membrane of human polymorphonuclear leucocyte lysosomes.

Sodium chromoglycate blocks the (or prevents the formation of) release of mediators by stabilizing mast cell membranes, by blocking calcium influx into mast cells.

Epinephrine and *theophylline* both block mediator release, though their mechanisms differ. Epinephrine stimulates the enzyme adenyl cyclase resulting in increased cAMP levels, which block degranulation of cells. Theophylline stimulates the enzyme phosphodiesterase, which inhibits the conversion of cAMP levels to AMP, so that the preserved levels of cAMP can block degranulation.

Antihistamines block H_1 and H_2 receptors on target cells. Diphenoxylate act as a H_1 mediator antagonist and block mediators from binding to target cells. However this class of drugs is ineffective against effects, mediated by primary mediators and symptoms of bronchial asthma, as they are primarily mediated by substances other than histamine.

A recent form of immunotherapy has been usage of humanized monoclonal anti IgE, which can bind IgE antibodies only if they have not bound to F_CE receptors. *Omalizumab* was the first anti IgE drug approved for usage in allergic asthma.

What provisional and confirmatory tests can be performed in this case to make a definitive diagnosis?

A.11 The tests for diagnosis of type 1 hypersensitivity disorder may be categorized as

- *Non-specific*: As β-tryptase levels (after reaction), total IgE levels, blood eosinophil counts (increased count may act as an indicator)
- *Specific*
  - 'In vitro' – Radioallergosorbent test (RAST), Radioimmunoabsorbent test (RIST)
  - 'In vitro' – ▪ Prausnitz Kustner test (PK test, historical value) ▪ Skin testing with specific allergens

One of the most important aspects in the work up of such a case is the elicitation of the history of the reaction. In a classic reaction, the onset of symptoms occurs within seconds to few minutes, after contact with the specific allergen. As many times the allergic manifestations can mimic the infectious conditions and the management of these entities is different, so it is important to diagnose some of the localized type 1 hypersensitivity disorders.

Elevation of *beta-tryptase* levels in serum indicate a mast cell activation. Elevation of total IgE levels in serum is another non-specific indication of involvement of type 1 hypersensitivity reaction. This test is often performed by the paper radioimmunosorbent technique (RIST). To detect the presence of specific IgE antibodies, a test known as radioallergosorbent test (RAST) is performed, which is radioactivity based. This test can indicate for instance, if specific IgE antibodies to 'rye groups' are present in the individual or not.

Another test that is of historical value is the *Prausnitz Kustner (PK) test.* It is a type of cutaneous anaphylaxis reaction, which is based on the specificity of IgE for the cells of the skin. In 1921, Kustner's serum which had gastrointestinal allergy to certain fish was introduced intradermally into the skin of Prausnitz (who was not hypersensitive to fish). After a latent period of 24 hours, the implicated fish allergen was introduced intradermally into the site of serum administration, the classic reaction of wheal and flare was manifested, which indicated the transfer of the hypersensitivity from Kustner to Prausnitz had occured. This test is not performed these days, due to risk of transmission of diseases by serum; as hepatitis B, C and HIV.

Skin testing with specific allergens: The test involves a panel of standardized antigens, which are introduced in small amounts intradermally or by superficial scratching, usually on the forearm of skin. If the case is allergic to any one of the antigens, local mast cell degranulation occurs, resulting in local wheal and flare reaction in 30 minutes. The advantage of this technique is that it is a simple and inexpensive test, which can screen a large number of allergens in short span of 20 minutes. The disadvantage of this technique is that it sometimes sensitizes the allergic individual to new allergens and rarely may induce systemic anaphylaxis.

What kit should this girl always carry with her?

A.12 She should always carry a kit, which mentions her name and the fact that she is allergic to some pollens. The kit should have a syringe and needle and an ampoule containing a drug as epinephrine and/or a steroid to be administered, if she has an anaphylactic attack.

What approaches could have been tried to prevent this problem in this girl?

A.13 Avoidance of the allergen is probably the best way to prevent these reactions. However such an approach is only possible with identified food allergens and not possible with environmental allergens.

Hyposensitization (Desensitization): It is a type of immunotherapy in, which increasing doses of identified allergen is given subcutaneously to achieve some clinical benefits; as decreased severity of clinical symptoms by preventing (decreasing) reaction between allergen, IgE and mast cells. It is a paradoxical approach in which one is preventing the reactions, by deliberately administering a sensitive person with increasing doses of extremely (homeopathic) low doses of the allergen. This type of therapy has been seen to be effective against some insect venoms and drug allergies.

How this therapy provides the benefit is not clear. *One of the mechanisms* to explain this the preferential shift of production of antibodies from the IgE to the IgG class antibodies with this therapy. These antibodies class are referred to as the 'blocking' antibodies, as they can bind to the incriminating allergen. They form a complex that is removed by phagocytosis and as a result decrease the availability of the allergen to bind to the fixed IgE antibodies on the mast cells. *Another, mechanism* to explain the benefit is the increased suppressor T cell activity (Treg cells) suppressing the production of IgE may be induced.

Integrated Clinical Case Based Study–2

As a part of the antenatal workup, Rh blood group of the pregnant woman is investigated and recorded. This is done to monitor the possibility of development of the hemolytic disease of newborn and its management, if need be. Let's study this clinical scenario with reference to hypersensitivity disorders.

What type of hypersensitivity reaction is the hemolytic disease of newborn (erythroblastosis fetalis)? Describe it.

A.1 It is a Type II Hypersensitivity [cytotoxic] reaction. This most commonly develops, when the Rh +ve fetus expresses Rh antigen on its RBCs, which the Rh –ve mother does not express on its RBCs. In such a condition, IgG maternal antibodies develop (specific for the fetal Rh +ve antigen), which cross the placenta and lead to destruction of the fetal RBCs.

Give other common examples of type II hypersensitivity disorders.

A.2
1. Blood transfusion reaction due to incompatibility between the donor (transfused) blood and the recipient blood, e.g., due to ABO system incompatibility or Rh group incompatibility.
2. Drug induced hemolytic anemia: Certain drugs; as penicillin,cephalosporins, and streptomycin can cause this type of reaction. Here the drug attach to the surface of RBCs forming a complex, which induce the formation of specific IgG antibodies. These antibodies can induce complement mediated lysis of RBCs leading to anemia.
3. Drug induced thrombocytopenic purpura: Certain drugs; as aspirin and sulfonamide can cause this reaction by a mechanism similar to drug induced hemolytic anemia.
4. Autoimmune haemolytic anaemia.
5. Goodpasture syndrome (lung and kidney basement membrane damage).

NB: Penicillin can induce all type of hypersensitive reactions, i.e., type I-IV (Clinical features can vary including the pathogenetic mechanisms.

Describe the mechanisms by which damage to host occurs in type II hypersensitivity disorders.

A.3 These are reactions mediated by antibodies usually IgG (sometimes IgM) against cell surface antigens see Fig. 2.13.2.

The mechanisms by which damage to cells occurs include:

1. IgG/IgM antibodies coating the host cell (pathogen with antigen) against which response initiated. These cells are termed as 'opsonized'. Their phagocytosis is enhanced, as Fc receptors on macrophages facilitate interaction with the Fc end of the antibody coating the cell bound antigen.
2. Enhanced phagocytosis; as a result of better interaction between C3b and C4b coated host cells and complement receptors CRI and CR3 on the phagocytic cells.

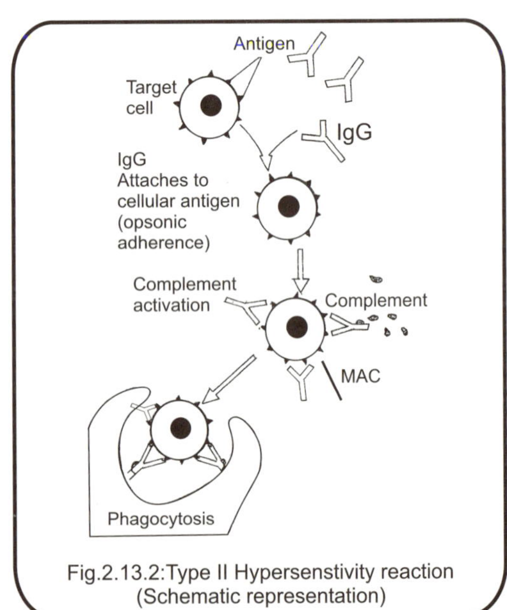

Fig.2.13.2:Type II Hypersenstivity reaction (Schematic representation)

3. Antibody dependent cell mediated cytotoxicity (ADCC), for instance interaction of Fc receptors on NK cells with Fc end of antibody on the antigen coated cell, resulting in enhanced cell destruction.
4. Complement fixing antibodies interacting with antigen and activating classical pathways, which results in formation of membrane attack complex, which can create pores in the bound cell with antigen.

NB: In some infectious diseases; as enteric fever and tuberculosis, antibodies may coat RBC and on subsequent exposure cause their lysis.

Outline the treatment and prevention modalities in the type II hypersensitivity disorders.

A.4 Treatment:

1. Withhold the offending drug: Once the drug is withdrawn, the hemolytic anemia or tissue damage disappears.
2. Plasmapheresis: The offending antibodies can be removed by exchange transfusion, as is done in hemolytic disease of newborn. In this the mother can be treated during pregnancy, using a cell separator machine. In this the machine, separates the mother's blood into two fractions, cells and plasma. The plasma containing the offending antibody (anti-Rh antibody) is discarded and the cells are reintroduced into the mother in a fresh-plasma solution.
3. The immune response may be suppressed with agents; such as corticosteroids.

Prevention:

1. Perform blood grouping, before transfusing blood.
2. Identify individuals hypersensitive to drugs and such individuals should carry identification tag (bracelet to prevent further administration of the same drug)

Integrated Clinical Case Based Study–3

'Serum sickness' a syndrome frequently seen in the pre-antibiotic era, when large doses of horse serum were used to protect individuals passively against infectious diseases; as diphtheria. The name 'serum sickness' was derived from the sickness that was observed in soldiers, after repeated injection of anti tetanus serum (raised in horses) to treat tetanus. Currently serum sickness is rare and may follow usage of some vaccinations and antibiotics (not confuse with drug allergy, which is not mediated immunologically).

What type of reaction is serum sickness? Describe the mechanism.

A.1 (a) It is a type of Type III hypersensitivity disorder (Immune complex mediated).

As the name indicates, these disorders are caused by immune complexes, formed by combination of antigen and antibody. Like type I and type II hypersensitivity disorders, these are caused after sensitization, i.e., when antigen exposure occurs for a second time. Unlike type II hypersensitivity disorder, the antigen here is not cell bound but is usually small and comprises soluble molecules. Another characteristic of this reaction is that they occur, after an exposure to high dose of the antigen, which could occur as a result of persistent infection, repeated exposure from environment or as a result of autoimmune reactivity.

The immune complexes that form in this disease, enter the circulation and are carried throughout the body. These eventually get deposited in blood vessels of the skin, heart, glomeruli of kidney and synovial membrane of joints. Depending on the organ involved, symptoms may be skin rashes, fever, swelling or joints pain. The primary pathology in this syndrome is vasculitis associated with destruction of vascular basement membrane.

The symptoms appear a few days to 2 weeks to appear after the second exposure of an antigen (horse serum in large dose). This syndrome is classified as an immediate type of hypersensitivity disorder as although extended time is taken for the antigen-antibody complexes to form, but once formed, the symptoms occur promptly.

Compare and contrast this syndrome with a type 1 hypersensitivity disorder.

A.1 (b) This syndrome may be contrasted with the type 1 hypersensitivity disorder.

	Type I	**Type III**
Onset	With few minutes	Within few hours to days
Mediated by	IgE	IgG, sometimes IgM
Major cells involved	Mast cells, basophils	Neutrophils
Mediators	Histamine, Leukotrienes, Prostaglandins	C3a, C5a

Give other examples of type III hypersensitivity disorders.

A.2 **Arthrus reaction:** It is a type of localized immune complex disease. It was another syndrome that was identified, in the early twentieth century (pre-antibiotic era) period, when antisera raised in animals were used in human. The syndrome is named after Dr. Arthur. This reaction follows repeated injection of the foreign serum introduced subcutaneously. The injection site becomes red, hot, swollen and painful in a few hours. This reaction is believed to be due to local immune complex deposition on the basement membrane of the blood vessels, which causes a vasculitis reaction mediated primarily by neutrophils.

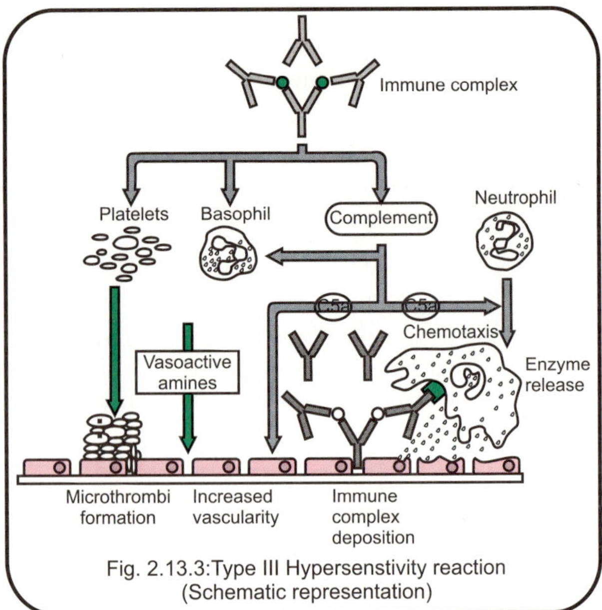

Fig. 2.13.3:Type III Hypersenstivity reaction (Schematic representation)

Other conditions; where circulating immune complexes contribute to pathogenesis of pathogenic conditions include:

- To inhalation of thermophilic actinomycetes – Farmer's lung.

*Post-streptococcal glomerulonephritis, Hepatitis, Infectious mononucleosis, Meningitis and Malaria.

ΔSystemic lupus erythematosus, ΔRheumatoid arthritis, Drug reaction to penicillin and sulfonamides and bacterial endocarditis.

NB: Type III hypersenstivity is also seen in patients, who received monoclonal antibodies of mice origin, the reaction developed was called human anti-mouse antibody response (HAMA).

Δ These entities have an autoimmune disease component also.

* an important component in the pathogenesis of those entities can be persistent and prolonged infectious diseases.

Describe the pathogenesis of type III hypersensitivity disorders.

A.3 When the free antigen enters the body for a second time, it can react with the antibodies to form antigen-antibody complexes (Fig. 2.13.3). Normally, large immune complexes are removed from the circulation in the liver and spleen by the process of phagocytosis. However soluble antigen-antibody complexes (especially in antigen excess) can escape the phagocytosis, penetrate endothelium and get deposited on its basement membrane. The clinical presentation depends on the amount of the complexes that are deposited and their distribution within the body. For instance, a distribution predominantly in the kidney would cause a glomerulonephritis like reaction; whereas a predominant deposition in the lungs would cause a hypersensitivity pneumonitis like reaction. The damage these complexes often cause is because they can fix complement, which elicit various inflammatory responses to eliminate the antigen-antibody complexes. The activated complement pathway, leads to generation of C3a and C5a, which cause mast cell degranulation, their product cause many effects including neutrophil attraction to the site. The neutrophils also get bound to these sites that have CRI receptor, which binds to C3b on the immune-complex. The neutrophils release their hydrolytic enzymes in an attempt to destroy these complexes, but also cause tissue damage that is acute but could become chronic, if antigenemia persists.

NB: The immune complexes adhere to specific antibody receptors on cells of the mononuclear phagocytic system and are engulfed and destroyed intracellularly.

Mention the diagnostic and treatment modalities for type III hypersensitivity disorders.

A.4 **Diagnosis:** Immune complexes can be detected by many techniques (in circulation and in tissues).

1. Immunofluorescence
2. Precipitation and measurement of IgG complex
3. Cryoprecipitation at 4°C

The formation of complexes can also be indicated indirectly by measurement of C3 and C3b levels (indicate complement consumption).

Treatment: The following approaches may be helpful:

1. Suppress immune response, for instance by azathioprine
2. Remove immune complexes by plasmapheresis

NB: Sequentially; different types of hypersensitivity reactions can occur following single antigen administration, for instance following insect bite there may be type I hypersensitive reaction to be followed in few hours by a type III reaction.

Integrated Clinical Case Based Study–4

A newborn mouse was injected with lymphocytic choriomeningitis virus (LCMV, a RNA virus). It remained healthy!! and grew into a healthy adult mouse. The virus got isolated from its tissue during its life without any sign and symptoms. However later, when it was injected intracerebrally with the same virus, the mouse became ill and died within a week. The autopsy revealed oedema and extensive inflammation in the brain with lymphocytic and monocytic infiltrates.

What would appear to be the cause of extensive cell (neuronal) damage and death of the animal?

A.1 It would appear that the cytopathic effect of the virus was responsible for the damage to neuronal cells. However the inflammatory infiltrate in the brain indicates, an immune mechanism to be responsible for the pathology

The above experiment was repeated; immunosuppressing the animal by irradiation, before the second administration of LCMV in the adult stage. The animal now survived happily.

How do you explain the animal remaining healthy?

A.2 It implied that the immunosuppression protected the animal, as the damage by immune mechanism was aborted.

The first experiment was repeated in a neonate mouse, which was thymectomized mice (nude mouse). The animal remained healthy even after the second intracerebral injection of LCMV. However if the second injection was preceded with administration of specific T_H1 lymphocytes to LCMV, the animal died.

What is the role of administration of specific T_{H1} lymphocytes to LCMV in mouse?

A.3 The specific TH1 lymphocytes to LCMV initiate the immune response mechanisms leading to host cell destruction.

How do you explain the ability of sensitized specific lymphocytes (which are often protective) to be harmful (even lethal) in the above experiment?

A.4 When the LCM virus is administered to the mouse, which is thymectomized, then it is not able to initiate a cell mediated immune response against the virus. However the adminstration of specific T_{H1} lymphocytes in the above experiment allows the hypersensitivity reaction.

Describe the evolution of type IV hypersensitivity disorder (concept).

A.5 Initially the type IV hypersensitivity type of reaction was described by Robert Koch in 1890, when he described a cutaneous reaction to mycobacterial antigen called tuberculin reaction. Later on it was found that this type of reaction like type I-III hypersensitivity reactions, also followed a second contact with many antigens (i.e., occurrence in a sensitized individual). This category of reactions were also called *delayed hypersensitivity reactions*, as these followed one to several days, after the second contact with antigen. One should not be mislead by the term hypersensitivity, which could mislead one into believing that their response is always detrimental. In many cases this response plays a key role in defense against intracellular pathogens. Contact dermatitis (not to confuse with atopic dermatitis) follows exposure to numerous agents; as skin cosmetics, jewelry hair dyes, poison ivy (urushiol, an oil from poisonous ivy plant) and elasticized undergarments (are probably the commonest examples of these type of reactions). These reactions are totally *unrelated* to any intrinsic toxicity of the eliciting chemicals, but are mediated by specific pathogenic mechanisms seen in this category of hypersensitivity.

Give an example of a classic human disease demonstrating extensive damage by type IV hypersensitivity reaction. Describe it.

A.6 Tuberculosis lesion; as *pulmonary cavitation*:

A Mantoux negative person contracting tuberculosis usually heals with little pulmonary (tissue) damage. However, if this sensitized person becomes again exposed to TB bacilli, then a type IV hypersensitivity reaction develops in the individual, the response in the lung tissue is much different, from what was initially (first time) a mild reaction. The damage in the lungs is extensive; leading to formation of cavities, and *M.tuberculosis* bacteria not remaining walled off and free to spread in the lungs and throughout the body.

Most individuals, who get *M. tuberculosis* infection the *first* time, remain *asymptomatic*. However, the same individuals *on subsequent* infection with *M. tuberculosis*, a DTH response (instead of being beneficial and protective) develops in the individual, if the antigenemia persists. Continuous secretion of cytokines from activated T_{H1} cells lead to accumulation of large number of macrophages, which may fuse to form giant cells. The formation of a granuloma is an attempt by the body to wall off a site of infection, which when fails leads to significant host tissue destruction; manifesting; as caseation and miliary spread of the infection.

Enumerate important examples of type IV hypersensitivity disorder. Describe tuberculin skin test and Contact dermatitis.

A.7 *Skin test*

- Tuberculin test
- 'Jones Mote' hypersensitivity (cutaneous basophil hypersensitivity)
- Lepromin test (early Fernandez reaction)
- Frei test (Lymphogranuloma venereum)
- Histoplasmosis, Toxoplasmosis
- Viral infections; as Herpes simplex, Mumps

Contact dermatitis

- Drugs – penicillin (topical application)
- Metals in jewelery form (as nickel)
- Chemicals – cosmetics, hair dyes, soap

Granulomatous reaction: Intracellular bacteria; as *M. tuberculosis* (pulmonary cavities developing in a tuberculin sensitive individual), *M. leprae* (Mitsuda reaction). *T. pallidum* (tertiary syphilis)

Intracellular fungi: Candida albicans,Cryptococcus neoformans

Tuberculin skin test:

It is based on the observation of an exaggerated skin reaction to an intradermal administration of tuberculin antigen (purified protein derivative) in an individual, who has been previously infected (exposed) with *M. tuberculosis* organism.

The characteristic skin lesion that develops at the site is described; as an indurated (hard) one, sometimes manifesting erythema. These lesions start developing 12-24 hours of the administration of the antigen and peaks at about 48 hours. It occurs due to initial neutrophil infiltration to be followed later by the mononuclear infiltration (lymphocytes and macrophages) at the site of lesion, which is responsible for the induration. The reaction is mediated by cytokines; as (MIF, MCF) which get released, when the tuberculosis antigen activates T_{H1} cells. This test is often used, as an indicator to know the infection status of concerned person i.e., in the past, if person got exposed to *M tuberculosis* organism (or to the BCG vaccine).

Contact dermatitis:

These occur in individuals to a wide range of substances, when they are exposed to the same substance, a second or a subsequent time. These reactions do not have any hereditary or genetic basis; unlike the atopic dermatitis. The skin lesion may present with itching, redness, papule/blister/eczema formation. It may be appreciated that the site of reaction is epidermal, unlike the delayed hypersensitivity reaction in which it is intradermal.

This reaction usually involves small molecules of the antigen (as drug, metal) combining with the skin antigen and getting internalized by antigen presenting cells of the skin, as Langerhan cells. The processed antigen along with class II MHC molecules activate the sensitized T_{H1} cells, which release various cytokines. Approximately 2-3 days after second exposure of antigen, the secreted cytokines cause macrophages to accumulate at the site. The release of various lytic enzymes from the activated macrophages result in the clinical lesions.

Describe the phases of the DTH response.

A.8 **Phases of delayed type hypersensitivity (DTH) response:** These untoward (undesired) reactions primarily involve the same limb ($CD4^+$ T_H cells of T_{H1} subtype), which is involved in the protective cell mediated responses, which gets mediated by T cells (Fig. 2.13.4). So, then how does one explain the tissue damage that is seen predominantly in this category of reactions? Presumably, the same machinery (that is usually protective), when it encounters the antigen under inappropriate circumstances, can lead to untoward events in the host. Generally, the pathogen is dealt effectively (i.e., destroyed) with minimal host tissue damage, however occasionally the antigen (pathogen) is not easily

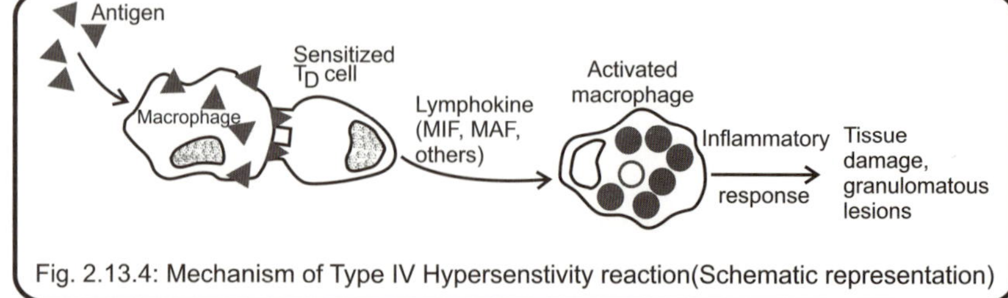

Fig. 2.13.4: Mechanism of Type IV Hypersenstivity reaction(Schematic representation)

cleared and the prolonged type IV response becomes destructive to the host, resulting in a granulomatous reaction. The T cell mediated response may be seen as a double edged sword, with a faint lime existing between the protective and the injurious response. What perpetuates either of the response is not totally clear. Three types of reactions are possible between sensitized T cell (specific antigen reactive) with specific antigen on an APC in host tissue, (i) predominant destruction of the pathogen/antigen with minimal damage to host tissue. This type of response would be desirable to the host and would represent the cell-mediated immune (protective) response (ii) predominantly host tissue damage response. This would represent an undesirable response and would represent the type IV hypersensitivity response (iii) both CMI and type IV hypersensitivity response occurying with varying degree of each.

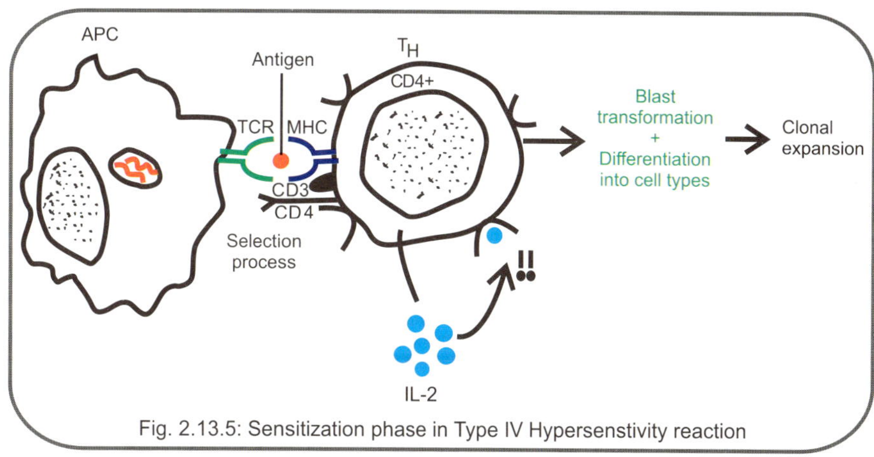

Fig. 2.13.5: Sensitization phase in Type IV Hypersenstivity reaction

There are two phases in this response, namely the sensitization phase and the effector phase. In the *sensitization phase*, primarily the Langerhan cells and macrophages act as the APCs and interact will the $CD4^+$ T_H cells to activate and differentiate them to TH1 cells, which then undergo clonal expansion (Fig. 2.13.5).

The *effector phase* comes into being on subsequent exposure to the same antigen. In this the macrophages are the key effector cells of the DTH response. In this the T_{H1} cells interacting with the macrophages secrete a variety of cytokines; as IFN-γ, TNF-β, IL-2 and MIF that recruit increased macrophages and other nonspecific inflammatory cells to the site. The macrophages are activated and they express increased levels of class II MHC molecules and cell adhesion molecules. The heightened phagocytic activity (manifested also by increased TNF receptors, increased oxygen radicals and increased nitric oxide) helps to clear the pathogens. But if the antigen doesn't clear readily, it can lead to significant inflammatory response; as granuloma formation, which could cause significant host tissue damage.

Describe the patch test and other strategies to diagnose type IV hypersensitivity disorders.

A.9 The diagnosis of contact dermatitis cases is *indicated* by taking the history of the eliciting allergen, for instance the case may give history of shifting to a new type of jewelery.

This role of the suspected allergen can be confirmed by the *patch test*. In it, the piece of gauze impregnated with the suspected allergen is placed on the skin under an adherent dressing. After 48 hours, the dressing is removed and examined for reaction as a reddening, itching or eczema formation, which if present; would indicate a hypersensitive response to the allergen.

Other tests see A6, p. 146

Mention the general approach to control the type IV hypersensitivity disorders.

A.10 Corticosteroids suppresses inflammed region by redistributing lymphocytes to the bone marrow and intravascular space. Antilymphocyte serum and cytotoxic immunosuppressive drugs; as azathioprine can modulate this response.

Aspects related to case theme/examination assessment

Describe Type V hypersensitivity reaction (Stimulatory hypersensitivity)

A.11 It is a *modification* of the type II hypersensitivity reaction, so it is mediated by an antibody. As the name of the reaction indicates, the antibody reacts with the cellular receptor, but instead of inhibiting, it activates the cell. The classic example of this is the *Grave's disease*. Here the 'long acting thyroid stimulator', an antibody against a determinant on the thyroid cell, stimulates excessive production of thyroxine, just as the action of TSH.

individual's B and/or T cells start reacting against the host cells? One of the key theories to explain this phenomenon is the presence of central and peripheral tolerance to self antigens in the healthy individual. According to it, in **central tolerance**, there is deletion of T or B cell clones, before they mature, if they possess receptors that recognize self antigens with a certain affinity (Fig. 2.14.1). This type of tolerance is seen in primary lymphoid organs; as thymus and bone marrow. There is need of **peripheral tolerance** in secondary lymphoid organs; as spleen, lymph nodes etc to deal with self-reactive lymphocytes that may escape central tolerance and get deposited at peripheral sites. Such self reactive lymphocytes are deleted by processes; as apoptosis or rendered inactive by other processes. Some self-reactive lymphocytes can escape both the tiers of regulation and may cause autoimmune disorder, i.e., persistence or development of forbidden clones.

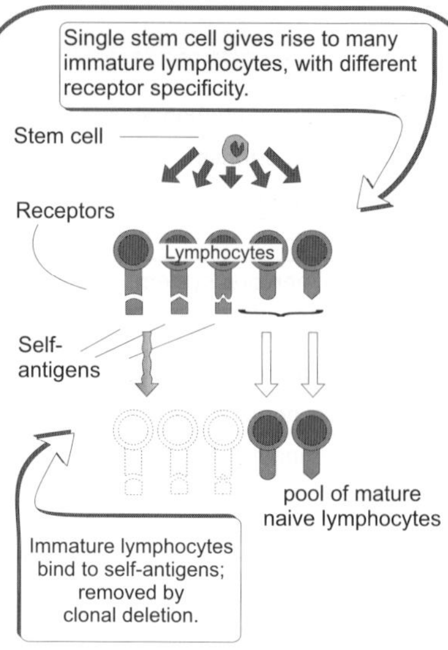

Fig. 2.14.1: Central tolerance theory to explain tolerance to self antigens

Then there is the theory of **sequestered (hidden) antigen**, according to which, if sequestered antigen is released, can cause autoimmune disease. According to it, there are certain immunological privileged sites in the body i.e. where B and/or T cells do not get a chance in the foetal stage to interact with self antigens, hence do not get deleted and/or inactivated. As a result, in later life, when the privileged sites become damaged by trauma and/or inflammation, these antigens are released into circulation and these local sites become target of B and/or T cell activation, example orchitis following vasectomy. As is known that sperms arise late in life, are treated as non-self and the B and/or T cells reactive to these antigen remain intact in the body. So sperms, when get released into circulation, following surgical trauma, initiate inflammation in the testis. Another similar example is the in mumps orchitis, where the viral infection causes damage to the testis. Another example as the sympathetic ophthalmia.[Δ]

Another theory that can have a role in the induction of autoimmunity is **molecular mimicry**. The basis of this is that many bacteria and viruses have antigenic determinants that resemble normal host cell antigens, hence the immune response generated against such microbes, becomes detrimental to the host. A classic example is the heart damage in rheumatic fever following *S. pyogenes* infection. This is believed to be due to antibodies to streptococcal antigen cross-reacting with the heart muscle. Another; example is the neuronal injury, following killed animal vaccine administration (as Rabies). Here the antibodies and activated T cells to the vaccine antigen (sheep brain component) cross react with human neurons. Another; classic example is the myocarditis (heart damage) occurring in Chagas disease following *T. cruzi* infection because of antigenic resemblance between antigenic components of *T. cruzi* and myocardium.

Another theory that has a role in the induction of autoimmune disorders is the **alteration of self antigens** by agents; as some drugs or microbes, which then become the target of the immune system e.g. drug induced anaemia's and thrombocytopenia.

Δ Sympathetic opthalmia: Inflammation of the uveal tract of the uninjured eye (sympathizing eye), some weeks after a wound involving the uveal tract of the other eye (exciting eye).

NB: Clonal anergy – functional suppression of a clone. • Clonal deletion – physical elimination of a clone.

Mention about the role of the cell mediated mechanisms in the occurence of autoimmune disorders.

A.4 (c) Broadly the autoimmune disorders can be mediated by either autoantibodies and/or T cells.

For *T cell mediated mechanisms* to have a role in the mediation of autoimmune disorders, the individual must have MHC molecules and T cell receptors, which are able to bind to self-antigen. Enhanced antigen presenting cell function because of altered co-stimulatory molecules and/or cytokine production, besides presentation of novel/cryptic epitopes can have a role in pathogenicity. Normally there is a balance between Th and Ts cell activity, so an under activity of Ts and over activity of Th can predispose to autoimmune disorders. Some autoimmune disorders that have a significant role of T cell mediation include multiple sclerosis, sympathetic ophthalmia, type I diabetes mellitus and rheumatoid arthritis. In multiple sclerosis and myasthenia gravis, there is evidence of restricted TCR expression.

NB: The classic rheumatoid factor is an auto antibody acting against Fc region of immunoglobulin G.

Describe the various laboratory tests indicative of an autoimmune disorder?

A.5 Making a laboratory diagnosis of an autoimmune disorder is a challenge, as auto antibodies that are indicative of autoimmune disorders are also present in some infections (non-autoimmune disorders). For instance, antinuclear antibodies present in many autoimmune disorders, may also be present in tuberculosis, fungal diseases; as histoplasmosis and many neoplasias; as malignant lymphoma. SLE is associated with antinuclear antibodies and rheumatoid arthritis is associated with rheumatoid factor, however both antibodies may be present in the normal population. In Hashimoto disease, auto antibodies to thyroid cell surface component and in Myasthenia gravis, auto antibodies to acetyleholine receptors on the motor end plates of muscles have been demonstrated. In SLE, antinuclear antibodies, directed against single stranded/double stranded DNA and other nuclear components have been demonstrated. In Indirect immunofluorescent test, staining with serum of SLE cases, elicits characteristic nuclear–staining patterns.

Some general features, indicative of presence of an autoimmune disorder include: (i) presence of various auto antibodies (ii) elevated levels of serum gamma globulins (iii) presence of immune complexes in serum and/or biopsies (tissue) (iv) decreased levels of serum complement (v) depressed levels of Ts cells.

What are the approaches available to treat an autoimmune disorder?

A.6 The aim of the treatment should be to minimize the autoimmune response, maintaining the rest of the immune response intact. However, achieving this state has not always been possible till now, although one is coming closer to this goal. Most of the immunosuppressants; as corticosteroids, azathioprine and cyclophosphamide used currently, only help in controlling the symptoms and do not lead to cure. These drugs suppress the immune system nonspecifically and cannot distinguish between a pathologic autoimmune response and a useful immune response. Because of this, such treated cases remain at risk of developing infections and malignancies. Recently more selective immunosuppressants, as *cyclosporine A and FK506* are available. These agents block signal transduction mediated by T cell receptor in only activated T cells.

In some automimune disorders, metabolic control is curative, as administering injectable B12 in pernicious anaemia cases and thyroid preparations in some thyroid disorders.

Drugs which target some sites that lead to reduction of inflammation have also been useful. For instance drug, as *Enbrel* that block TNFα receptor are widely used and are beneficial in rheumatoid arthritis, Crohn's disease and ankylosing spondylitis. Anakinra (Kineret) that blocks IL-1 receptor has been successfully used in rheumatoid arthritis.

In future monoclonal antibodies that target appropriate MHC molecules may be beneficial by retarding autoimmune response.

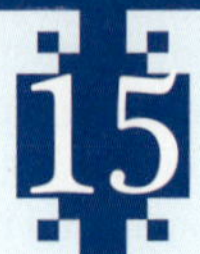

Immunology of Transplantation

- *'Leave a legacy of life. Be an organ donor'*
  - *'The fact is, redefinition of death has been going on ever since organ transplants have become more and more possible and successful'.* — *Jay Boyd*

Forty five year old, Sukhdeep was on renal dialysis for the last four years. Recently, he received a renal transplant from his cousin brother. All functions remained normal for two weeks after the transplantation. But after that, tenderness appeared at the operative site, creatinine levels rose and the renal biopsy revealed increased lymphocytic infiltrates in the renal cortical region.

What type of graft (transplant), has the case received?

A.1 (a) Allograft (graft between two genetically nonidentical members of the same species).

What are the other categories of transplants?

A.1 (b)
- **Autograft:** Graft (tissue/organ) taken from one part of an individual to another site of the same individual, e.g., skin from healthy site to a burns site, saphenous vein from leg to blocked artery in heart (in coronary artery bypass operation)
- **Isograft:** Graft between genetically identical (syngeneic individuals), e.g., monozygotic (identical) twins, inbred strains (as in mice) where sufficient brother/sister mating through generations results in homozygosity in vast majority of >98% of gene loci.
- **Xenograft:** Graft between different species e.g. human being given a pig heart

What are the common transplantations carried out in man?

A.1 (c) The common transplantations include kidney, liver, skin, cornea, bone marrow, heart, lung, small intestine and pancreas.

Which are the common grafts that can be taken from a deceased (dead) person?

A.1 (d) It includes kidney, cornea, liver, small intestine, heart and lung.

How are grafts from deceased donors rapidly transported to the needy individual?

A.1 (e) Depending on circumstances; commercial airplanes, privately chartered jets or air ambulances (helicopters) are used.

What type of clinical graft rejection has occurred in this case?

A.2 (a) It is an acute rejection occurying for the first time.

What are the other types of clinical graft rejections?

A.2 (b) In the *Hyperacute category*, the rejection is so fast that grafted tissue never gets vascularized and the pre-existing antibodies, cause rejection within one day of transplantation. Such antibodies may be present on account of prior transplantation, pregnancy (multiple) and blood transfusions.

In the *chronic category*, the rejection occurs months to years after transplantation, with humoral and cell mediated immune responses participating in the rejection process.

What is allograft rejection?

A.3 (a) *Allograft rejection* refers to the rejection of the graft by the recipient (which has genetical non-identity with the graft tissue). Initially the graft gets vascularized and appears to be accepted but by about the 4th day, gets invaded by the lymphocytes and macrophages. The vascularity in the graft diminishes and by about the 10th day, it gets sloughed off. This event is known as the *first set response* (also first set rejection). Cell mediated mechanisms are responsible for this reaction.

When a second allograft from the same donor is grafted to the sensitized recipient, the graft reaction occurs in an accelerated fashion within 5-6 days. Antibodies play a key role in the graft rejection. This type of rejection is known as 'second set response'.

What is the cause of allograft rejection? Describe transplantation (histocompatibility) antigens present in man.

A.3 **(b)** If the grafted tissue has antigens that are absent in the recipient, then the grafted tissue is recognized as foreign and immune response is generated against the graft, which may result in its rejection. Antigens that may participate in graft rejection are called transplantation or *histocompatibility antigens*. These antigens are specific for each individual and are under genetic control. The term major histocompatibility system refers to a system of cell antigens that play a critical part in the allograft rejection (or acceptance).In man this system is called the human leucocyte antigen (HLA) system.

How important is good matching between donor and recipient in successful transplant action?

A.4 **(a)** A good match improves the survival of the graft, but perhaps not enough to justify the longer period that a patient would have to spend waiting for a well matched transplantation. This scenario has resulted due the availability of the new generation immunosuppressants; as Cyclosporines.

What compatibility is donor and recipient screened for before performing HLA typing?

A.4 **(b)** ABO blood group compatibility is carried out, as blood group antigens are strong histocompatible antigens. This is important in all transplantations.

Describe tissue typing (histocompatibilty testing) techniques commonly performed?

A.4 **(c)** The HLA typing and tissue matching technique identify the HLA antigen on the surface of leucocytes.

(i) *Cytotoxic test* (for class 1&11 antigens)

Lymphocytes of donor in microwells of tissue typing tray

+

Add panel of standard* sera for HLA antigens

↓

Incubate (when lymphocytes have appropriate antigen will react with cytotoxic antisera)

↓

Add rabbit complement

% of cell death is assessed by dye (trypan blue) uptake into cells (dead cells are stained)

*Standard sera are got from a recipient of multiple blood transfusions and multigravida women, who have antibodies to HLA of husband.

(ii) *Mixed lymphocyte reaction*/culture (MLR/MLC)

This reaction detects MHC class II antigens. In it lymphocytes from both donor and recipient are cultured together, i.e., co-cultivated. The test is based on the principle that T lymphocytes, when exposed to incompatible HLA antigen, undergo blast transformation and take up thymidine (radioactive) and divide, which can be measured.

In a common version of the test called one way MLR, the donor cells are irradiated or treated with mitomycin to hinder (destroy) their capacity to divide but remain viable. To the mixture of donor and recipient lymphocytes, radioactive DNA precursor (having tritiated thymidine) is added. After adequate incubation, the radioactivity in the cells is measured by measuring the ratio of average counts per million (cpm) in experimental culture and average cpm in control cells.

Note—One way MLR is most useful, when one set of cells is permitted to respond.

– Control cultures are those in which responder cells are cultured with mitomycin treated cells from same or syngeneic donor.

Mention about immunosuppressant agents used to improve survival of graft?

A.5 These have reduced the long waiting that was previously required for a good matching, which is not totally justified currently, as effective immunosuppressive therapy leads to success. These include steroids (Prednisone, Dexamethasone), mitotic inhibitor drugs; as cyclophosphamide, azathioprine, new generation cyclosporine A (derived from fungus; as *Trichoderma polysporum*), FK-506 and Rapamycin.

Describe graft-versus host (GVH) reaction.

A.6 It is an interesting situation, where the graft (tiny) mounts an attack against the host (large) instead of the common host versus the graft reaction, which occurs usually in a transplantation case.

Such a situation occurs when the host (recipient) does not reject the graft,possesses transplantation antigens absent in the graft and sensitized immunocompetent T cells present in the graft. The allograft is usually not rejected, when specific immunological tolerance has been induced, the host is immunologically deficient or has been immunosuppressed, as in a case of bone marrow transplant.

The immunocompetent T lymphocytes in the graft recognize the (different) MHC antigens of the recipient, get activated and produce an immune response mediated by lymphokines, cytotoxic T cells and antibodies. This leads to the *GVH reaction*, which is primarily cell mediated. In animals; this syndrome is called *'runt disease'* and is characterized by growth retardation, emaciation, hepatosplenomegaly, anaemia and sometimes death.

Aspect related to case theme/examination assessment

Discuss the concept of tumor immunology including immune surveillance and tumor antigens.

A.7 **Tumor immunology** is an interesting concept because if it is true, then the immune response can be exploited to prevent and cure malignancies.

Concept: When a cell is transformed to a malignant one, it may acquire new antigens (including on surface) and may lose some constitutional antigens. Due to this phenomenon, the tumor mass may be immunologically distinct from the normal tissue mass. Hence the tumor may be considered as an allograft by the body and an immune response may be generated against it.

Clinical evidence:

(i) Cases are on record, where a tumor regressed spontaneously. In it, an immune response is likely to have played an role.

(ii) Initiation of chemotherapy leading to complete cure. In such a scenario, immune response may be playing a major role.

(iii) Post mortem records often document tumors that were never mentioned by the case; when alive, indicating that immune response may have been responsible for keeping them in check.

(iv) A high rate of malignancies have been reported in cases, that have malignancies or disease (infectious) of the immune system; as AIDS; implying inability of the immune system to conduct optimal immunological surveillance. The concept of **immune surveillance** was first proposed by Paul Ehrlich, a German scientist.

Tumor antigens: The tumor antigens; against which the immune response is generated can be classified into two categories, namely Tumor specific antigens (TSAs) and Tumor associated antigens (TAAs).

Tumor specific antigens, as the name indicates are antigens present only on the tumor cells and not on the normal cells. TSAs of viral induced tumors are virus specific.

Tumor associated transplantation antigens (TAAs) are present both on the tumor and the normal cells. These can be categorized into:

(i) Tumor associated carbohydrate antigens, e.g., some pancreatic and breast cancers.

(ii) Oncofetal antigen-present on embryonic and malignant cells but not in normal adult cells, e.g., Alpha-fetoprotein (AFP) in hepatomas and carcinoembryonic antigen (CEA) in some colonic cancers.

(iii) Differentiation antigens, e.g., Prostrate specific antigen (PSA) in prostatic malignancies.

Immune response: Both specific and non-specific immune defense mechanisms participate in the response against the tumor cells. Notable amongst it is the NK cell activity, antibody dependent cellular cytotoxicity (ADCC) and cytotoxic mediated immunity (CD8) of the cell-mediated immunity. The key cytotoxic factors include tumor necrosis factor (TNF).

Challenges: Immune response against tumors may be unsuccessful due to many reasons:

(i) Poor immunogenicity of the tumor, resulting in ineffective immune response

(ii) Masking of the tumor antigens by substances; as sialomucin

(iii) Immunosuppression by tumor cells (activation of Ts cells) and production of blocking antibodies.

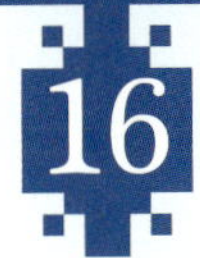

Immunodeficiency Diseases and Evaluation of Immune Status

A two year old male child Shitij, presented with history of repeated bacterial and fungal infections. Routine investigations are within normal limits.

What is your differential diagnosis?

A.1 **(a)** (i) Immunoglobulin deficiency

(ii) Complement deficiency

(iii) Other lymphoid cell disorder

(iv) Myeloid cell disorder affecting phagocytic function; as Chronic granulomatous disease

(v) AIDS.

Classify the immunodeficiency syndromes.

A.1 **(b)**

Table 2.16.1: Classification of Immunodeficiency syndromes

PRIMARY (resulting from genetic or developmental defects)
A. *Humoral immunodeficiencies* (B cell defects)
(i) X-linked agammaglobulinemia (Bruton's disease), all classes of immunoglobulins depleted
(ii) Transient hypogammaglobulinemia of infancy (is only a delay)
(iii) Common variable immunodeficiency (manifests late in life)
(iv) Selective immunoglobulin immunodeficiency (for instance only IgA deficiency)
(v) Immunodeficiencies with hyper – IgM (elevated IgM and low IgA and IgG, associated with infections)
(vi) Transcobalmin II deficiency (signs of vitamin B12 deficiency observed)
B. *Cellular immunodeficiencies* (T cell defects)
(i) Thymic hypoplasia (Di-George's syndrome)-developmental defect
(ii) Chronic mucocutaneous candidiasis
(iii) Purine nucleoside phosphorylase deficiency (PNP)
C. *Combined immunodeficiencies* (B and T cell defects)
(i) Cellular immunodeficiency with abnormal Ig synthesis (Nezelof syndrome)
(ii) Ataxia telangectasia (autosomal recessive disorder associated with cerebellar ataxia and telangectasia)
(iii) Wiskott-Aldrich syndrome (X-linked recessive disease)
(iv) Severe combined immunodeficiencies (deficiencies of both humoral and cell mediated immunity)
D. *Disorders of complement*
(i) Complement component deficiencies
(ii) Complement inhibitor deficiencies (refer the clinical problem at pg. 120)
E. *Disorders of phagocytosis*
(i) Chronic granulomatous disease (refer to current clinical problem)
(ii) Myleoperoxidase deficiency (deficiency of myeloperoxidase observed)-see A6, p.168
(iii) Chediak-Higashi syndrome (autosomal recessive disorder)
(iv) Leucocyte G6PD deficiency (deficiency of Glucose-6 Phosphate dehydrogenase in leucocytes)
(v) Job's syndrome see A 6, p. 168
(vi) Tuftsin deficiency
SECONDARY (acquired loss of immune function to disease states; as malignancy, malnutrition and others)
(i) Depression of humoral immunity
(ii) Depression of cell-mediated immunity

A thorough investigation of the case revealed the case to be HIV non reactive with immunoglobulin and complement levels to be within normal range.

What is your presumptive diagnosis?

A.2 Chronic granulomatosus disease (CGD)

What test can help to support diagnosis of CGD?

A.3 (a) Nitroblue tetrazolium (NBT) reduction test

What is the basis of this test?

A.3 (b) The leucocytes of the CGD cases have an approximate 50% reduction in the ability to reduce NBT.

Is the phagocytic function normal in CGD cases?

A.3 (c) The phagocytes of these cases can phagocytose normally the bacteria but cannot effectively kill the microbes.

CGD cases usually succumb to infections caused by less virulent microbes but are able to resist virulent organism as Neisseria spp. and S. pneumoniae. How can this be explained?

A.4 Organisms; as *S. pneumoniae* produce H_2O_2 but lack catalase (to reduce H_2O_2), hence the microenvironment of these phagocytes provide an environment that can lyse microbes. The feebler organisms have high level of catalase, so their level of H_2O_2 is minimal.

How do you therapeutically approach a case of CGD?

A.5 Adminstration of IFN-r has been seen to restore the function of granulocytes and monocytes of CGD cases.Antimicrobials may have to be often administered and surgical drainage of abscesses performed; whenever necessary.

Aspects related to case theme/examination assessment

Describe Myeloperoxidase deficiency and Job's syndrome.

A.6 **Myeloperoxidase deficiency:** It is a disease associated with deficiency of enzyme myeloperoxidase in leucocytes, involved in lysis of microbes. The disease often goes unnoticed, as other microbicidal mechanisms in the cell may compensate for this deficiency. However these individuals are susceptible to candidiasis.

Job's syndrome: It is an autosomal dominant hyper-IgE syndrome, affecting several body systems; especially the immune system. It is believed due to be due to decreased production of interferon gamma by the helper T cells. Elevated IgE levels in the serum is a hallmark of this disease. Recurrent staphylococcal infection is common in this condition.

What are secondary immunodeficiencies? Enumerate common causes.

A.7 These immunodeficiencies are designated such; as these occur secondary to many conditions and if these are corrected, the deficiency also gets reversed. The factors associated with these are diverse including malnutrition, infections, metabolic disorders, drug therapy and X-ray irradiation. The secondary immunodeficiencies are more common than the primary immunodeficiencies.

These deficiencies can be categorized either due to impairment of the humoral immune response or due to impairment of the cell mediated immunity. In the former category; the common causes include lymphoid malignancy (as chronic lymphatic leukemia), multiple myeloma (abnormal immunoglobulins get produced) and nephrotic syndrome (increased loss of immunoglobulins). Amongst the latter category, the common causes are AIDS, Hodgkins's lymphoma and lepromatous leprosy. Acquired immunodeficiency syndrome is a very common condition in this category, the details of it may be seen in chapter 15, pages 484-496.

Give two animal experimental models of immunodeficiency.

A.8 The animal models form an important resource in the study of immunodeficiency diseases. Two of the common genetically altered animals include *nude mouse* and *severe combined immunodeficiency (SCID) mouse*. The nude mouse lacks cell-mediated immunity and is unable to synthesize the antibodies to most of the antigens. The SCID mouse has been named, due to its resemblance to the human severe combined immunodeficiency. This model is useful in studies of cellular immunology; especially graft studies. The details are beyond the undergraduate curriculum.

Outline the tests commonly performed in the evaluation of host defense status in an individual.

A.9 *Initial screening*

- Complete blood count with differential smear
- Serum immunoglobulin levels including IgM, IgA, IgG and others

Other assays

- Quantification of blood mononuclear cells (markers used)
  T cells-CD2, CD3, CD4, CD8
  B cells-CD 20, CD21
  NK cells-CD16
- T cell functional assays
  DTH skin tests (with PPD, Candida etc.)

Proliferative response to mitogens (as PHA, Concanavalin)

- B cell functional assay
  Natural and commonly acquired antibodies (to influenza, DT, TT)
- *Complement levels*
  C3, C4
  CH 50
- *Phagocyte function*
  Reduction of nitroblue tetrazolium
  Chemotaxis assay
  Bactericidal assays

What is the basic approach in treating immunodeficiency disorders?

A.10 One has to initially characterize the immunodeficiency. If it is a secondary type, then the precipitating factor has to be dealt with. For example, if it is severe nutritional deficiency, then one has to correct it. If it is a severe infection, antimicrobials have to be administered.

If there is a deficiency of lymphocyte cell function, transfer factor therapy or bone marrow transplantation may be beneficial.

Section II: Immunology

17 Assessment/Examination Questions

Chapter 1

1. What makes the study of immunology so exciting? A 1a., p. 93
2. Give an example to illustrate how immunologic principles was even practiced by Kings in olden times. A 2a., p. 93
3. Describe briefly contribution of Edward Jenner A1b,c., p. 93

Chapter 2

1. Describe innate response and the role of anatomical, physiological, biological substances and cellular barriers in it. Vignette, A 2a,c., p. 96
2. Describe NK cells. A 4a., p. 99
3. Describe T cell receptor A 4a., p. 99
4. What is acute phase response? Describe how C reactive protein help in providing innate response? A 5., p. 100
5. Discuss the role of pattern recognition receptors (PRRs) and pathogen-associated molecular patterns (PAMPs) in providing innate immunity. A 6c., p. 100-101
6. Describe signal conduction pathway. A 7., p. 101

Chapter 3

1. Define immune response and describe its characteristics. A 1., p. 102
2. Tabulate the differences between innate, active and passive immunity. A 5., p. 104
3. Depict the activities associated with spectrum of immune reactivity. A 4., p. 103-104
4. Describe immunological tolerance and give classic examples. A 2a, e; p 102-103
5. Depict diagrammatically in detail the process of immune response. A 3b., p. 103
6. What is herd immunity? Discuss its possible role in outbreak causation. A 6., p. 104-105

Chapter 4

1. Define antigen. A 1., p. 106
2. What are the two key properties of antigen? Describe with special reference to haptene. A 2., p. 106
3. Describe the factors affecting antigenicity. A 4., p. 107-109
4. Describe briefly Forsmann antigen, superantigen and heterophile antigen. A 4., p. 109, A 11., p. 110
5. Describe adjuvant, including its inclinical application emphasizing their role in immune response. A 4., p. 108
6. Describe antigen presenting cells A 11, 12., p. 110

Chapter 5

1. Enumerate the various classes of immunoglobulins. Describe the structure and properties of IgG, IgM, IgA and IgE. A 4b., p. 112-114
2. Diagrammatically depict IgG, IgM and IgA. Fig. 2.5.3a, 2.5.4, 2.5.5., p. 112-113
3. Diagrammatically illustrate the development of B cell and formation of immunoglobulins. A 4a., p. 112
4. Describe the three levels of immunoglobulin antigenic determinants namely isotypic, allotypic and idiotypic. A 5., p. 114-115
5. Diagrammatically illustrate the mechanisms by which immunoglobulns act in the body. A 6-7., p. 115-116

Chapter 6

1. Describe monoclonal antibody, including a line diagram depicting its synthesis. A 3a, b, A4., p. 117-118

2. Enumerate the drugs based on monoclonal antibodies that are in clinical usage Table 2.7.1., p. 119
3. Compare and contrast the terms monoclonal antibody and polyclonal antiserum A 3a., p. 118

Chapter 7

1. Describe the classical complement pathway. A 6b., p. 122.123
2. Describe the alternate complement pathway. A 6b., p. 122
3. Write briefly on the lectin complement pathway. A 6b., p. 122
4. What are the key functions of the complement? A 5., p. 121
5. Enumerate the key complement deficiency diseases and associated syndromes. A 6c., p. 123

Chapter 8

1. What are the features of the antigen antibody reaction? Define the terms affinity, avidity, sensitivity and specificity with reference to antigen-antibody based tests. A 2b, A 5., p. 124-125.
2. Describe the prozone phenomenon and mention its importance. Vignette, A 2b, A 3., p. 124-125
3. Enumerate the stages of interaction in the antigen antibody reactions and give examples. A 6b., p. 125
4. Define precipitation reaction and mention the various categories; giving examples. Mention the difference of this category of reaction from the agglutlnation reactions. A 7a, b., p. 126-127, and A10a., p. 130
5. Describe VDRL test, radial immunodiffusion, Oucterlony's procedure (Elek's test for toxigenicity of *C. diphtheriae*), rocket electrophoresis, immunoelectrophoresis and Immunoelectroblot (Western blot technique) Vignette p. 125, A 7b., p. 126, 127, A16, p. 134
6. Mention about radioimmunoassay and its current status. A 7c., p. 128
7. Describe ELISA test with special reference to the common types with their usage A 8., p. 128-130
8. Briefly describe the immunofluorescence tests mentioning the difference between the direct and the indirect IFAT. A 9., p. 130-131
9. Define agglutination reactions and mention the various categories giving examples. Mention the difference between flocculation and the agglutination reactions. A 10a, b., p. 130-133
10. Write briefly on latex agglutination reaction, coagglutination, Coomb's test, Rose–Waaler test and conglutination test. A 10b., p. 132.
11. Describe Complement function test including its current status. A 11-12., p. 133-134
12. Categorize the various types of neutralization reactions; giving examples. A. 13., p. 134
13. Describe the chemiluminescence immunoassays. A. 14., p. 134

Chapter 9

1. Describe the two key theories to explain antibody production. A 9., p. 136-137
2. Describe the pathway involved in activation of the resting B cell to the synthesis of antibody. A 7-8., p. 136
3. Describe the primary and secondary immune responses and tabulate the differences between the two. A 11., p. 137-138
4. Enumerate and describe the factors affecting the antibody production. A 12., p. 138-139
5. Describe humoral immunity, including immunosuppressive agents. A 11-12, p. 137-139
6. Describe clonal selection theory. A 9., p. 136

Chapter 10

1. How are cytokines defined and mention their differences from interleukins and hormones? A 1, 2, p. 140
2. What are the key cells involved in cytokine synthesis? Mention their key attributes. Illustrate the action of cytokines diagrammatically. A 4a, b, c., p. 141
3. How are cytokines classified? Enumerate the cytokines involved in adaptive immunity and mention their key functions. A 5a, 4b., p. 141
4. Enumerate examples of cytokine related diseases and mention some important diseases in which cytokines play a role. A 5b, 5c., p. 141

Chapter 11

1. Diagrammatically illustrate the HLA complex, depicting the three MHC classess, genes and gene products. A 2., p. 143
2. Describe the characteristics, transport and evolutionary significance of MHC molecules. A 3., p. 142-143
3. What is MHC restriction? Describe its relevance. A 3., p. 143

Chapter 12

1. What is the need of a cell mediated immune defense mechanism? Mention the reason for terming this type of immunity; as cell mediated? A 2 b,c., p. 144
2. What are the steps involved in induction of CMI with reference to tuberculosis? Describe the processes of primary and secondary CMI response. A 5., p. 145-146
3. Enumerate and describe the tests to evaluate CM (delayed hypersensitivity) A 6., p. 146
4. Describe transfer factor. A 2d., p. 144-145

Chapter 13

1. Classify the hypersensitivity disorders and tabulate the differences between them. A 5., p. 149
2. Classify type I hypersensitivity disorders. A 6., p. 149-150
3. Describe clinical aspects of generalized anaphylaxis. A 8., p. 151-152
4. Describe pathogenesis and mediators of generalized hypersensitivity reactions. A 7., p. 152-153
5. Describe briefly Atopic disorders, Prausnitz-Kustner reaction and Schultz–Dale reaction. A 9, All., p. 152-153
6. Describe common localized type I hypersensitivity disorders. Table 2.13.2., p. 150 and A 9., 152
7. Describe desensitization. A 13., p. 154
8. Describe type II hypersensitivity disorders. Vignettle A1-A4., p. 154-155
9. Write briefly on arthrus reaction. A 2., p. 156
10. Describe serum sickness. A 1a., p. 155
11. Describe the pathogenesisof type III hypersensitivity disorders. A 3., p. 156
12. Describe type IV hypersensitivity disorders. Vignettle, A 5, 6., p. 157
13. Enumerate disorders related to type IV hypersensitivity disorders with special reference to contact hypersensitivity. A 7., p. 158
14. Describe tuberculin reaction. A 7., p. 158
15. Describe pathogenesis of type IV hypersensitivity disorders A 8., p. 158-159
16. Describe stimulatory hypersensitivity disorders. A 11., p. 159

Chapter 14

1. Define autoimmune disorders. Enumerate the autoimmune diseases mediated primarily by autoantibodies and mention the mechanism of action of these antibodies (pathogenesis). A 1a, A2., p. 160-161
2. Mention about the role of cell mediated mechanisms in the pathogenesis of autoimmune disorders. A 4c., p. 162
3. How are autoimmune disorders classified according to organ specific and non organ specific (localized) diseases. Table 2.14.1., p. 161
4. Describe the various theories to explain the occurrence of autoimmune antibodies. A 4b., p. 161-162
5. What is molecular mimicry and mention the role of sequestered antigens in autoimmunity. A 4b., p. 162
6. Describe Hashimoto's disease, Systemic lupus erythematosus, Rheumatoid arthritis, Grave's disease and Myaesthenia gravis. A 3., p. 161

Chapter 15

1. Define the various types of transplants. Describe the features of allograft rejection. A 1b, A 3a., p. 164-165
2. What is major histocompatibilty complex and mention the various histocompatibilty antigens. A 4c., p. 165
3. Describe the procedures for histocompatibility testing/Methods of HLA testing. A 4b, c., p. 165-166
4. Describe briefly Graft-versus hist reaction (GVH). A 6., p. 165-166
5. Describe briefly immunotherapy of cancer. A 7., p. 166
6. Enumerate and describe various tumor antigens. A 7., p. 166
7. Write briefly on tumor escape mechanisms and immunosurveillance. A 7., p. 166

Chapter 16

1. What are immunodeficiency diseases? Classify them and mention about differences between primary and secondary immunodeficiencies. A 1b., p. 167
2. Enumerate primary immunodeficiency disorders based on defects of phagocytosis and describe chronic granulomatous syndrome; including its diagnosis and treatment. Table 2.16.1 and A2-A5., p. 167-168
3. Describe primary immunodeficiency disorders based on combined B and T cell defects. Table 1.16.1., p. 167
4. Describe chronic granulomatous disease, Myeloperoxidose deficency and Job's syndrome A 2, A 6., p. 168

Section III: Gram Positive Cocci

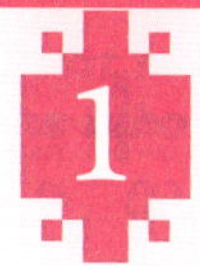

Classification, Metabolic and Microscopic Features of Gram Positive Cocci (GPC)

Algorithm for identification of Gram positive cocci

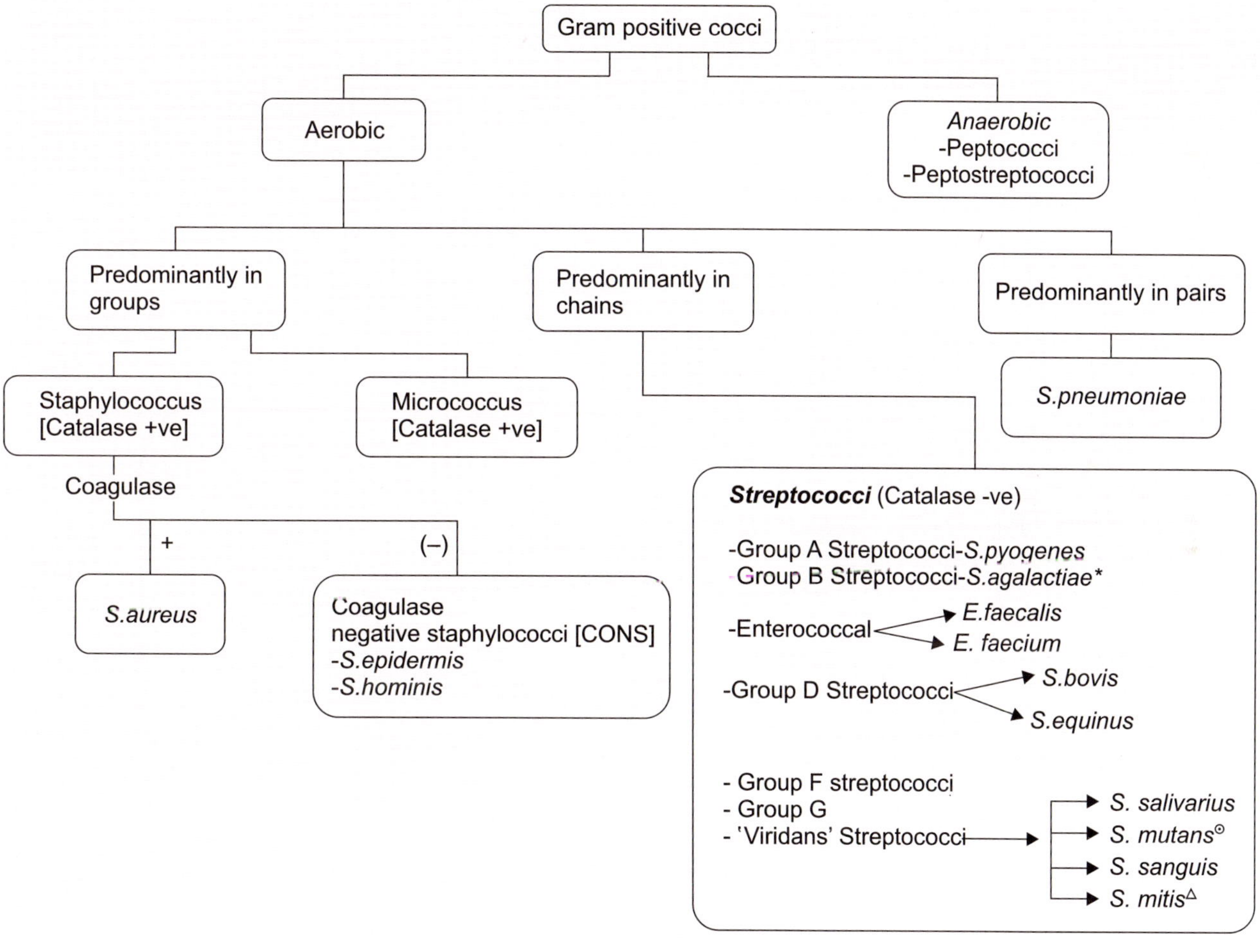

- Gram positive cocci
  - Aerobic
    - Predominantly in groups
      - Staphylococcus [Catalase +ve]
        - Coagulase
          - + → *S.aureus*
          - (–) → Coagulase negative staphylococci [CONS]
            - -*S.epidermis*
            - -*S.hominis*
      - Micrococcus [Catalase +ve]
    - Predominantly in chains
      - ***Streptococci*** (Catalase -ve)
        - -Group A Streptococci-*S.pyogenes*
        - Group B Streptococci-*S.agalactiae**
        - -Enterococcal → *E.faecalis*; *E. faecium*
        - -Group D Streptococci → *S.bovis*; *S.equinus*
        - - Group F streptococci
        - - Group G
        - - 'Viridans' Streptococci → *S. salivarius*; *S. mutans*[⊙]; *S. sanguis*; *S. mitis*[△]
    - Predominantly in pairs
      - *S.pneumoniae*
  - *Anaerobic*
    - -Peptococci
    - -Peptostreptococci

* agalactia = 'want of milk' original isolate caused bovine mastitis.
⊙ mutans = 'changing' cocci may appear rodlike (initially), when isolated from culture.
△ mitis = 'mild' falsely thought to cause mild infection

Metabolic and Microscopic Features of Gram Positive Cocci

Organism	Growth Requirements							Cellular Morphology and Staining Characteristics					
	O2 Requ.	Optimal	CO2	Incubation Period			Shape	Gram	Arrangement	Capsule	Motility	Spore	Special Staining/ microscopy/Special Features
		Temp.	Requ.	Days	Weeks	Months							
Staphylococcus aureus	Facultative anaerobic	37°C	–	1	–	–	Cocci	+ve	In clusters (Fig. 3.1.1)	+ (many)	–	–	–
Micrococcus sps	Strictly aerobic	37°C	–	1	–	–	Cocci	+ve	In small groups of four/eights	–	–	–	–
Streptococcus pyogenes (group A)	Facultative anaerobic	37°C	+	1	–	–	Cocci	+ve	In short/long chains	+	–	–	–
Peptoccoccus niger	Strictly anaerobic	37°C	–	Few	–	–	Cocci	+ve	In singles/pars/ clumps	–	–	–	–
Peptostreptococcus sps.	Strictly anaerobic/aerotolerant (some strains	37°C	–	5	–	–	Cocci	+ve	–	–	–	–	–
Sarcinia sps.	Strictly anaerobic	37°C	–	Few	–	–	Cocci	+ve	In groups of 8 or more.	–	–	–Δ	–
Streptococcus agalactiae (group B Streptococci)	Facultative anaerobe	37°C	–	1	–	–	Cocci	+ve	In short chains	+	*–	–	–
Enterococcus sps. (group D strept)	Facultative anaerobe	37°C	–	1	–	–	Cocci	+ve	Oval cocci in pairs and short chains	±	–*	–	–
Streptococcus 'viridans'	Facultative anaerobe (some microaerophilic)	37°C	+	1	–	–	Cocci	+ve	In short chains	–	–	–	–
Streptococcus pneumoniae	Facultative anaerobic	37°C	+	1/typcal mophology may take few days	–	–	Cocci (lanceolate shaped in pairs with broad end opposite) (Fig. 3.1.2a,b)	+ve	In pairs	+	–	–	–

* Enterococci are non-motile except *E. gallinarum* and *E. casseliflavus*

Δ In Sarcinia spores reported, but not usually seen.

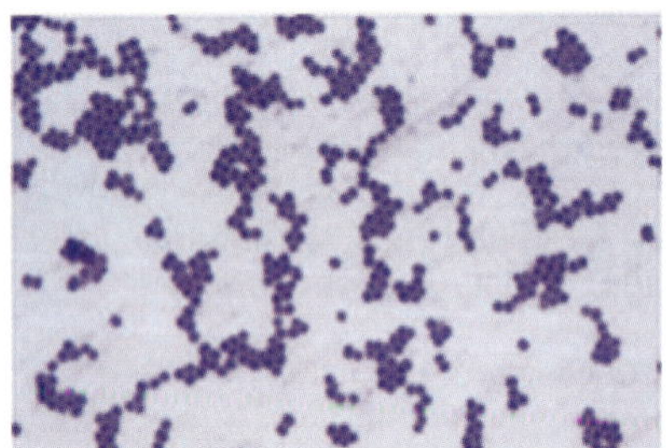

Fig. 3.1.1: Gram positive cocci: Gram stained smear demonstrating gram positive cocci in pairs, tetrads and small clusters

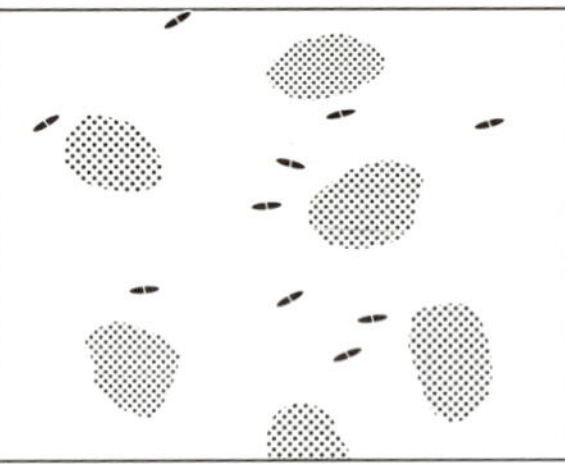

Fig. 3.1.2(a):Diplococci;Schematic representation of gram positive cocci in pairs with broad ends facing each other and pointed ends facing outwards

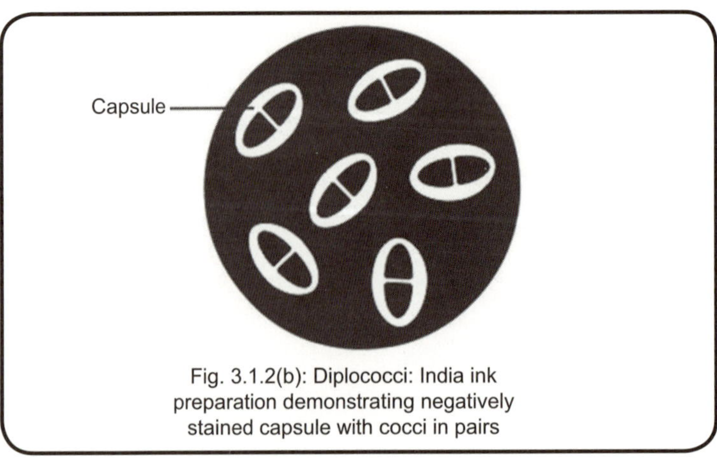

Fig. 3.1.2(b): Diplococci: India ink preparation demonstrating negatively stained capsule with cocci in pairs

An Overview of the Media Requirements, Colonial Characters and Diagnostic Characteristics of Key Gram Positive Cocci

	Basal	Enriched	Selective / indicator	Characterization & confirmation of isolate
S. aureus	Nutrient agar: large, golden yellow, circular colonies	Blood agar: large, β. haemolytic colonies (Fig. 3.2.1)	- Mannitol-salt agar - Salt milk agar & broth containing 8-10% NaCl - Ludlam's medium containing LiCl, tellurite & polymyxin Above three media used for isolating bacteria from specimens; as faeces - MacConkey: Tiny lactose positive colonies	- Smear & staining characteristic - Catalase test (Fig. 1.9.10) (+) - Coagulase test (Fig. 3.2.2) (+) - Mannitol fermentation (+) - DNase production (+) - Phosphatase production (+) - Glucose metabolism (fermentative) - Presence of teichoic acid (+) - Phage typing

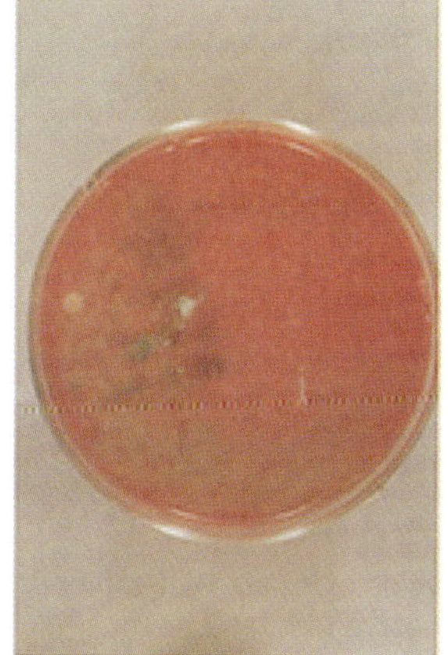

Fig.3.2.1: Pin head, large (2-4 mm) haemolytic colonies of *S.aureus*

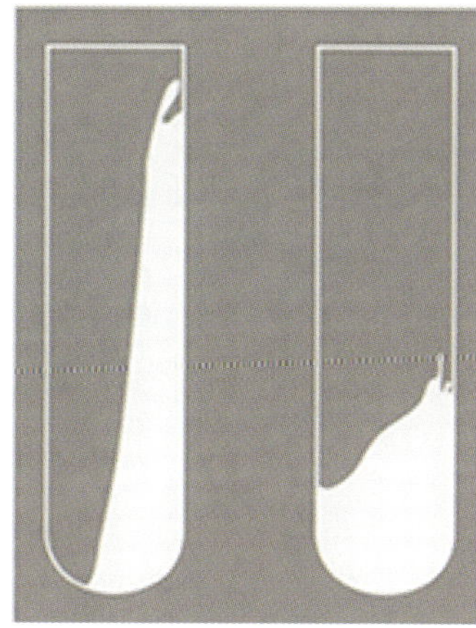

Fig.3.2.2: Tube coagulase test

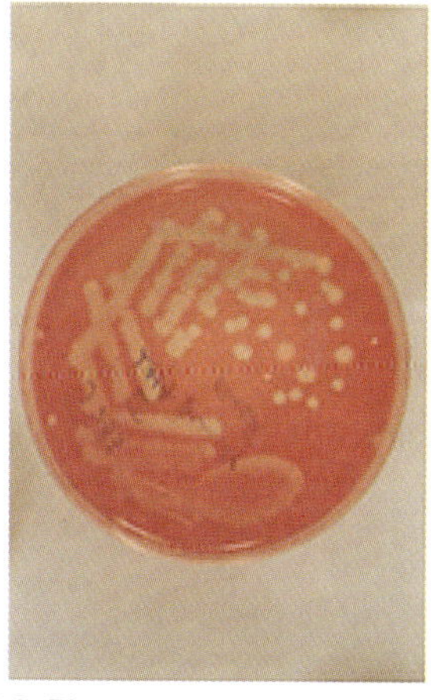

Fig.3.2.3: Pin point colonies on Blood agar: Small colonies (1-2 mm) beta haemolytic colonies of *S.pyogenes* on blood agar

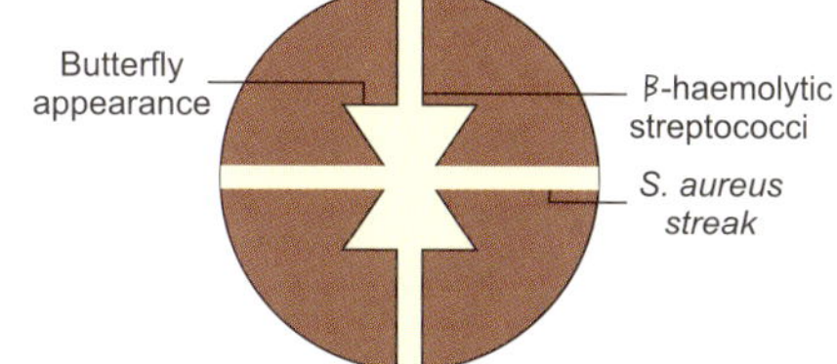

Fig. 3.2.4:CAMP test:Arrow head suggestive of Group B streptococci. CAMP test named after Christie, Atkins and Munch –Petersen. It is based on the production of CAMP factor by Group B streptococci that enhance lysis of sheep erythrocytes by staphylococcal B- lysin (evident as arrow head haemolysis, when group B streptococcus is inoculated at right angles to *S. aureus* streak on blood agar plate)

	Basal media; as Nutrient agar	Enriched media	Selective/ others	Characterization and confirmation of isolation
S. pyogenes [*Group A Streptococcus*]	No growth (poor)	• Blood agar: small pin-point, β haemolytic colonies (Fig. 3.2.3) • In serum/glucose broth, growth appears as granular turbidity	• Crystal violet blood agar: growth +ve (medium inhibits other gram positive cocci) • MacConkey: No growth (NG)	• Smear & staining characteristics • Catalase: negative • Ferments sugars producing acid only (no gas) • Bacitracin sensitive • Presence of group A antigen • Hydrolysis of pyrrolidonyl napthalamide (PYR test) • M-typing (about 100 Griffith types) • T. typing • Not ferment ribose (helps to differentiate *S.pyogenes* from other streptococci)
S. agalactiae [*Group B Streptococcus*]	Poor growth	Blood agar: β haemolytic colonies	-	• Hippurate hydrolysis +ve • CAMP test +ve (Fig. 3.2.4)
Enterococcus spp.	Grow easily	Blood agar: Usually non-haemolytic	On MacConkey: tiny pink colonies	• Bile aesculin hydrolysis test +ve, PYR test +ve • Heat resistant (60°C – 30 mins) • Ability to grow at 45°C and in presence of 6.5% NaCl • Resistant to trimethoprim – sulfamethoxazole
S. 'viridians'	Easily grow	Good growth	-	• Catalase: negative • Facultative anaerobe • Alpha haemolysis (often)
S. pneumoniae	NG (scanty growth)	Blood agar: haemolytic, dome shaped colonies, which later become flat with central umbonation (draughtsman colony) Chocolate agar: +ve (growth)	• MacConkey- NG • Mice intraperitoneal inoculation (rarely performed, if organism expected to be scanty in specimen, animal dies in 1-3 day) (isolate organism from various sites)	• Catalase: negative • Optochin sensitive • Bile soluble • Ferments inulin • Pathogenic to animal (animal pathogenicity test +ve) • Ferments several sugars with acid but no gas (Hiss's serum water / agar slopes) • Typing of isolate with appropriate antisera (routinely not possible, nor required)

Clinical (Pathogenicity) Profile of Infection Caused by Gram Positive Cocci

ORGANISM			
Staphylococcus aureus	Invasive	• Superficial	As pustules, folliculitis, boils, carbuncles, styes, impetigo, abscesses, furuncle (Fig. 3.3.1) cellulitis (Fig. 3.3.2) • Case: pgs 179-182
		• Deep	Osteomyelitis, pneumonia, empyema and others
	Toxinoses	• Food poisoning • Toxic shock syndrome • Scalded skin syndrome	
S. epidermidis	Opportunistic pathogen in prosthetic devices; as urinary catheters, prosthetic valves		
S.saprophyticus	Urinary tract infection in sexually active females and an opportunistic pathogen		
Micrococcus sps.	rarely opportunistic infections		
Streptococcus pyogenes (group A Streptococci) (Fig. 3.3.3)	Suppurative	Local	Sore throat (pharyngitis), pyoderma (localized skin infection with vesicles/pustules) Case: pgs 188-193
		Spreading	Impetigo, Erysipela (Fig. 3.3.3), Scarlet fever, necrotizing fascitis, cellutitis
		Others	Puerperal infection, sepsis, wound infection, abscesses
	Non suppurative (post streptococcal sequelae)	• Acute Rheumatic fever • Acute glomerulonephritis	
Peptococcus niger	Skin, soft tissue, respiratory tract and female genita tract infections		
Streptococcus agalactiae (group B Streptococci)	New born (infants)	• Early birth onset-sepsis, pneumonia and meningitis (few days to a week of birth)	
		• Late onset syndrome (occurs 3-8 weeks after birth) Often nosocomial, has decreased complications	

Contd.

Contd.

Adults	• Puerperal infection and infections associated with gyanecologic surgery and abortion
Streptococcus groups C,G. and *S. dysgalactiae*	• Respiratory infection , skin infections, endocarditis, meningitis
Enterococcus sps.	• Urinary tract & biliary tract infections, Septicaemia, endocarditis & intra-abdominal infections • Case: pg 193
Streptococcus group F, G (*S. anginosus* group)	• Abscesses
Streptococcus 'viridans' (S. *mutans*, *S. salivarius*, *S. mitis*)	• Subacute bacterial endocarditis (associated with 'salivarius and 'mitis), Dental caries (associated with 'mutans'), Brain and liver abscess • Case: pg 195
Streptococcus pneumoniae	• Pneumonia (Lobar) & bronchopneumonia, meningitis (all ages), sinusitis, otitis media, arthritis, septicaemia and others • Case: pgs 196-198

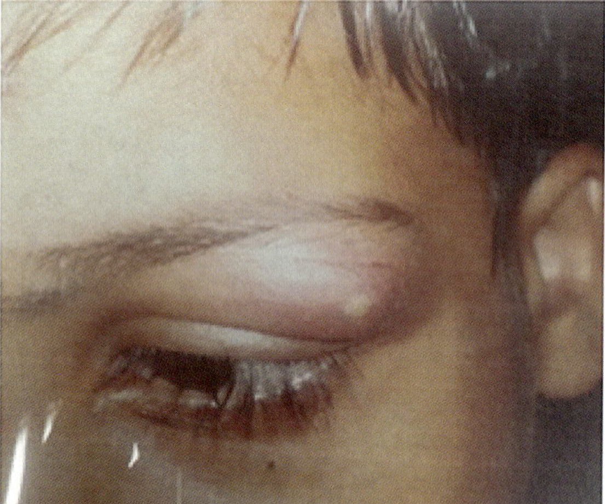

Fig. 3.3.1: Furuncle: on upper left eye lid

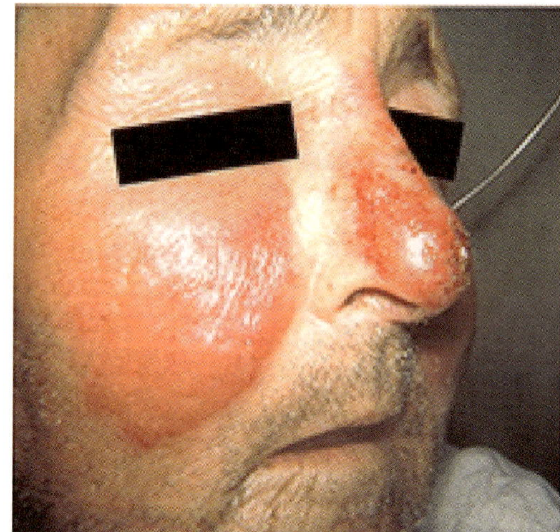

Fig. 3.3.3: ERYSIPELAS (Facial)

Courtesy: Dr. Thomas F. Sellers, Emory University/CDC, USA

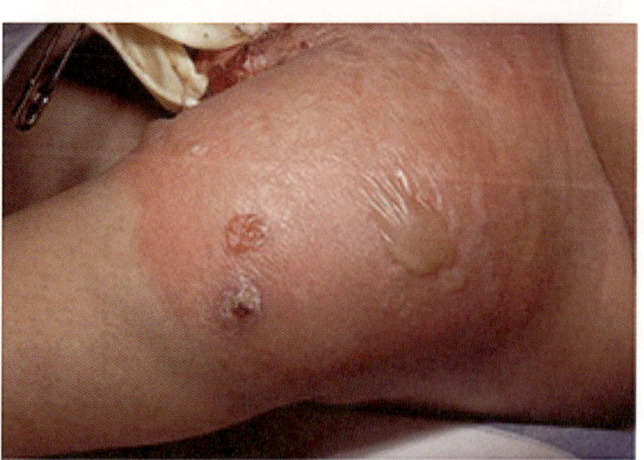

Fig. 3.3.2: CELLULITIS

Courtesy: Allen W. Mathies, MD/CDC

Integrated Clinical Based Study of Staphylococcus/Abscess

A 40 year man, Sohan Lal presented with an abscess on the right upper gluteal region He gave a history of having received an intramuscular infection at the site, 10 days back Fig. 3.4.1. The aspirated pus was gram stained, revealed gram positive cocci. The growth of the organism on blood agar medium is depicted in Fig. 3.2.1. (p. 175)

Linkages: Pg. 173-175, 177, chapter 5, 199, 200

What is the provisional diagnosis, as to the most likely organism causing the infection in this case?

A.1 (a) The infection is most likely caused by *S.aureus*.

Which are the important tests that can be performed on the isolate to confirm its identity?

A.1 (b) Catalase and coagulase tests can help in confirming the identity of this isolate. DNAase test can further help (if the test is available) in assessing the virulence of the isolate.

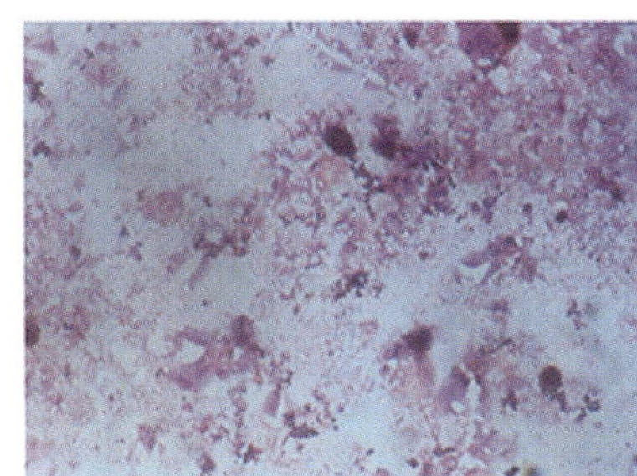

Fig. 3.4.1: Smear of gram–stained abscess demonstrating degenerating pus cells and gram positive cocci

Who gave the nomenclature of Staphylococcus?

A.1 (c) (i) The name Staphylococcus was given by Sir Alexander Ogston (1880), who also studied its role in suppurative lesions.

To which family does Staphylococcus belong?

A.1 (c) (ii) Staphylococcus belongs to the family Micrococcaceae.

What are the other genera that belong to this family?

A.1 (c) (iii) The other three genera in this family are Micrococcus, Planococcus and Stomatococcus.

Is it possible for this infection to be endogenous in origin? If so, how would this individual have acquired infection with this organism?

A.2 Yes. About 10-20% of adults can be nasal carriers of *S.aureus* and about 10% of a population can be carriers of this organism on perineum. The case could have acquired the organism from any of these sites. The probability of acquiring such organisms, would be increased, if the case had infections; as folliculitis etc.

Enumerate the virulence factors of S. aureus?

A.3 (a) These can be categorized into antigenic structure (of the organism). toxins and enzymes of *S aureus*. The key components of the *antigenic structure* include capsule (in some strains), peptidoglycan, teichoic acid and protein A. The key *toxins* are haemolysins (alpha, beta, gamma and delta), leucocidins, enterotoxins and exfoliative (epidermolytic) toxin. The important *enzymes* include coagulase, deoxyribonucleases and phosphatase (described at A3, Pg 184-185, Case 5).

Compare and contrast the virulent factors of S.aureus, S.pyogenes and S.pneumoniae.

A.3 (b)

	S.aureus	*S.pyogenes*	*S.pneumoniae*
Cell associated (antigenic structure)	Capsule (polysaccharide)	Capsule (hyaluronic acid)	Capsule(polysaccharide)Keyvirulentfactor, about 90 serotypes (refer A.4c, Case 9, pg 197)
	Teichoic acid (facilitate adhesion, are protective)	Fimbriae	
	Protein A	M, T&R protein	
Enzymes	Coagulase	Streptokinase	
	Deoxyribonuclease	Deoxyribonuclease	
	Phospatase	• Nicotinamide adenine dinucleotidase (NADase) • Hyaluronidase • Others	
Toxins	Haemolysins (alpha, beta, gamma and delta)	Streptolysins (O&S)	Toxins have little role
	Leucocidins (Panton-Valentine toxin)	Pyrogenic toxin (responsible for scarlet fever)	Hemolysins
	Toxic shock syndrome toxin		Leucocidin
	Exfoliative toxin (epidermolytic)		Pneumolysin

Describe the epidemiology of S.aureus infections.

A.3 (c) It is very important to study the epidemiology of *S. aureus* (including MRSA), as they are responsible worldwide for causing nosocomial infections (including outbreaks), being a common cause of surgical wound infections. Currently; *S. aureus* (including MRSA) has been reported to be an important pathogen, even in community acquired infections. So, it is important to understand, how these infections may be controlled.

S. aureus is a part of the normal human flora. Shortly after birth, the neonate may be colonized, by organism from neighbouring human surroundings. These sites include the umbilical stump, perineal area and skin. Later on in life, the carriage rate of the organism in healthy person varies between 25-50%, depending on the area, season and local epidemiological factors. The colonization may be transient or persistent. The commonest site for colonization is the anterior nares (nasal vestibule), to be followed by skin, perineal area, oropharynx and vagina (the latter site was evaluated, after reporting of the outbreak of toxic shock syndrome in adult premenopausal women).

Source of infection: Human cases and carriers.

Mode of transmission:

- Direct contact with infected patient/carrier (commonest mode)
- Indirect contact with environment; as fomites (bed linen, blankets, door knob) or airborne (droplets having desquamated epithelial cells).

Type of infection:

- In a hospital setting, the infection are often exogenous, often acquired from the hospital care giver.
- In a community setting, infections are often endogenous, i.e., acquired from self colonized strain present on the desquamated cells, from the skin or nose.

Some groups of individuals have been reported to have higher rates of colonization with *S. aureus* than the general population, as the doctors, nurses and hospital ward attendants. The patients with increased rate of colonization include insulin dependent diabetics, HIV infected patients, injection drug users and individuals (patients) with various dermatologic conditions.

In a hospital setting, infection often occurs by transient colonization of hands of hospital personnel, who transfer strains from one patient to another.

The reasons for *S. aureus* to be an important nosocomial agent include:

(i) Ability to survive harsh environment, as with high salt concentration
(ii) Presence of numerous virulent factors in the organism
(iii) Ability to persist intracellularly in certain phagocytes
(iv) Potential to acquire resistance to antimicrobials.

The nosocomial strains in an hospital usually belong to certain phage types (e.g., phage type 80/81) and are usually multidrug resistant. This makes them have the potential to cause outbreaks.

What is the primary modality of management of this case (pyogenic abscess)?

A.4 (a) The primary modality of management of such a case is surgical, i.e., incision and drainage of the lesion, to be followed by antimicrobial therapy.

Is the administration of antimicrobial, sufficient to resolve the infection in this case?

A.4 (b) Administration of antimicrobial alone is not be able to resolve this infection, as this agent won't be able to reach the interior of the lesion, in an adequate concentration level to be effective

This case was started on oral cephalexin, but the treatment was changed after the availability of the antibiotic susceptibility report, which categorized the isolate to be a methicillin resistant *S. aureus*.

What is this process (of changing antimicrobials) called?

A.5 (a) 'De-escalation'

What is the likely resistance mechanism in the incriminated pathogen, that could be responsible for this scenario?

A.5 (b) The presence of *mec A* gene in a *S.aureus* isolate, results in acquistion of new penicillin$^{\Delta}$ binding protein (PBP), which makes it as a methicillin resistant *S.aureus* (MRSA). These isolates are resistant to penicillinase stable penincillins. The latter antibiotics were developed, when this organism started developing resistance to penicillin, due to production of β-lactamase enzyme, that degrades the beta-lactam ring of penicillin, making this antibiotic ineffective. Currently; around 30% *S.aureus* of isolates produce this enzyme. The MRSA isolates have a modified cell wall protein termed penicillin binding protein 2 (PBP-2), which has significantly reduced affinity for all beta lactam antimicrobial agents, making these isolates resistant to all penicillins, cephalosporins, monobactams (as aztreonam) and carbapenems (as impenem). This makes the elimination of these isolates difficult.

Δ Penicillin resistance in Streptococcus pneumoniae is by modification of existing PBP.

What does GISA stand for? Explain.

A.6 'GISA' stands for Glycopeptides intermediate *S.aureus*. These isolates have reduced susceptibility to vancomycin.

Describe genome of S.aureus. Mention its role in pathogenicity especially antibiotic resistance.

A.7 Size: 2800 kbp, 'circular', with prophage, plasmid and transposon

They are: • Lysogenized

- Have unique 'pathogenicity' or 'genomic islands', which are mobile genetic elements, containing clusters for enterotoxins and antibiotic resistance.
- Have Staphylococcal cassette chromosome mec (SCC mec), are islands, containing methicillin resistance (*mec A gene*).

The expression of virulence determinant (both toxin and non-toxin mediated) is dependent on series of regulatory genes (e.g., accessory gene regulator). Also see A.5b.

What toxin mediated syndromes, can a case infected with S.aureus infection develop?

A.8 (a) Food poisoning,Toxic shock syndrome and Staphylococcal scalded skin syndrome.

Describe the pathogenesis of toxic shock syndrome.

A.8 (b) Toxic shock syndrome develops, when the *S.aureus* starts producing an exotoxin called toxin shock syndrome toxin 1 (TSST-1). About 20% of *S.aureus* isolates causing bacteremia contain the TSST-1 gene, but only a small fraction express it in a clinical setting.

Describe the role of Staphylococcal enterotoxin, Toxic shock syndrome toxin (TSST) and exfolative toxin in S. aureus pathogenicity.

A.8 (c) **Enterotoxin:** About one-third of *S. aureus* strains, produce one of the at least six (A-F) serologically distinct enterotoxins, responsible for staphylococcal food poisoning. Most of these strains belong to bacteriophage group III.

The *gene* for this toxin appears to be chromosomally mediated but is regulated by a plasmid borne protein. The molecular weight of these toxins vary from 26-30 kDa. The toxins are heat-stable, so the heating of the food may destroy the bacteria, but not the toxin. So; laboratory processing of such food may not yield the organism.

The toxins are superantigens and act by stimulating a subset of T lymphocytes, producing large amounts of interleukins. These can increase the intestinal persistalsis and can have an emetic effect.

The foods *often implicated* is milk products (as milk, sweets), potato salad and meats. These foods promote the growth of *S. aureus*. A tiny amount of enterotoxin; as small as few microgram can cause food poisoning.

The *common symptoms* of the illness include nausea, vomiting, diarrhea and at times dehydration and hypotension may occur. The absence of fever, rapidity of onset and epidemic nature of the illness can be a pointer to the illness, to be due to this entity.

The *diagnosis* of this entity is by demonstration of the enterotoxin and/or bacteria in the implicated food and/or vomiting/stool. The toxin can be detected by serological tests; as latex agglutination and ELISA.

The *treatment* is essentially supportive and symptomatic. The illness can be prevented by screening and isolating a food handler, who may be carrier of toxigenic *S. aureus*.

TSST (Toxic shock syndrome toxin):

This is a toxin produced by *S. aureus,* which is distinct from the enterotoxins, previously described in *S. aureus* food poisoning. This toxin; which also acts as a superantigen, may produce enteritis but does not produce food poisoning and instead produces a distinct syndrome called *toxic shock syndrome*. The strains often belong to phage group I. The toxin has a M.W. of 22 kDa and resembles enterotoxin F. The toxin induces production of interleukin-1, TNF α and other cytokines; which produce leakage and cellular damage of endothelial cells resulting in widespread organ damage.

This syndrome gained recognition in the early 1980s, when a national *outbreak in USA*, occurred in young, apparently healthy, menstruating women. Epidemiological investigations revealed a strong association between syndrome and use of a recently introduced high absorbent tampon in the market. The withdrawal of the tampon; resulted in marked decline of these cases. Apparently, the TSST producing *S. aureus* isolates had contaminated the tampon, which had resulted in the absorption of the toxin from the female genital tract.

This *syndrome* is currently seen in both sexes. The syndrome begins with non-specific 'flu' like symptoms. Evidence of a clinical *S. aureus* infection is not a prerequisite for development of this illness. The multisystem illness is characterized by high fever, headache, subcutaneous oedema, vomiting, diarrhea and erythroderma. Severe cases can go into acute renal failures, D.I.C., brain encephalopathy, shock and death.

The *diagnosis* of this entity is essentially clinical. The diagnosis is based on a constellation of findings rather than on one specific finding. The case should be negative serologically for diseases; as measles, leptospirosis and Rickettsial diseases. Culture of blood and/or cerebrospinal fluid should be negative for organisms other than *S. aureus*. TSST can be demonstrated by latex agglutination test/ELISA. TSST genes can be demonstrated by PCR based tests.

Exfoliative (Epidermolytic) toxin:

This toxin is a group of two antigenically distinct antigens, namely toxin A (M.W.-30 kDa) and toxin B (M.W.-29 kDa). These toxins act as superantigens. Toxin A is of chromosomal origin, heat stable (100°C – 30 min) whereas toxin B is of plasmid origin and heat labile. These toxins are responsible for staphylococcal scalded skin syndrome (SSSS), which affects mainly newborns and children. The pathogenic role of the exfoliative toxin in this syndrome is demonstrated, by the presence of specific antibodies; protective in nature in both man and mice. The toxin causes separation and loss of most superficial layers of the epidermis. The disease can vary from the localized form; in which blister formation is seen to a generalized form of the staphylococcal scalded skin syndrome. The severe from of SSSS is known as Ritter's disease in newborn.

Enumerate the principles and describe the treatment of cases infected with S. aureus.

A.9 CASES:

Gen-principles:

- Surgical incision and drainage is essential for suppurative lesions
- Device removal may be necessary, in infected ones
- No conclusion on duration of treatment but invasive lesions may require 4-8 weeks of parenteral (I/V) treatment.

Antimicrobials have adjunctive role, if lesions are abscesses.

I: If isolate is *penicillin sensitive* → PnG (however many reports have found > 80% isolates resistant to this antibiotic.

II: If isolate is *penicillin resistant, but methicillin sensitive*, i.e., MSSA → Naficillin, oxacillin–semi synthetic penicillinase resistant penicillins (SPRPs).

(Methicillin* was withdrawn after about 1 yr of usage)

III: If isolate is *Methicillin resistant *S.aureus* (MRSA), Vancomycin is drug of choice (MRSA).

Alternatives

Quinupristin/Dalfopristin

Linezolid, Tigecycline, Levofloxacin, Doxycycline, Daptomycin, Teicoplanin, Ceftobiprole

Some groups have advocated combination of ciprofloxacin and rifampicin to deal with the possibility of emergence of drug resistance.

IV: If isolate is *Vancomycin Intermediate susceptible S. aureus/Vancomycin resistant* (VISA/VRSA)Δ-----------limited options, as Linezolid, daptomycin and quinupristin/dalfopristin.

* The cause of MRSA is mec A novel gene (acquired likely from *S. sciuri*), which alters penicillin-binding protein (PBP) on *S. aureus* cell membrane. The altered PBP2a of these strains have decreased affinity for β lactam antibiotics. Such isolates are often resistant to other groups of antimicrobials; as quinolones, aminoglycosides and macrolide.

Δ The cause of VRSA is Van A gene, acquired from a Vancomycin resistant strain of *Enterococcus faecalis* by conjugation (VISA is due to increase of cell wall thickness of *S. aureus*)

Approach and treatment of *S. aureus* carriers, see A.7, Pg 187, Case 5.

Aspects related to case theme/examination assessment

Enumerate Coagulase negative staphylococci (CONS). Describe the epidemiology, pathogenesis, laboratory diagnosis and treatment of infections caused by CONS.

A.10 These are staphylococci, which are other than *S. aureus* and are coagulase negative, hence designated as CoNS in short

- Co-coagulase
- N – Negative
- S – Staphylococci

There are about 32 species which come in this category. Out of it, half have been associated with human infection.

The common species isolated from pathogenic lesions are:

- *S. epidermidis* – most common CoNS isolate, therefore many laboratories designate all CoNS as *S. epidermidis,* a practice that needs to be discouraged.

S. saprophyticus, S. hominis (causes bacteremia in malignancy cases), *S. saccharolyticus* (causes endocarditis)

S. lugdunensis, S. schleiferi (cause native valve endocarditis and osteomyelitis)

Note: Original valve is term used in comparison to implanted/artificial valve

- **Epidemiology:** Of all the CoNS, *S. epidermidis* is most frequently isolated. It is a normally found on the skin. Carriage rate of it is exceedingly high, for this reason, it is commonly isolated; as an contaminant from clinical cultures. Similarly, this organism has also been found to contaminante other specimens; as CSF, respiratory samples, hence their isolation should be interpreted carefully.

  In the past they were rare cause of significant infections, but now they are increasingly linked to human infections. This is likely to be due to increased population that is immunocompromised/debilitated and has artificial devices; as implanted catheters (I/V catheters, dialysis catheters), prosthetic devices (as artificial joint) and cardiac related devices (heart valves, stents, pacemakers). The bacterium is transmitted by contact with infected persons and hospital personnel. For this reason, it is an important nosocomial pathogen.

  S. saprophyticus is a commensal of the skin and genital mucosa. It causes urinary tract infection in young women.

- **Pathogenesis:**

  CoNS are opportunistic bacteria. Cell envelope factors that help attachment to plastic (artificial) surfaces act as virulent factor. Following initial adherence of the organism to the surfaces, further adherence is provided by the polysaccharide glycocalyx (slime), produced in significant quantities by this organism. Biofilm appears to act as barrier protecting the organism. The resistance of many CoNS to multiple antimicrobial agents, contributes further to their persistence in the body. The capacity of *S. saprophyticus* to cause UTI in young women, appears to be related to its enhanced capacity, to adhere to uroepithelial cells (related to 160 kDa haemagglutinin/adhesin).

- **Pathogenicity:**

  Commonly cause infections in immunocompromised/debilitated patients as:

  Bacteremia (as in premature infants, diabetic patients, patients on steroids, transplant recipients),

  UTI and Osteomyelitis.

Infections also in patients with indwelling devices (see epidemiology above).

- **Laboratory diagnosis:**

  The isolation is not difficult using standard bacteriological media, however their interpretation is difficult, i.e., giving significance to their isolation. Following aspects need to be given importance, while reporting this.

  (i) Presence of clinical relevant features and laboratory parameters, increases the significance of the isolation.

  (ii) Repeated isolation of the organism adds significance to the isolation

  The isolate repeatedly cultured should have same antibiogram and/or a closely related DNA fingerprint. *S. saprophyticus* is novobiocin resistant.

- **Treatment:**

Frequently, the removal of the infected indwelling device, if possible is helpful. This is easily possible in i/v catheters etc. but is difficult to perform in implants; as artificial hip joint. However; sometimes chronically infected devices don't respond to antimicrobials and there is no choice than to remove them.

Vancomycin is the drug of choice for infections caused by *S. epidermidis*. These isolates often can be multidrug resistant. Trimethoprim – Sulfamethoxazole or norfloxacin (quinolone) is effective in treatment of *S. saprophyticus* infections.

Describe Micrococcus.

A.11 This belongs the family Micrococcaceae. These are commensals, free living, coagulase negative, but catalase positive. Their pathogenic significance is doubtful.

Egs: *Micrococcus ^roseus, Micrococcus luteus* and *Micrococcus varians*

On culture, they often produce beautiful colonies with red, yellow or orange pigments. Their identification is important, as their isolation from a clinical specimen would indicate the isolate to be of minimal importance, as it would mostly indicate specimen contamination. Micrococci appear as gram positive cocci, stain darker and non uniformly (than staphylococci), appear in groups of four (tetrad) or eight and size of coccus is larger than that of staphylococcus. They break down carbohydrates oxidatively in comparison to fermentative breakdown by staphylococci.

^Named so, because of red pigment it produces.

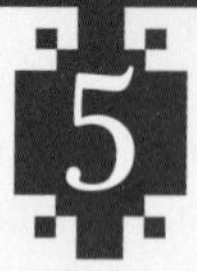

Integrated Clinical Case Based Study of Staphylococcus/Cellulitis

A 40 year old man presented with acute pain in right arm and shoulder. Examination of the affected part revealed swelling with glistening erythema and purplish discoloration of the skin with pus discharge.

Linkages: Pg 173-175, chapter 4, 199, 200

What is the clinical differential diagnosis of the above case?

A.1 (i) Abscess (burst) (ii) Cellulitis of the affected part
(iii) Erysipelas (iv) Necrotizing fascitis

What are the likely pathogens that can be implicated in this case?

A.2 (i) S.*aureus* (ii) Streptococci
(iii) Anaerobes; as Bacteroides (iv) Coliforms
(v) Pseudomonas species (vi) Mixed infection

What is the typical pathological finding in a case of S.aureus infection? Describe the pathogenesis of pyogenic S.aureus infections.

A.3 It is presence of abscess. Leukocytes constitute the primary host defense mechanism against *S. aureus*. Migration of leukocytes to site of infection, results from orchestrated expression of molecules on endothelium; is initiated by TNF α, IL-1 and IL-6. The initial intense polymorphonuclear response (PMN), is followed by infiltration of fibroblasts and macrophages. The host cellular response (which includes deposition of fibrin and collagen) usually contains infection, but if not controlled, infection spreads to neigbouring tissue or blood.

The degree of virulence of *S. aureus* is considered to be modest. It would be interesting to compare the pathogenicity of this to coagulase negative staphylococci, which is believed to be low but with increased use of implanted catheters and prosthesis, have emerged as important iatrogenic pathogens.

So the significance of diminution of host defense, when it occurs is of importance. The following are the key factors (i) breech skin/mucosa (ii) neutropenia (acquired defect) and (iii) presence of foreign body.

Pathogenesis

The virulence factors of *S. aureus* can be categorized into

Cell wall associated factors

- **Capsule:** A few strains of *S. aureus* contain polysaccharide capsule, which is antiphagocytic (inhibits phagocytosis) and protects the organism.
- **Protein A:** It is present in cell wall of 90% of strains (especially Cowan 1). It binds to Fc moiety of IgG, exerting an antiphagocytic effect. It is used in coagglutination category of antigen-antibody reactions, as it can bind to the Fc portion of IgG leaving the Fab portion of the antibody to bind to antigen.
- **Teichoic acid:** It is a polymer of ribitol phosphate and forms major antigenic determinant of cell wall of *S. aureus*. It mediates adhesion of the organism to host tissue and is anticomplementary (protects organism from complement). It is absent in coagulase negative staphylococci and micrococci.
- **Peptidoglycan:** It is a polysaccharide polymer, which activates complement and may participate in inflammatory reactions.

Toxins:

They are categorized as toxins, as they affect host cell function and/or morphology. Their action may be mediated by enzymes or by inducers, by acting as superantigens

(1) **Cytolytic exotoxins** (haemolysins): As the name indicates; these cause lysis of red blood cells of several species. These cytolytic exotoxins, also act on a wide variety of other cell types; as platelets, leucocytes and cells of the skin (dermonecrotic). Four types of these namely, alpha, beta, gamma and delta have been characterized.

Of these, **alpha (α) toxin** is the most important in pathogenicity. It is chromosomally mediated. Chemically; it is a protein with

MW of 33 kDa. It is inactivated at 60°C, however its activity is regained paradoxically, if it is heated to between 80-100°C, due to the heat labile inhibitor getting inactive at higher temperature. The alpha toxin can be toxoided but neither toxoid nor anti-α-haemolysin has been shown to be of any value in the treatment or prevention of chronic staphylococcal infection.

Beta-haemolysin is also active on a variety of cells. It has a molecular weight of 35 kDa and exhibits hot-cold phenomenon, i.e., haemolytic properties of toxin on RBC's become evident at 37°C, after the RBC's have been exposed to cold temperature.

(2) **Leucocidins:**

These damage leucocytes and macrophages, as the name of toxin indicates. This toxin is also named 'Panton-Valentine' leucocidin, after its discoverers.

(3) **Exfoliative toxin, enterotoxin** and **toxic shock syndrome toxin** (TSST-1) also have superantigen activity. (See A 8c, pg. 181-182).

Enzymes:

- **Coagulase:** It is an enzyme, which can convert fibrinogen of the plasma (not serum) into fibrin. The fibrin can coat the staphylococci and make it resistant to opsonization and phagocytosis. However; it's deposition around the pathogenic lesion, may result in its localization. There are two forms of this enzyme, whose differences are given in the table 3.5.1. For the methods for their performance, refer page 67-chapter 9, Section 1. This enzyme is present in almost all isolates of *S. aureus* and its presence helps to differentiate *S. aureus* from the less virulent staphylococci, often designated as coagulase negative staphylococci (CONS).

Table 3.5.1: Differences between *free* and *bound* coagulase

Free coagulase	Bound coagulase (clumping factor)
- Secreted free into culture medium	- Is constituent of cell wall
- Heat labile	- Heat stable
- Detected by tube test	- Detected by slide test
- One antigenic type identified	- 8 antigenic type (A-H) identified
- Considered more diagnostic of *S. aureus*	- Less diagnostic
- Requires coagulase-reacting factor for its action	- Does not require CRF

- **Catalase:** Staphylococci produce this enzyme, which converts hydrogen peroxide into nontoxic H_2O and oxygen.
- **Fibrinolysin** (staphylokinase)-role not clear
- **Nucleases,** lipases and protease-role not clear
- **Penicillinase:** As many as 80% of *Staphylococcus aureus* strains are resistant to penicillin. This is because of the presence of enzyme, penicillinase (beta-lactamse), which is often plasmid mediated in these strains (gene also present on chromosome). The enzyme inactivates penicillin and cephalosporins, by splitting the beta lactam ring. Staphylococci produces four types (A-D) of penicillinases. These plasmids are transmitted amongst the staphylococci strains both by transduction and conjugation. These plasmids may also carry resistance to some heavy metals; as mercury, arsenic and some antibiotics; as erythromycin.
- **Penicillin binding protein (PBP-2a):** Is a membrane bound enzyme (contrast with beta lactamase, which is extracellular). Some multiresistant *S. aureus* strains widely referred to as methicillin resistant *S. aureus* (MRSA) are resistant to penicillinase resistant penicillins, cephalosporins and some other groups of drugs. There were designated as MSRA, as the strains were resistant to methicillin, which was used to treat the penicillinase resistant staphylococci. The resistance is mediated by *mec A* gene, which is a part of the mobile genetic element termed staphylococcal cassette chromosome mec (SCC mec). This chromosomal mediated resistance gene is hypothesized to have been acquired by horizontal transfer from a related staphylococcal species, *S. sciur*. This gene is responsible for production of low affinity penicillin binding proteins on the cell wall (instead of normal PBP), which have less binding to many antibiotics, making them ineffective.

The steps involved in the pathogenesis are:

(1) Inoculation and asymptomatic colonization of tissue surface site. The anterior nares is the principal site of staphylococcal colonization in man. The biology of the colonization process is poorly understood. Staphylococci are opportunists. For the initiation of the infection, a breech in the cutaneous or the mucosal barrier is necessary. The presence of microcapsule (in some strains), protein A and the ability to internalize, helps the organism to evade host defense mechanisms and is critical in invasion.

Once the infection is initiated, the pathogenesis of Staphylococcal infection is complex and obscure.

(2) Invasion of tissue because of organism enzymes; as cytotoxins, lipase, proteases, hyaluronidases and thermonucleases. The enzymes facilitate the spread of infection across tissue surfaces but their precise role is not clear.

(3) This can lead to bacteremia, which may be asymptomatic or symptomatic.

(4) This can lead to metastasis of infection to sites; as bones, lungs.

(5) Evasion and host defense.

The immunity is not strong or long testing, as is evident by the continuous susceptibility of the individual to infections throughout life. The reasons for this are not understood.

What relevant investigations would you like to perform in this case?

A.4 (a) (i) Pus culture with antimicrobial susceptibility testing

(ii) Blood culture

(iii) Appropriate radiologic investigation to delineate the extent of infection.

Tabulate the characteristics of S. aureus, S. epidermidis and S. saprophyticus.

A.4 (b)

Table 3.5.2: Characteristics of Three Species of Staphylococcus

	S. aureus	*S. epidermidis*	*S. saprophyticus*
Coagulase test	+	–	–
Mannitol fermentation	+	–	–
Production of			
DNAase	+	–	–
Phosphatase	+	–/+	–
Protein A in the cell wall	+	–	–
Lysostaphin sensitivity	+	–	–
Novobiocin resistance	–	–	+

What is the role of bacteriophage in typing of S.aureus? Describe the technique.

A.5 Purpose: Strain typing

Principle: Strains of *S. aureus* are lysed by more than one specific phage, the pattern of lysis serves as marker for the strain. An international set of 23 standard phages of *S. aureus* are used. Susceptibility of *S. aureus* strains to various temperate phages, provides the basis for a phage typing system.

Most strains of *S. aureus* are lysogenic, but they are immune to them. These can lyse some other strains. The bacteriophages are propagated on special strains of *S. aureus,* which also serve as controls for the specificity of bacteriophages.

Benefit:

- Provides epidemiologic information
- No help in treatment

Limitation of technique:

- Is an phenotypic typing system, so less valuable than genotypic typing systems; as DNA fingerprinting and ribotyping
- Technique is
  - Complex
  - Time consuming
  - Requires trained personnel
- Non specific results can be due to
  - Spontaneous lysis by phages
  - Activation of latent phages

Procedure:

- Lawn culture of *S. aureus* strain to be typed is prepared

- One RTD of 23 standard typing phages applied on the lawn culture
- Plate incubated overnight and read subsequently

The National reference center for staphylococcal phage typing in India is located at department of Microbiology, Maulana Azad Medical College, New Delhi.

Interpretation:

Phage type of strain is expressed by the designation of the phages that lyse it.

The commonest phage type prevalent in most parts of India is 52/52A/80/81 (which means that it is lysed by these phages). If two *S. aureus* strains have same phage type, one cannot conclude that they are identical or same. However if two *S. aureus* strains have two different phage types, one can be sure that the two strains are 'different'. So the typing help to distinguish *S. aureus* strains.

How should this case be managed?

A.6 The lesion should be surgically explored and managed; appropriately. Appropriate antimicrobials should be started empirically and then 'de-escalated' [changed, if indicated]; if necessary.

Classify S.aureus carriers. How are they treated?

A.7 CARRIERS

- Skin
- ^Nasal
- Others

^often accompanied with skin carriage

Indication of treatment: Surgeons, nurses, healthcare workers; especially if carry MRSA

Skin: Local cream with antimicrobials

Nasal carrier:

- Locally: neomycin and bacitracin
- Intranasally: mupirocin
- Systemic: rifampicin can be considered in chronic nasal carriers

  Complication (of treatment): Some consider such regimes useless, as these encourage replacement of susceptible *S. aureus* strains with multidrug resistance ones.

How are S.aureus infections controlled?

A.8 (i) Screening of hospital staff; as surgeons, nurses and health care workers for *S. aureus* (especially MRSA). If found positive, may be given non-clinical duties, until negative for *S. aureus* spontaneously or with treatment. Intranasal mupirocin may be helpful in carriers.

(ii) Monitoring of the nosocomial *S. aureus* strains in the hospital (by antibiotic susceptibility pattern, phage type etc.).

(iii) Isolation and effective treatment of infected cases. Topical application of antimicrobial agent can prevent dissemination of infection to others.

(iv) Reinforcement of health-care associated policies in the hospital; as mandatory hand hygiene.

(v) Monitoring of sterilization of instruments etc. in the hospital.

Integrated Clinical Based Study of *S.pyogenes*/Sore Throat

A 6 year old girl, Ashima presented to a medical *practitioner* with sore throat and fever. He did not order for any microbiological investigation and prescribed drugs for providing symptomatic relief, only.

Linkages: Pg 173, 174, 176, 177, 199, 200

Which is the essential investigation that the practitioner should have ordered for the above scenario? Justify it.

A.1 (a) It is essential to get a throat swab culture performed on every case (of child) of sore throat, to rule out group A streptococcal infection (identifying the cause of pharyngitis is not possible clinically). The practitioner should have requisitioned this investigation. In case culture test is not feasible, antigen detection for group A streptococcus, in throat swab specimen may be performed. Definitive treatment for group A streptococcal infection is necessary and penicillin prophylaxis is also recommended to prevent long term post-streptococcal sequelae; as rheumatic heart disease.

Enumerate the key non-suppurative complications of S. pyogenes infection. Compare and contrast them in a tabular fashion.

A.1 (b)

Table 3.6.1: Comparison of Acute rheumatic fever and acute post-streptococcal glomerulonephritis

	Acute rheumatic fever	**Acute post-streptococcal Glomerulonephritis**
Preceding infection	Sore throat	Skin infection/sore throat
Prior sensitization	Essential	Not necessary
Latent period	Longer 2-4 weeks	Shorter (1-3 weeks)
***S. pyogenes* (serotypes implicated)**	Any, but some are more associated	Pyoderma types and throat infection types
Hereditary tendency	Present	Not known
Pathology	Characteristic lesion is 'Aschoff nodule'	Antigen-antibody complexes on glomerular basement membrane and increased PMN infiltrate
Pathogenesis	Most likely due to cross-reactivity between antigens of organism and myocardium/heart valves	May be due cross reactivity between nephritogenic streptococci and glomerular antigen or due to immune complexes deposition, leading to activation of C3 and C5, leading to tissue destruction
Complement level	Unaffected	Lowered
Serological response	Elevated ASO (titer > 200) and anti DNAase titres	ASO titres may not increase Anti DNAase levels increased (titer>300)
Clinical profile	Often dependent on inflammation of joints and heart	Albuminuria, haematuria, oedema
Course	Progressive or static	Usually spontaneous resolution
Prognosis	Variable	Good (in 80-90%)
Antimicrobial prophylaxis	Indicated (beneficial)	Not indicated

Describe the procedure for taking throat swab?

A.2 (a) The case is made to sit on a stool and asked to lift the head back and preferably close the eyes. The throat is well illuminated and the tongue is depressed with a tongue depressor and the patient is asked to say 'Ah'. The throat (including the tonsillar and the inflamed area) is swabbed vigorously with the swab and placed in the tube to be transported to the lab (procedure done with gloved hands)

It is important to collect it properly, so that the specimen does not get contaminated with the commensal flora of oral cavity, while collecting sample, which could result in a fallacious report.

What medium can be used to transport the throat swab, if delay in the transport of the clinical sample to the laboratory is expected?

A.2 (b) Pike's medium

The growth that has occurred on the blood agar plate inoculated with the throat swab (pin point size colonies with beta hemolysis) Fig. 3.2.3.

Enumerate the likely pathogens based on the mentioned colonial characteristics.

A.3 (a) Beta haemolytic colonies on blood agar in context with the current clinical picture could be *S.pyogenes, Haemophilus haemolyticus and Listeria monocytogenes.*

Describe the classification of beta hemolytic streptococci.

A.3 (b) *Rebecca Lancefield* in 1933 classified β-haemolytic streptococci into distinct serogroups, a study that helped tremendously in understanding the epidemiology of streptococcal infections. The streptococci can be classified on the basis of oxygen requirements into aerobes, facultative anaerobes and obligate anaerobes (Fig. 3.6.1). Most streptococci which cause human pathogenicity are facultative anaerobes, although some are obligate anaerobes.

The streptococci can be further classified on the basis of their haemolysis on blood agar into α, β and γ streptococci. The diferentiating features of haemolysis is given in table 3.6.2. Most streptococci that are human pathogens are β haemolytic.

Table 3.6.2: Differentiating features of alpha, beta and *gamma haemolysis

Alpha-haemolysis	Beta-haemolysis
- Zone of *partial haemolysis* seen around the colony (unlysed RBCs seen in the zone)	- Zone of *complete haemolysis* seen around the colony (all RBCs in the zone are lysed)
- Zone of lysis is *narrow* (1-2 mm in width)	- Zone of lysis is *wide* (2-4 mm in width)
- Zone has *indefinite margin*	- Zone has *definite* margin
- Zone is *greenish* in color (as RBCs are incompletely digested)	- Zone is *colorless* (as complete haemolysis occurs)

*Gamma haemolysis implies no haemolysis (NH)

The β-haemolytic streptococci are classified by the Lancefield system. The serologic grouping based on reactions of specific antisera with cell wall carbohydrate antigens of the organism, identifies 20 groups, A to V (without I and J). Out of these groups, group A streptococci are of most human importance. The group A streptococci (GAS) are further divided; on the basis of M protein precipitin reaction, T protein agglutination method and R antigens on the cell surface.

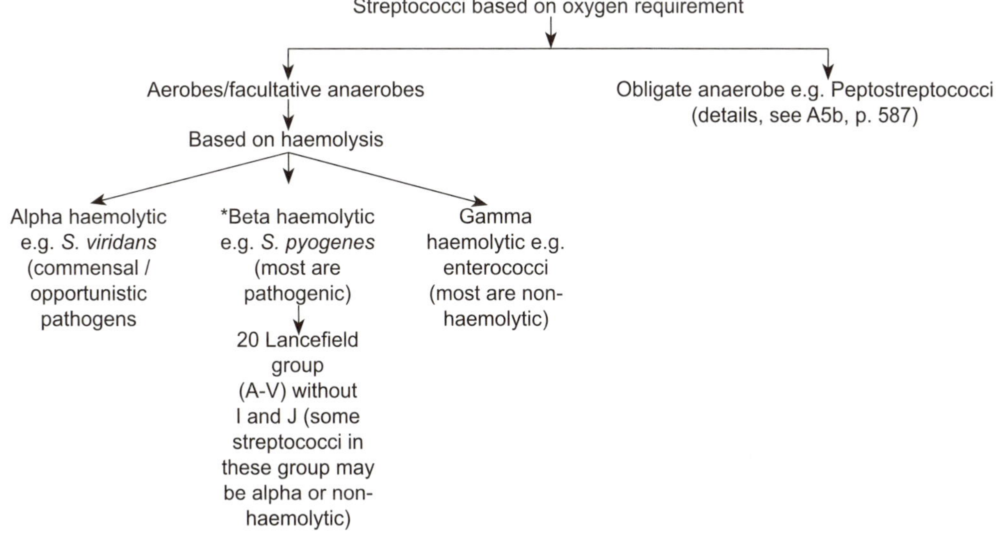

Fig. 3.6.1: Classification of Streptococci

What is the reservoir of group A streptococcus (GAS)?

A.4 (a) The upper respiratory tract of man including the throat, nasopharynx and nose is the primary reservoir for GAS.

Describe the epidemiology of group A streptococcal pharyngitis.

A.4 (b) **GAS pharyngitis:**

Agent: *S. pyogenes*

Any serotype can cause acute rheumatic fever, but M type 5 is more associated with this entity. Acute glomerulonephritis is associated with certain pyodermal types; as 49, 53-55 and pharyngitis strains; as 1 and 12.

Source of infection:

Human upper respiratory tract (including throat, nasopharynx and nose) of cases and carriers.

- Occasionally even anal carriers.
- Food, also source (less common) of outbreaks.
- Non human source of infection include bovine mastitis, through milk.
- Serotyping and molecular typing is important in epidemiological study.
- Control measures include early detection of carriers, cases and early antibiotic therapy.

Mode of transmission:

- It is spread by respiratory secretions, which can be acquired by direct contact with the mucosa, through contaminated dust/fomites or through large droplets produced by coughing, sneezing or even conversation. Droplet transmission is effective at short distances of 2-5 feet. Fomites is not important in spread, though GAS survive for short period in dried secretions.

Host:

The infections occur worldwide. The respiratory infections are commonest in children amongst 5-8 year age group. For this reason, rheumatic fever is common in 5-15 year age group. Immunity occurs following infection is type specific and is associated with antibody to the M protein. However; reinfection is common due to multiplicity of serotypes.

- Asymptomatic carrier rate is usually low (sometimes carriage rates of greater than 10% is documented in children)
- Throat carriers outnumber nasal carriers, but nasal carriers have greater infectivity than throat carriers.
- Acute cases are most important in spread of infection (much more than carriers).

Environment:

Infection is common in closed places. Outbreaks of infection are common in boarding schools and military camps.

Describe erysipelas.

A.4 (c) It is an acute and diffuse infection of the skin, involving the superficial lymphatics (subcutaneous tissue). It affects all age groups, including adults and often involves the face. It is characterized, by lesion having fiery red advancing erythema; with swollen, red and indurated skin.

Describe scarlet fever.

A.5 (a) It is a complication of streptococcal pharyngitis caused by some strains of *S. pyogenes* that produce certain pyrogenic exotoxins (erythrogenic toxin). The disease is uncommon in the tropics and does not occur in India. The disease has become less common in recent years for unknown reasons. The cases have fever, pharyngitis and characteristic rash that may occur due to hypersensitivity reaction and requires prior exposure to toxin.

Is scarlet fever prevalent in India? What are the possible reasons for the prevalent scenario?

A.5 (b) Scarlet fever has not been reported from India, despite common occurrence of GAS infections in the country. The reason for this could be the absence of strains in this area, having the temperate bacteriophage, responsible for the erythrogenic toxin.

Describe the pathogenesis of group A streptococcal pharyngitis.

A.6 (a) The attachment (pharyngitis) of GAS to epithelial cells of the host is the first step. The organism may come in an inhaled droplet. The attachment of the organism occurs by the M protein, lipoteichoic acid and F protein of the organism with the fibronectin on epithelial cells of the host. This leads to bacterial colonization stage.

In some cases, the bacteria proliferates, secretes various toxins, causing damage to surrounding cells, invading the mucosa and eliciting inflammatory response. The enzymes; as streptokinase, deoxyribonucleases and hyaluronidase lead to spread of the infection. The organism may result in spread of the infection causing cellulitis, fascitis and other manifestations.

The virulence is determined by the ability of the organism to adhere, avoid phagocytosis (mediated by capsule, M and M like proteins) and production of toxins.

Describe the role of S. pyogenes antigens, enzymes and toxins in it's pathogenicity.

A.6 **(b)** The schematic representation of the organism is depicted in Fig. 3.6.1.

Capsule on the outer side

- Present in some strains
- Composed of hyaluronic acid, production of excessive amount of capsule gives a mucoid appearance to the colonies.
- Is weakly antigenic/non-immunogenic, antibodies to it have not been shown to be protective. The possible reason for this is the resemblance of the hyaluronic acid of human connective tissue to that of the capsule.
- The capsule can prevent the organism from ingestion and killing by phagocytes (also prevents complement action by preventing binding of complement components).

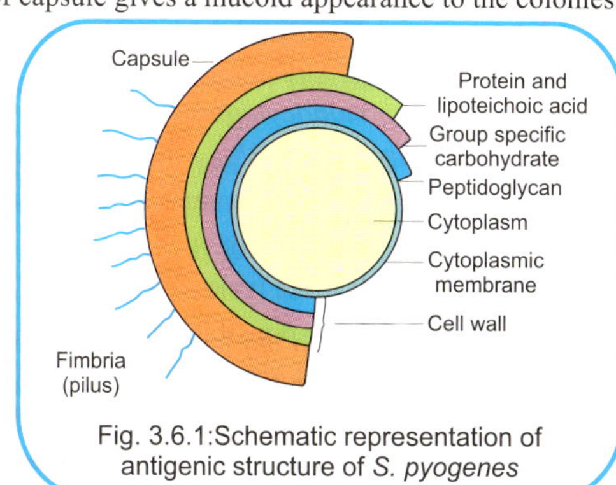

Fig. 3.6.1:Schematic representation of antigenic structure of *S. pyogenes*

Fimbriae:

- They extend from the cell membrane (where they are anchored) passing through the cell-wall and capsule to be extending outside it (so may be the outermost structure).

M. Protein:

- It is a major protein of cell wall of group A streptococci.
- It is a fibrillar protein, which extends from the peptidoglycan to the outside cell surface.
- More than 100 M types are known and it is the basis of *Griffith* typing
- M. protein is a major virulence factor (bacterium is non-infectious, in the absence of M. protein).
- It is antiphagocytic and facilitates the attachment of the organism to the epithelial cells.
- Antibodies to M protein (overcome resistance to phagocytosis) are opsonic/protective. Thus, persons with antibodies to a specific M type acquired due to prior infection are protected against subsequent infection with Group A streptococci of the same type but not against different M types. So; individuals may have numerous GAS infections in their life-time, as they encounter new M protein types, for which they have no antibodies.
- The carboxy terminal of the M protein is attached to the peptidoglycan of the cell wall and the amino terminal extends towards the surface.
- The antigenic specificity of the M protein lies in the amino terminal portion, which is the most variable portion of the molecule and is available for immune surveillance.
- The resistance of the organism (with M protein) to phagocytosis may partly be due to the binding of the fibrinogen to M protein molecules on streptococcal surface, which could interfere with the deposition of opsonic and complement fragments and its activation on the organism surface.
- Typing of strains on the basis of M protein is done conventionally in a few reference labs by antisera.
- Typing for assignment of M protein type is also done by PCR, which is based on amplification of variable region of M protein gene.

Lipoteichoic acid:

It is also associated with the M protein and the complex play a role in the adhesion of the organism to the (host) oral epithelial cells.

T and R protein:

These are the two other major proteins of the cell wall of the organism. T typing of the strains has value in the epidemiological surveillance of infection.

Group specific carbohydrate (polysaccharide):

The major component of the cell wall of the organism is the peptidoglycan, which provides rigidity to the organism. Within this matrix, lies the group specific antigen (polysaccharide), which is composed of a polymer of rhamnose and N-acetyl glucosamine. On the basis of these antigens, *S. pyogenes* is divided into 20 groups (A to V) without I and J (Lancefield groups). The specific 'C' antigen can be extracted by numerous techniques. One of the commonest extraction method is done with hydrochloric acid (Lancefield's acid extraction method) and typing done with type specific antisera.

Protein F (fibronectin-binding protein):

It mediates attachment to fibronectin in the pharyngeal epithelium.

Extracellular Products/Toxins/Other virulence factors:

Streptolysin O:

- As name indicates, it causes lysis of cells, and is antedated 'O', as it is oxygen labile (is active only in its reduced form).

7 Integrated Clinical Based Study of Enterococcus/Septicaemia

A 6 year old girl, Sabeena admitted in a PICU (paediatic ICU) was on central venous line for 15 days. She received ceftazidime and gentamicin. She remained stable, but subsequently presented with high spikes of fever Her blood culture yielded *Enterococcus faecalis.* Without waiting for the antimicrobial susceptibility result, she was started on a presumptive treatment with vancomycin. The case did not respond to the administered antimicrobial and repeat blood culture again yielded *Enterococus faecalis.*

Linkages: Pg. 173, 174, 176, 177, 199, 200

What infection has this child likely developed?

A.1 The case has most likely developed a central venous line induced nosocomial septicaemia.

What is your microbiological diagnosis?

A.2 Her clinical condition is most likely due to vancomycin resistant enterococci (VRE)

What are the risk factors for developing enterococal infection?

A.3 Old age, prolonged hospitalization, prolonged antimicrobial adminstration, debility or conditions in which mucosal and/ or epithelial barriers have been disrupted.

What are the characteristics of an isolate that suggest it to be an enterococcal one?

A.4 (i) microscopically appear as gram positive cocci in pairs and small chains, (ii) growth on MacConkey appear; as tiny pink colonies and as black colonies on tellurite blood agar, (iii) ability to grow in presence of 40% bile, 6.5% NaCl and pH 9.6, (iv) Heat test positive (ability to withstand heat at 60°C for 30 mins)

What is the combination of drugs used for treating enterococcal infection?

A.5 Penicllin or ampicillin is often used in combination with an aminoglycoside. The combination of these drugs gives synergistic activity, i.e., either of the above two classes of drugs used individually, cannot achieve a therapeutic effect, as achieved by their combination.

What does high level aminoglycoside resistance in enterococcus convey?

A.6 Common regime for treatment of serious enterococcal infections, as septicemia involve combination of cell wall inhibitors; as penicillin, ampicillin or vancomycin with aminoglycosides as; streptomycin or gentamicin.The addition of the cell wall inhibitor agent helps in the penetration of the aminoglycoside into the bacterial cytoplasm, making the intrinsically resistant organism; aminoglycoside susceptible. The presence of high level aminoglycoside resistance (HLAR) in enterococci makes the combination of cell wall inhibitors and aminoglycosides ineffective. HLAR in enterococci is defined, as the minimum inhibitory concentration of aminoglycoside for the isolate to be greater than 2000 μg/ml. Amongst the many mechanisms for the resistance of these isolates, is the secretion of enzymes by these isolates, which inactivate the aminoglycosides by different mechanisms; as adenylation or phosporylation

What antimicrobials are commonly used for treating vancomycin resistant enterococci (VRE)?

A.7 Quinupristin/dalfopristin, Linezolid or combination of ciprofloxacin and rifampicin.

Prolonged therapy is required for resolution of most infections, which may be 6-8 weeks.

Integrated Clinical Based Study of *S.viridans*/Infective Endocarditis (I.E.)

A 60 year old man, Sohrahudin presented with a 2 month history of low grade fever and facial swelling. He is a known diabetic and has long standing hypertension. Echocardiography has revealed vegetations on the implanted Valve.

Linkages: Pg 173, 174, 176, 178, 199, 200

What is your differential diagnosis?

A.1 Infective endocarditis, connective tissue disorders and chronic infection (as brucellosis, tuberculosis, etc).

What are the common microbes that are implicated in Infective endocarditis?

A.2 *Staphylococcus epidermis, Streptococcus 'viridians', S.aureus, Enterococcus spp., C. burnetii*

Which criteria are commonly used for making a diagnosis of Infective endocarditis (I.E.)?

A.3 Modified Duke criteria are often used for diagnosis of endocarditis, which has major and minor criteria. The cases get mainly categorized into definitive I.E, possible I.E. and IE excluded.

Classify endocarditis and enumerate the common microbes associated with the different categories?

A.4 Subacute, Acute and *Prosthetic valve endocarditis are the common types of endocarditis. These are most commonly associated with *S.viridans, S.aureus and S.epidermidis,* respectively.

Which is the most important microbiological investigation that can be done to make a diagnosis of I.E.? Describe the procedure.

A.5 Blood culture is the most important microbiological investigation. Briefly, a minimum of three blood cultures should be performed in the first twenty four hours. 5-10 ml of blood each should be inoculated to a set of two blood culture bottles, used for each of three blood cultures. Such procedure is employed, so that the intermittent release of organisms that may occur in this disease can be detected.

Which is the most useful test to establish a diagnosis of I.E.?

A.6 Echocardiography is the most useful diagnostic tool for IE. Transesophageal echocardiography has been demonstrated to be more sensitive and specific than transthoracic echocardiography to demonstrate valvular vegetations.

Mention the key principles that should be utilized in initiating antimicrobial therapy for I.E.?

A.7 The incriminated microbe should obviously be susceptible to the antimicrobial being instituted. Besides this, the levels of adminstered antimicrobials should exceed the MIC level for the incriminated microbe. Lastly, prolonged therapy is required for resolution of most infections, which may be 6-8 weeks .

Mention one preventive strategy in relation to I.E.

A.8 Person with I.E. must have minor procedures; as dental extraction performed under antimicrobial cover.

If Streptococcus bovis had been isolated from this case, what system (organ) in the case was likely to be source of this etiological agent?

A.9 Gastrointestinal lesions; as polyps or malignancies; as carcinoma are associated with *S.bovis* endocarditis.

Integrated Clinical Based Study of *S.pneumoniae*/Pneumonia

A 55 year old man, Ghanshyam Singh presented to the ICU with high grade fever and respiratory distress. He had a long history of alcohol intake. Sputum sample was not available from this case, as he had only non-productive cough. Blood culture was performed, which grew alpha haemolytic colonies, whose, microscopy revealed gram positive cocci; predominantly in pairs. His chest X-ray revealed infiltrates in upper and middle lobes of right lung.

Linkages: Pg 173, 174, 176, 178, 199, 200

What is the clinical diagnosis in the above case?

A.1 Community acquired pneumonia. The case under discussion has developed this pathology, while being in the community (and not during stay in the hospital). The etiological agent is likely to be pneumococcus.

Which screening test can be done on the isolated suspected pneumococal colonies to have its presumptive diagnosis?

A.2 (a) Bile solubility test and Optochin sensitivity can be performed on the isolated colonies to arrive at a presumptive diagnosis of *S.pneumoniae* (this isolate is susceptible to ethyl dihydrocuprein). Because of typical growth of pathogen on blood agar medium, fungal, viral or tubercular causes of pneumonia are unlikely.

What is Quellung reaction? Mention its historical role.

A.2 (b) Quellung reaction (Latin 'quellung': swollen) was described by Neufeld in 1902. The test consists of the addition of a drop of homologus antiserum to a suspension of capsulated bacteria; as pneumococci, resulting in apparent capsular swelling; capsule becoming clearly delineated and refractile.

This test was used in the past, for identification, when specific antisera were used, as part of the treatment protocol.

Can S.pneumoniae be present in an individual, without causing any morbidity?

A.3 (a) Yes. The normal colonization rate of this organism in the human throat (upper respiratory tract) is about 5-10%.

Who is credited with the discovery of S. pneumoniae?

A.3 (b) Louis Pasteur and Sternberg in 1881

Describe the epidemiology of pneumococcal infections.

A.3 (c) *S. pneumoniae* colonies the nasopharynx. The organism colonizes the infant at about 6 month of age. Later on the organism can be isolated from about 20-40% of healthy children and 5-10% of healthy adults. The infection has a seasonal incidence, being more common in winter (pneumococcal pneumonia). No significant animal reservoir for this pathogen exists.

Pneumococcal infection is leading cause of deaths worldwide. Infections due to serotype 3 are most virulent. Cases are seen more often in the two extreme age groups. The incidence of pneumococcal bacteremia is high in children up to two years of age.

Infection with *S. pneumoniae,* usually result in carriage of the organism for few months. Disease results; when the host resistance is lowered due to stress, malnutrition viral infection, alcoholism etc.

The organism spreads from one individual to another, as a result of direct contact and respiratory droplet transmission. It is for this reason that closed and crowded spaces as military camps, day care centers, crowded wards are associated with pneumococcal outbreaks.

There are two systems for the classification of more than 90 serotypes (based on distinct capsular composition) of *S. pneumoniae*. In the American system, serotypes are numbered in the sequence in which they were identified. The strains that frequently cause disease were generally the earliest to be identified and therefore tend to have lower numbers. The Danish system places serotypes into groups, based on antigenic similarities.

Serotyping was useful in the 1930s, when type specific antisera were administered as part of treatment protocol and again in the 1990s, when used to track the source of outbreaks. Capsular switching, which has reported to occur in pneumococcus, limits the epidemiological reliability of strain serotyping. Currently; molecular techniques; as pulsed –field gel electrophoresis and multilocus sequence typing are used to type these strains.

Which predisposing factor in this case likely led this case to the present condition?

A.4 (a) Consumption of alcohol of long standing duration.

What is the possible mechanism by which this factor (alcohol consumption) likely played a part in the pathogenesis of the current case?

A.4 (b) Inhibition of the ability of polymorphonuclear neutrophils (PMNs) to ingest the organism.

What are the key virulent factors of S. pneumoniae?

A.4 (c) Polysaccharide capsule (the various vaccines are based on this) and cytolysin (pneumolysisn), which acts on both alveolar epithelial cells and pulmonary endothelial cells.

Describe the pathogenesis of pneumococcal infections.

A.4 (d) The first essential step is the bacterial adherence (colonization) to human pharyngeal cells through the specific interaction of bacterial surface adhesins; as pneumococcal surface antigen A and epithelial cell receptors. The latter are glycoconjugates containing specific disaccharides.

Once colonization has occurred, infection occurs, if the organisms are carried into anatomically contiguous areas; such as the eustachian tube or the nasal sinuses or the lungs and their clearance does not readily occur. The normal non-specific defense mechanisms; as cough reflex, epiglottal reflex, mucociliary movement and patency of eustachian tube and sinuses help in the organism clearance. So; conditions; as otitis media and pneumococcal pneumonia usually result, when the non-specific defense and specific defense mechanisms are lacking.

It is important to study the conditions that predispose to pneumococcal infection because they not only help to understand the pathogenesis of the disease but also help in deciding, which individuals are to be vaccinated. Following are the conditions that frequently predispose to pneumococcal infections:

Increased likelihood of exposure:

- Day care centers
- Homes for the eldery
- Military training camps
- Prisons

Defective antibody formation:

- Primary deficiencies; as selective IgG deficiency.
- Secondary deficiencies due to diseases; as HIV infections, lymphoma, multiple myeloma etc.
- Complement deficiencies

Insufficient number of PMN:

- Drug induced neutropenia
- Aplastic anemia

Defective clearance of bacteremia:

- Hyposplenia/asplenia
- Splenectomy

Respiratory infection:

- Air pollution
- Allergy
- Cigarette smoking
- Asthma

Multifactorial:

- Infancy and aging
- Stress
- Glucocorticosteroid treatment
- Malnutrition
- D.M.
- Alcoholism
- Cirrhosis
- Renal insufficiency
- Chronic disease hospitalization

S. pneumoniae produces few toxins unlike *S. pyogenes* and *S. aureus,* which produce a variety of tissue damaging substances. The chief virulent factor of the pneumococcus is the capsule. It is made up of repeating oligosaccharides, that are synthesized within the cytoplasm. Nearly; every clinical isolate of *S. pneumoniae,* contains a capsule and only rarely have uncapsulated isolates been implicated in infections. Anticapsular antibody provides the best specific protection against pneumococcal infection. In the absence of anticapsular antibody, the phagocytic cells have limited capacity to ingest and destroy pneumococci. The role played by pneumococcal toxins; as haemolysin, leucocidin and pneumolysin is limited. However pneumolysin may be considered as a virulent factor, as it has cytotoxicity potential.

The capacity of pneumococci to cause disease, depends on its capacity to replicate (extracellularly) in host tissue (escaping ingestion and killing by host phagocytic cells) and ability to generate an intense inflammatory response; damaging tissues. The cell wall components of pneumococcus; as teichoic acid, peptidoglycan, phosphorylcholine etc. may play a part in the pathogenesis process.

The principal site of pneumococcal clearance from the blood stream is believed to be the spleen. It is for this reason that overwhelming pneumococcal infection occurs in children and adult after splenectomy. The incidence of pneumococcal infections also occur many fold in this population.

Numerous studies have shown that specific antipneumococcal antibodies can occur following infection with the organism. These antibodies appear approximately a week after infection and are type specific, i.e., immunity is only against the serotype with which infection has occurred.

After two days of hospitalization, the consciousness of the case deteriorated. The case also developed neck stiffening. Lumbar puncture revealed CSF, which had cloudy appearance.

What is your clinical diagnosis?

A.5 Acute meningitis.

What could be the reasons for cloudy appearance of CSF?

A.6 The CSF can be cloudy either due to increased number of leucocytes and/or microbes.

What microbiological tests can be done to make a presumptive diagnosis in this case?

A.7 Gram stain of the CSF can throw light on the type of infection Emphasis during smear reporting should be given on the type of leucocytes, bacteria/yeast present in the CSF. Empiric therapy can be started based on these findings.

Latex agglutination test on the CSF can also be done to detect the presence of antigen of common pathogens. Culture of the CSF and/or blood is a time consuming investigation.

What are the differentiating features between S.pneumoniae and 'S.viridans'?

A.8 **Distinguishing features of key alpha haemolytic streptococci i.e., S. *pneumoniae* and 'S. *viridans*':**

	S. pneumoniae	***'S. viridans'***
→Microscopic features		
Shape	Lanceolate with broad ends facing each other	Round/oval
Arrangement	Pairs/sort chain	Chains
Capsule	Present (mostly)	Absent
Quellung reaction	Positive	Negative
→Growth (cultural) characteristics		
On blood agar	Alpha haemolytic, transparent, draughtsman colonies	Alpha haemolytic
In liquid media	Uniform turbidity	Granular turbidity
→Identification tests		
Bile solubility	+	-
Insulin fermentation	+	-
Optochin sensitivity	+	-
→Animal pathogenicity test		
Intraperitoneal mouse inoculation	Fatal	Non fatal

What is the treatment protocol in managing pneumococcal infections with special reference to meningitis?

A.9 Pencillin had been the drug of choice till the 1970s, when increasing number of penicillin resistant strains started getting isolated. Currently about 10-15% of pneumococcal strains are penicillin resistant (have altered bacterial penicillin binding proteins with lowered affinity for penicillin) and some other beta lactams antibiotics also demonstrate resistance.

Strains with susceptibility (sensitivity) to penicillin are defined as those, which have MIC value of < 0.1 µg/ml, intermediate susceptible with MIC 0.1-1 µg/ml and resistant with MIC ≥ 2.0 µg/ml. These definitions are based on drug levels achievable in CSF during treatment of meningitis. The drug concentration achievable in the blood, lung, sinuses and middle ear are actually much higher than CSF, thus the MIC needs to be interpreted with reference to the infections being treated. The beta lactam antibiotics are successful in treatment of otitis media, sinusitis etc. but not meningitis, if the cause is penicillin resistant pneumococci.

The appearance of resistance in pneumococcal isolates is worrisome and is likely to arise via horizontal transfer of genetic material, as resistance to other antibiotics; as chloramphenicol, erythromycin and clindamycin is often present. Resistance in penicillin intermediate susceptible strains is likely due to spontaneous mutation, which necessitates higher concentration of penicillin to saturate the penicillin binding proteins.

Penicillin susceptible pneumococci are susceptible to all commonly used cephalosporins. Penicillin-intermediate susceptible strains are likely to be susceptible to many third-generation cephalosporins including cefotaxime and ceftriaxone. Meningitis due to penicillin resistant strain is not likely to respond with third generation cephalosporins. Vancomycin is the drug of choice, if the pneumococcus is ceftriaxone resistant.

Could this episode in this individual have been prevented?

A.10 Yes. If this individual had taken the pneumococcal vaccine (if the strain, which caused this episode was included as one of the antigens in the components of the vaccine). Details see page 629.

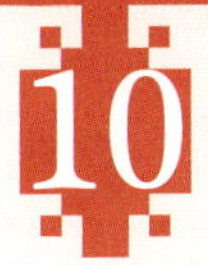

10 Laboratory Diagnosis and Treatment (Overview)

An Overview of the Comparative Approach in Laboratory Diagnosis of Key Gram Positive Cocci (Aerobic) Organisms

Organism / Disease	Specimen	Stain enhanced microscopy	Detection of microbial antigen/ metabolite/ genome	Serological Tests	Culture of Organisms in Media/ Characterization and Confirmation of isolate	Differential Diagnosis	Antimicrobial Susceptibility Tests
Staphylococcus aureus	- exudates - anterior nare swab (in carriers) - food, vomitus, stool (in food poisoning) - blood (in septicaemia) - serum	Gram staining; gram positive cocci in clusters	-	- Antistaphylolysin titre may help in detecting deep infection in body; as osteomyelitis (titre>2 units/ml) considered to be significant	Nutrient agar: large, golden yellow circular colonies Details see in characterization and confirmation of isolate: pg 175	- *Staphylococcus saprophyticus* - other coagulase negative staphylococci - Anaerobic cocci - Micrococcus species - Streptococcus species	- usual tests antibiotics tested usually are Penicillin , Vancomycin, Ampicillin, aminoglyco-sides,erythromycin, chloramphenicol, trimethoprim-sulphamethoxazole, ciprofloxacin For detecting methicillin resistance, can use, cefoxitin disc screen test
Streptococcus pyogenes	- exudates throat swab - blood culture - serum (for antistreptolysin O & antiDNase level in Rheumatic heart disease & acute glomeru-lonephritis, respectively - sputum	Gram staining (cocci in chains)	Latex agglutination, coagglutination & enzymes immunoassays techniques available for detecting microbial antigen in sample (antigen is extracted from specimen)	- Antistreptolysin 'O' titre (A6b, see p. 191-92) - levels greater than 200 todds units indicative of active infection, Anti-DNase B levels also estimated	Nutrient agar : NG Details see in characterization and confirmation of isolate, p 176	- Other Streptococcal groups namely B,C,&G - Streptococcus 'viridans'	- Organism is uniformly sensitive to Penicillin G & Erythromycin, so susceptibility tests not routinely put up
Streptococcus pneumoniae	- exudates - cerebrospinal fluid - blood	- Gram staining (diplococci lanceolate shaped with broad ends facing each other - India Ink preparation (capsule demonstration) - Quellung test (addition of antiserum makes capsule swell apparently)	- Latex agglutination, coagglutination and counter immunoelectro-phoresis techniques available to detect the antigen from various samples; as cerebrospinal fluid		- Nutrient agar: NG (scanty growth) Details see in characterization and confirmation of isolate	- Streptococcus 'viridans'	- Special protocol to be followed for performing the antimicrobial susceptibility test on special media, as blood agar

An Overview of the Antimicrobial options in the infections caused by Gram Positive Cocci

	Cell Wall Inhibitors	Cell-Membrane Inhibitors	Amino Acid Synthesis Inhibitors	Nucleic Acid Synthesis Inhibitors	Other
ORGANISM					
Staphylococcus aureus (non penicillinase producer)	• Penicillin G (DOC) • Cefazolin (if penicillin allergy)		• Erythomycin (DOC) (if penicillin allergy)		
Staphylococcus aureus (penicillinase producer) (but methicillin susceptible)	• Cloxacillin (oral)		• Clindamycin	Fluoroquinolones	
	• Nafcillin (parentral)		• Linezolid		
	• Cephalosporins				
	• Pn +β lactamase [Δ] inhibitors; as amoxicillin + clavulanic acid (DOC)				
	• Carbapenems; as Meropenem				
	• Daptomycin				
Staphylococcus aureus (methicillin resistant)	• Vancomycin (DOC) • Daptomycin		• Linezolid • Quinupristin-Dalfopristin	Fluroquinolone	• Vancomycin(DOC) ± Gentamicin ± Rifampin
Staphylococcus aureus (VISA/VRSA)	• Daptomycin		• Linezolid • Quinupristin-Dalfopristin		
Nasal Staphylococcal colonization			• Mupirocin		
S. epidermidis (coagulase negative Staphylococci)	• Cloxacillin • Naficillin • Vancomycin				
Streptococcus pyogenes (group A)	• PnG (DOC), PnV • Cephalexin (if penicillin allergy)		• Erythromycin (if patient is allergic to penicillin)		
	Antimicrobial prevention is required for cases with history of rheumatic fever, before procedures; as dental, that may induce bacteremia Adequate therapeutic levels of drug must be maintained for 10 days to prevent development of acute rheumatic fever				
	Drugs have no role on acute rheumatic fever and acute glomerulonephritis (established cases). But persons who have recovered from ARF, must be given prophylactic treatment to prevent recurrences. Acute GN does not recur, so no use of prophylactic antimicrobials in it.				
Streptococcus groups (hemolytic B, C & G)	• PnG (DOC), PnV • Ampicllin • Cephalosporins (3rd generation) • Daptomycin • Vancomycin		• Erythromycin • Azithromycin • Clarithromycin • Clindamycin		
**Streptococcus group D (General)*	• PnG	+	Aminoglycosides (as gentamicin) (DOC)		
**Enterococcus faecalis*	• Ampicillin	+	Gentamicin (DOC)		
	• Vancomycin	+	Gentamicin		
**Enterococcus faecium*	• Vancomycin	+	Gentamicin (DOC, if isolate is vancomycin susceptible) • Linezolid (DOC, if isolate is vancomycin resistant • Quinupristin-Dalfopristin (DOC, if isolate is vancomycin resistant)		
Streptococcus 'viridans'	• PnG • Cephalosporins • Vancomycin	+	Gentamicin (DOC)		
Streptococcus pneumoniae	• PnG (DOC), PnV • Cephalosporins • Carbapenems • Vancomycin		Erythromycin Azithromycin Clindamycin	• Trimethoprim-Sulfamethoxazole • Fluoroquinolone	
Anaerobic cocci; as Peptococcus	• PnG		• Clindamycin • Metronidazole		

Δ. β- Lactamases are enzymes that hydrolyze the β - lactam ring of the β-lactam category of antimicrobials, inactivating the drug. Such enzymes are specific for penicillins, cephalosporins and carbapenems, designated as penicillinases, cephalosporinases and carbapenemases; respectively.

* Synergistic combinations are essential.

11 Assessment/Examination Questions

1. Classify the lesions caused by *S. aureus*. p. 177
2. Describe in detail the epidemiology of *S. aureus* infections. A 3c., p. 180
3. Classify the *S. aureus* carriers. Mention their importance and treatment. A7., p. 187
4. Enumerate the virulence factors of *S.aureus*. Compare and contrast the virulence factors of *S. aureus*, *S. pyogenes* and *S. pneumoniae.* A3., p. 184-185, A3b., p. 179
5. Describe the pathogenesis of *S. aureus* infections. Mention the role played by the genome of *S. aureus* in antibiotic resistance. A 3., p. 184-86, A 7., p. 181
6. Tabulate the key differences between *S. aureus, S. epidermis and S.saprophyticus. Describe coagulase test.* A 4b., p. 186, p. 185, p. 67
7. Describe in detail the laboratory diagnosis of *S. aureus* infections. p. 173-175
8. Enumerate coagulase negative staphylococci (CONS). Describe the epidemiology, laboratory diagnosis and treatment of CONS infections. A. 10., p. 182-183.
9. Describe Micrococcus. A 11., p. 183
10. Outline the morphology and cultural characteristics of *S. aureus.* p. 173-175
11. Describe the importance and treatment of infections caused by Methicillin resistant *S. aureus* (MRSA). A 9., p. 182, p. 200
12. Describe bacteriophage typing. A 5., p. 186-187
13. Enumerate toxin mediated syndromes, *S. aureus* can cause. Describe Staphylococcal food poisoning and Staphylococcal scalded skin syndrome. A 8b, c., p 181-182
14. Outline the treatment of *S. aureus* infections. p. 200, A 9., p. 182
15. How are *S. aureus* infections controlled? A 8., p. 187
16. Classify the lesions caused by *S. pyogenes.* Compare and contrast the non-suppurative complications of *S. pyogenes* in a tabular fashion. p. 177 and A 3b., 179
17. Describe the classification of beta hemolytic streptococci. A 3b., p. 189
18. What is the reservoir of group A streptococcus? Describe the epidemiology of group A streptococcal pharyngitis. A4a, b., p. 190
19. Describe the pathogenesis of group A streptococcal pharyngitis. A 6a., 190 and A 6b., p. 191-193
20. Describe the role of *S. pyogenes* antigens, enzymes and toxins in the pathogenicity. A 6b., p. 191-193
21. Outline the morphology and cultural characteristics of *S. pyogenes.* p. 174, 176
22. Describe the laboratory diagnosis of streptococcal sore throat. p. 199, p. 174, 176
23. Can a case of streptococcal sore throat be treated without performing the antibiotic susceptibility testing? Describe the treatment guidelines of group A streptococcal infection including antimicrobial prophylaxis. A 7a., p. 193, p. 200
24. Describe antigenic structure of *S. pyogenes.* Diagramatically depict cell wall of *S. pyogenes.* Discuss the relevance of cell wall antigens to virulence and classification. A 6b., p. 191
25. Describe the laborarory diagnosis of rheumatic fever. A 1b., p. 1888
26. Is Scarlet fever prevalent in India? What are the possible reasons for this scenario? A 5b., p. 190
27. Describe Lancefield grouping. A 3b., p. 179
28. Describe Group B streptococci, Group D streptococci, Enterococci, Streptococcus 'viridians'. p. 176, cases 7, 8., p. 194-195
29. Describe Streptolysins, Streptokinase and Streptodornase. p. 191-192
30. Describe Heat test and CAMP test. p. 176
31. Outline the morphology and cultural characteristics *of S. pneumoniae.* p. 174, 176
32. What are the key virulent factors of *S. pneumoniae*? Describe the pathogenesis of pneumococcal infections. A 3a., p. 196
33. Can *S. pneumoniae* be present in an individual without causing any morbidity? Describe the epidemiology of pneumococcal infections. A 3a., p. 196, A3c., p. 196
34. Describe the laboratory diagnosis of pneumococcal infections. p. 199, p. 173-176
35. Tabulate the differences between *of S. pneumoniae* and *S. viridans* in a tabulated fashion. A 8., p. 198
36. Describe quelling reaction, bile solubility test and optochin sensitivity test. A 2a,b., p. 196, A 8., p. 198
37. Describe *Pneumococcal* vaccine. p. 629

Section IV: Gram Negative Cocci

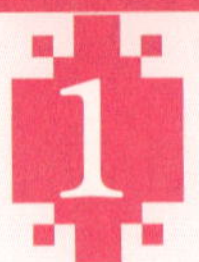

Classification, Metabolic and Microscopic Features of Gram Negative Cocci (GNC)

Algorithm for Identification of GNC

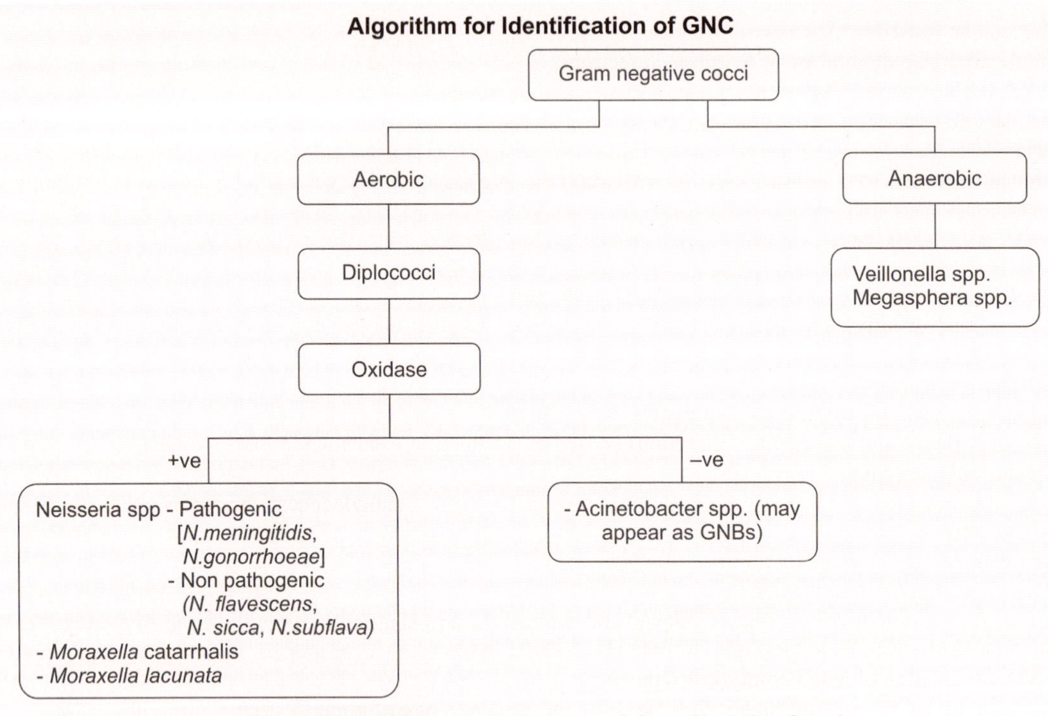

Metabolic and Microscopic Features of Gram Negative Cocci

Organism	Growth Requirements						Cellular Morphology and Staining Characteristics						
	O2 Requ.	Optimal Temp.	CO2 Requ.	Incubation Period			Shape	Gram	Arrangement	Capsule	Motility	Spore	Special Staining/ microscopy/ Special Features
				Days	Weeks	Months							
Neisseria meningitidis	Strictly aerobic	37°C	+	1	–	–	Bean shaped cocci	–ve	In pairs Fig. 4.1.1	+	–	–	–
N. gonorrhoea	Strictly aerobic	35-37°C	+	1-2	–	–	Bean shaped cocci	–ve	In pairs Fig. 4.1.2	+	–	–	–
Acinetobacter spp. [Common spp. are baumanii and Iwofii]	Strictly aerobic	37°C	–	1	–	–	Cocco-bacilli	–ve	In pairs, singly, chains	+	–	–	May appear as diplococci and cause diagnostic confusion
Moraxella catarrhalis	Aerobic	37°C	–	1	–	–	diplococci (adjacent sides flattened)	–ve	–	±	–	–	–
Moraxella lacunata	Aerobic	37°C	–	1	–	–	Bacilli	–ve	–	±	–	–	–
Veillonella spp.	Anaerobic	37°C	–	1	–	–	Cocci	–ve	pair, chains, clumps	(–)	–	–	–

±: More research is necessary to definetly demonstrate the presence and define its role.

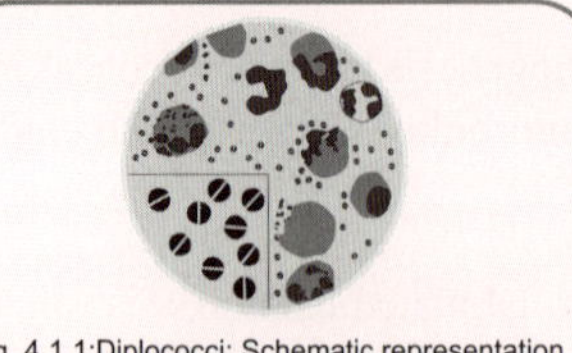

Fig. 4.1.1:Diplococci: Schematic representation of diplococci of *N.meningitidis*(gram negative) demonstrating adjacent edges to be flat

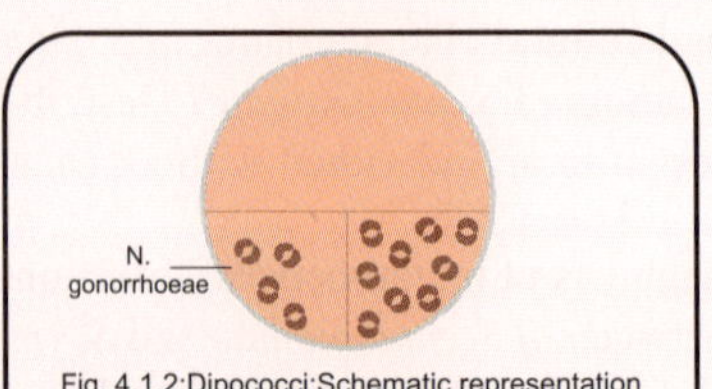

Fig. 4.1.2:Dipococci:Schematic representation of diplococci of *N. gonorrhoeae* (gram negative) demonstrating adjacent edges to be concave

2 An Overview of the Media Requirement, Colonial Characters and Diagnostic Characteristics of Key Gram Negative Cocci

	Basal media	Enriched media	Selective/others	Characterization and confirmation of isolate
N. meningitidis	No growth	- Blood agar: Small (1-2 mm), translucent, haemolytic colonies - Choclate agar & Mueller - Hinton media also used for isolation	- MacConkey: No growth - Thayer Martin medium with antibiotics used (Vancomycin, colistin, trimethoprim and nystatin)	- Microscopic and staining characteristics - Catalase +ve - Oxidase +ve - Sugar fermentations (using serum sugars) - Ferments glucose and maltose with acid only but no gas - Serogrouping (using poly and monovalent sera)
N. gonorrhoeae	No growth	- B.A.-Small, translucent colonies (five types) known, T1-T5 - Chocolate agar and Mueller Hinton media used	- MacConkey-no growth - Thayer Martin medium with antibiotics used - Mueller Hinton medium (also used)	- Microscopic and staining characteristics - Catalase +ve - Oxidase +ve - Sugar fermentation using serum sugars (Fig. 4.2.1) - Ferments glucose with acid only but no gas - Aerobe (can grow anaerobically)
Moraxella catarrhalis	N.A. (+)	+	–	- Microscopic and staining features - Catalase +ve - Oxidase +ve - Doesn't ferment sugar
Moraxella lacunata	N.A. – NG	- B.A- (+) - Serum agar (+) (pitting colonies)	–	- Microscopic and staining features - Catalase +ve - Oxidase +ve - Doesn't ferment sugars
Veillonella spp.	Anaerobic	(details beyond U.G. level) B.A. (+)		- Microscopic and staining features - Sugars oxidatively utilized
**Acinetobacter sps* (baumanii & lwofii are two key species)	N.A. (+)	(+)	MacConkey (+) (pinkish)	- Microscopic and staining features - Obligate aerobe - Oxidase negative - Characterized as glucose oxidizer/Nil fermenter. - Acid produced without gas from glucose (in *A. baumanii)*

NB: (i) NA is Nutrient agar, (ii) NG indicates no growth, (iii) (+) indicates growth, (iv) *also characterized as an gram negative bacilli by some authorities, as has features of both cocci and bacilli, i.e., is a cocco-bacilli.

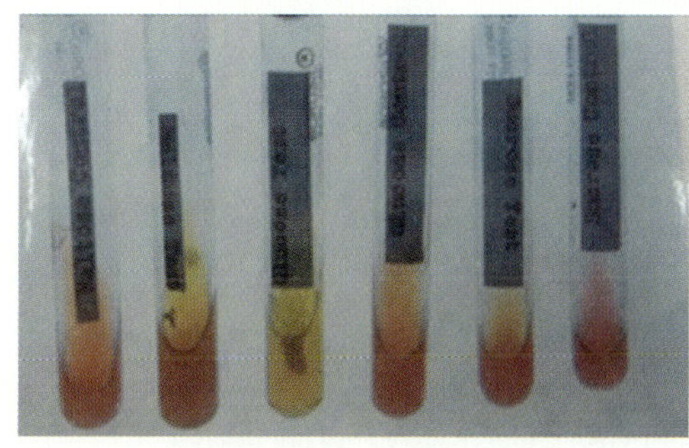

Fig. 4.2.1: Biochemical reactions of *N. gonorrhoeae* fermenting only glucose with acid production (but no gas production)

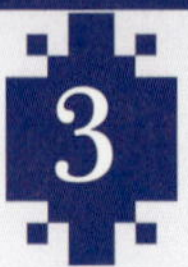

Clinical (Pathogenicity) Profile of Infections Caused By Gram Negative Cocci

Neisseria meningitidis	Carrier state (localized infection in nasopharynx)
	Meningococcaemia, Meningitis • [Case: pg 205-206]
	Waterhouse Friderischen syndrome (DIC shock, damage to adrenal gland), chronic meningococcal bacternia
N. gonorrhoeae	Carrier state in women
	In Men
	- Acute gonorrhoea (primarily urethra involved) (Fig. 4.3.1)
	- Sometimes epididymitis and prostatitis
	- Other lesions less common; as arthritis, meningitis etc.
	In women
	- Acute gonorrhoea (primarily urethra involved), sometimes PID.
	- Other lesions less common
	In children
	- Ophthalmia neonatorum
	- Conjunctivitis
	- Gonorrhoea [Case: pg. 207-208]
Moraxella catarrhalis	Lower respiratory tract infection (Organism is part of normal flora of upper respiratory tract and genital tract
Moraxella lacunata	Conjunctivitis (angular and other)
Veillonella spp.	Bacteremia
Acinetobacter spp.	Opportunistic and healthcare associated infections; as pneumonia, septicaemia and meningitis and soft tissue infections

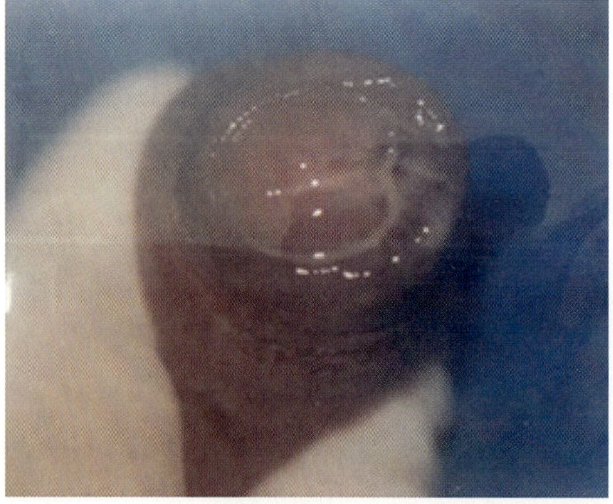

Fig. 4.3.1: Gonorrhoea:Profuse purulent discharge per urethra

Integrated Clinical Based Study of *N. meningitidis*/Meningitis

A seven year old girl Sameena, presented to the paediatric emergency with history of fever, headache, stiff neck and double vision. She had all the routine immunizations on schedule. CT scan revealed mild cerebral oedema.

Linkages: Pg. 202-204, 209, 210

What is your differential diagnosis of this case?

A.1 Meningitis, encephalitis, brain abscess, cerebral neoplasm or any space occupying lesion of the brain.

A L.P. is done on the child. The C.S.F. when gram stained revealed presence of polymorphs and numerous gram negative diplococci in pairs (Fig. 4.4.1).

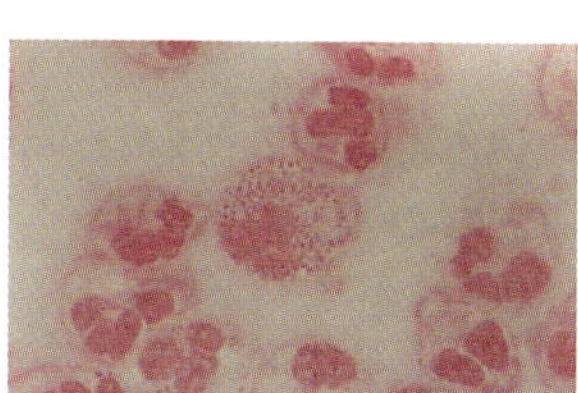

Fig. 4.4.1: Diplococci: Gram stained smear of cerebrospinal fluid from a case of acute meningitis demonstrating gram negative diplococci in leucocytes

What is the likely pathogen based on these findings?

A.2 (a) *N. meningitidis* (first isolated by Weichselbaum in 1887)

Name some commensal Neisseria of the respiratory tract.

A.2 (b) *N. flavescens*, *N. sicca*

How are they differentiated from N. meningitidis?

A.2 (c) The commensal Neisseria are characterized by their ability to grow on ordinary media (non enriched), producing pigmented colonies and fermenting a number of carbohydrates. (see Pg 203, Chapter 3)

What is the reservoir of N. meningitidis?

A.3 (a) Man is the only reservoir for meningococcus. This fact is employed in control of meningococcal outbreaks by isolation of the cases.

Are asymptomatic carriers known with N. meningitidis?

A.3 (b) The asymptomatic carrier rate is about 5-10%. This rate often rises before an impending epidemic. Hence, sometimes trends of the nasopharyngeal colonization rate are used for intervention in a community.

Describe the epidemiology of meningitis caused by N. meningitidis.

A.3 (c) **Epidemiology:**

Agent: *N. meningitidis*

- Agent serogroups A, B, C, Y, and W-135 responsible for > 90% of meningococcal infections worldwide.
- Group A strains have the potential to cause epidemics (in past; epidemics have occurred at intervals of 8-10 years)
- Group A meningococcus epidemic occurred in Delhi in 1985
- Serogroup B strains have been associated with epidemics in developed countries
- Techniques; as PFGE (classifies bacteria into electrophoretic types-ETs), bacterial genome sequences amplification by PCR and multilocus enzyme electrophoresis help in strain identification.

The organism is unique among the major bacterial agents to cause both epidemic as well as endemic (sporadic) disease.

Reservoir infection: Human nasopharynx is the primary reservoir of human infection (cases and carrier)

Source of infection: Nasopharyngeal and Bronchial secretion (infective).

- Carriers are the most important source of infection.
- In interepidemic periods, approximately 10% of healthy individuals are colonized as carriers of meningococcus. This rate may exceed 80% in close communities during epidemics.

Transmission occurs through inhalation of respiratory droplets from a carrier or a patient (in early stages of disease). It is less often by fomites. The transmission requires close contact and susceptibility (lack of specific antibodies).

Host

- It predominantly causes disease in children and adult of both sexes.
- Attack rate is higher among children than among adults (although one-third to one half of all cases of sporadic meningococcal disease are reported in adults)

- Carriers of *N. meningitidis* rarely contract the illness themselves
- All ages are susceptible, although younger age groups are more susceptible than older age groups, as immunity in them is lower.
- The meningococcal disease occurs more commonly among household contacts of primary cases than in general population.
- Most cases occur within 2 weeks of the occurrence in the primary case, although some cases can occur several months later.

Environmental factors: Outbreaks occur more frequently in the dry and cold months of the year.

Outbreaks (epidemics) occur commonly among the poorest groups, where crowding and lack of sanitation are common. The places of outbreaks include schools (day care centers), prisons and army camps. During epidemics, both chemoprophylaxis; which gives short term protection and vaccination for long term protection is indicated, (if a case occurs in a family setting). Recently; epidemics have been reported from Australia, China, Netherland and Africa.

How many serogroups are known for this pathogen?

A.4 It is divided into 13 serogroups. Some serogroups are associated more frequently with causation of epidemics. Typing of isolate helps in characterizing the outbreaks, which occur differently in the various parts of the world. The vaccine is constituted by those serogroups that are prevalent in a geographical region. Serogroup B is poorly immunogenic, hence not included in common polyvalent vaccine.

Why does an outbreak with N. meningitidis cause so much fear?

A.5 **(a)** Because meningococcal meningitis is associated with severe morbidity and high mortality, sometimes (upto 70% mortality has been reported in some outbreaks).

Outline the pathogenesis of meningitis caused by N. meningitidis.

A.5 **(b)**

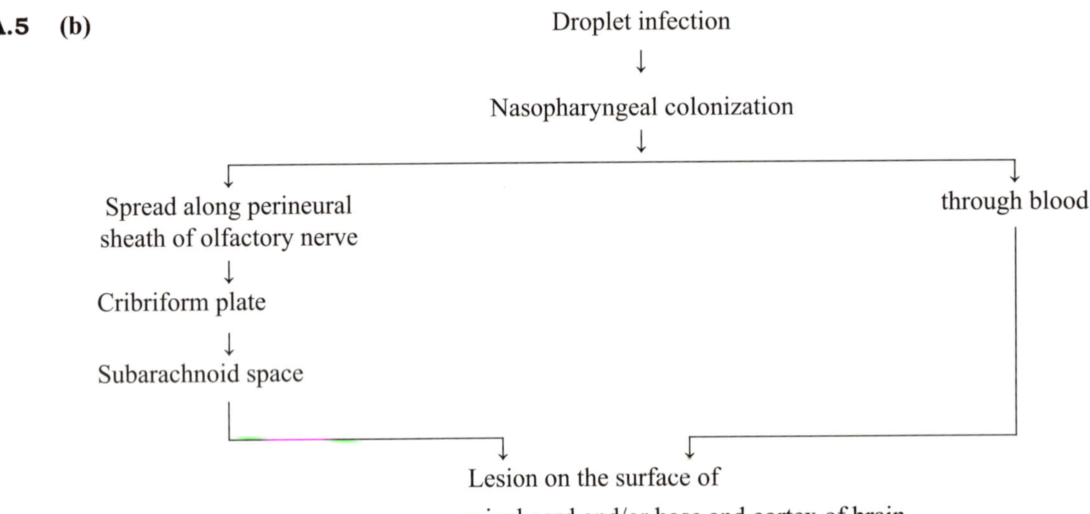

What measures are taken to control a meningococcal meningitis outbreak? Does immunization and chemoprophylaxis have any role in the control of an outbreak?

A.6 Control measures; include isolation of cases, chemoprophylaxis and immunization of contacts. The latter two have a role; unlike in some disease outbreaks, as cholera, where their role is minimal.

What pharmacokinetic aspect of antimicrobial is to be considered, when administering drugs for treatment of meningitis?

A.7 The antimicrobial should be able to cross the blood-brain barrier (meninges) to reach the brain

What are the current challenges in the study of N. meningitidis?

A.8
- To understand, why certain populations are susceptible to *N. meningitidis* meningitis.
- To understand the sporadic (endemic) nature of the disease, which sometimes occurs with this agent.
- To understand the mechanism, by which some persons become carrier with this pathogen and the mechanism of the eradication of the organism.
- To make group C vaccine more immunogenic in children under 2 years of age (not clear, why it is less immunogenic).
- Development of group B polysaccharide vaccine (not clear, why this group is less immunogenic).

Integrated Clinical Based Study of *N. gonorrhoeae*/Gonorrhoea

A 20 year college going male student Shahid, reported to the medical OPD with complaints of burning micturition, dysuria and profuse seropurulent urethral discharge (Fig. 4.3.1, p. 204). A history of having sexual relation with three female partners in the past three months was elicited. A gram stain of the urethral discharge revealed PMNS with intracellular diplococci, Fig. 4.1.2. (p. 202). Urine culture did not reveal any pathogens.

Linkages: Pg. 202-204, 209-210

What is your provisional diagnosis in the above case?

A.1 (a) Urethritis (acute) most likely due to *N. gonorrhoeae.* This organism was first described by Neisser in 1879; in exudates.

How is urethral specimen collected?

A.1 (b) A fine, flexible swab is inserted about 4 cm into the urethra, rotated twice and removed. If fresh exudate is available, then the surface exudate is discarded and the freshly expressed one can be utilized for processing. The patient should not have urinated, at least one hour before collection of this sample.

What is the sensitivity of gram stain in diagnosing gonococcol urethritis in males?

A.1 (c) Approximately 95% in males.

What is the reliability of this technique in diagnosing gonococcal cervicitis in females?

A.1 (d) The reliability of gram stain in detecting the infection in females is low, as it is difficult to distinguish commensal Neisseria in genital flora from pathogenic *N. gonorrhoeae*. The positivity of Gram stain of cervical specimen for this pathogen is only about 50 to 60%, making it an unreliable tool. In females, smears should be prepared from urethral discharge and/or cervical swab.

What are the non gonococcal (NGU) causes of urethritis?

A.1 (e) It includes C.*trachomatis, Ureaplasma urealyticum, Mycoplama genitalium, Trichomonas vaginalis*, Human Herpes viruses and Adenoviruses

What microbiological test can be done to isolate N.gonorrhoeae from clinical specimen suggestive of gonorrhoea?

A.2 (a) Conventionally, the urethral exudate can be cultured onto Chocolate agar/Thayer Martin medium for extended period (of at least 36-48 hrs) in environment of 5% CO_2 for isolation of *N. gonorrhoeae.*

What rapid diagnostic techniques can be employed on a clinical sample with suspected N. gonorrhoeae infection?

A.2 (b) The gonococcal antigen in clinical specimens, as urethral discharge and endocervical discharge can be detected utilizing assays, utilizing direct fluorescent antibody or enzyme linked antibody principles.

Molecular amplification techniques based on PCR, LCR and TMA (transcription based amplification) technology for detection of this pathogen are also commercially available.

Is it unusual for the urine culture of this case not to reveal any pathogen in this case?

A.2 (c) In urine, this pathogen can be demonstrated, using antigen detection or genome amplification detection techniques. However a conventional culture using blood agar medium incubated for only 24 hrs in an environment without increased CO_2 concentration is unlikely to lead to isolation of this pathogen.

What is the reservoir of N. gonorrhoeae?

A.3 (a) The reservoir of this pathogen is infected men and women, who are cases and carriers. In men, the commonest site is urethra and in the women; endocervix. Women play a bigger role in the transmission of this infection, as they are often asymptomatically infected, so go undetected. Infection of rectal and pharyngeal regions has also been seen especially in individuals, who practice uncommon sexual practices.

Is it possible for an woman infected with N. gonorrhoeae to be asymptomatic?

A.3 (b) Yes.

What is the mode of infection for gonorrhoea? Mention its epidemiology.

A.3 (c) It is primarily venereal. This may be contrasted with Ophalmia neonatorum, which is a non-venereal gonococcal infection.

Agent: *N. gonorrhoeae* (types T1-T4)

An Overview of the antimicrobial Options for Infections caused by key Gram Negative Cocci (Key)

	Cell Wall Inhibitors	Cell-Membrane Inhibitors	Amino Acid Synthesis Inhibitors	Nucleic Acid Synthesis Inhibitors	Others
Neisseria meningitidis	• PnG (DOC) • Cephalosporins		Chloramphenicol (in penicillin sensitive cases)	Fluoroquinolones	
Neisseria meningitidis *Carriers*, for eradication of organism			Rifampicin (given at end of therapy to eradicate organism)		
N.gonorrhoeae (most penicillinase producing)	[Ceftriaxone or cefixime	+	Azithromycin or doxycycline (DOC)]	• Ciprofloxacin • Ofloxacin • Gatifloxacin	
Moraxella catarrhalis (previously Branhamella catarhalis)	Cephalosporins as cefuroxime (DOC)		Doxycyline	• Fluoroquinolones • TMP-SMZ	
Moraxella lacunata	PnG				
Acinetobacter spp.	• Carbapenems (DOC) • Piperacillin tazobactam • Ceftazidime	Polymyxin B	• Doxycycline • Minocycline • Aminoglycosides often combined with imipenem/ ceftazadime for serious infections.	Fluroquinolones TM-SMZ	

- Treatment should be administered based on antimicrobial susceptibility testing, however the choices mentioned are general indications.
- DOC is Drug of first choice
- TMP-SMZ is Trimethoprim-Sulfamethoxazole

7 Assessment/Examination Questions

1. Outline the morphology and cultural characteristics *of N. meningitidis.* p. 202-203
2. What is the reservoir of *N. meningitidis*? Are asymptomatic carriers known to occur with this pathogen? Describe the epidemiology of *N. meningitidis* infections. A 3a,b,c., p. 205-206
3. Describe the pathogenesis of meningitis caused by *N. meningitidis.* A 5b., p. 206
4. Describe the laboratory diagnosis of meningococcal meningitis. p. 209, p. 202-204
5. Describe the antigenic structure of *N. meningitidis* and describe the meningococcal vaccine. A 3c., p. 205, p. 629
6. Outline the morphology and cultural characteristics *of N. gonorrhoeae.* p. 202-203
7. What is the reservoir of this pathogen? Describe the epidemiology of gonorrhoea. A 3 a-d., p. 207-208
8. What virulent factors are responsible for the pathogenicity of this pathogen? Describe the pathogenesis of gonorrhoea. A 5a, b., p. 208
9. What does PPNG stand for? What are some of the factors that promoted the development of this entity? A 4b. p. 208
10. Describe the laboratory diagnosis of gonorrhoea. p. 209, 202-204
11. Should aymptomatic women infected with this pathogen be treated? Explain. A 4a., p. 208
12. Enumerate the differences between *N. meningitidis* and *N. gonorrhoeae.* p. 202-203
13. Describe non gonococcal urethritis. A 8., p. 208
14. Describe *Moraxella catarrahalis.* p. 203-204
15. Name a gram negative bacilli that may appear as gram negative cocci. p. 202
16. Describe Acinetobacter spp. p. 202-204

Section V: Gram Positive Rods/ Bacilli

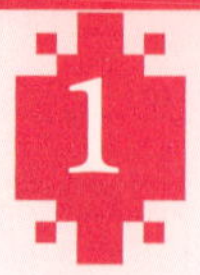

Classification, Metabolic and Microscopic Features of Key Gram Positive Bacilli

Algorithm for identification of Gram Positive Bacilli

Gram positive bacilli

- *Aerobic (see p. 213)
- Anaerobic
  - *Sporing* (Spore +ve)
    - *Clostridium perfringens*,
    - *C. septicum*, *C.oedematiens*
    - *C.tetani*
    - *C.botulinum*, *C.difficile*
  - *Non-Sporing* (Spore -ve)
    - Lactobacillus spp.
    - Bifidobacterium spp.
    - Propionibacterium spp. (brachi, nodatum)
    - Actinomyces spp. Eubacterium spp.
    - Mobiluncus spp.

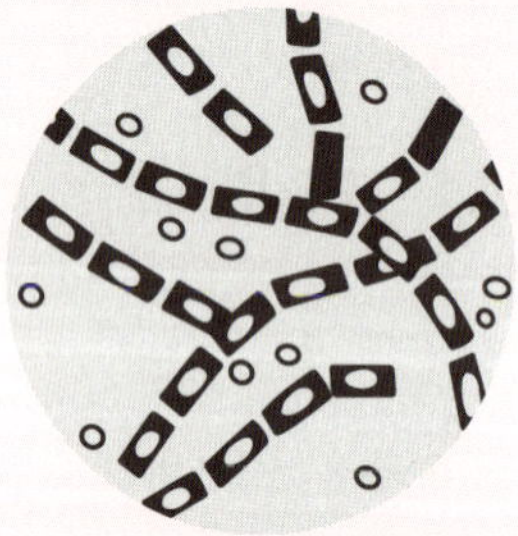

Fig. 5.1.1: Anthrax: Diagrammatic representation of gram positive bacilli (Bamboo stick appearance with spores). Spores not usually seen in smears from clinical samples

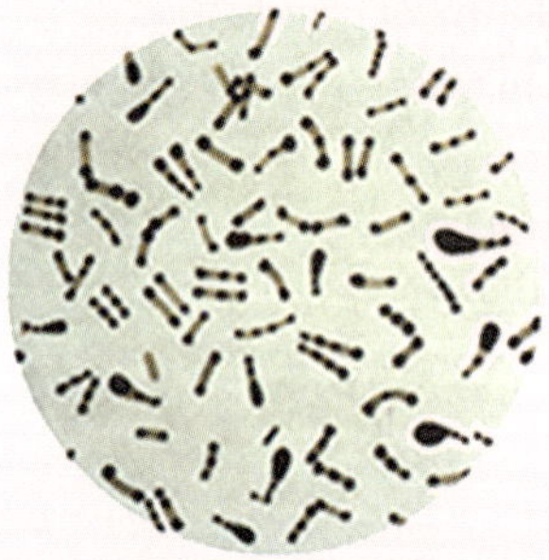

Fig. 5.1.2: *Corynebacterium diphtheriae*: Photomicrograph of *C.diphtheriae* (magnification 1200X)

Courtesy: Centers for Disease Control and Prevention, Atlanta, USA

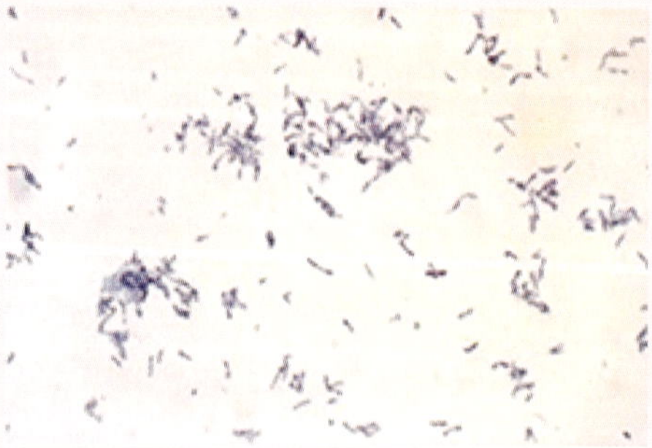

Fig. 5.1.3: Diphtheroids: Gram stained smear demonstrating gram positive bacilli with palisade appearance

Courtesy: CDC

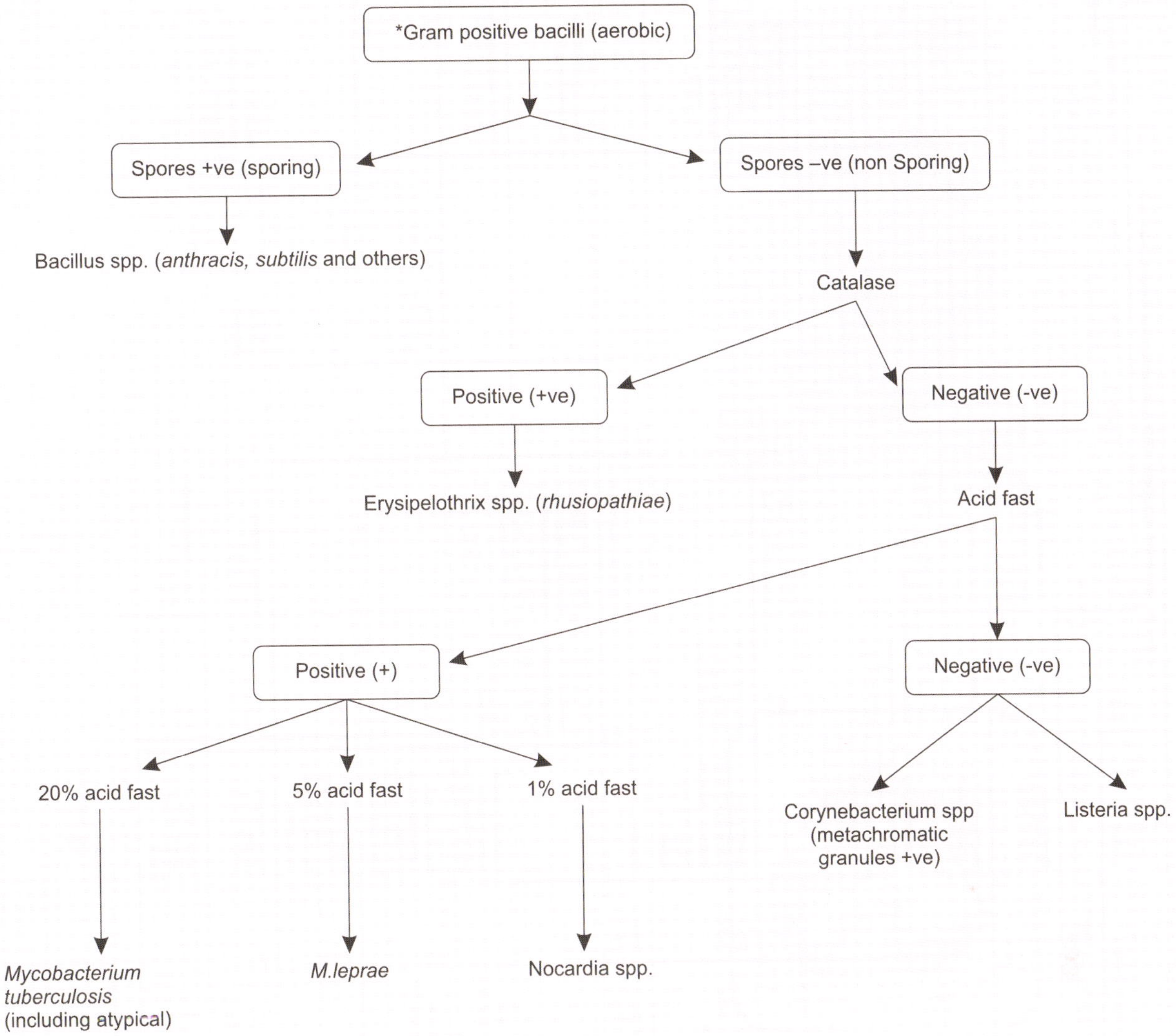

Note: many gram positive bacteria can appear as gram variable and even gram negative due to overdecolourization, phagocytosis, antimicrobial effect, aging etc.

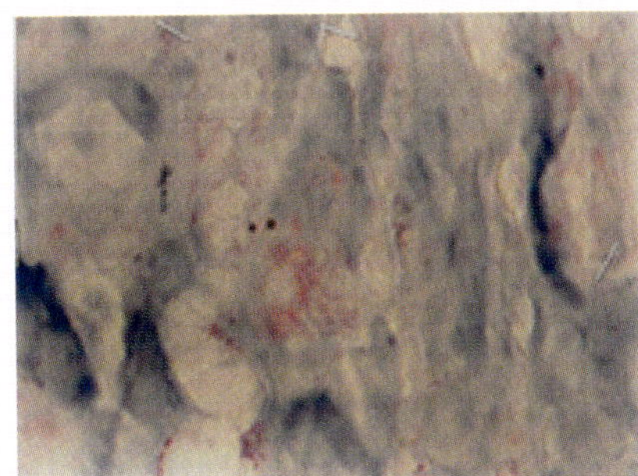

Fig. 5.1.4: Leprosy: Acid fast staining of tissue demonstrating acid fast bacilli in groups (globi), designated as 'cigar bundle' appearance

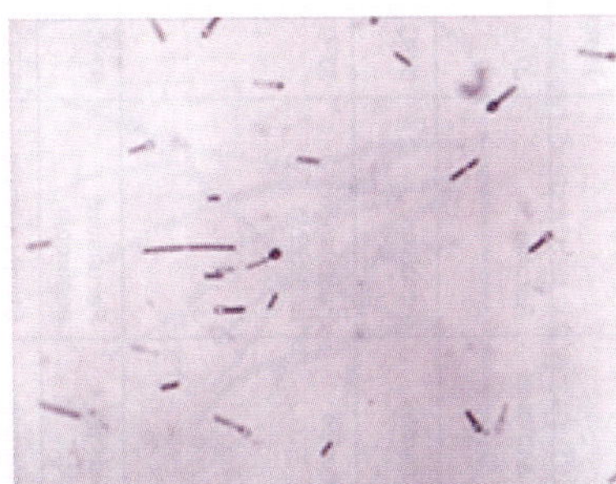

Fig. 5.1.5: Tetanus: Gram stained smear demonstrating gram positive bacilli with terminal spherical spores (drum stick appearance)

Courtesy: Centers for Disease Control and Prevention, Atlanta, USA

	Basal media	Enriched media	Selective/ others	Characterization and confirmation of isolation
Clostridium perfringens (based on 4 major toxins namely alpha, beta, epsilon and iota, categorized into 5 types, A to E.	Nutrient agar: + (incubated anaerobically)	• Blood agar (with neomycin, which inhibits gut bacteria & aerobic spore bearers: + • Egg yolk agar medium with half plate having *Clostridium perfringens* anti-toxin (to demonstrate the Nagler reaction i.e. half plate with no antitoxin has opacity because of lectithinase activity while the other half with antitoxin has no opacity, as antitoxin (anti-alpha toxin antibody) neutralizes alpha toxin (Fig. 5.2.8) • Robertson cooked medium (4 tubes are inoculated & heated at 100°C for 5, 10, 15 and 20 min. Then incubated for 24-48 hrs & sub-cultured on to blood agar plates • Marshal's medium–black colonies (medium has polymyxin, neomycin & iron citrate) • Note: Incubation at 45°C for 4-6 hrs can serve as enrichment (as this temperature is optimal for this organism). Later subculture to blood agar plates is done (this organism has low generation time of 10 minutes)	-	• Microscopy (gram staining) p. 300 **Target haemolysis on B.A.* **narrow zone of complete haemolysis caused by theta toxin & wider zone of incomplete heamolysis caused by alpha toxin* • RCM: meat pink, as organism predominant saccharolytic, reaction, culture has predominant acid reaction • Litmus milk: Stormy reaction (lactose fermented, so litmus turns red from blue, casein coagulate is disrupted by gas produced (stormy fermentation) *Biochemical characterization* • Most strains reduce nitrate • Ferments many sugars with acid & gas • MR+ve,VP(-), H_2S produced • Gas liquid chromatography (confirms species) • Reverse CAMP test: +ve (Fig. 5.2.9) • Typing of staining is done on type of toxins produced by different strain Note: Different methods; as neutralization test, specific antitoxin & intracutaneous injection in guinea pig or intravenous injection in mice are used for further characterization
Clostridium tetani (ten serological types, I to X	• NA:+ • Gelatin stab culture: Fir tree type growth	• Blood agar: haemolytic (because of tetanolysin), swarming, except type VI which is non-flagellate • (Horse) blood agar with tetanus antitoxin on half plate to demonstrate tetanolysin, part with antitoxin has no haemolysis, 4% agar plates used to inhibit swarming • Robertson cooked medium: Specimen inoculated into 3 test tubes of RCM, one is heated at 80°C for 15 mins, second is heated at 80°C for 5 minutes and the third in not heated. The principle is to kill the vegetative bacteria & leave tetanus spores, which vary in heat resistance. These are incubated at 37°C & then subcultured to blood agar daily for 4 days (At 80°C tetanus spores get killed)	MacConkey:+	• Microscopic character (gram staining) • 'drum stick' appearance • Motile (swarming+) • Biochemical characterization (tests put in anaerobic condition utilizing specialized techniques • Slightly proteolytic • Not ferment any sugar (no saccharolytic property) • Toxigenicity testing (tests only tetanolysin) • Animal pathogenicity test: (demonstrates tetanospasmin in isolated organism) culture in RCM is injected into tail of two mice, one acts as test and control receives tetanus antitoxin one hour earlier. If test is +ve, test animal develops stiffness of tail, which ascends to leg and other parts. Control animal shows no change.
Clostridium botulinum (8 types: A,B, C1, C2, D, E, F and G based on distinct toxins	NA: +	• Blood agar: + • Egg yolk agar: + • Robertson cooked medium (two bottles incubated one is heated at 80°C for 10 min to act on resistant spores)		• Gram staining (subterminal, oval, bulging spore) p. 300 • Toxigenicity test for toxin in mice • Biochemical characterization • Fluorescent antibody test • Testing of specific toxin in isolated strain after appropriate incubation in liquid media
Clostridium difficile	NA: NG	• Blood agar: + • Robertson cooked medium: (saccharolytic reaction)	• CCFA (cycloserine, cefloxitin fructose agar) is selective medium • Yellow colonies formed due to fructose fermentation	• Microscopic (gram staining-oval, subterminal, large spore) • For epidemiological purposes, divided into 7 types (slide agglutination, bacteriophage typing, bacteriocin typing done)
Actinomyces israelli	N.A.: NG	• B.A.:+ve • BHI agar: molar tooth appearance • Thioglycollate broth (specimen inoculated anaerobically for few weeks)	MacConkey: NG	• Gram positive, branching bacilli • Non acid fast • Anaerobic organism • Biochemical tests helpful

NB: – + indicates growth
– NG indicates no growth
– BHIA is Brain heart infusion agar
– SDA is Sabouraud's dextrose agar

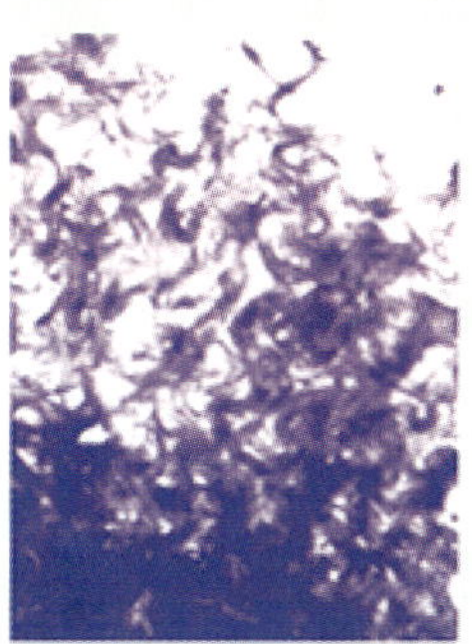

Fig. 5.2.1: Anthrax: Medusa head appearance of *B. anthracis*

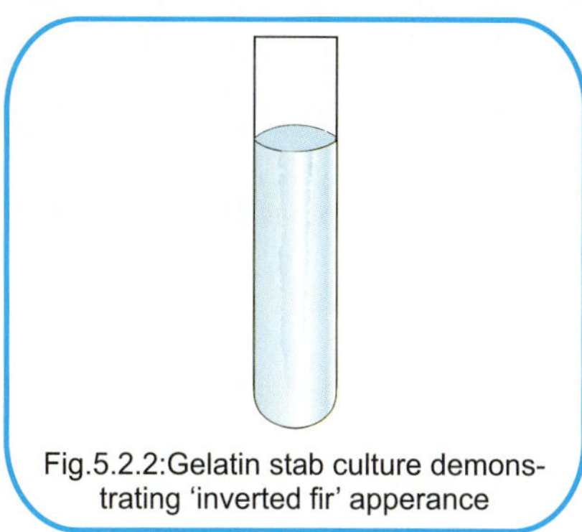

Fig.5.2.2:Gelatin stab culture demonstrating 'inverted fir' apperance

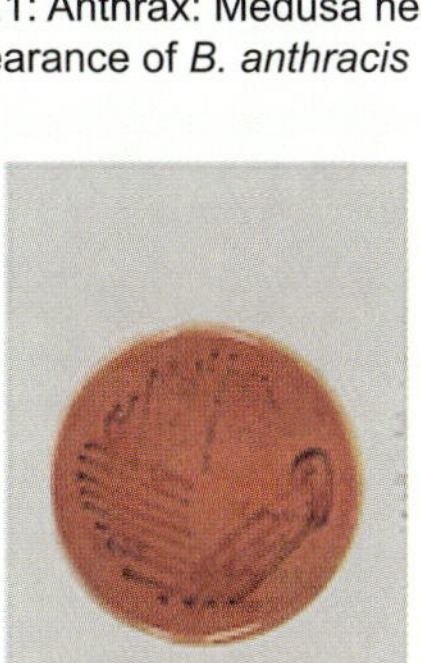

Fig. 5.2.3: DIPHTHERIA: Colonies of *C. diphtheriae*, gravis biotype on potassium tellurite blood agar

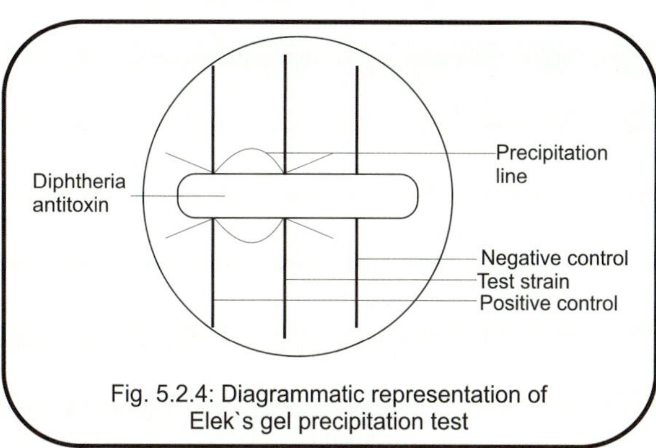

Fig. 5.2.4: Diagrammatic representation of Elek`s gel precipitation test

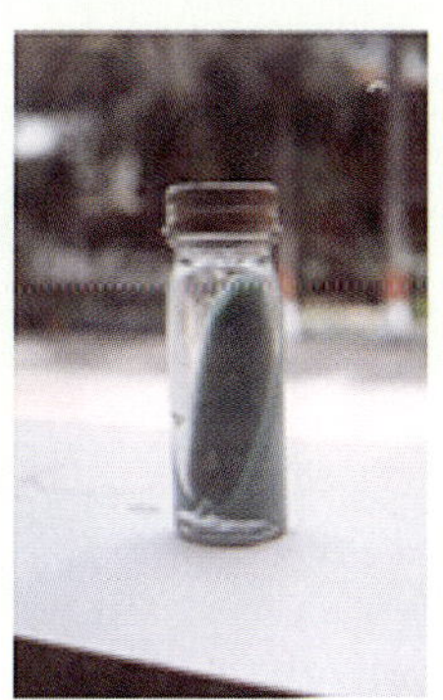

Fig. 5.2.5: Lowenstein-Jensen medium

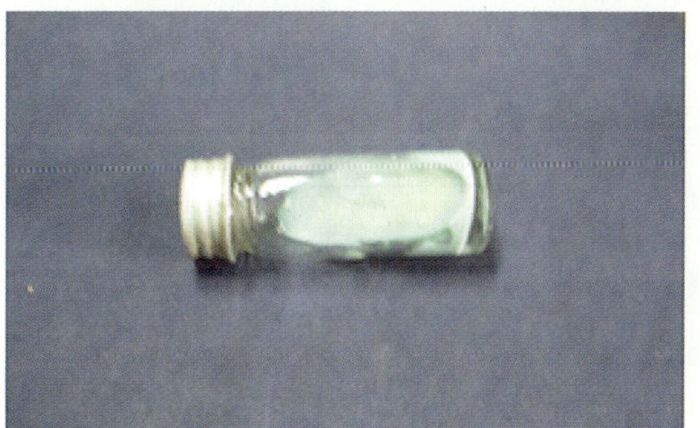

Fig. 5.2.6: Macroscopic appearance of *M. tuberculosis* on L.J. medium

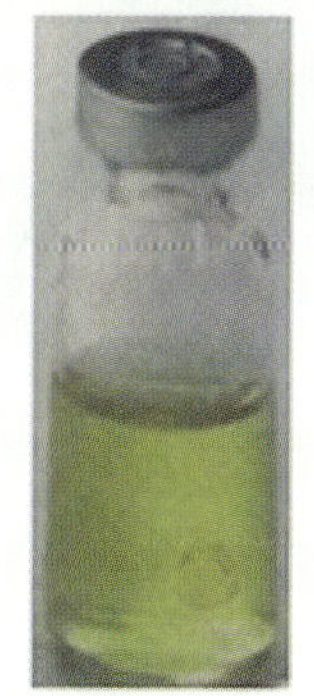

Fig. 5.2.7: Niacin test

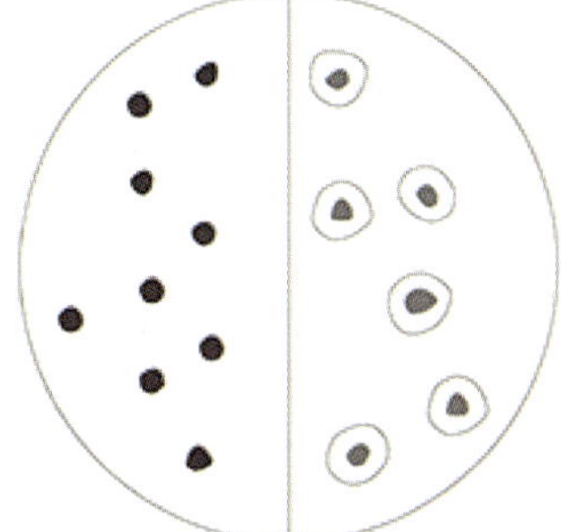

Fig. 5.2.8: *C.perfringen*: Nagler reaction

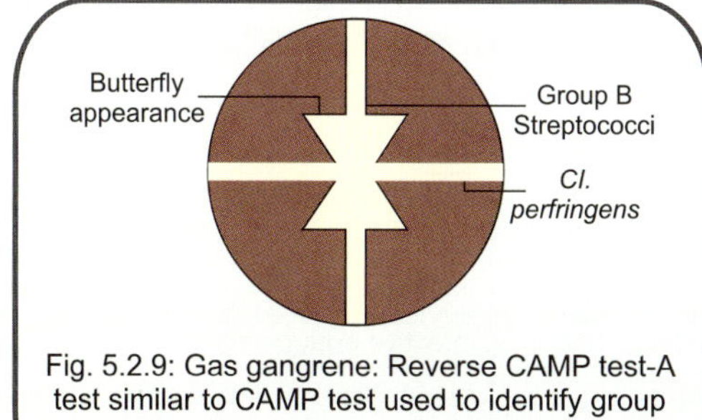

Fig. 5.2.9: Gas gangrene: Reverse CAMP test-A test similar to CAMP test used to identify group B streptococcus. Here group B streptococcus *(S .agalactiae)* streaked instead

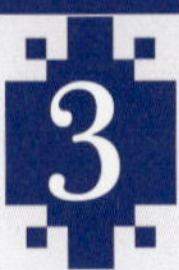

Clinical (Pathogenicity) Profile of Infection Caused By Gram Positive Bacilli

Bacilus anthracis	Cutaneous anthrax (malignant pustule), hide porters' disease) (Fig. 5.3.1) • Case: pg 224-225
	Pulmonary anthrax (wool sorter's disease) • Case: pg 223
	Intestinal anthrax
	Septicaemic anthrax
Bacillus subtilis	Opportunistic infections
Bacillus cereus	Food poisoning (emetic and diarrhoeal types, details see 4d. p. 225) ocular infections, bactermia
C. diphtheriae	Carrier state (significant number)
	Diphtheria most common - upper respiratory (pharyngeal/tonsillar), the pseudmembrance on it may extend to larynx, trachea and cause respiratory obstruction (Fig. 5.3.2) • Case: pgs 226-229
	Cutaneous diphtheria (toxin production is not significant) (Fig. 5.3.3)
	Diphtheria of others sites - rare and usually secondary to above lesions e.g., conjunctival, otitic, corneal etc.
	• Diphtheria toxin can cause: myocarditis - manifest as (weakness, dyspnoea, arrythmia and cardiac enlargement and C.H.F. during 2nd, 3rd week of severe infection • Peripheral neuropathy, cranial nerve palsy - paralysis of palate, oculomotor (eye) muscle or other group; also observed

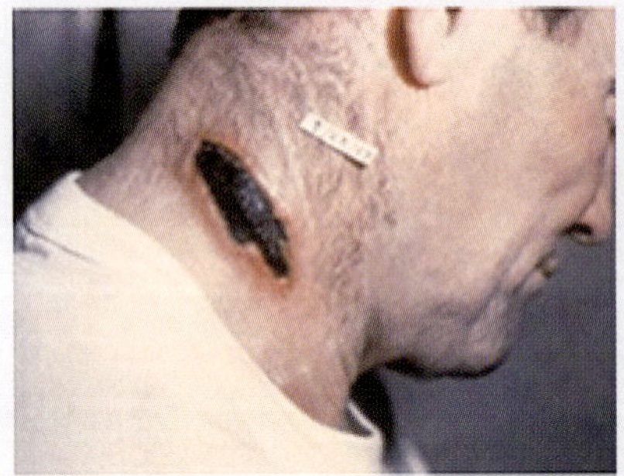

Fig. 5.3.1: CUTANEOUS ANTHRAX: Classic lesion on the neck

Courtesy: Centers for Disease Control and Prevention, Atlanta, USA

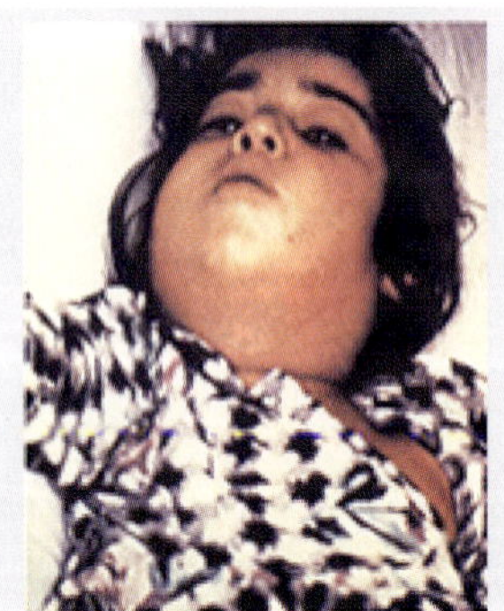

Fig. 5.3.2: DIPHTHERIA: Child with diphtheria presented with typical swollen neck, occasionally referred to as bull neck

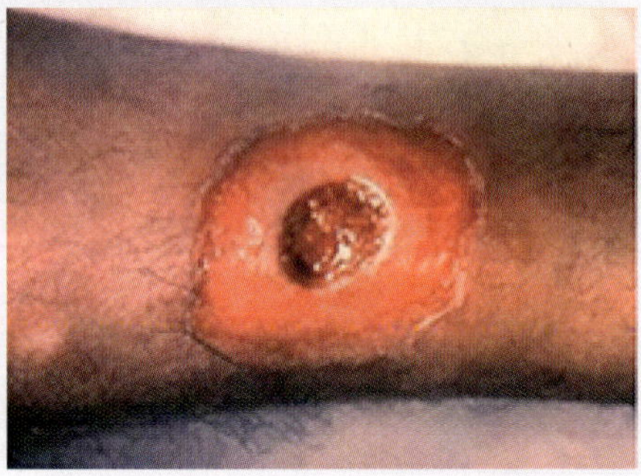

Fig. 5.3.3: DIPHTHERIA: Rarely diphtheria affects the skin where it can manifest as ulcer

Courtesy: Centers for Disease Control and Prevention, Atlanta, USA

Corynebacterium sps other than *C.diphtheriae* as *C.ulcerans*, *C.jeikeium*, & others	See A.10, pg 229	
Arachnobacterium haemolyticum	See clinical problem 6, A11, pg 229	
Rhodococcus equi	Infections in immunocompromised individuals	
Rothia dentocariosa	Infective endocarditis	
Diptheroids e.g.. *C. xerosis*	rarely associated with human disease	
Mycobacterium tuberculosis	Pulmonary tuberculosis Cases: pgs 230-232 and 233-236	- Primary infection - Post-primary (secondary tuberculosis) usually by endogenous reactivation - usually in apex of lungs

	Extrapulmonary tuberculosis		
	Tuberculous lymphaderitis (common presentation in children)		
	Tuberculous enteritis	(Usually post primary)	
	CNS	- Small cortical lesion (Rich's focus), - Tuberculous abscess (tuberculoma) - Other types	
	Urinary system	- Tuberculous pyonephritis, - Tuberculous pyonephrosis, - Others	
	Genital tract	- Tuberculous prostatitis, - Tuberculous epidymitis, - Tuberculous salpingitis, - Tuberculous endometritis	
	Skeletal system	- Synovitis, arthritis, - Pott's disease of spine - Psoas abscess (along fascial planes)	
	Skin	- Lupus vulgaris	
		- Scrofuloderma (involvement of the skin, direct extension from underlying lymph gland)	
		- Papulo-necrotic tuberculide probably represents extreme hypersensitive reaction to infection elsewhere in body	
	Serous cavities	- Tuberulous pleurisy, - Tuberculous pericarditis, - Tuberculous peritonitis	
	Eyes	- Phlyctenular conjunctivits, - Iridocyclitis - Tubercles in the choroid (in miliary spread)	
Non-Tuberculous mycobacteria			
M.kansasii (photochromogen) *M.marinum*		Chronic pulmonary disease (resembles TB) • Case: pg, 237-238 Swimming pool granuloma See A.7, p. 238	
M.scrofulaceum (scotochromogen) *M. gordonae*		- Cervical adenitis (Scrofula) - Contaminant of clinical sample as present in tap water (rare cause of pulmonary disease M. avium-intracellular ?one word)	
M.avium-(Non photochromogen) *M. intracellulare* *M.ulcerans*		- Chronic pulmonary disease - Renal infection - Lymphadenopathy, - Disseminated disease, - Buruli ulcer - Chronic lung disease	
M.chelonae, *M.fortuitum*		Chronic abscesses, outbreaks following parenteral adminstration of injections reported	
Mycobacterium leprae	Tuberculoid leprosy (Fig. 5.3.4)	Skin - few, non-elevated. hypo/hyper pigmented macular anaesthetic patches involving the faces, trunk & Limbs • Case: pgs 239-241	
		Nerve - peripheral & bigger nerve trunks (hard, thickened & tender) may be involved leading to deformities of hand & feet	
	Lepromatous leprosy (Figs. 5.3.5, 5.3.6)	See A2b(ii), pg 239	
Nocardia sps (asteroides & brasilensis)	- Pulmonary lesions (bronchopneumonia is common), - Brain abscess, - Others including mycetoma, cellulitis		
Listeria monocytogenes	*In neonates* - Sepsis - Meningitis - Granulomatosis infantiseptica	*In pregnant women* - Febrile illness - Spontaneous abortions - Still-births (granulomatis infantiseptica) - Puerperal sepsis	*Adults* - Sepsis/meningitis/others especially in immunocompromised
Erysipelothrix rhusiopathiae	Erysipeloid		
Actinomyces israelii	- Cervicofacial actinomycosis (most common Fig. 5.3.7), - Thoracic actinomycosis (rare) - Abdominal actinomycosis (rare) • Case: pgs 248-249		

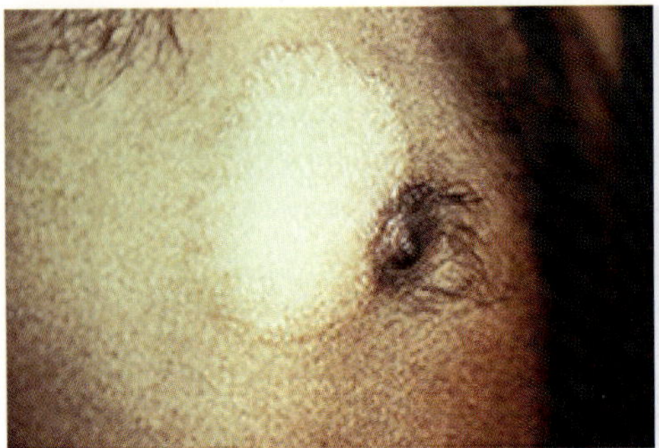

Fig. 5.3.4: TUBERCULOID LEPROSY: Case with hypopigmented cutaneous lesion known as plaque, lateral to his right nipple

Courtesy: Arthur E. Kaye/DC

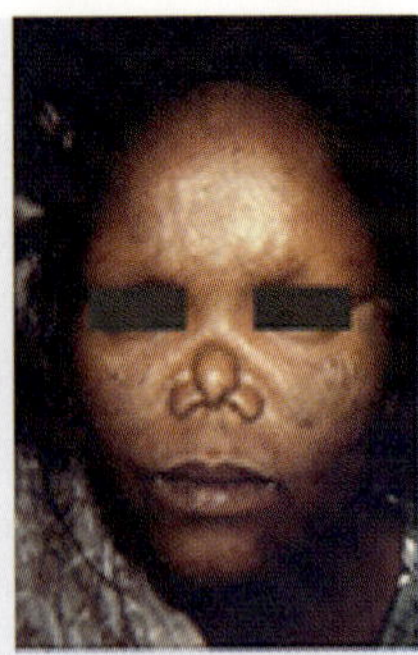

Fig. 5.3.5: LEPROMATOUS LEPROSY: Case with depressed nasal bridge known as saddle-nose deformity, lack of eye brows and mottled discoloration of sclera bilaterally

Courtesy: Dr. Andre J. Lebrun/CDC

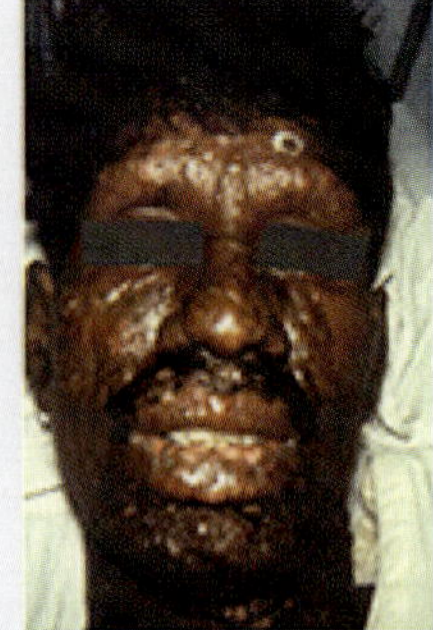

Fig. 5.3.6: LEPROSY: Male case with lepromatous leprosy. Nodules dispersed over face and eyebrows missing

Courtesy: Dr. Andre J. Lebrun/CDC

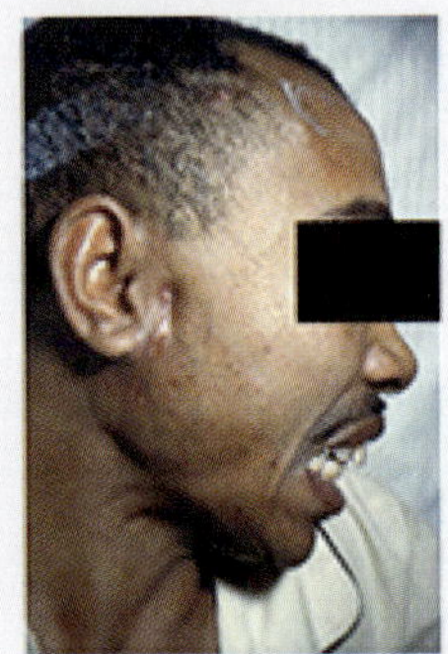

Fig. 5.3.7: ACTINOMYCOSIS: A patient with classic lesion on the right side of the face

Courtesy: CDC/Dr. Thomas F. Sellers/Emory University

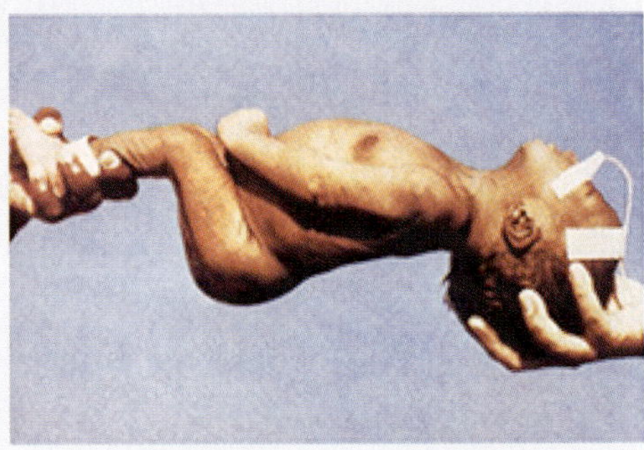

Fig.5.3.8: TETANUS: Neonate displaying characteristic rigidity of tetanus

Courtesy: Centers for Disease Control and Prevention, Atlanta, USA

Actinomadura madurae & pelletieri	Mycetoma (bacterial)
Streptomyces somaliensis	Mycetoma (bacterial)
Lactobacillus spp.	Commensals & non pathogenic, however may be involved in serious infections & dental caries
Eubacterium spp.	Commensals, however may be involved in periodontitis
Bifidobacterium spp.	Commensals however may be involved in dental caries
Propionibacterium spp. as *P. acnes* (anaerobic diphtheroids)	Commensal, pathogenic role not clear although regularly isolated from acne and some other lesions
Mobiluncus spp. (as *curtisii*)	Isolated from bacterial vaginosis site along with *Gardnerella vaginalis* & Bacteriodes species.
Clostridium perfringens	- Simple saprophyte contamination of wound (Upto 80-90% of isolates in this category) - Anaerobic cellulitis, - Gas gangrene, - Food poisoning (some of type A), - Necrotising enteritis - Others as clostridial endometritis, gangrenous appendicitis. Case: pg. 242 and 243
Clostridium tetani	Generalized tetanus (as muscle spasm, lock jaw (trismus), risus sardonicus (sardonic smile) Other types–neonatal tetanus (Fig. 5.3.8), uterine tetanus & otogenic tetanus.
Clostridium botulinum	- Food borne botulism (by improperly canned or preserved food), - Wound botulism, - Infant botulism
Clostridium difficile	- Pseudomembranous colitis (diarrohea), - Antibiotic associated colitis. Case: pg. 247

Integrated Clinical Based Study of *B.anthracis*/Anthrax

In September 2001 in USA, an adult presented with bronchopneumonia to the medical emergency. An odd history of opening a postal envelope containing some powder like material was available. The powder was tested and it was found to contain some spores.

Linkages: Pg. 212, 214, 216, 219, 220, 250, 252

What is the provisional diagnosis of this case?

A.1 It is a likely a case of microbial bioterrorism, which followed exposure to anthrax spores. The case is likely to have inhaled the infective spores and developed bronchopneumonia.

What makes B. anthracis a bioweapon?

A.2 Anthrax is easily spread by spores, has a low LD50 value, is stable, has a long life and is difficult to destroy. In fact Gruinard island near Scotland in 1940s, deliberately contaminated during bacteriological warfare (anthrax bomb), is still considered to be uninhabitable.

The disease, this agent causes resembles clinical disease and is likely to be taken as a routine sickness; unless a suspicion of bioterrorism is considered. This agent can also be genetically engineered to make it multidrug resistant, so would be difficult to treat.

What impact the postal bioterrorism incidents had in U.S. in 2001?

A.3 In the September 2001 postal bioterrorism incidents, 11 patients acquired inhalational (pulmonary) anthrax, out of which 5 died. Eleven cases of cutaneous anthrax were also reported, all of which survived.

What is the LD50 (lethal dose, 50%) for anthrax spores?

A.4 Animal studies in 1950s conducted in monkeys; using aerosolized infective material, suggested that 10,000 spores could produce lethal disease in 50% of animals exposed.

What are the virulent factors for B. anthracis?

A.5 There are two key virulent factors. One is the capsule, which is unique, being composed of polypeptide. It inhibits phagocytosis and the non-capsular strains lack this virulence factor. The second factor is the toxin produced by the organism, which is plasmid mediated.

What was the basis of the original Pasteur anthrax vaccine?

A.6 (a) It was based on encapsulated strain, which was repeatedly subcultured at 42-43°C to be make it non-virulent. At that time, the mechanism of the vaccine strain was not clear, but now we know that strain lost the virulence due to loss of plasmid, which controls the toxin production.

Describe the currently used anthrax vaccine for human use.

A.6 (b) **Composition:** Alum precipitated toxoid from protective antigen

Indication: In individuals occupationally exposed to anthrax infection

Dosage: Three doses intramuscularly at intervals of 6 weeks and 6 months. A booster dose may be administered, after one year.

Why do extra precautions have to be undertaken, while handling clinical specimens with suspected bioweapons? Mention the reason chemoprophylaxis may be ineffective in such a scenario.

A.7 Extreme precautions have to be taken, while handing a specimen suspected to be infected with anthrax, as transmission by aerosol formation can occur. Biosafety level-3 (BSL-3) facility has to be used for sample handling and microbiological work.

The strain used for bioterrorism could be genetically engineered to make it multidrug resistant. Hence, one has to be extra cautious, while handling it, as this factor would make the microbe resistant to commonly used antimicrobials in chemoprophylaxis.

Enumerate antimicrobials to be administered and the duration in post-exposure anthrax cases?

A.8 Ciprofloxacin or Doxycycline can be administered for 60 days. Such regime is followed, as *B. anthracis* isolates can express penicillin resistance.

Integrated Clinical Based Study of *B.anthracis*/Pustule

A veterinarian Dr V. Salunke after handling a sheep, developed a pustule on his hand. Gram stained smear of the lesion revealed gram positive bacilli in long chains.

Linkages: Pg. 212, 213, 214, 216, 219, 220, 250, 252

What is your diagnosis of this case?

A.1 (a) **Cutaneous anthrax.** It follows entry of anthrax spores through skin, for instance in dock workers carrying loads of hides through their back.

What are the other two other common forms of anthrax?

A.1 (b)
- **Pulmonary anthrax:** It is commonly called 'wool sorter's' disease, as it is common in wool factory workers, due to inhalation of dust from infected wool. The common presentation is of haemorrhagic pneumonitis, with a complication of haemorrhagic meningitis.
- **Intestinal anthrax:** It is a rare form of anthrax, seen commonly in communities, who eat improperly cooked infected meat especially of animal carcasses. Bloody diarrhea is a common presentation.

Which rapid technique can be performed on the blood smear from an animal; with suspected anthrax infection?

A.2 Polychrome methylene blue staining of the blood smear. If it demonstrates amorphous purplish material (representing capsule), it would indicate infection by *B. anthracis*. This finding, if present is indicative of Mc Fadyean's reaction.

Highlight the historical importance of Anthrax?

A.3 (a) Robert Koch established the Koch postulates by his studies on *B. anthracis*. He was able to grow this organism in pure culture (first organism to be grown so), demonstrated it to have an endospore (first organism to have this demonstration) and produced experimental anthrax by infecting animals (first time). It was the first pathogenic bacterium to be demonstrated under the microscope (Pollender, 1849). It was the first bacterium to be used for the preparation of live attenuated vaccine by Louis Pasteur in 1881.

B. subtilis is used as a model in bacterial genetic studies.

Describe the epidemiology of anthrax.

A.3 (b) Anthrax is enzootic in India. It commonly involves herbivores; as goat, sheep and cattle. The source of infection is spores in soil, which enter the animals through unrecognized breaks in skin and mucus membrane. Outbreaks of anthrax have been reported from A.P., Tamil Nadu, Karanataka and West Bengal. These episodes are responsible for human infections, especially the cutaneous type. In September 2001, postal bioterrorism incidents were reported from USA.

What is the importance of culturing the exudate of the clinical lesion of the above case (with suggestive microscopic features of anthrax infection)?

A.4 (a) Isolation of typical 'medusa head' colonies on nutrient agar medium along with performance of other appropriate tests on it, can help in confirming the identity of the isolate. Further strain characterization is performed, if necessary using molecular techniques; as amplified fragment length polymorphism.

With which group of organisms, can B. anthracis be confused with?

A.4 (b) This organism can be confused with aerobic spore bearers (anthracoid bacteria), which are common laboratory contaminants.

Tabulate the differentiating features between anthrax bacilli and anthracoid bacilli.

A.4 (c)

		Anthrax bacilli	Anthracoid bacilli
Microscopic features	*Capsule*	+	-
	Motility	Non motile	Motile
	Length of chain	Long	Short
	McFadyean reaction	+	-
Cultural characters	*Medusa head colony*	+	-
	Gelatin stab culture	'Inverted' fir appearance	Rapid liquefaction
	Broth	No turbidity, but floccular growth	Turbidity
	Growth at 45°C	No growth	Growth
Identification tests	*Salicin fermentation*	-	+
	Direct fluorescent antibody test	+	-
	Gamma phage	Susceptible	Not susceptible
	Pathogenic to guinea pig	Pathogenic	Not pathogenic

Compare and contrast the two types of B. cereus food poisoning.

A.4 (d)

	'Emetic' type	'Diarrhoeal' type
Food	Fried rice (especially from Chinese restaurant)	Meat, vegetables
Incubation period	Short (1-5 hrs)	Long (8-16 hrs)
Pathogenicity	Nausea and vomiting common	Abdominal pain and diarrohea
Mechanism	Emetic toxin (by serotypes 1, 3 & 5)	Enterotoxin (by serotypes 2, 6, 8, 9, 10 &12)

Enumerate uses of organisms belonging to Bacillus genus.

A.5 *Geobacillus. stearothermophilus* (previously genus Bacillus) – used in sterility testing of autoclaves

B. pumilus – used to test efficacy of ionizing radiation for sterilization

B. globigii – used to test efficacy of ethylene oxide (biological control)

B. thuringensis – Malaria (larval) control

B. subtilis and licheniformis – Bacitracin synthesis

B. polymyxa – polymyxin synthesis

B. brevis – gramicidin synthesis

B. coagulans – biological controls in assay of Folic acid

B. megaterium – biological control in assay of aflatoxin

B. subtilis – biological control in assay of hexachlorophane

B. subtilis – model in bacterial genetic studies

What processes are employed to disinfect common animal products, infected with anthrax spores?

A.6 For disinfecting wool, it can be exposed to 2% formaldehyde at 30-40°C for 20 minutes (duckering). Animal hair can be disinfected by exposure to 0.25% formalin solution at 60°C for 6 hours.

Mention general prophylactic aspects for anthrax.

A.7
- Improvement of hygiene, wherever meat processed
- Sterilization of animal products, as wool and hide
- Carcasses of animals suspected to have died of anthrax to be buried deep with lime
- Vaccination of humans (at risk) and animals

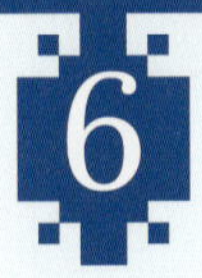

Integrated Clinical Based Study of *C.diphtheriae*/Diphtheria

An 8 year girl, Nasreena presented with fever and cervical lymphadenopathy. Her oral examination revealed a greyish membrane on right tonsil extending to the posterior pharyngeal wall.

Linkages: Pg. 212-214, 216, 219, 220, 250, 252

Enumerate the microbes that can produce a membranous lesion, like the one in this case? What is your presumptive clinical diagnosis?

A.1 *C.diphtheriae*, *Candida albicans*, *Streptococcus pyogenes*, *Treponema vincentii* and *Lepotrichia buccalis*.

Diphtheria. The diphtheria bacillus was first described by Kleb in 1883 and cultivated by Loeffler in 1884, hence also known as Klebs-Loeffler bacillus.

Why is this membrane like structure in a diphtheria case called a 'pseudo membrane'?

A.2 It is called a pseudomembrane (False membrane), as it doesn't have an epithelial layer.

Enumerate the differences between three biotypes of C. diphtheriae.

A.3 (a) Differences between three biotypes of *C.diphtheriae* (on *potassium* tellurite *blood agar*)

	Gravis	**Intermedius**	**Mitis**
Morphology			
(i) Form	Short rods (uniform staining)	Long barred forms (irregular staining)	Long curved forms (pleomorphic) ww
(ii) Granules	Few	Few	Significant
Culture			
(i) Haemolysis	Variable	Non-haemolytic	Haemolytic
(ii) Size	1-2 mm	1 mm	variable
(iii) Shape	Grey with raised center	Grey-black with granular center	Shiny back, circular and smooth
(iv) Edge	Crenated	Glistening periphery	Smooth
(v) Appearance	'Daisy head' colony	'Frogs egg' colony	'Poached egg' colony
(vi) Consistency	Brittle	Intermediate (between gravis and mitis)	Soft, buttery
Biochemical reactions			
Glycogen and starch fermentation	+	–	–
Virulence	Severe	Intermediate	Mild

Which Corynebacterium species other than 'diphtheriae' can cause a clinical picture similar to above case?

A.3 (b) Tox+ strains of *C.ulcerans*. Some believe this organism to be a subgroup of diphtheria bacilli. It resembles the gravis biotype of diphtheria bacillus but varies biochemically. It is susceptible to erythromycin and diphtheria antitoxin is protective.

Should the pediatrician wait for a microbiology report, before the treatment is initiated?

A.4 The paediatrician shouldn't wait of the microbiologic confirmation of the diagnosis, as delay in the initiation of treatment can compromise with the positive outcome in a case. He should immediately start the treatment on clinical suspicion and initiate the laboratory processing of the specimen for confirmation of the clinical diagnosis. The microbiological diagnosis is more of epidemiological importance.

What is the major virulent factor for C. diphtheriae?

A.5 (a) The virulent factor is the presence of phage in the isolate, which incorporates the diphtheria toxin gene (tox) responsible for production of exotoxin (Diphtheria exotoxin, discovered by Roux and Yersin,1888).

Can you have a C. diphtheriae strain, which is non virulent?

A.5 (b) Only lysogenized strains of *C. diphtheriae* can cause the disease. Non lysogenized strains of *C. diptheriae* strains are non-virulent.

What is the mechanism of action of diphtheria toxin?

A.5 (c) The exotoxin coded by the bacteriophage has two fragments. Fraction B; aids in binding of the toxin to certain tissues and has increased affinity for myocardium, adrenal glands and nerve endings. Fragment A; is active and inhibits protein synthesis in host cells by inactivating elongation factor (EF-2), required for elongating polypeptide chain in presence of nicotinamide adenine dinucleotide. So, the exotoxin is like a eukaryotic protein synthesis inhibitor, just like some antibiotics are prokaryotic protein synthesis inhibitors.

What are the rapid techniques to detect the diphtheria toxin?

A.6 (a) PCR based tests to demonstrate the diphtheria toxin gene are available. This test give results from the clinical specimen, before culture results are available. As an alternative to Elek's test, enzyme-linked immunosorbent assay is available to detect diphtheria toxin from clinical *C.diphtheriae* isolates.

Describe the conventional techniques, which determine virulence in an diphtherial isolate?

A.6 (b) Virulence tests

'In vivo':	*'In vitro'*
(i) Subcutaneous test	(i) Elek's gel precipitation test
(ii) Intracutaneous test	(ii) Tissue culture test

- *Subcutaneous test:* Broth emulsion is prepared from the test isolate and injected subcutaneously into two guinea pigs. One guinea pig is protected with 500 units of ADS (anti-diphtherial serum)18-24 hours before the test. If the test strain is virulent, the unprotected guinea pig dies, whereas the protected animal survives. The autopsy of the dead animal demonstrates classical findings including enlarged lymph nodes (at draining site of inoculation) and enlarged haemmorhagic adrenals (pathognomic finding). This procedure is wasteful of animals.
- *Intracutaneous test:* This test is so devised that death of animal does not occur and many strains (isolates) can be tested on one animal. The broth emulsion is prepared from the test isolate and injected into two guinea pigs. One of these acts as control and receives 500 units of ATS, the previous day and the other gets 50 units of ATS intraperitoneally four hours, after the test to prevent the death. If the test isolate is virulent, inflammatory reaction occurs at the site of injection in the test animal; progressing to necrosis in 48-72 hours and in the control animal, the infection site remains unaffected.
- *Elek's gel precipitation test:* It is a variant of a 'double diffusion in double dimensions' of precipitation reaction. Filter paper strip (rectangular) impregnated with diphtheria antitoxin is placed on surface of solid enriched medium (horse serum agar), when it is in fluid state
  - When it solidifies, test strain along with positive and negative strains are inoculated at right angles to the paper strip zone.
  - Plate incubated at 37°C for 24-48 hours
  - Presence of arrowhead shaped precipitate (Fig 5.2.4, pg 219) around the test strain, indicates the strain to be toxigenic (toxin diffuses obliquely, where it meets antitoxin in optimum concentration, it produces a precipitate). Nontoxigenic strains do not produce precipitation lines
- *Tissue culture test:* This is performed by incorporating the test strains into an agar overlay of cell culture monolayers. If the strain is toxigenic, the diffused toxin kills the underlying cells.

What are the key mechanisms; by which C. diphtheriae can cause human mortality (death)?

A.7 (a) The organism can cause death by the following mechanisms:

(i) Expanding and sloughing membrane on the throat, can cause respiratory obstruction leading to asphyxia

(ii) Myocarditis can lead to heart failure

What are the complications, a case with diphtheria infection can develop?

A.7 (b) (i) Polyneuropathy and post-diphtheric paralysis of palatine and ciliary muscles.

(ii) Septic complications; as localized ulceration and cellulitis (around pseudomembrane)

(iii) Degenerative changes in adrenal, kidney and liver. The pseudomembrane also serves as a base from which the toxin is secreted.

How is antidiphtheric serum (ADS) produced?

A.8 (a) Diphtheria antitoxin (anti-diphtheria serum) discovered by von Behring (1890) is produced by hyper-immunizing the horses with the diphtheria toxin, following a standard protocol and then collecting the horse serum; which is subsequently standardized.

What is the role of ADS?

A.8 (b) As the antitoxin is effective only against unbound toxin, it should be administered at the earliest suspicion of the disease. The administration of this antitoxin results in reduction of complications; as myocarditis, neuropathy and in reducing the mortality.

The *skin or conjunctival test* should be performed (giving a test dose) before its administration. This is to rule out immediate hypersensitivity to this product, as it is raised in an animal. If the individual is hypersensitive to the serum, the patient should be desensitized, before the antitoxin is administered.

Is Diphtheria a notifiable public health infectious disease? Mention about the control measures.

A.9 (a) It is a nationally notifiable disease in our country. An active search for cases and carriers should be done. All cases (included suspected and carriers) should be isolated for at least 14 days or until proved free of infection. The carriers should be treated with 10 day course of oral erythromycin. Vaccination measures should be strengthened.

Describe the epidemiology of diphtheria.

A.9 (b)
- *Agent:*
  - Toxigenic (tox$^+$) *C. diphtheriae* is responsible for the respiratory diphtheria.
  - Non Toxigenic (Tox$^-$) *C. diphtheriae* often causes cutaneous diphtheria and other forms of diphtheria.
  - Growth of this pathogen under low-iron conditions mimics 'in vivo' conditions of host and induces production of the diphtheria toxin

Four types of diphtheria biotypes are known namely; gravis, mitis, and intermedius and belfanti.

- *Reservoir of infection:* It can be a case or carrier. Carriers are important sources of infection. The carriers may be throat/nasal or cutaneous carrier. In endemic areas, 3-5 percent of healthy individuals may harbour this pathogen in the throat. Skin infection can be an important silent reservoir of infection and has been responsible for several epidemics in the West.
- *Sources of infection:* Nasopharyngeal secretions and infected cutaneous lesions
- *Mode of transmission:* It spreads primarily by droplets. The transmission can also occur directly to susceptible persons by fomites; as pencils and toys contaminated by infected nasopharyngeal secretions.
- *Host factors:*

  Age: Children primarily aged 1 to 5 are affected. Before immunization was introduced, this was primarily a disease of childhood. Currently; older age groups including adults are reported to be getting infected.

  Immunity: Infants born to immunized mothers are protected for a few weeks.

  Vaccination and natural infection provide protection from the infection for many years.

  A herd immunity of over 70 percent is believed to be necessary to prevent outbreaks.
- *Environment:*

  The disease occurs throughout the year with increased incidence in colder months, crowded areas especially with people belonging to poor social economic status. It has been seen that diphtheria outbreaks occur at gaps of 10 years or more. A massive diphtheria outbreak occurred during the 1990s in the Russian federation (former Soviet Union).

What is the utility of the Schick test? Describe it.

A.9 (c) *Schick test* was introduced in 1913 to determine, if a person is susceptible to infection by *C.diphtheriae* and if it requires diphtheria vaccination. However; this test is no longer in use, as the availability of a safe, cost effective vaccine has obviated this need. It was a test to measure the level of immunity by an 'in vivo' method.

The test is an example of an *'in vivo' neutralization test*, where a very minute amount of diphtheria exotoxin (0.2 ml containing 1/50, minimum lethal dose (MLD) is injected intradermally on the left (passive) forearm (test area) and a similar dose of inactivated toxin is injected into right forearm (control area). The results are read after 1, 4 and 7 days. The four type of reactions that can occur are depicted in the table 5.6.1.

Table 5.6.1: Interpretation of Schick test

Type	Reaction	Interpretation
Positive	No reaction in control area,but erythema and swelling reaction peaking in the test area between 4th and 7th day	Person is susceptible to diphtheria
Negative	No reaction in the test and control area	Immune to diphtheria
'Pseudo' reaction	Erythema occurying in a few hours but disappearing within 4 days. Same reaction in both areas. (test and control)	Immune and also hypersensitive to diphtheria bacilli components
Combined reaction	Initial reaction is of 'pseudo' reaction, but in the test area the reaction progresses to a positive reaction	Susceptible to diphtheria and hypersensitive to bacilli components

Aspects related to case theme/examination assessment

Which are the non-diphtherial corynebacteria (Corynebacterium species other than C. diphtheriae) associated with human diseases?

A.10

Table 5.6.2: Key Non-Diphtherial corynebacteria and diseases (in man) associated with them

Organism	Disease
C. ulcerans	Acute pharyngitis (clinically indistinguishable from pharyngitis)
C. jeikeium (group JK)	Wound infection and septicaemia (in immunocompromised)
C. pseudotuberculosis (ovis)	Systemic infections; as endocarditis, pneumonia in immunocompromised individuals
C. urealyticum (group D2)	Urinary tract infections (as; pharyngitis, cystitis)
C. xerosis, C. bovis	Infective endocarditis
C.minutissum, C.tenus	Superficial skin infections

Name some Coryneform genera other than Corynebacterium, associated with human disease.

A.11

***Arachnobacterium haemolyticum* (formerly *C. haemolyticum*)**	Pharyngitis, peritonsillar abscess, cervical lymphadenitis and skin ulcers
***Rhodococcus equi* (formerly *C.equi*)**	Infections in immunocompromised individuals

What are diphtheroids?

A.12 (a) Are commensal corynebacteria normally found in sites; as skin,throat swab and conjunctiva, rarely associated with human disease.

Name some common diphtheroids.

A.12 (b) *C. xerosis* (found in throat, formerly called *C.hofmanii*) – *C. pseudodiphtherticum*

How do you differentiate C. diphtheriae from diphtheroids?

A.12 (c)

Table 5.6.3: Differences between *C.diphtheriae* and *Diphtheroids*

Feature	*C.diphtheriae*	Diphtheroids
1. Morphology	(i) Thin bacilli	Short and thick bacilli
	(ii) Metachromatic granules* present	few/absent
	(iii) Chinese letter pattern	Pallisade arrangement
	(iv) Pleomorphism present	Minor pleomorphism
2. Culture	Grow on enriched media	Can grow on basal media
3. Biochemical tests	Ferments glucose only	Ferments both glucose and sucrose
4. Toxin production	Toxic (mostly)	Nontoxic
5. Virulence test	Positive	Negative

* Also termed as Volutin/Babes-Ernst granules

Compare active, passive and combined immunization in diphtheria.

A.13 – *Active* immunization consists of administration of a full course of diphtheria toxoid vaccine.

– *Passive* immunization consists of administration of antidiphteritic serum (ADS) subcutaneously (500-1000 units) in a susceptible person exposed to diphtheria, as an emergency measure. The aim is to minimize the binding of the diphtheria exotoxin to the host receptors, so that pathogenicity may not occur and it may be life saving. For this reason, it is administered on clinical ground, without waiting for the microbiology results.

– *Combined* immunization consists of adminstration of toxoid on one arm and ADS on the other arm.

Integrated Clinical Based Study of *M.tuberculosis*/Pulmonary Tuberculosis 1

A 25 year old destitute, Sharanam presented with 3 week history of fever, cough with expectoration and night sweats. Chest X-ray revealed cavitation in right upper lobe. Z.N staining of sputum revealed acid fast bacilli.

Linkages: Pg. 212-214, 216, 219-221, chapter 8, 250, 252

What provisional clinical diagnosis can be made in this case?

A.1 Pulmonary tuberculosis

What is the habitat of M. tuberculosis?

A.2 Primarily the respiratory tract of the infected human host

What are the risk factors for tuberculosis?

A.3 **(a)** (i) HIV infection
- (ii) any condition that leads to immunosuppression; as steroid therapy etc
- (iii) Undernutrition
- (iv) Overcrowding with living in poorly ventilated rooms
- (v) genetic predisposition

What is the natural history of pulmonary TB?

A.3 **(b)** As it is currently understood, only 30% of the exposed cases get *infected*. Of those infected, 90% remain in a condition called *latent tuberculous* infection and only 10% develop *progressive primary T.B.*

Classify Mycobacteria (including atypical and leprae)

Table 5.7.1: Classification of Mycobacteria

A.3 **(c)**

Tubercle bacilli	Atypical Mycobacteria (opportunistic Mycobacteria	Lepra bacilli	Saprophytic mycobacteria
(i) *M.tuberculosis* (Human)	I. Photochromogens (require light for production of light) (i) *M. kansasii,* (ii) *M.marinum*	(i) *M.leprae* (Human)	(i) *M.butyricum*
(ii) *M.bovis* (Bovine)	II. Scotochromogens (produce pigment even in dark) (i) *M.scrofulaceum* (ii) *M.gordonae*	(ii) *M. lepraemurium* (Murine)	(ii) *M.phlei*
(iii) M. africanum	III. Non photochromogens (do not produce any pigment) (i) *M.avium,* (ii) *M.intracellulare* (iii) *M.ulcerans*		(iii) *M. smegmatis*
	IV. Rapid growers (grow within 7 days, even on basal media) (i) *M.chelonae,* (ii) *M.fortuitum*		

NB: Refer Table 5.9.2, pg 238 also.

Why is it important to initiate ATT (antituberculous) treatment, while awaiting culture results in a case with provisional diagnosis of T.B.?

A.4 Traditional culture of sample for cultivation of *M. tuberculosis* requires that the sample be incubated for at least 8-12 weeks, before considering a sample negative for tuberculosis (positive result usually take a minimum of few weeks). Waiting for this long time would lead to systemic spread of the infection, if the case is infected, which needs to be checked out.

Why is long period required for isolating Mycobacteria?

A.5 (a) The generation time for *M. tuberculosis* is about 14-15 hours in contrast to about 20 minutes for *E. coli*. This increased period mandates prolonged incubation period for isolating this organism on inanimate media.

What is the need of rapid identification of M.tuberculosis? Mention the techniques that can result in rapid identification of M.tuberculosis complex?

A.5 (b) The conventional technique of mycobacteria culture using L.J. medium has number of constraints. For instance; it is very time consuming, the organism may be lost to contamination or to the concentration techniques and it may not be able to detect small number of acid fast bacilli in specimens; as pleural fluid.

Following are the various techniques that can result in rapid identification of *M. tuberculosis* complex. **(i)** *MGIT method* (Mycobacterial growth indicator tube) is an automated growth detection system to detect presence of growth by appearance of fluorescence in a silicone plug at the bottom of the tube. It is superior to the radiometric method of Bactec 460TB, as it is a non radiometric technique and can even detect drug resistance. **(ii)** *Nucleic acid amplifications technique*, as PCR have the advantage of giving the result in 6-8 hours but errors as false positivity may occur. In India sequences; as 16S rRNA are preferred over IS 6110, as some strains in India do not have the latter sequence. **(iii)** *Quantiferon gold TB* gold test is performed using whole blood specimen and based on cell mediated immune response. However, it can not distinguish between tuberculosis disease and infection. **(iv)** *Interferon gamma test* is based on measuring significant r-interferon (produced by CD4 lymphocyte) level (in serum). **(v)** *Measurement of adenosine deaminase* (produced by T lymphocyte) enzyme levels can also be helpful in a case, such as diagnosis of tuberculous pleural effusion cases. **(vi)** *GeneXpert* MTB/RIF is a cartridge based nucleic acid amplification test (NAAT) to identify *M. tuberculosis* and resistance to Rifampicin.

What specific precautions needs to be taken to transport specimen with suspected tubercle bacilli to a distant referral laboratory for nucleic acid amplification studies?

A.5 (c) It is important to transport the specimen in dry ice or ice pack.

What is the role of serodiagnosis in the diagnosis of tuberculosis?

A.6 Tuberculosis is a chronic disease, with a large population being infected with *M. tuberculosis,* which is an facultative intracellular pathogen. In such a scenario, one can't rely on a diagnosis based on demonstration of specific antibodies, as these would be often present and one can't make out, if their presence represents a current infection. The antigenic composition of *M. tuberculosis* is also complex, making cross-reactivity a common feature, that may lead to false positive tests. However; in the market many type of serological tests, based on different *M. tuberculosis* and *M. bovis* antigens are available, due to commercial reasons. The Government of India vide their letter dated 7th June 2012 has banned all serodiagnostic tests by kits manufactured in India as well as all types of imported kits.

Are all laboratories competent to perform mycobacteria susceptibility testing?

A.7 (a) (i) No, only labs with necessary expertise and adequate volume of work and biosafety provisions can generate quality reports.

Discuss the aspect of drug resistance in M.tuberculosis.

A.7 (a) (ii) The aspect of drug resistance in *M. tuberculosis* has been dealt in, Section 1, Pg. 34 Clinical vignette 2 and section 17, case 1, Pg. 614.

What are the techniques available for performing mycobacteria drug susceptibility testing?

A.7 (b) The conventional techniques available are absolute concentration method, resistance ratio method and proportion method. The newer techniques include *radiometric method* (Bactec 460), non radiometric techniques based on *Luciferase reporter* (containing firefly luciferase enzyme) *mycobacteriophage* (containing firefty luciferase gene) and molecular techniques to detect *resistance genes* in the organism, as detection of mutation in rpoB gene to detect rifampicin resistance.

Why does the physician not wait for the results of mycobacterial susceptibility testing, before initiating ATT?

A.7 (c) Mycobacterial susceptibility testing tests can be usually performed after isolation of *M. tuberculosis*. The process of isolation, usually takes few weeks and performing conventional susceptibility testing also takes another few weeks, as this organism is slow growing. For this reason, the physician initiates the treatment, but changes the therapy, if required, after the results of the susceptibility testing are available. This process of change in administered antimicrobials is designated 'de-escalation'.

Describe the epidemiology of tuberculosis.

A.3 **(a)**
- **Agent:**
  - *M. tuberculosis* is the most important agent of the M. tuberculosis complex
  - Other important members of the complex include *M. bovis* and *M. africanum*
  - Evidence of *M. bovis* in causation of T.B in the Indian population is lacking
- **Reservoir of infection:** Infected human case
  - *Source of infection:* The most important source of the infection is the case, whose sputum is positive for tubercle bacilli. The other source of questionable importance is the infected milk of the bovine group.
- **Host factors**

  Age: All ages are affected

  Sex: Males are more commonly affected than females.

  Heredity: Individuals with some characteristic genes may be more prone to infection.

  Immunity: Cell mediated immunity acquired, as a result of natural infection or BCG vaccination, provides some degree of resistance to severe disease. Malnutrition is believed to predispose to this infection.

  One third of the world population is infected with *M. tuberculosis*. More than 40% of the Indian population is infected with this pathogen.
- **Environment:** A number of social factors; as overcrowding, poor social housing lack of awareness etc contribute to the occurrence and spread of this infection. This has-been a reason of the two to three fold increase in the cases in the former Soviet Union. The HIV epidemic has resulted in the doubling or tripling of the cases in many regions; especially the sub-Saharan Africa.

Enumerate the morphological differences between M.tuberculosis and M. bovis.

A.3 **(b)** Differentiating features between *M.tuberculosis* and *M.bovis*

	M. tuberculosis	***M. bovis***
Morphology	Long, slender, slightly curved	Short, stout and straight
Staining characteristics	Barred/Beaded appearance	Uniformly stained
Growth character on L.J. medium	• Eugonic (luxuriant) • Growth enhanced by glycerol	• Dysgonic • Growth inhibited by glycerol
Colony morphology	Dry, rough, raised and buff colored	Moist, smooth, flat and white colored
Biochemical reactions		
Niacin test	+	–
Nitrate test	+	–
Animal pathogenicity test (historical value)		
In guinea pig	Pathogenic(+)	Pathogenic(+)
In rabbit	Non pathogenic(–)	Pathogenic(+)

Depict the conventional approach made in a Lab for TB diagnosis.

A.4

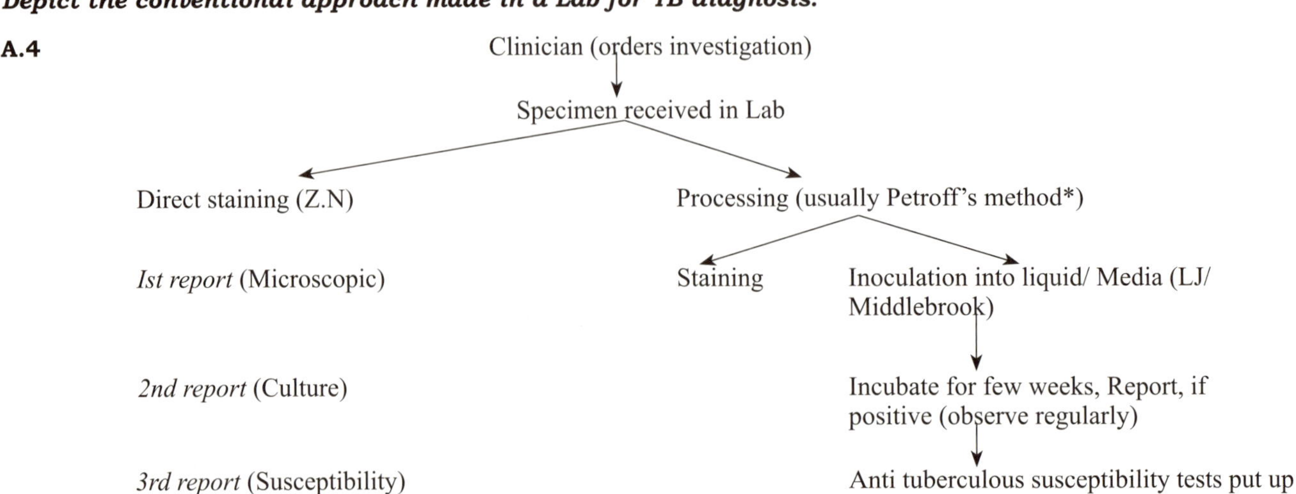

* A concentration technique involving exposure of sample to sodium hydroxide followed by centrifugation and using the deposit for processing

What invasive sample can be taken in a suspected pulmonary TB case to make a definitive diagnosis?

A.5 Bronchoalveolar lavage taken with the help of fibreoptic bronchoscopy.

Culture of BAL fluid by conventional LJ medium gave negative result in this case, however PCR test for tuberculosis was positive in the BAL fluid. Explain.

A.6 (a) For a conventional culture to give a positive result, the clinical sample has to have infection quantum in the range of few thousand bacilli per ml of sample. The sample in this case was likely to have lesser quantum of infection, hence not detectable.

Describe the automated culture methods to diagnose TB.

A.6 (b) Automated culture methods

I. *Radiometric:* BACTEC 460 was the first mycobacterial method for rapid culture and drug susceptibilty. The system contains radiolabelled 14C labeled substrate. The ratio and amount of $^{14}CO_2$ produced in the absence and presence of drugs is measured and compared. This method has been abandoned due to radioactive concerns.

II. *Non–radiometric*

(i) Mycobacterial growth indicator tube method (MGIT)

(ii) BacT/ALERT: This is a non radiometric method, which is colorimetric based (measures color) and has a carbon dioxide sensor in the bottle to measure the levels of the gas in the bottle. It uses liquid media with and without drugs. The advantage of this method over conventional LJ medium culture is rapid report within 2-3 weeks, higher sensitivity and lower contamination.

Describe tests based on molecular biology principle to diagnose TB.

A.6 (c) Tests based on molecular biology:

(i) *Conventional PCR:* It detects specific DNA sequences from samples and can give a report in few (6-8) hours

(ii) *DNA probe:* 'Accuprobe' identification system can identify MTB complex from isolates (in liquid or solid media) in 2 hours.

(iii) *Trancription based amplification (TMA) test:* It is a FDA approved test, which detects *M.tuberculosis* complex rRNA quantitatively from clinical samples

(iv) *GeneXpert MTB/RIF* is a cartridge based nucleic acid amplification test (NAAT) to identify *M. tuberculosis* and resistance to Rifampicin.

(v) *Combined multiplex PCR and DNA strip* hybridization assay (Hain Life science, Germany): In the test multiplex PCR is followed by hybridization to specific probes to detect mutations in genes conferring resistance to rifampicin (rpoB), high–level INH (katG) and low level INH resistance (inhA). The multidrug resistant status of the strain can be provided to the clinician in 24 hours.

Aspects related to case theme/examination assessment

What is Koch phenomenon?

A.7 This was described by Robert Koch, a phenomenon which depicts a combination of immunity and hypersensitivity. If a normal guinea pig is injected subcutaneously, virulent tubercle bacilli, a nodule forms at the site of injection after 10-14 days of inoculation. This latter forms a ulcer which persists, draining lymph node gets enlarged and caseous, and the animal dies of progressive tuberculosis.

On the other hand if a sensitized (which had received avirulent tubercle bacilli, 4-6 weeks earlier) guinea pig is injected a virulent tubercle bacilli subcutaneously, an indurated lesion appears at the site in a day or two, which heals without involvement of draining lymph nodes. The quick tissue damage response is indicative of hypersensitivity, whereas the faster healing and no spread of disease (to lymph nodes) are indicative of immunity.

Mention the morphology of M.tuberculosis and role of M.tuberculosis antigens in pathogenesis of tuberculosis.

A.8 (a) *M.tuberculosis* is a facultative intracellular pathogen, which is non motile, non piliated, non capsulated, produces no exotoxin or endotoxin (has lipopolysaccharide but no lipid A)

(i) *Lipid:* Cord factor and long chain fatty acids called mycolic acid are virulent factors. Mycolic acid in complex with peptidoglycan is responsible for granuloma formation.

(ii) *Proteins:* Are responsible for delayed hypersensitivity

(iii) *Polysaccharide:* Role is not clear.

Describe pathogenesis of M.bovis and M.tuberculosis infections.

A.8 (b) The outcome of infection has a wide spectrum; varying from subclinical and just tuberculin sensitive at one end to fatal disseminated disease at other extreme. Some of the factors can accelerate healing by fibrosis, whereas others which lead to rapidly spreading fatal disease include dose, virulence of organism, age, general health, occupation (as miners are prone) and previous infection.

The sequence of events can be depicted as below:

(i) *M.bovis*

Bacilli excreted in milk of animals; as cow

↓

Ingestion of raw milk by man (consumption of boiled milk, eliminates this infection)

↓

Primary infection in tonsillar, cervical and mesenteric lymph nodes

(if infection, not contained)

↓

Miliary spread

(ii) For *M.tuberculosis*

Entry of bacilli into lung by inhalation

↓

Initiation of *primary TB in lung (*Infection occurying in a person never previously exposed to *M tuberculosis*)

↓

Exudative lesion (bacilli usually destroyed by alveolar macrophages)

↓

Ghon focus/Primary tuberculosis (here tuberculous sensitivity develops)

Containment of bacilli usually occurs at this stage (including regional L.N)

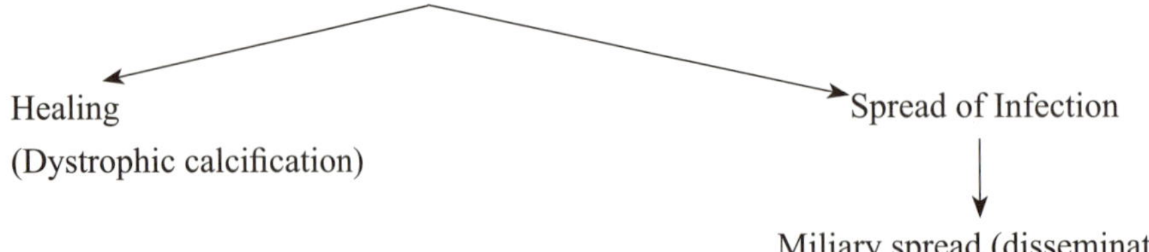

- Secondary (Post–Primary) tuberculosis: caused by reactivation of primary lesion (endogenous) or exogenous reinfection
- Tubercle (hard) undergoes necrosis and cavities may develop in it. Protective immunity is mediated by CD4+T cells, which secrete cytokines; as interferon (gamma), IL2 and TNF alpha. Tissue damage and disease progression is mediated by TH-2 cytokine profile reactions.

Integrated Clinical Based Study of Non-Tuberculous Mycobacteria/Pulmonary Tuberculosis

A 45 year old man, Kshitij who received a renal transplant 3 years back, presented with severe cough and fever of 3 weeks duration. Chest X-ray revealed diffuse infiltrates in the right lung. The sputum was cultured on L.J. medium and it grew few colonies in few days, whose smear examination revealed presence of acid fast bacilli.

Linkages: pg. 212-214, 217, 221, 250, 252

What could be the probable factor in the above case, that made him prone to chest infection?

A.1 This case would be receiving immunosuppressants to prevent the rejection of the renal allograft, which would make him prone to opportunistic infections.

What is the clinical diagnosis in the above case?

A.2 (a) The case is having a pulmonary disease similar to pulmonary tuberculosis.

How do you explain the rapid growth of acid-fast bacilli in few days. (as M. tuberculosis takes few weeks to produce colonies)?

A.2 (b) This case has been most likely to have been infected by group IV of non –tuberculous mycobacteria (NTM), i.e., rapid growers. The members of this group are characterized by rapid growth within few days of incubation.

How do you classify non-tuberculous mycobacteria (atypical mycobacteria), i.e., mycobacteria other than tubercle bacilli?

A.3 (a) According to Runyon classification, they are categorized on the basis of pigment production and rate of growth into four groups namely Photochromogens, Scotochromogens, Non photochromogens and Rapid growers (Table 5.9.2). Table 5.7.1, pg. 230 also to be consulted. These are also categorized as anonymous mycobacteria.

Tabulate the differences between tubercle bacilli and non-tuberculous mycobacteria.

A.3 (b) **Table 5.9.1:** M. tuberculosis and non-tuberculous mycobacteria (NTM)-Differentiating characteristics

	M. tuberculosis	***Non-tuberculous mycobacteria (NTM)***
Growth characteristics		
Rate of growth	Slow	Slow/rapid
Optimal temperature	37°C	25-45°C
Growth on L.J. medium	Eugonic	Dysgonic
Colony characteristic	Dry, buff (colored), rough and tough	Dry, cream/yellow/orange colored
Biochemical reactions		
Niacin test	+	–
Nitrate reduction test	+	–
Source	Infected person	Soil/water
Drug resistance	Occasional to anti-TB drugs	Often resistant to anti-TB drugs

What is the usual habitat of non-tuberculous mycobacteria?

A.4 (a) They mostly exist as saprophytes and are commonly found in soil and water.

Describe the common features of non-tuberculous mycobacteria.

A.4 (b) (i) are opportunistic pathogens with low virulence, so commonly seen as pathogens in immunocompromised individuals.

(ii) Infections caused by them, are more common in developed countries than developing countries.

(iii) are difficult to treat, as many of them are resistant to many antituberculous drugs, so require alternative drugs for prolonged periods.

(iv) cause more calcification and necrosis than *M.tuberculosis.*

(v) Must be repeatedly isolated about 3-4 times from multiple (repeat) samples, to incriminate them as a cause of a lesion.

(vi) Cause sensitization in individuals, so can give false positive tuberculin reaction and may reduce efficacy of BCG vaccine.

Name a saprophytic mycobacteria that can result in a false positive diagnosis in a case of tuberculosis. How can this error be prevented?

A.4 (c) *M. smegmatis*. If the smear used for diagnosis is decolorized with acid-alcohol, then this problem can be avoided, as this organism is acid fast, but not alcohol fast.

Name a key biochemical test that is diagnostic of M.tuberculosis and helps to differentiate it from non tuberculous mycobacteria?

A.5 (a) Niacin test is positive in *M. tuberculosis* and negative in non tuberculous mycobacteria. Aryl sulphatase test is positive in many non-tuberculous mycobacteria and negative in *M. tuberculosis*.

Tabulate the key characteristics of atypical mycobacteria, which help in their identification.

A.5 (b) **Table 5.9.2:** Differentiation between tubercle bacilli and different species of atypical mycobacteria

	M. tuberculosis	*M. bovis*	*M. kansasii*	*M. scrofulaceum*	*M. intracellulare-complex*	*M. fortuitum/ chelonae*
Growth within 7 days	–	–	–	–	–	+
Growth at 25°C	–	–	+	+	±	+
Growth at 37°C	+	+	+	+	+	+
Growth at 45°C	–	–	–	±	±	–
Pigment production in light	–	–	+	+	–	–
Pigment production in dark	–	–	–	+	–	–
Niacin production	+	–	–	–	–	–
Nitrate reduction	+	–	+	–	–	±
Urease production	+	+	–	+	–	+

NB: Table 5.7.1, pg. 230 to be referred to also.
+–: indicates reaction can be positive or negative

What is the difficulty in treating non-tuberculous mycobacterial infections?

A.6 Many of the non tuberculous mycobacteria are resistant to most of the antituberculous drugs 'in vitro'. These infections commonly require combination of drugs (often toxic) for prolonged periods of many months for successful treatment.

Aspects related to case theme/examination assessment

Compare and contrast key charactenstics of Buruli ulcer and swimming pool granuloma.

A.7 The differentiating features are depicted in table 5.9.3.

Table 5.9.3: Differentiating features between Buruli ulcer and swimming pool granuloma

	***Buruli ulcer**	**Swimming pool granuloma**
Etiological agent	*M. ulcerans*	*M. marinum*
Distribution	Tropics (Africa, America and S.E. Asia)	Temperate zone
Clinical course	Chronic, progressive ulcer, involves bones	Self-limited ulcer (acquired from water sources)
Rate of growth	Slower, 4-8 weeks	Faster, 1-2 weeks
Growth at 25°C	–	+
Growth at 37°C	–	+
Pigment production in light	–	+

* Buruli is a district of Uganda, where an outbreak of this disease has occured

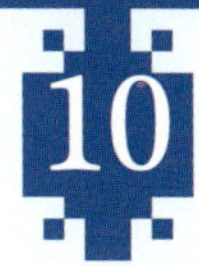

Integrated Clinical Based Study of *M.leprae*/Leprosy

An adolescent male, Shameen presented with few circular, hypopigmented skin patches with no sensation (senstivity) on the right forearm. Examination of the case revealed the right ulnar never to be thickened. Skin biopsy from the edge of the skin lesion was negative (didn't yield) for acid fast bacilli. The lepromin test was positive in this case.

Linkages: pg 212-214, 217, 221-222, 251, 252

What is the differential diagnosis of this case?

A.1 (a) Leprosy, Lupus erythematous, Lupus vulgaris, Sarcoidosis and Yaws.

What is the diagnostic approach that needs to be taken to make a clinical diagnosis of leprosy?

A.1 (b) The suspected case should be stripped and the whole body be examined for 3 cardinal signs namely; hypopigmented patches, loss of sensation and thickened nerves.

What is the likely diagnosis in this case? Discuss.

A.2 (a) The case is likely to be having leprosy, as the skin patches have loss of sensation. The leprosy is likely to be of the tuberculoid type, as the case has thickened nerves, with skin lesions not demonstrating acid fast bacilli and the case is lepromin positive. The lepra bacilli were first observed by Hansen in 1868.

Outine a common classification systems to categorize leprosy and mention its importance.

A.2 (b) (i) Ridley and Jopling (1966), on the basis of clinical,histopathological & immunological findings devised a scale to categorize the spectrum of leprosy into five groups, as depicted in the Figure 5.10.1 with Tuberculoid (TT) at one end and Lepromatous (LL) at other end.

TT	BT	BB	BL	LL
Tuberculoid	Bordeline Tuberculoid	Borderline	Borderline lepromatous	Lepromatous

Fig. 5.10.1: Spectrum of Leprosy

The groups are not fixed for an individual, for example a case with BL category, when responds to treatment changes towards BT, this phenomenon is called 'reversal phenomenon'.

(ii) The WHO has divided leprosy into two groups, namely paucibacillary and multibacillary leprosy. Paucibacillary leprosy includes all cases of TT and some cases of BT, whereas multibacillary leprosy includes all cases of LL and some cases of BL.

The classification helps in the management of the cases. It helps in determining the drugs to be administered and duration of treatment, besides predicting prognosis of a case. The differences between the tuberculoid and lepromatous leprosy are depicted in the table 5.10.1.

Table 5.10.1: Differentiating features between *Tuberculoid* and *Lepromatous* leprosy

	Tuberculoid Leprosy	**Lepromatous Leprosy**
Cell-mediated immunity	- Good	- Deficient
Prevalence	- More	- Less
Appearance	- Minimal Disfigurement	- Significant Disfigurement (as 'leonine facies')

Contd.

Contd.

Lesions	- Few - Macular - Significant loss of sensation	- Many - Nodular - Minimal loss of sensation
Infectivity	- Usually non infective	- Highly infective
Microscopy of infected tissue	- Paucibacillary (few leprosy Bacilli in lesion) - Granuloma common - Plasma cell infiltration: Minimal	- Multibacillary (plenty of bacilli) - No granuloma - Present significantly
Antibodies to *M.leprae*	+/-	+++
Diagnostic criteria	Sensory loss	Bacilli in smear
Lepromin test	+++	-
Therapeutic response	Effective	Sluggish
Prognosis	Good	Poor
Duration of treatment	6 months	24 months

Can M. leprae be cultivated on inanimate media?

A.3 Till now, *M. leprae* has not been successfully cultivated on inanimate media.

What are the animal models used for cultivation of M. leprae?

A.4 Commonly; foot pad of mice, nine banded armadillo (*Dasypus novemcinctus*), chimpanzee, monkey and Indian pangolin are used as models.

Describe immunopathogenesis of tuberculoid leprosy.

A.5 (a) The lymphocytes from patients of tuberculoid leprosy easily recognize *M.leprae* and its constituent antigens; unlike the untreated LL patients, which often fail to recognize these antigens. The tuberculoid leprosy cases have positive lepromin test with a strong T cell activity and macrophage activation, which results in localizing of the infection. The leprosy infected tissue has a 2:1 predominance of helper CD4+ to CD8+ T cells. The involved tissue have a predominant T_{H1} cytokine profile with high concentration of mRNAs of interleukin 2, interferon gamma and interleukin 12. This pattern is in contrast to the untreated LL cases, which have a predominantly T_{H2} response.

As lepromatous leprosy case are lepromin test negative (indicative of decreased C.M.I), are these cases more prone to other infections, besides leprosy?

A.5 (b) The lepromatous leprosy cases are believed to have specific anergy (limited reactivity) of their T_{H1}cells to *M.leprae* antigens. Hence these cases are not prone to other infections.

Grade (roughly) the infectivity of the case being discussed.

A.6 (a) The case under discussion is likely to be having tuberculoid leprosy. The infectivity of a tuberculoid leprosy case is low.

What is the likely reservoir of M.leprae?

A.6 (b) The main reservoir of this organism is probably only man.

How does leprosy spread?

A.6 (c) The spread of this infection is *believed to* occur from mainly the respiratory secretions of lepromatous leprosy and borderline cases.

Describe the epidemiology of leprosy.

A.6 (d)

- **Agent:** *M. leprae*
- **Source of infection:** The lepromatous leprosy and borderline lepromatous human cases are the important sources of infection. Some wild animals; as armadillos and chimpanzees have also been recently found to have this infection.
- **Mode of transmission:** It is likely to spread from person to person by contact. Lepers were in the past shunned on the false belief that leprosy was a very infectious disease. In fact; this is a minimally contagious disease and prolonged contact is necessary for the transmission to occur. The generation period of this organism is in the range of 12-13 days and the incubation period of the disease averages a few years. Nasal secretions is the most important specimen; as far as the excretory load of bacilli is concerned. The mode of the entry of the infection may be the respiratory tract or the skin.

- **Host Factors:** The disease is now confined to the tropics and the southern hemisphere. In India, the disease is present in all the states and union territories, though the prevalence varies in them. Orissa and Bihar have the highest prevalence of > 3 per 1000 population. Infection can occur in any age. Presence of cell mediated immunity, acquired naturally; provides certain degree of resistance to infection.

Which is the key antigen used for the serodiagnosis of leprosy?

A.7 (a) Phenolic glycolipid-1 (PGL-1) is a key antigen used for the serodiagnosis of leprosy using ELISA technique. Serological test using antibodies to this unique antigenic determinant has good specificity but sensitivity is lacking in tuberculoid leprosy cases.

As tuberculin test is used to detect tuberculosis infection, why does the lepromin test not have similar role?

A.7 (b) (i) Many healthy individuals in non endemic areas give positive lepromin test

(ii) Lepromatous leprosy cases give a negative lepromin test, hence this category of cases would be missed out, if a diagnosis was only done only on the basis of this test.

Describe the lepromin test and its role.

A.7 (c)

- **History:** First described by Mitsuda in 1919
- **Procedure:** Intradermal injection (0.1 ml) of antigen (currently lepromin A, derived from armadillo used) in forearm. Observe for classic reaction at the end of 48 hrs and at the end of 3 weeks.
- **Reaction:** Classically; a biphasic reaction is observed, a early Fernandez reaction and a late Mitsuda reaction. The Fernandez reaction consists of erythema and induration at the site of reaction developing in 24-48 hours, a reaction analogous to tuberculin rection. The Mitsuda reaction consists of development of a nodule at the site of the development (which may ulcerate) and appear after 1-2 weeks and peaks at four weeks.
- **Interpretation:** Mitsuda reaction is given more importance than the Fernandez reaction, which indicates the ability of the individual to induce cell mediated immune response against the lepra antigen
- **Uses:**
  (i) *Classification of leprosy:* The test is positive in tuberculoid leprosy and negative in lepromatous leprosy cases.
  (ii) *Monitoring of treatment:* A change of reaction from lepromin negative to positive indicates effective treatment.
  (iii) *Assessment of prognosis:* A positive lepromin test indicates a good prognosis in contrast to a negative one.
  (iv) *Assessment of resistance to leprosy:* Lepromin positive cases have resistance to leprosy, hence only such individuals are recruited in leprosy homes and for field work.
  (v) *To verify* candidate lepra bacillus to be used as a vaccine.

Outline the approach to perform laboratory diagnosis of leprosy.

A.7 (d) See pg 251 and the case discussion in this chapter

What is the regimen used to treat tuberculoid leprosy case?

A.8 Multiple drug therapy regime comprising Rifampicin (600 mg once monthly) and Dapsone (100 mg once daily) is to be administered for six months.

What is the aim of the leprosy vaccines? Name the vaccines used for this purpose.

A.9 The aim is to seek an antigen, which cross reacts with *M.leprae*, can activate T cells but lacks the suppressor epitopes resonsible for anergy.

The vaccines that have been tried include:

(i) BCG vaccine (limited protection)

(ii) Heat killed *M. leprae* antigen

(iii) BCG vaccine + heat killed *M.leprae* antigen (Convit vaccine)

(iv) Cultivable mycobacteria [Mycobacteria 'W' of GP Talwar and ICRC bacillus-(Indian cancer research center.)]

Currently 'Leprovac', a leprosy vaccine has been marketed by Cadila Ltd.

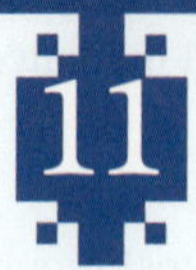

Integrated Clinical Based Study of *C.perfringens*/Gas Gangrene

A soldier, Swatantar Singh during the 1971 Indo-Pak war, reported with severe pain in his left wrist region. He had sustained a bullet injury in the area, 2 days back. Local examination revealed a localized tender area with skin disruption and crepitus. X-ray of the local part, revealed gas in the muscle. Administration of ceftazadime was started.

Linkages: pg. 212, 213, 215, 218, 219, 251, 252

What is your clinical diagnosis of this case?

A.1 Gas gangrene of the left arm.

What is the likely pathogenesis in this case?

A.2 (a) The bullet caused a wound in the arm, which got contaminated by pathogenic clostridia from the soil. The release of various toxins; especially alpha and the tissue degradative enzymes from the invading clostridia, resulted in the lesion.

What is the composition of the gas in the lesion?

A.2 (b) It is largely composed of hydrogen and carbon-dioxide.

What is the role of laboratory diagnosis in the management of a gas gangrene case?

A.3 (a) The role of the laboratory is to confirm the presumptive clinical diagnosis, which has been made. The treatment in the case has to start without waiting for the result of the laboratory diagnosis. Delay in treatment can have fatal consequences.

What are the likely pathogens that could play a role in this case?

A.3 (b) Clostridal spp, Streptococcus spp and mixed aerobic and anaerobic organisms. If in a wound, the oxidation reduction potential is low, the *C.perfringens* spores can germinate and multiply rapidly. Infection is often mixed. Amongst the Clostridia spp., *C.perfringens* (60%) is most frequently associated with gas gangrene, to be followed by *C.novyi;* (30%) and *C.septicum* (10%). *C.histolyticum* and *C.fallax* play a lesser pathogenic role.

Classify C.perfringens.

A.3 (c) *C. perfringens* is classified into 5 types A to E, depending on the production of the four major toxins (alpha, beta, epsilon, and iota). Gas gangrene is primarily caused by type A strains. Some strains of type A also produce food poisoning, while necrotizing enteritis is caused by type C strains. Types B, D and E of *C.perfringens* are animal pathogens.

The case is shifted to the closest hospital. The operating surgeon explored the site and amputated at a level just above the left elbow joint.

Justify the action of amputating at a level which was healthy. Would the administration of antimicrobials not have been sufficient to manage this case?

A.4 Once gas gangrene occurs, there is little role of conservative treatment. Wide surgical debridement has to be undertaken, as toxaemia can spread like 'wild fire', despite administraton of antimicrobials. A delay in following an aggressive approach may cost the life of the patient. So; a part of the healthy anatomical part often needs to be sacrificed on the ground that observing grossly the affected part, it may not be possible to distinguish between clostridial infected tissue and healthy tissue. This is a decision of the treating surgeon based on his judgement.

Which antimicrobials are usually chosen in management of a case of Clostridial myonecrosis?

A.5 Metronidazole and clindamycin are antimicrobials of choice, which may be administrated intravenously.

What other modalities could have been tried, while managing this case?

A.6 Surgical treatment would have aimed at radical excision of affected part. Introduction of hyperbaric oxygen into depth of the wound may have a beneficial role. There may not be much role of antigas gangrene serum in this case, as there may be only minimal soiling.

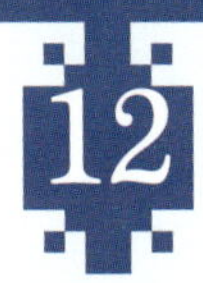

Integrated Clinical Based Study of *C.perfringens*/Clostridial Myonecrosis

A forty year old fat female, Savita underwent laparoscopic cholecysteomy at a district hospital. On day 4 of her surgery, the operating site developed dehiscence of the surgical wound. Local examination revealed wound dehiscence with wound edges having blackish discoloration and crepitus at the site.

Linkages: pg. 212, 213, 215, 218, 219, 251, 252

What is the differential diagnosis of this case?

A.1 Clostridial myonecrosis, *Pyomyositis, Intraabdominal infection

*In anaerobic myositis, gram stained smear of specimen shows pus cells and streptococci.

What is the likely pathogenesis in this case?

A.2 *C.perfringens* can sometimes be present in the bile of cases and can cause gas gangrene of abdominal muscles, if bile is spilled during operation. So; this is an example of endogenous infection. Similarly clostridial endometritis can occur following uterine surgery (*C. perfringens* is also at times present as commensal of the female genital tract), especially after conducting abortion with unsterilized instruments.

What is the key virulent factors of C. perfringens?

A.3 **(a)** Alpha toxin is a very important toxin produced by all types of *C. perfringens*. It has lecithinase activity that can split lecithin (an important component of cell membrane) to phosphoryl choline and diglyceride. Lysis of erythrocytes, leucocytes and platelets is also caused by this toxin. The specific effect of this toxin is utilized in the development of Nagler reaction.

Describe reverse CAMP test.

A.3 **(b)** See Fig. 5.2.9, p. 219

How do you make a diagnosis of clostridial endometritis?

A.4 To make a diagnosis of clostridial endometritis, history of instrumentation of the uterus would be available in most of the cases. Isolation of the *C. perfrigens* from the endometrial tissue would be helpful but would not be as useful as demonstrating bacilli in a frozen section biopsy of the endometrium. A characteristic pathologic finding of gas gangrene is near absence of polymorphonuclear cells, despite extensive tissue necrosis.

Is isolation of C. perfringens enough to incriminate it, as an etiological agent in C. perfringens food poisoning?

A.5 As *C.perfringens* is a commensal of the gastrointestinal tract, just isolation of this organism from the food is not enough. Isolation of greater than 10^5 organisms per gram of ingested food is considered significant.

Aspects related to case theme/examination assessment

What is necrotizing enteritis.

A.6 Necrotizing enteritis (jejunitis) is a serious type of food poisoning caused by type C strain of *C. perfringens*. Outbreaks of such bowel disease with high mortality have been reported from New Guinea and Germany

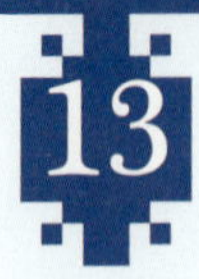

Integrated Clinical Based Study of *C.tetani*/Neonatal Tetanus

A 10 day old male infant, Nitin presented with irritability, poor feeding, body rigidity and occasional spasms. The delivery history revealed birth in a village home, facilitated by a 'Dai'.

Linkages: Pg. 212-213, 215, 218, 219, 22, 251, 252

What is the likely clinical diagnosis of this case?

A.1 Neonatal tetanus

What Indian customs may have a possible role in the pathogenesis of tetanus in this case?

A.2 (a) In the rural areas, *'Dai's' who conduct the deliveries, sometimes use unsterile blade to cut the umbilical cord. There is also the custom of placing soil on the umbilical wound, believing that it would have a therapeutic role. Both these actions can lead to the neonate getting infected with *C. tetani* spores.

*Female health workers in rural areas trained to facilitate child delivery.

Describe the predisposing factors for development of tetanus.

A.2 (b) The predisposing factors are not known exactly. It may be low oxidation–reduction potential and presence of foreign body at the trauma site. Surprisingly the injury may be trivial and the patient may not be able to recall it. The bacterial proliferation occurs at the site with toxin production, with no damage or invasion of the adjacent tissue.

Describe the epidemiology of tetanus.

A.2 (c)

- **Agent:** *C. tetani* (Kitasato-1889 isolated pure culture of this organism)
  Genome-2,799,251 bp circular DNA including plasmid (pE88) with 61 ORFs
- **Reservoir of infection:** – Soil
  – also intestines of animals and occasionally man
- **Mode of transmission:** it is acquired by contamination of wounds with tetanus spores. The latter may be a cause for rare outbreaks of tetanus in OTs. Agricultural workers are at increased risk. Even immunized individuals, who haven't received vaccine booster and if antitoxin levels are < 0.15 units/ml may be susceptible to the disease. It is for this reason that immunization is important even after the occurence natural infection, as the episode may not result in a protective antitoxin titers.
- **Age:** It is a disease of active life (5-40 years), when a man is exposed to different kinds of trauma. The risk of development of disease is highest among elders. No age is immune, unless recently immunized.
- **Sex:** A higher incidence is found in males, though females have periods when exposed excessively to this agent; as during delivery and abortion.
- **Environment:** The disease is an environmental hazard. The disease is more common in warm areas, when soil is cultivated during summer.

It is very important to know the conditions that are associated with tetanus, as then a clinician can suspect this clinical entity, when the suspected case presents. These include ulcer, abscesses, burns, gangrene and frost bite. Even trivial injuries, which the patient may not recall can result in tetanus. Other conditions include illicit i/v drug abuse, middle ear perforation (otogenic), septic abortion, delivery conducted with 'dais', (inexpert placenta removal), neonatal procedure (when umbilicus cut uncleanly) and surgery with unsterile equipment, as circumcision.

Which virulent factor product produced by C.tetani is responsible for the symptomatology in this case?

A.3 (a) Tetanospasmin (neurotoxin) exotoxin formed by the organism is responsible for all the clinical manifestations of tetanus. The gene encoding it resides in the plasmid (pE88). So, if this organism is devoid of this plasmid, the organism loses it's virulence. This toxin is synthesized as a 150-kDa peptide that undergoes post translation proteolytic cleavage. It enters presynaptic nerve cytosol by receptor -mediated endocytosis and is transported via retrograde axonal transport to the nerve cell bodies in the brain stem and spinal cord. It causes presynaptic blockade of the release of inhibitory neurotransmitters, as glycine and γ-aminobutyric acid (GABA). The suppression of the inhibitory nerve function results in increased activation of nerves innervating muscles, resulting in spasm and increased muscle rigidity.

The other toxin namely, tetanolysin (haemolysin, can lyse RBCs of some species) does not appear to have a pathogenic role.

Describe the laboratory tests to detect the two key toxins of C. tetani.

A.3 (b) The two distinct toxins are tetanolysin and tetanospasmin (also discussed at p. 218).

The role of the tetanolysin in the pathogenicity is not clear. This toxin can cause lysis of erythrocytes of many animal species. For its detection, 'in vitro' toxigenicity testing is performed, using blood agar plate (horse RBCs and 4% agar to inhibit the swarming) with anti tetanus toxin serum on half of the plate. The plate is incubated anaerobically for 3 days. If the strain is tetanolysin producing, haemolysis would be seen only in the half of the plate without the antitoxin, as there the toxin produced by the strain would not be neutralized by the added antitoxin. The limitation of this test is that, it only detects tetanolysin.

For detection of the tetanospasmin, animal pathogenicity ('in vitro' toxigenicity) is performed. Two mice are taken, one is protected with antitoxin administered intraperitoneally, one hour earlier to injection administration. Approximately; 0.2 ml each of culture isolate to be tested is injected into root of the tail each of the of two mice. In case, the strain is tetanospasmin producing, stiffness develops in the unprotected mouse in about 12 hrs. It is followed by development of ascending tetanus and the animal dies in about 2 days.

In adults, which clinical features, if observed are indicative of tetanus?

A.4 (a) In adults, usually the first indication of the disease is the trismus (lock jaw), produced as a result of spasm of masseter muscle and usually manifests; as difficulty in swallowing. Muscle spasm and rigidity may also develop due to simultaneous contraction of agonist and antagonistic muscles.In later stages, opisthotonus may occur due to contraction of the back muscles.

Mention the causes of death in tetanus.

A.4 (b) Death may occur due to paralysis of chest muscles, resulting in respiratory failure.

What is the role of serum antitoxin levels in the diagnosis of tetanus?

A.4 (c) The diagnosis of tetanus is unlikely, if the case is vaccinated and antitoxin levels exceed 0.15 units/ml.

Which agent, if administered early in tetanus can be life saving?

A.5 Human tetanus immunoglobulin, if administered early in the disease, i.e., before the neurotoxin (tetanosposmin) has bound to the neuronal receptors can be life saving, i.e., the patient's life can be saved and recovery occurs. Human tetanus (TIG) immune globulin (750 units) may be administered intramuscularly on one arm. The aim is to neutralize immediately unbound toxin in wound and circulation. The other arm is used for active immunization. Unlike diphtheria antitoxin (immunoglobulin) which is raised in horses, this is a human product and safe (non allergic).

Can neonatal tetanus be eradicated from India?

A.6 Yes, if pregnant women, which is a relatively small population is targeted for tetanus immunization. If all this population is immunized, then this form of disease can be eradicated.

Integrated Clinical Based Study of *C.botulinum*/Food Poisoning

A 25 year old housewife, Savita presented with blurred vision and constipation, after eating home canned apple. This was followed by weakness and hypotonia of the upper body. She also had difficulty in eating and breathing. She was intubated because of respiratory difficulty.

Linkages: Pg. 212, 213, 215, 218, 222, 251, 252

What is the presumptive diagnosis of the above case?

A.1 (a) The case is likely to be one of food borne botulism, as the presentation followed consumption of home canned fruit; which is known to be contaminated with *C. botulinum*. Such cases usually begin with cranial nerve involvement. [here effect in vision]

What is the differential diagnosis of this case?

A.1 (b) The differential diagnosis includes Myasthenia gravis, Guillain Barré syndrome and central nervous system infection.

Enumerate microbes that can be incriminated in the above case.

A.2 (a) Commonly *C. botulinum* types A, B, and F are involved (of the eight types known).

Describe the epidemiology of botulism.

A.2 (b) The disease occurs worldwide. Botulism is due to non–invasive, preformed toxin. The botulism described in this case is of food borne type. In *infant botulism*, infants below 6 months are usually infected by ingestion of contaminated food with spores in food (often honey). The child has flaccid paralysis, with loss of body tone ('floppy body' syndrome. *Wound botulism* is an extremely rare condition occurying, due to contamination of wound with spores of *C. botulinum*.

What are unique clinical features of botulism?

A.3 Botulism cases are usually afebrile. It is also a unique food poisoning not to have diarrhoea, but has constipation as a presentation.

The cases are mentally intact but have areflexia, which could be seen; as dilated pupils not responding to light. The paresis is symmetrical and descends downward.

Describe an 'in vivo' test performed to detect botulinum toxin?

A.4 'Mouse lethality' assay is a test often performed to detect botulinum toxin in various samples; as serum, food items and faeces. The saline filtrate of the specimen is injected intraperitoneally into mice, which are observed over a 96 hour period, for the development of paralysis. The paralysis usually begins in the hind legs and progresses to the death of the animal. To confirm that the paralysis is specifically due to botulinum toxin, control mice are administered the saline filtrate of the specimen, which is preincubated with polyvalent antiserum against common botulinum toxin types and observed. Such control animals do not develop the paralysis.

Discuss the role of antimicrobial administration in the management of botulism?

A.5 Administration of antimicrobial won't have a significant effect in a case of food borne botulism, as the neurotoxin is already present in the food, responsible for the manifestations. However, if the consumed food has proliferating *C. botulinum*, then the antimicrobial administration may have a role in minimizing the exotoxin production.

What specific therapy, if administered early in disease in this case, may result in a dramatic recovery in a few days?

A.6 Early administration of polyvalent antiserum against common *C. botulinum* types A, B, and F can have a life saving effect in this case, if the administration occurs, before substantial botulinum toxin has bound to the neuronal receptors.

Aspects related to case theme/examination assessment

Mention about the bioterrorism aspect of this organism.

A.7 Botulinum toxin has been one of the most toxic toxins known to mankind. In this background, it is believed that this exotoxin had been manufactured by certain countries; as Iraq. This toxin can be delivered as food or even as an aerosol. This infection is a matter of concern, as it's medical management requires ventilator for respiration, which would be a constraint in a routine medical set-up.

Mention one use of the botulinum toxin that this housewife may have utilized in a beauty clinic.

A.8 'Botox' could have been used as part of anti-wrinkle therapy.

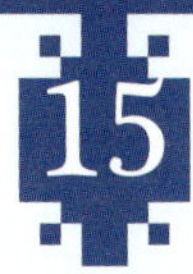

Integrated Clinical Based Study of *C.difficile*/Diarrhoea

An 80 year old man, Suraj Prakash had a prostrate biopsy done 10 days back, after which he developed UTI. He received a seven day course of cefuroxime for it. Five days after he finished the course of antimicrobial, he developed diarrhoea, abdominal pain and vomiting. Stool microscopy didn't reveal any significant finding and stool cultures did not yield any pathogens; as Salmonellae, Vibrio, Yersinia or Campylobacter.

Linkages: Pg. 212, 213, 215, 218, 222, 251, 252

What is the likely diagnosis of this case?

A.1 Antibiotic (*Clostridium difficile*) associated diarrhoea. *C. difficile* was first isolated from the faeces of a newborn by Hall & O`Toole.

What microbiological investigations can help to clinch the diagnosis in this case?

A.2 (a) Detection of *C. difficile* toxin, using a tissue culture cytotoxicity assay. Cytotoxicity is neutralized in cell cultures, by antitoxin to *C. sordelli*. This assay is very sensitive and highly specific but is technically demanding and requires 1-2 days to complete it. As an alternative to it, an enzyme immunoassay can be performed, which lacks sensitivity, but is highly specific and can be completed in a few hours. However; it can't distinguish between *C. difficile* strains that are toxigenic and those that are non toxigenic. Toxigenic strains (i.e., which produce the toxins A & B for pathogenicity) have genes in the region of the chromosome of this organism called the 'pathogenicity locus' for toxins. This organism has toxin A (responsible for diarrhea) and toxin B (cytotoxin).

What are the problems (limitations) in using the culturing technique to make diagnosis of C.difficile infection?

A.2 (b) There are two problem using culture; as a technique to diagnosis *C. difficile* associated diarrhoea. One, the organism is difficult to culture, but can be cultured using CCFA medium. Secondly, about 20% of individuals can also be carrying this organism asymptomatically.

What makes C.difficile a difficult to manage nosocomial agent?

A.3 *C. difficile* is a spore forming bacterium. Its spores are a source of infection for many weeks, even after the patient is discharged from the hospital. Also they are difficult to be destroyed, as they are more resistant to disinfectants than the vegetative forms.

What is the normal carriage rate of C.difficile?

A.4 (a) The normal carriage role of this organism is about 40-50% in gut of healthy infants and about 3-5% in gut of healthy adults.

How does man acquire C.difficile infection?

A.4 (b) The disease can be acquired from the persons own flora (i.e., endogenous) or from cross infection during the stay in a hospital (i.e., nosocomial)

What are the approaches in managing a case of C.difficile associated diarrhoea?

A.5 (a) *One approach* is to stop all antimicrobial agents being administered to the patient. This option is feasible in cases having mild disease, where the diarrhoea may resolve, however it isn't possible in cases having severe infection.

The *second approach* is to give oral metronidazole or vancomycin. Administration of oral metronidazole is preferred by some as they believe that administration of vancomycin, may encourage the development of VRE (vancomycin resistant enterococci).

The *third approach* would be to encourage the development of indigenous flora of the gut, hoping that it would inhibit the growth of *C. difficile*.

Can the antimicrobial which is useful in the treatment of C.difficile associated diarrhoea, itself may be responsible for the causation of this disease?

A.5 (b) Yes, surprising though it may sound, administration of vancomycin or metronidazole itself could be responsible for causing *C. difficile* associated diarrhoea.

In what form are recurrences seen in case of C.difficile associated diarrhoea?

A.6 Recurrences in this disease can be due to either relapse or reinfection. In relapse, the spores of this organism, which are resistant to antimicrobial agents can become active, after varying periods of dormancy and give rise to disease.

In reinfection, another strain of *C. difficile* is responsible for the disease.

What characteristic complication can occur in the case being discussed, for which a gastroenterological invasive technique is required to make the diagnosis?

A.7 Rarely, pseudomembranous colitis can develop in *C.difficile* associated cases. It is a fulminant, life threatening condition. Colonoscopy can help in demonstrating the yellowish membranous lesion in the colon. This membrane is composed of polymorphonuclear leucocytes, fibrin and mucin and is attached to the mucosal surface. Rarely, the case can have perforation of the bowel.

Integrated Clinical Based Study of Actinomyces/Actinomycosis

A 45 year old man, Ghanshyam reported to a surgical OPD with a 5 by 6 cm swelling at the angle of the right jaw. He gave history of dental extraction 2 months back. Recently yellowish granules discharge was reported from the lower portion of the swelling. Microscopic examination of the yellow granules, when crushed (as between two slides) and gram stained, revealed central zone of gram positive hyphal fragments surrounded by peripheral zone of swollen radiating club shaped structures, giving a sunray appearance (Figs. 5.1.6b, 5.1.6c at pg. 215).

Linkages: Pg. 212, 213, 215, 218, 221, 222, 251, 252

What is your diagnosis of this case?

A.1 (a) Cervicofacial actinomycosis

To which family does Actinomyces genus belong?

A.1 (b) It belongs to family Actinomycetes.

Besides Actinomyces the three other important genera in this family are Streptomyces, Nocardia and Actinomadura (responsible for bacterial mycetoma)

Why is Actinomycetes sometimes confused with fungi?

A.1 (c) Actinomycetes is classically considered as transitional forms between bacteria and fungi. Like fungi they form mycelial network of branching filaments (Fig. 5.1.6a, pg. 215).

What are the features the actinomycetes possess, because of which they are classified as bacteria?

A.1 (d) It possesses the following prokaryotic characters: (i) Possesses cell wall containing muramic acid, which can be gram stained; (ii) has prokaryotic nucleus; (iii) multiply by binary fission; (iv) antigenically related to Mycobacteria; (v) Susceptibe to antibacterial antimicrobials; (vi) antifungals have no effect.

With which entities is actinomycosis usually associated with?

A.2 (a) The infection is often associated with facial trauma, tooth extraction and poor dental hygiene.

What is the likely origin of actinomycosis in this case?

A.2 (b) This infection is most likely endogenous in origin i.e., in this case, patient's normal flora is responsible for this infection. It is believed that *A. israelli* requires other bacteria; as streptococci and *Eikenella corrodens* to cause this lesion.

Can Actinomyces cause bacterial mycetoma? Enumerate the other bacterial agents that can cause bacterial mycetoma.

A.2 (c) Yes. The numerous agents that cause bacterial mycetomas include

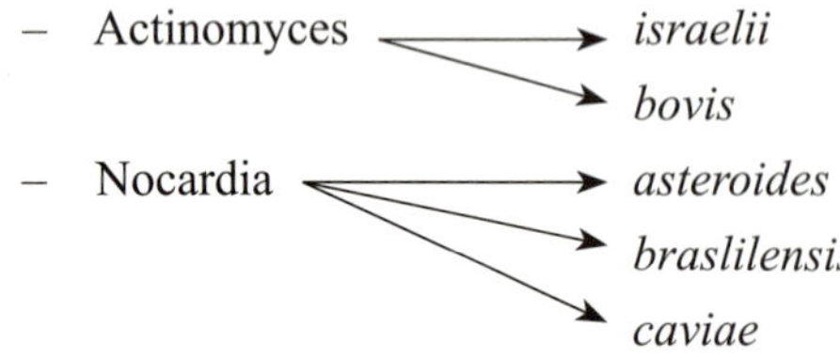

– *Streptomyces somalensis*

It is important to differentiate mycetomas caused by fungi from those caused by bacteria; due to difference in drug of choice and occasional requirement of radical surgery for eumycotic mycetomas. In actinomycotic mycetomas, the granules are white to yellow (called sulfur granules) in contrast to often black granules in eumycotic mycetomas. In the latter, the filaments are thicker about 4-5µm in diameter in contrast to the former, where they are about 1 µm in diameter.

How can you cultivate Actinomyces?

A.3 Actinomyces is grown best in brain heart infusion agar or thioglycollate broth, in anaerobic or microaerophilic conditions with 5-10% CO_2 at 37°C. This organism is slowly growing, so it can take a few days for growth.

Describe the epidemiology of Actinomycosis.

A.4
- **Agent:** *A. israelli* (Commonest)
- **Reservoir of infection:** The organism is normal flora of the mouth, respiratory tract, and genital tract.
- **Mode of transmission:** It is usually an endogenous infection, so disease isn't communicable. Under some conditions, the organism becomes invasive and cause damage to the underlying structure.
- **Host:**
  - The disease occurs worldwide, though the incidence has declined in the developed countries.
  - Young males are commonly affected.
  - The disease is common in agricultural workers in the rural areas.
- **Risk factor:** Condition that produce low oxygen tissue tension; as trauma, poor oral hygiene, tooth extraction and fracture of jaw.

How can you differentiate Actinomyces from Nocardia?

A.5 (a) Both Actinomyces and Nocardia on gram staining appear as branching, beaded, gram positive rods. They can be differentiated by modified acid fast staining in which Nocardia appear as partially acid fast while actinomyces do not. The growth conditions also vary, with Nocardia sps being strictly aerobic, where as Actinomyces prefer anaerobic conditions.

Describe the epidemiology of Nocardiosis.

A.5 (b)
- **Agent:** (i) *Nocardia asteroides* (usually for pulmonary nocardiosis); (ii) *Nocardia brasiliensis* (usually for subcutaneous infections, as myetoma)
- **Reservoir of infection:** These organisms are environmental saprophytes.

  (Unlike actinomycosis, this infection is exogenous)
- **Sources of infection:** Contaminated air/soil.
- **Modes of transmission:** Pulmonary nocardiosis is acquired by inhalation into the lungs whereas subcutaneous nocardiosis usually occurs following trauma to skin. These organisms are believed to be opportunists having low infectivity, so there is no case to case transmission.
- **Host:** The infection occur worldwide. Pulmonary nocardiosis usually occurs in individuals, who have some underlying disease as leukemia, lymphoma, chronic pulmonary disease or are receiving immune suppressive agents.

  It is important to differentiate Actinomyces from Nocardia, as though both infections require prolonged therapy extending to months, sulfa drugs are drug of choice for Nocardia infections whereas penicillin G is drug of choice for actinomyces infection.

How do you manage an actinomycosis case?

A.6 If the lesion is large, surgical intervention is necessary, besides prolonged antimicrobial administration, as the drug alone won't be able to penetrate throughout the lesion, to inhibit or kill the microbe.

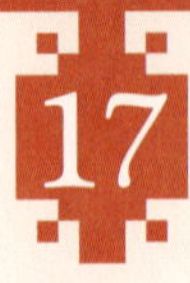

17 Laboratory Diagnosis and Treatment (Overview)

An Overview of the Comparative Approach in Laboratory Diagnosis of Key Gram Positive Bacilli

Organism / Disease	Specimen	Stain enhanced microscopy	Detection of Microbial • Antigen • Metabolic *products* • *Genome*	Serological/ Hypersensitivity Tests	Culture of Inanimate Organism In Media / Characteri-Zation of Isolate	Differential Diagnosis	Antimicrobial Susceptibility Test
Bacillus anthracis	• Fluid from vesicle (in malignant pustule) • Material beneath edge of black eschar • Sputum (in pulmonary anthrax) • Blood • Gastric aspirate • Faeces • Food (The lesion may be colonized with other bacteria, which may cause confusion in the diagnosis)	• Gm stain: Gram positive bacilli • Polychrome methylene blue: (Mc Fadyean reaction) amorphous purple material represents capsule • Giemsa stain: Blue stained bacilli with irregular purple colored capsule	• Can be demonstrated by ELISA • Ascoli's thermoprecipation test (ring ppt test, if sample is putrid, can extract antigen & layer anti-anthrax serum on it)		• Characterization and confirmation of isolate, see p. 216	• *Bacillus cereus* • Anthracoid bacilli (e.g., B.subtilis)	–
Bacillus cereus	• Food • Faeces • Vomitus	• Gram staining	-	-	• Mannitol-egg yolk-phenol red-polymyxin agar (MYPA):+	-	-
Corynebacterium diphtheriae	Exudate (pseudomembrane) at various sites • Fauces • Larynx • Nasal • Other sites as otitic, conjunctival (two swabs can take one for staining and other for culture)	• Gram stain (gram positive bacilli) • Albert stain (green bacilli with purplish granules arranged in 'chinese letter formation'		• Schick test - done in individuals to asses if they have been exposed to diphtheria & if are hypersensitive to diphtheria antigen details see A.9c, pg. 228-229	• Nutrient agar: No growth • Characterization and confirmation of isolate see p. 216	• Coryneform organism (e.g., *C.xerosis* • *C.pseudodipth-eriticum* • *C.ulcerans* (resembles gravis type of *C.diphtheriae* but liquifies gelatin, ferments trehalose slowly, does not reduce nitrate to nitrite	• Not performed as organism is sensitive to Penicillin & Erythromicin
Mycobacterium tuberculosis	• Sputum (in pulmonary tuberculosis) • C.S.F (in tubercular meningitis) • Lymph node Aspirate, • Biopsy (tubercular lymphadenitis, common in children • Gastric aspirate (as alternative to sputurn in patients unable to produce sputum, uncooperative patients as children or those too ill to expectorate • Laryngeal swab (indication as above) • Urine (in renal tuberculosis) • Tissue biopsies (e.g. skin lesion) • Body fluids synovial ascites • Exudates • Blood (in AIDS patients, circulating mycobacteria have been detected)	• Gram staining: bacilli usually does not take stain • Ziehl Neelsen staining (advantage taken of heat & increased incubation for making the dye penetrate the mycolic acid rich cell wall): • Pink/red colored bacilli seen, different grading schemes exist for grading the magnitude of AFB infection • This technique has the limitation of detecting AFB, if sample has 10,000 to 100,000 bacilli per ml of sample. • It may also not discriminate saprophytic mycobacteria from pathogenic • Fluorescent stain with Rhodamine auramine available (AFB fluoresce brightly against dark background	• Latex agglutination & ELISA test available for detecting antigen in CSF • PCR also available to detect the DNA in samples as sputum • DNA probe available to detect the DNA bacterial in samples as sputum • Details A.6b, pg. 235, case 8	• ELISA & other tests commercially available to measure different classes of antibodies to different antigenic fractions as 32kDa, 64kDa of *M.bovis* • However, clinically, no serologic test is acceptable so far. see A6., p. 231 • Tuberculin test (details see pg. 158, section 2)	• Nutrient agar: No growth • Characterization and confirmation of isolate (see pg.216) and see A5b, A6 (p.231)	• *M.bovis* (Niacin negative, does not reduce nitrate and is resistant to Pyrazinamide) • A typical Mycobacteria (MOTT) • *M.leprae* (globi appearance • Nocardia spp. (branching filament, less acid fast (1%) grow on ordinary media)	• With the emergence of multi drug resistant *M.tuberculosis*, susceptibility testing is essential • Special protocols have to be followed • Tests avaiable are: • Absolute concentration method • Resistance ratio method • Proportion method • Radiometric method (eg. *Bactec*) • - other see. A.7b,c, (p. 231), case 8 A6a,b,c (p. 235)

Contd.

Contd.

Mycobacterium leprae	• Skin slit smear (of affected sites usually ear, chin, hypopigmented sites lacking sensation • Nasal mucosa smear (over inferior turbinate) • Biopsy of: skin lesion: thickened nerve(partial); Lymph node	• Ziehl Neelsen staining (5% H_2SO_4 instead of 20% used for decolorization • Different indices calculated as Bacterial index grades the number of Acid fast bacilli in smear (determines infectivity) of patient & classifies leprosy cases • Morphological index: calculates percentage of uniformly stained bacilli (assess progress of patient to chemotherapy)	test being developed to detect specific anitigen in blood (using monoclonal antibody to phenolic glycolipd-1)	• Antibodies to PGL1 (specific phenolic glycolipid of leprosy bacillus) can be determined by ELISA & fluorescent technique • Lepromin test developed by Japanese, Mitsuda in 1916 based on delayed hypersensitivity. Lepromin injected intra-dermally & reaction read at 48 hours & 21 days. A positive test can occur in leprosy patients & even healthy individuals. It indicates presence of comparative resistance to disease as compared to non-reactors (details see A7c., pg. 241)	• Not possible so far to grow them on inanimate medium • Characterization and confirmation of isolate (see pg. 217	• Atypical mycobacteria	• Research tool: available to predict response to drug
Listeria monocytogenes	• Cervical/vaginal secretion • Cord blood • Sputum • Tissue biopsy	Gram staining (gram positive rods)	-	-	• Nutrient agar: No growth • Characterization and confirmation of isolate (see pg. 217)	• *Erysipelothrix rhusiopathiae* • Corynebacterium species	-
Clostridium tetani	• Wound exudate/ tissue from deeper parts of wound (as organism survives better in deeper parts, which are anaerobic in nature)	• Gram staining (may show drum stick appearance bacilli, gram posiive • Direct immunoflourescence test with conjugated immunoglobulin can demonstrate the bacilli	-	-	Nutrient agar: + Characterization and confirmation of isolate (see pg. 218)	• *Clostridium tetanomorphum* • *Clostridium sphenoides* (resembles C.tetani bacillus morphologically)	-
Clostridium perfringens (welchii)	• Exudate from depth of wound • Tissue from muscles at junction of affected area and normal • Necrotic tissue & muscle fragment • Blood (*Clostridium perfringens* bacteremia, may also occur without gas gangrene)	• Gram stain (large gram positive bacillus without spore)	-	-	• Nutrient agar:+ Culture in RCM s/c on to B.A. after 24-48 hr • Characterization and confirmation of isolate (see pg. 218	• *Clostridium septicum* (pleomorphic boat/ leaf shaped bacilli with irregular staining) • *Clostridium oedematiens* (large bacilli with oval, subterminal spore) • *Clostridium histolyticum* • *Clostridium fallax* • *Clostridium bifermentans*	-
Clostridium difficile	• Fresh faeces • Rectal swab (should be immediately processed, as organism is obligate anaerobe & gets killed on exposure to air)	Gram stain (gram variable bacilli with oval and terminal spore)	• Toxins can be detected by ELISA & latex agglutination technique, Toxin has two parts: toxin A (enterotoxin): toxin B (cytotoxin)	-	• Nutrient agar: No growth • Characterization and confirmation of isolate (see pg. 218.	Other clostridia	-
			Note: Faecal supernatant can be tested for cytotoxin by effect on human fibroblast (rounding effect on cells, can be neutralized by specific antitoxin)				
Clostridium botulinum (Food poisoning)	• Food (suspected) • Gastric fluid • Vomitus • Faeces • Wound exudate • Serum • Environmental sample • Sample must be handled with extreme precaution, as toxin is extremely potent	• Gram stain (gram positive sporing bacilli) • (Direct) immunofluorescent test available	• Toxin can be demonstrated in food & other samples by specific neutralization test in mice or guinea pig	• Serologic not much role, however retrospective diagnosis can be made by detection of antitoxin in patient's serum in some cases (A4, p. 246)	Nutrient agar: No growth - RCM: + - BA: + (haemolytic) Characterization and confirmation of isolate (see pg. 218)	• Other clostridia	-
Actinomyces israelli	• Pus from lesions as sinus tract & fistula • Sputum(in pulmonary lesions) • Tissue biopsy	Gram staining: whitish/ yellowish specks about 5mm in sample may be crushed between slides, stained & examined. Then gram positive filaments surrounded by peripheral zone of radiating club shaped structures (sun ray appearance) can be observed	-	Not significant	• Nutrient agar: No growth • Characterization and confirmation of isolate (see pg.218)	• Propiniobacterium species (anaerobic diphtheroid which may also have tendency to branch)	

An Overview of the Antimicrobial Options for Infections caused by Gram Positive Bacilli (Key)

	Cell Wall Inhibitors	Cell-Membrane Inhibitors	Amino Acid Synthesis Inhibitors	Nucleic Acid Synthesis Inhibitors	Others
Bacillus anthracis	PnG, Amoxicillin (for cutaneous form), Imipenem		Doxycycline (DOC) Clindamycin	Ciprofloxacin(DOC) Levofloxacin	
Bacillus cereus	Vancomycin PnG		Erythromycin Gentamicin	Ciprofloxacin	
C. diphtheriae	PnG		Erythromycin (DOC) Drugs to eliminate pathogen, stop toxin protection		
C.jeikeium	Vancomycin [PnG	+	Erythromycin]		
Mycobacterium tuberculosis	Multidrug therapy with Different combinations of bactericidal & bacteriostatic drugs are available as Rifampicin plus INH plus Pyrazinamide and/or Streptomycin or ethambutol, details see in medicine text book				
Non_Tuberculous mycobacteria	most strains resistant to usual anti-TB drugs, treatment to be based on combination of drugs, using drug susceptibility testing.				
Mycobacterium leprae				Rifampicin + Dapsone (for paucibacillary leprosy) Clofazimine added to above for multibacillary leprosy	
Listeria monocytogenes	Ampicillin Cephalosporins are ineffective	+	Gentamicin (DOC)	TM-SMZ	
Erysipelothrix rhusiopathiae	PnG, Ampicillin Piperacillin		Clindamycin	Ciprofloxacin	
Actinomyces israelii	PnG (DOC)		Clindamycin Tetracycline		
Nocardia spp. (*asteroides* & *brasilensis*)	Carbapenems Cephalosprins		Minocycline Linezolid	TM-SMZ Sulfisoxazole	
Clostridium perfringens	PnG, Carbapenems (DOC) (Surgical debridement is key)		Doxycycline Chloramphenicol Clindamycin (DOC)	Metronidazole	
Clostridium tetani	PnG (DOC) Carbapenems (Wound debridement is important)		Doxycycline Chloramphenicol Clindamycin (DOC)		
Clostridium botulinum	No role of antimicrobials, though organism susceptible to PnG/metronidozole (give anti-toxin)				
Clostridium difficile	Stop the incriminating antimicrobial Vancomycin (may)			Metronidazole (may)	
Mobiluncus spp	Pn G		Erythromycin Gentamicin Clindamycin		

NB: *DOC-refers to drug of choice*

18 Assessment/Examination Questions

1. What makes Bacillus genus of considerable historical importance? A 3a., p. 224
2. Describe the epidemiology of anthrax. A 3b., p. 224
3. What makes *B. anthracis* a bioweapon? A 2., p. 223
4. Why do extra precautions have to be undertaken while handling clinical specimens with suspected bioweapons? Why can chemoprophylaxis be ineffective in such a scenario? A 7., p. 223
5. Classify zoonotic diseases, giving examples. Describe epidemiology and laboratory diagnosis of any one. A 5., p. 223
6. Mention about virulence factors of *B. anthracis*. What was the basis of the original Pasteur anthrax vaccine? Describe the currently used anthrax vaccine for human use. A 6a,b., p. 223 and p. 632
7. Describe malignant pustule. p. 220, a 1b., p. 224
8. Enumerate the diseases caused by Bacillus species. p. 220
9. What processes are used to disinfect common animal products?
10. Describe laboratory diagnosis of anthrax. p. 250, chapter 4., p. 223, chapter 5., p. 224
11. What antimicrobials are administered in post exposure cases of anthrax Mention the duration of administration. A 7., p. 223
12. Tabulate the differences between anthrax bacilli and anthracoid bacilli (aerobic spore bearers). A 4c., p. 225
13. Compare and contrast the two types of *B. cereus* food poisoning. A 4., p. 225
14. Describe anthracoid bacilli. A 4b., p. 224-225
15. Enumerate the microbes that can produce a membranous like lesion; in a case of sore throat. A 1., p. 226
16. What are the non–diphtherial corynebacteria (Corynebacterium species other than *C. diphtheriae*) associated with human disease? A 10., 228
17. Is Diphtheria a notifiable disease? Describe the epidemiology of diphtheria. Mention the control measures of diphtheria. A9a,b, A3., p. 228-229
18. Enumerate the differences between three biotypes namely; gravis, intermedius and mitis of *C.diphtheriae*. A 3a., p. 226
19. What are the virulent factors of *C.diphtheriae*? What is the mechanism of action of diphtheria toxin? What are the conventional and rapid techniques (toxigenicity tests) used to detect this toxin in a diphtheria toxin (including the Elek's test)? A 5a,b,c, A6a,b, p. 227
20. What are the mechanisms by which *C.diphtheriae* can cause death in an infected case? What are the other complications the diphtheria infection can cause in a case? A 7a,b., p. 227-228
21. Describe the laboratory diagnosis of diphtheria. Describe the Schick test and mention its utility. p. 250, A 9c., 228-229
22. Should a physician wait for a microbiologist's report before a treatment is initiated, in a case of suspected case of diphtheria? Compare active, passive and combined immunization in diphtheria. A 4., p. 226, A 13., p. 229
23. Name some Coryneform genera resembling but other than Corynebacterium, associated with human disease. A 11., p. 229
24. What are diphtheroids? Name some common diphtheroids. How is *C. diphtheriae* differentiated from diphtheroids? A 12a,b., p. 229
25. Classify mycobacteria (including atypical and leprae). Describe Lowenstein–Jensen medium. A3c., p. 230, p. 56
26. What is the habitat of *M. tuberculosis*? Describe the epidemiology of tuberculosis. A 2., p. 230, A 3a., p. 230
27. What is the natural history of pulmonary tuberculosis? What are the risk factors for this disease? A 3b., p. 230, A3a., p. 234
28. What is Koch phenomenon? Describe pathogenesis of *M.bovis* and *M.tuberculosis* infections. Mention the role of antigens of *M. tuberculosis* in the pathogenesis. A 7., p. 235, A 8b., p. 236, A8a, p. 235-236
29. Enumerate morphological differences between *M.bovis* and *M.tuberculosis*. A 3b., p. 234
30. Describe laboratory diagnosis of pulmonary tuberculosis. p. 250 and see chapters 6, 7, 8
31. Describe Mantoux test. What is the diagnostic role of this test in India in comparison to the developed countries; as USA. A 2d., p. 233
32. Enumerate and describe the automated culture methods and molecular biology based tests to diagnose TB. A 6b,c., p. 235
33. What is the role of serodiagnosis in the diagnosis of tuberculosis? A6., p. 231

34. Why does the physician not wait for the results of mycobacteria susceptibility testing before initiating ATT (anti tuberculosis treatment)? Are all labs competent to perform mycobacteria susceptibility testing? What are the techniques available to perform mycobacteria susceptibility testing? A 7c., p. 231
35. Describe MDR and XDR–TB. See case., p. 614
36. Mention about the RNTCP programme/DOTS programme. A 13a,b,c., p. 232
37. Describe BCG vaccine. pg 630
38. How do you classify non-tuberculous mycobacteria (atypical mycobacteria) i.e. mycobacteria other than tubercle mycobacteria. A3c., p. 230, A5b., p. 238
39. Tabulate the differences between tubercle bacilli and non-tuberculous mycobacteria. Outline a flow diagram to identify the different mycobacteria. A 3b., p. 237
40. What is the usual habitat of non-tuberculous mycobacteria? Describe common features. A 4a., p. 237, A4b., p. 237-238
41. Describe Photochromogens, Scotochromogens and Mycobacterium avium–intracellulare complex. A 3c., p. 230, A5b., p. 238
42. Compare and contrast two skin lesions, namely Buruli ulcer (caused by *M. ulcerans*) and swimming pool granuloma. A 7., p. 238
43. What is the difficulty in treating infections caused by non-tuberculous mycobacteria (atypical mycobacteria)? A 6., p. 238
44. Describe the morphology of *M.leprae*. p. 213-214
45. What is the likely reservoir of *M.leprae* and how does leprosy spread? Describe the epidemiology of leprosy. A 6b,c,d., p. 240
46. Describe the differences between tuberculoid and lepromatous leprosy. Table 5.101., p. 239-240
47. Describe immunopathogenesis of leprosy with focus on tuberculoid leprosy. A. 5a., p. 240
48. Can *M.leprae* be cultivated on inanimate media? Describe animal models to cultivate this organism. A3, pg. 240
49. Describe Laboratory diagnosis of leprosy? p. 251, chapter 10
50. What is the key antigen used for the serodiagnosis of leprosy? Describe the lepromin test. A 7a., p. 241, A7c., p. 241
51. What is the regimen to treat tuberculoid leprosy? p. 252
52. Classify *Clostridia perfringens.* A3c., p. 242
53. Enumerate the microbes incriminated in gas gangrene A 3b., p. 242
54. Describe virulence factors including alpha toxin of *C. perfringens*. Explain Nagler reaction, stormy clot reaction and reverse CAMP test. A 3a., p. 243, p. 218
55. Describe pathogenesis of gas gangrene A 3b., p. 242, A2., p. 243
56. Describe the role of laboratory diagnosis in management of a gas gangrene case. A 3a., p. 242
57. Is isolation of *C. perfringens* from clinical samplesenough to incriminate it as a etiological agent in *C. perfringens* food poisoning? A5., p. 24
58. Describe necrotizing enteritis. A 6., p. 243
59. Describe the morphology of *C. tetani.* p. 215
60. What Indian customs have a possible role in the pathogenesis in neonatal tetanus? A 2a., p. 244
61. Describe in detail epidemiology of tetanus. A 2c., p. 244
62. Mention role key of virulent factors in pathogenesis of tetanus. A 3a., p. 245
63. Describe laboratory diagnosis of tetanus. p. 25 and case at p. 244
64. Describe laboratory tests to detect two key toxins of *C.tetani.* A 3b., p. 245
65. Mention the role of Human tetanus Immunoglobulin in management of early tetanus case. Describe prophylaxis against tetanus. A5., p. 245
66. Describe the epidemiology of botulism. A 2b, p. 246
67. Outline the laboratory diagnosis of botulism. p. 251, case at p. 246
68. Mention about the exotoxins of *C. botulinum* and bioterrorism aspect of *C. botulinum.* chapter 14., p. 246
69. What is the normal carriage rate of *C. difficile*? How does man acquire infection with this microbe? A 4a,b., p. 247
70. Describe laboratory diagnosis of *C. difficile* associated diarrohea. p. 251, case at p. 247
71. Can the antimicrobial which are used in the treatment of *C. difficile* associated diarrohea itself be responsible for the causation of this disease? Mention the approaches and challenges in treating this disease. A 5b, A5a., p. 247
72. Enumerate the pathogens that cause bacterial mycetomas. A 2c., p. 248
73. Describe the epidemiology of actinomycosis. A 4., p. 249
74. Describe laboratory diagnosis of actinomycosis. p. 251 and case at p. 248
75. Describe Sulfur granules. clinical vignette p. 248
76. Describe Nocardia spp. A 5b., p. 249

Section VI: Gram Negative Bacilli–Enterobacteriaceae

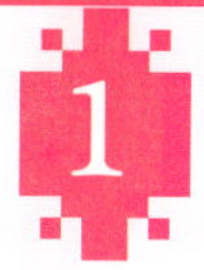

Classification, Metabolic and Microscopic Features of Gram Negative Bacilli (GNB)

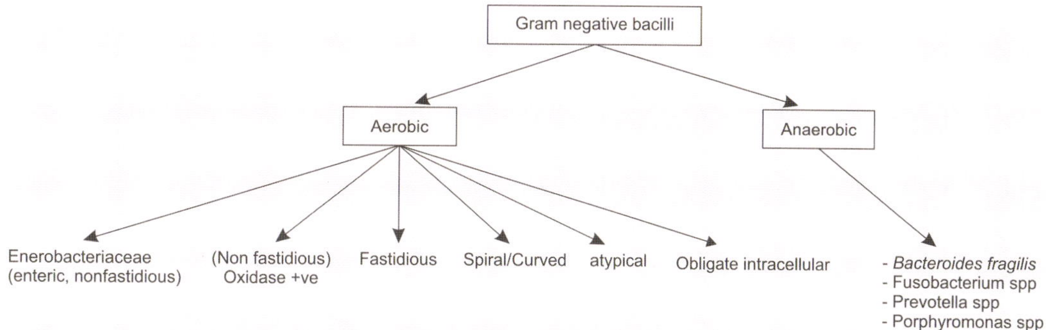

Fig. 6.1.1: Broad categories of Gram Negative Bacilli

Note: Demarcations are not absolute, as in fastidious category, oxidase +ve organisms exist and in other categories, exceptions also exist

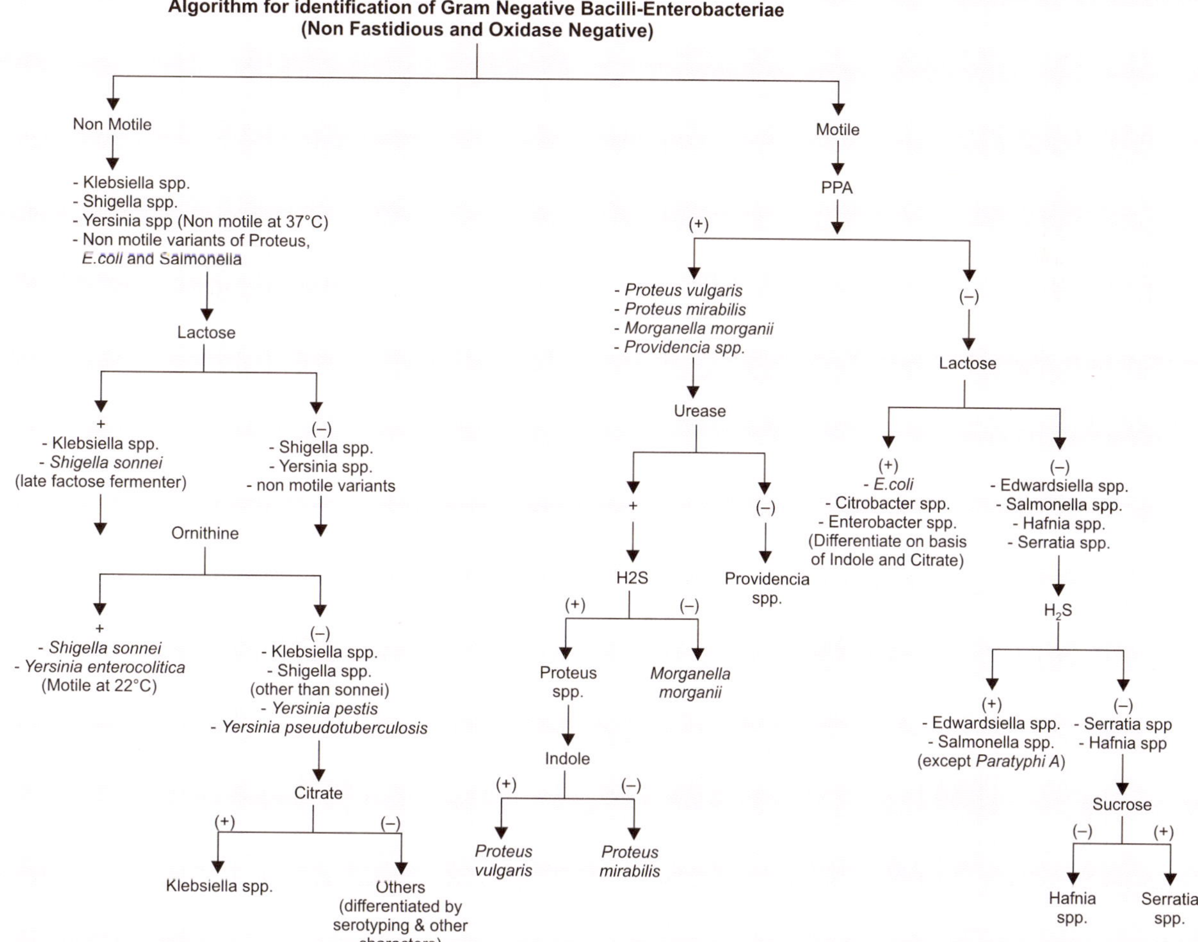

Fig. 6.1.2

Contd.

Salmonella Paratyphi A & B	Enteric fever
Salmonella NT (Typhimurium, Senftenberg, Enteridis, Cholerasuis & other serotypes)	Salmonella gastroenteritis (Food poisoning) Septicaemia and focal suppurative lesions, as osteomyelitis, pneumonia, endocarditis, abscesses and meningitis may occur may occur with these serotypes • Case: pg 271-272
Yersinia pestis	Plague
	In man, three forms seen:
	(i) Bubonic plague _regional lymphadenopathy at site draining infected rat flea bite, bubo may form later (Fig. 6.3.1)
	(ii) Pneumonic: plague_ usually secondary to bubonic plague (rarely primary) • Case: pg 273-275
	(iii) Septicaemic: plague_ involvement of blood vessels in skin and mucosa can result in haemorrhages (purpuric lesions) named 'black death' because of extensive involvement of blood vessels resulting in cyanosis and gangrene in terminal cases
Yersinia pseudotuberculosis	Mesentric lymphadenitis (fever and abdominal pain resembling acute appendicitis or septicaemic illness)
Yersinia enterocolitica	Enterocolitis: (common presentation) presenting as fever, diarrohea and abdominal pain, sometimes present a picture of mesentric lymphadenitis
Plesiomonas shigelloides	Gastroenteritis: (in immunosuppressed, a cholera like illness) Associated with cellulitis, septicaemia and neonatal meningitis)
Bacteriodes spp.	Most common non sporing anaerobe involved in pathogenicity, Often involved in mixed infections Involved in peritonitis following bowel surgery and pelvic inflammatory disease. Also in pulmonary, abdominal and brain abscesses (infections often polymicrobial).
Prevotella melaninogenica	Associated with oral and intestinal lesions, mastoiditis, pulmonary and liver abscesses
Fusobacterium spp. (as nucleatum, necrophorum)	Dental and peridontal infections Cerebral abscess and other infections of head and neck
Leptotricha spp.	Acute ulcerative gingivitis (Vincent's angina), *B. vincentii* associated with this lesion
Porphyromonas gingivalis	Gingival disease
Porphyromonas endodontalis	Root canal (dental) infections

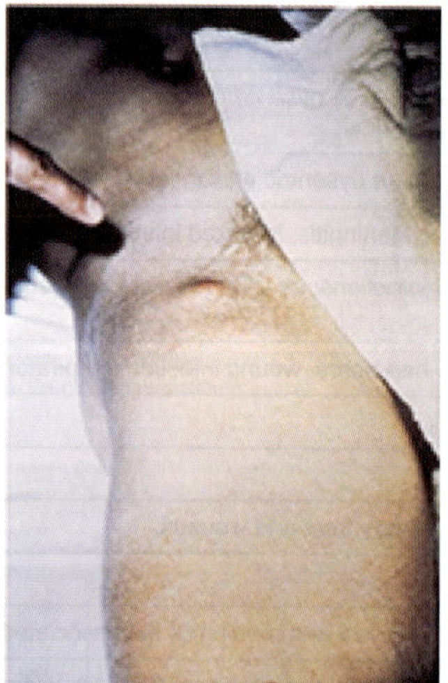

Fig. 6.3.1: PLAGUE: Case with bubo (swollen inguinal lymph node)

Courtesy: CDC, Atlanta

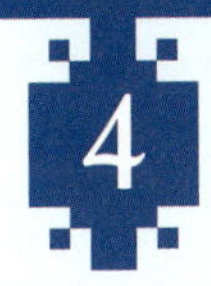

Integrated Clinical Based Study of *E.coli*/Diarrhoea

A traveller, Mr Michael from United Kingdom to Delhi, presented with history of passage of 7-8 loose stool, since the past one day. Direct stool examination did not reveal any ova, trophozoites or cysts. Stool culture revealed growth of large lactose fermenting colonies on MacConkey agar.

Linkages: Pg. 256-259, 276, 278

What is the likely clinical diagnosis of this case?

A.1 The likely clinical diagnosis is travellers' diarrhea.

What is the microbiological differential diagnosis?

A.2 (a) Large lactose forming colonies growing on MacConkey medium, can be of *E. coli*, Klebsiella sps, Enterobacter spp. or Citrobacter species.

Based on the clinical history of this case, *E.coli* is the most likely organism to be isolated from this case.

What do the terms 'coliform' bacilli and 'paracolon' bacilli convey?

A.2 (b) 'Coliform' bacilli refers to lactose fermenting members of the family enterobacteriaceae, whereas 'paracolon' bacilli refer to the late lactose fermenters; as *Shigella sonnei*, Edwardsiella, Serratia, Citrobacter, Providencia and Erwinia.

Outline the important tribes of Enterobacteriaceae and common tests to differentiate them.

A.2 (c) The various tribes are as follows:

I.	ESCHERICHIEAE-Escherichia, Shigella.	V.	KLEBSIELLEAE-Klebsiella, Enterobacter, Hafnia, Serratia
II.	EDWARDSIELLEAE	VI.	PROTEEAE
III.	SALMONELLEAE	VII.	YERSINIEAE
IV.	CITROBACTEREAE	VIII.	ERWINIEAE (not included in table below, as clinically not of much significance)

	Tribe I	Tribe II	Tribe III	Tribe IV	Tribe V	Tribe VI	Tribe VII
Acid from lactose	±	-	-	-	±	-	±
Motility	±	+	+	+	±	+	- (at 37°C)
Indole test	±	+	-		-	±	-
Methyl Red test	+	+	+	+		+	+
Voges Proskaeur test	-	-	-	±	+	-	±
Citrate test	-	-	+	+	+	±	-
Phenyl pyruvic acid production	-	-	-	-	-	+	-
H_2S production	-	+	±	±	-	+	-
Urease test	-	-	-	±	+	±	-

Is Escherichia coli a pathogen or commensal?

A.3 (a) Most of the *E.coli* (named after *Escherich*, who first isolated it) present in the human GIT are commensals. It is important to know; if the isolated *E.coli* is a pathogenic one. The commensal *E.coli* acquires virulent genes by conjugation or lysogeny or other means and acquires virulence (pathogenicity)

Which type of pathogenic diarrhoeagenic E.coli is involved in this case?

A.3 (b) The clinical picture in the case is one of diarrhoea and not dysentery. So; in this case, the isolated *E.coli* is likely to be an enterotoxigenic or a enteropathogenic one.

To which family does E. coli belong?

A.3 (c) Enterobacteriaceae

What are the characteristics of the bacteria, which belong to Enterobacteriaceae?

A.3 (d) They are gram negative bacilli, non acid fast, non sporing, non fastidious (grows on basal media), aerobic and facultative anaerobic metabolism, motile by peritrichous flagella or non motile, ferment glucose with production of acid or acid and gas, reduce nitrates to nitrites, oxidase negative and catalase positive.

Name some organisms which belong to Enterobacteriaceae, but do not fulfill all its criteria.

A.3 (e)
- Erwinia and Yersinia spp. (some strains) do not reduce nitrate to nitrite
- Tatumella spp. is not motile by peritrichate flagella (but by polar and sub-polar flagella)
- Tatumella spp. has poor growth on ordinary media
- *Shigella dysentriae* type 1 is catalase negative

Enumerate commonly used systems used to classify Enterobacteriaceae. Outline the approach.

A.3 (f) There are three widely used classification systems for Enterobacteriaceae, namely Bergey's manual, Kaufmann's and Edward –Ewing. There are certain differences amongst them but the basic approach is the same. The family is first categorized into groups or tribes. Each tribe consists of one or more genera and each genus consists of one or more sub genera and species. The species is further categorized into types as serotypes, biotypes and phage types.

What is the commonly followed system used to classify Enterobacteriaceae in the laboratory?

A.3 (g) Enterobacteriaceae are divided on the basis of lactose fermentation (on MacConkey plate) into lactose fermenters, late lactose fermenters and non lactose fermenters. The lactose fermenters (rapid) include *E.coli*, Enterobacter and Klebsiella spp. The late lactose fermenters include Edwardsiella, Serratia, Citrobacter, Providencia, *S.sonnei* and Erwinia; wheras the non lactose fermenters include Shigella (except sonnei), Salmonella and Proteus species.

What tests are required to confirm the isolate (in this case), as one belonging to Enterotoxigenic Escherichia coli (ETEC)?

A.4 (a) Serotyping of the isolate, using O antisera (targeting 'O' somatic antigen) would help in making the diagnosis. If is important to test at least ten isolated colonies, as more than one serogroups could be present in one sample. Commonly strains of ETEC belong to serogroups as 06,08, etc. The flagellar antigen are designated as 'H' antigen and capsular antigen as 'K' antigen.

Describe a classical animal test done to demonstrate labile toxin of ETEC.

A.4 (b) Classically, Rabbit ileal loop assay is performed to demonstrate enterotoxin of *E.coli*. Briefly, in it, the animal`s abdominal wall is dissected, to isolate 3-4 ileal loops about 5 cm in length. Culture fluid to be tested (including control), 1ml each (containing about $1X10^8$ cells) is introduced into each of the loops. After 18 hours, the animal is killed. The loops are taken out, the volume and length of each is measured. The ratio of volume of loop (ml)/length (cm) is calculated. If it is more than one, then the isolate is considered to be positive for presence of enterotoxin. i.e., the isolate likely belongs to ETEC.

Enumerate tests to differentiate between heat labile toxin (LT) from heat stable toxin (ST) of ETEC.

A.4 (c)

Test	Heat-labile toxin (LT)	Heat-stable toxin (ST)
'IN VITRO' TESTS		
Ligated rabbit ileal loop assay Reading at 6 hours	±	+
Reading at 18 hrs	+	-
Infant mouse intragastric test	-	+
'IN VIVO' TESTS		
Rounding in Y1 adrenal cell culture	+	-
Elongation of Chinese hamster ovary (CHO) cells	+	-
ELISA test	+	+ (ST type)
DNA probes (varying)	+	+

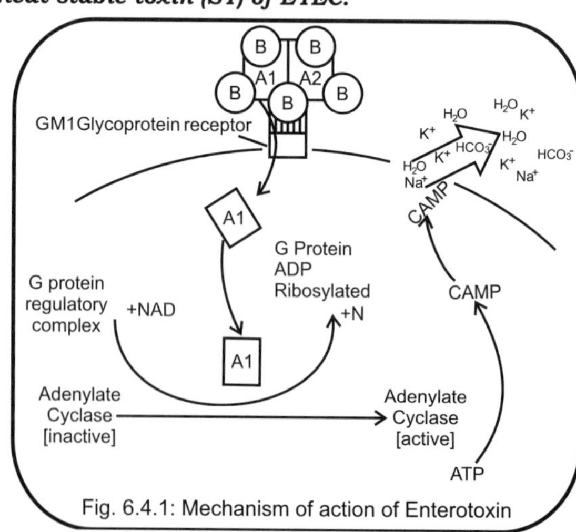

Fig. 6.4.1: Mechanism of action of Enterotoxin

What is the mechanism by which ETEC causes diarrohea?

A.4 (d) These strains possess colonization factors that may be pili or specific type of protein K antigen. These promote the virulence of these strains, by enhancing their adherence to small intestinal mucosa. These strains form a heat labile enterotoxin (LT) or a heat stable toxin (ST) or both. The structure and function of LT is similar to that of the vibrio toxin, though significantly less potent (Fig. 6.4.1). The heat stable (ST) toxin is, as the name indicates, resistant to heat and act by activation of the guanylate cyclase. It stimulates the formation of cGMP leading to fluid accumulation in the gut.

Aspects Related to Case Theme/Examination Assessment

What infections does E.coli cause; besides gastroenteritis?

A.5 *E. coli* causes UTI (this agent is commonest organism, responsible for this syndrome), septicaemia and pyogenic infections; as wound infection, neonatal meningitis, peritonitis, brain abscess etc.

Compare and contrast the pathogenicity of the different types of diarrhoeagenic E.coli.

A.6 Pathogenicity of different types of diarrhoeagenic *E.coli*

	Enteropathogenic *E.coli* (EPEC)	Enterotoxigenic *E.coli* (ETEC)	Enteroinvasive *E.coli* (EIEC)	Enterohaemorrhagic *E.coli* (EHEC)
Epidemiology	Infantile and childhood diarrhoea	Childhood diarrhoea Traveller's diarrhoea	Uncommon dysentry presentation	In developed countries, Haemorrhagic colitis, H.U.S. (Haemolytic Uremic Syndrome)
Primary site	Small Intestine	Small intestine	Large intestine	Large intestine
Mucosal picture	Microvilli destruction	Normal, hyperaemia	Ulceration, inflammation, necrosis	Destruction of microvilli
Genetic control	Plasmid associated	Plasmid associated	Plasmid associated	Lysogenic (phage)
Pathogenetic mechanism	Adherence to enterocyte	LT/ST	Invasion and epithelial damage	VT-1.VT-2 (SLT)
Clinical picture	Diarrhoea	Diarrhoea	Dysentry	Dysentry
Fever	Frequent	Absent	Common	Absent
Stool **Nature**	Watery	Watery	Purulent, scanty	Bloody, copious
Pus (WBCs) in stool	Scanty	Absent/scanty	Significant	Insignificant

NB: Recently Enteroaggregative *E.coli* have been described, which form 'stacked brick' appearance on HE_P-2 cell and form enteroaggregative heat stable enterotoxin-1 (EAST-1)

What is the habitat of E.coli?

A.7 (a) Most pathogenic strains for causing human disease reside in the human intestine.

To which category, do most of the E.coli infections belong, i.e., endogenous or exogenous?

A.7 (b) Most *E.coli* infections except those causing neonatal meningitis and gastroenteritis are endogenous, i.e., patients own flora is the cause of the infection.

Mention about the pathogenicity and diagnosis of EIEC infections.

A.7 (c) Enteroinvasive *E.coli* (EIEC) strains have the potential of invading the intestinal mucosa and causing a dysentery like illness, just as Shigella species does. The serogroups belonging to this category include: O112, O124 and O136. The ability to invade the cells is determined by a large plasmid, which codes for outer membrane antigens called the virulence marker antigens (VMA). EIEC causes keratoconjunctivitis when introduced into eye of guinea pig. This is basis of sereny test.

The EIEC strains are suspected by the atypical biochemical reactions, given by them; as being late lactose fermenter/non-lactose fermenter, anaerogenic and/or being non motile. The VMA antigen can be tested by the ELISA test. DNA probes are also available to screen these strains from the faeces specimen.

Which serotype of E.coli is commonly associated with causation of haemolytic uremic syndrome?

A.8 (a) Strains belonging to serogroup O157H:7, also known as Enterohaemorrhagic *E.coli* (Verotoxin producing *E.coli*)

Is there any role of antimicrobials in preventing development of H.U.S?

A.8 (b) No, as it is a post-infective syndrome.

Describe the epidemiology and diagnosis of EHEC infection.

A.8 (c) In 1982, the importance of EHEC was realized, when this organism was isolated from cases with two syndromes of unknown etiology namely; hemorrhagic colitis and hemolytic uremic syndrome (HUS). At that time, a multistate outbreak of hemorrhagic colitis in Michigan, USA related to eating of hamburgers, from a fast food chain (McDonald) restaurant had occurred. The implicated food item was the used beef. These strains did not have the characteristics of EPEC,toxins of ETEC or had the invasive character of the EIEC strains, hence were declared the fourth type of *E. coli*. Subsequently a large outbreak in Nevada, USA was reported, in which 41 cases of HUS occurred and four deaths were reported. Majority of these strains produced 'verotoxin' (affecting vero cells), so are also designated as verotoxin producing *E. coli*.

Sorbitol fermentation is used to select out these strains, as majority (95%) of these strains do not ferment this sugar. As majority of these stains are of type O157:H7; 055:B5, O and H antisera can also identify these strains. Other tests; infrequently used to identify them include demonstration of Shiga - like toxin (cytotoxicity on Vero cell lines) and PCR for Shiga-like toxin gene (including DNA probe for toxin genes).

Outline a diagnostic pathway for identification of Enterobacteriaceae

A.9 See Table 6.1.2, p. 255

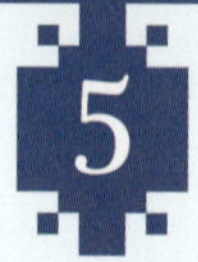

Integrated Clinical Based Study of Shigella/Dysentery

A mother brought a five year old male child, Sonu to the clinic, with history of frequent passage of stool, with his shorts being smeared with feces. On examination, he was found to be febrile. There was no history of recent antibiotic use and no one in the family was ill at the time of the incident.

Linkages: Pg. 256-259, 276, 279

What rapid test can be done on the bedside in this case, to get a clue to the type of diarrhoea in the above case i.e., whether enterotoxigenic or invasive pathogenetic mechanisms?

A.1 (a) One can grossly examine the faeces for the presence of any blood and/or pus. If both are absent, one can stain the faeces for presence of leukocytes and also examine for the presence of occult blood in the faeces. If either of two is present, the case is likely to have an invasive type of diarrhoea.

What is the importance of demarcating diarrhoea on the basis of pathogenetic mechanism?

A.1 (b) Demarcating the type of diarrhoea narrows down the list of implicated pathogens and helps in determing the treatment.

Classify the bacterial pathogens on the basis of enterotoxigenic and invasive pathogenicity mechanisms in the bowel wall?

A.1 (c) The known *enterotoxin producers: V. cholerae, E. coli* (certain types), *B. cererus, S. aureus* (some)

The *enteroinvasive organisms:* Shigella sps excepting *S. dysentriae* (serotype 1), Salmonella, Campylobacter, *E coli* (some), *C.perfringens*, *B. cereus, Y. enterocolitica and V. parahaemolyticus.*

What is the most important microbiological investigation that should be done in this case?

A.2 Stool culture. Rectal swab can also be cultured, if stool is not available.

The stool culture of the case yielded non lactose fermenting colonies on MacConkey agar. Inoculated Triple sugar agar medium demonstrated an alkaline slant, acid butt with no H_2S or gas. The urease test was negative. On these findings, what is the likely organism that has been isolated from this case?

A.3 (a) Shigella spp. The genus Shigella is named after Shiga, who isolated this agent from a dysentery outbreak in Japan.

Can Shigella be cultivated on a basal medium? If yes, what is the role of specialized media; as enrichment and selective medium in the isolation Shigella spp.?

A.3 (b) The organism can grow on basal media. Enrichment and selective media are required, so that this organism can be isolated from the predominant commensals, which are prevalent in the faeces specimen.

Using a genetic definition for species, the four species of Shigella would be regarded as serologically defined anaerogenic biotypes of E. coli (i.e., E.coli and Shigella are very close genetically and even resemble on DNA hybridization. Why is then a separate nomenclature maintained for E.coli and Shigella?

A.3 (c) A separate nomenclature is maintained largely for medical purposes of the useful association of Shigella with a distinct disease; as shigellosis (for epidemiologic reasons)

Which tests can help to speciate and type Shigella isolate into serotypes?

A.4 Typing using Shigella polyvalent and monovalent antisera.

What is the natural habitat of Shigella?

A.5 Human gastrointestinal tract. Unlike many Salmonella and *E.coli* isolates, which have many animal reservoirs, the bacterium in question has no such reservoir.

What is the importance of 'the history of no recent antibiotic uptake' and no history of similar family illness, in the workup of this case?

A.6 No, history of recent antimicrobial intake reduces the probability of diarrhoea being due to *C.difficile* or *C. albicans*

The history of no one in the family being ill, indicates that the child has likely acquired this infection from outside the house.

How has the child likely acquired this infection?

A.7 As his family members are healthy, the child is likely to have acquired the infection from his playmates or outside environment.

Why are fomites important in the spread of Shigella infection?

A.8 (a) This organism can have a low infective dose, of as low as 100 organisms, so inanimate object; as toilet taps, door handles of toilets, and toys can become colonized with this organism and be responsible for outbreaks by this organism.

Describe the epidemiology of Shigellosis.

A.8 (b) • **Agent: Shigella species have four species with characteristics as depicted below:**

Subgroup	Fermentation of			Indole test	Ornithine decarboxylase activity	Serotypes
	Lactose	Mannitol	Sucrose			
Shigella dysentriae	-	-	-	d	-	15
Shigella flexneri	-	A	-	d	-	6+2 variants
Shigella boydii	-	A	-	d	-	19
Shigella sonnei	A-late fermenter	A	A-late	-	+	1 (has numerous colicin types)

NB: A indicates acid production, d-variable

The epidemic strains depict plasmid borne multiple drug resistance.

In India, *S. flexneri* is the predominant species (50-85%) with *S. boydii* (0-8%), being the least frequently isolated species.

- **Reservoir of infection:** It is a pathogen of only humans and higher primates. Cases and carriers both have a role. Chronic carriage is rare except in some malnourished children and cases with AIDS.
- **Source of infection:** Faeces (infective) infected water, food and fomites; as door handle of toilet. It is spread primarily by faecal-oral route. The incubation period is 1-7 days (usually 2days).
- **Mode of transmission:** The modes may be as,
  - (i) Hand to mouth, directly by contaminated finger
  - (ii) through contaminated food and drinks
  - (iii) Fomites, as door handles should be considered; as modes of transmission. Such a mode in possible, as the infective dose can be as low as 100 organisms.

    For this reason outbreaks frequently occur in picnic camps, resorts and hotels, where hygiene gets compromised.
  - (iv) Flies can also transmit infection by acting as mechanical vectors.
  - (v) A recent mode of transmission has emerged because of change of sexual practices. In young male homosexuals, gay bowel syndrome has been reported.

  Note-mnemonic with 5 f′ s-finger, fomite, food, faeces and flies.
- **Host Factors:** The disease occurs worldwide, though differences in type and extent of infection occur.

  In the industrialized world, *Shigella sonnei* is the predominant agent. In India, the predominant species is *S. flexneri* and the least common species being *S. boydii.*

  The infection is commonest in children. It is often symptomatic in children but asymptomatic picture in adults occurs, probably due to acquired immunity in them. Males and females are equally affected; except women aged 20-39 are affected more probably because of their greater contact with children. Malnourished children have severe and recurrent infection, often resulting in malnutrition.

- **Environment:** Where ever the sanitation is poor; as in poor colonies, slums day care centers, the infection is common and the chances of outbreak are high. Several localized outbreaks in India have been reported recently. Outbreaks do get reported in war; as occurred in the recent Rwandan civil war in 1994.

Blood culture perfomed in this case did not yield any growth, i.e., was sterile. Is such a finding consistent with this case?

A.9 (a) The finding is consistent with this case, as mostly this organism is locally invasive and systemic spread does not occur.

Describe the pathogenesis of Shigellosis.

A.9 (b) All species of Shigella are strict human pathogens. The minimum infective dose is in the range of 100-1000 bacilli. The spread is through food or drink contaminated with faeces of infected cases. The organism can survive low pH, so can pass through stomach acid barrier. It multiplies to high numbers (10^8/ml) in distal small intestine in about 12 hours. It invades the large intestine in 1-4 days. *S dysentriae type 1* (*S.shigae*) is the only shigella to act by exotoxin (neurotoxicity also demonstrated). A cytotoxin (verocytotoxin, VT) has also been recognized, which is produced by certain strains of *S dysentriae,* which is similar to VT of ETEC. It comprises of two subunits A and B. Subunit A is active and binds to 60S ribosome, resulting in inhibition of protein synthesis, leading to cell death. The subunit B is the binding unit. Genes for this toxin are located in the bacterial chromosome.

The ingested Shigella enter intestine by endocytosis via M cells. The shigella escape endocytic vesicle and multiply in the cell protected from the macrophage. Shigella are non motile but move within the cell by forming a tail of polymerized host actin, created by microbial protein. The bacterium comes out of the vacuole and invades the adjacent cell, by lateral membrane. The invasion of and destruction of the neighbouring cells results in a mucosal abscess.

The invasive properties of the Shigella is related to the presence in the organism of a large plasmid, responsible for coding outer membrane proteins, required for host cell penetration. These proteins are called virulence marker antigens (VMA). This shigella has the abilty of invading Hela cell lines. Detection of this antigen by ELISA, serves as virulence marker for Shigella.

How should this case of Shigellosis be managed?

A.10 The fluid and electrolyte loss in this case should be replaced. Antimicrobials should be used only in severe cases.

Is a prolonged carrier state commonly associated with Shigella infected cases?

A.11 No. This infection is usually self limiting unlike many salmonella infections.

Is it possible to prevent shigellosis?

A.12 Theoretically this disease can be prevented using public health measures; as proper sewage treatment, clean water supply and other measures; as hand hygiene. But practically, it is difficult to implement this, as clean drinking water is not available to large population and it is difficult to implement hygienic measures in children. No vaccine is currently available and prophylactic antimicrobials are usually not recommended.

6 Integrated Clinical Based Study of Salmonella/Enteric Fever

A United Kingdom businessman, Mr. Philip presented with fever and abnormal behavior, after his return to London from a 10 day business trip to Jaipur. He gave history of eating at local eatery a week back and subsequently developing gastointestinal disturbance. His examination; revealed a mildly enlarged spleen, palpable (2 cm below left costal margin) and blood examination revealed leucopenia. On blood culture, no organism could be isolated. Widal test revealed significantly raised specific antibodies against *S.* Typhi antigens.

Linkages: Pg. 255, 256, 258, 259, 277-279

What is the provisional clinical diagnosis of this case?

A.1 (a) Fever (likely represents a systemic infection) following a GIT disturbance, with spenomegaly, leucopenia and visit to an endemic area; makes enteric fever a provisional diagnosis.

What does the term 'enteric fever' convey?

A.1 (b) 'Enteric fever' includes typhoid fever (by S.Typhi) and Paratyphoid fever (by S.Paratyphi A/B/C).

Why was the term 'enteric fever' preferred over 'typhoid fever'?

A.1 (c) The term 'Typhoid fever' caused confusion with Typhus fever. The term enteric (enteron-'intestine') fever conveys pathology in intestine, which is a correct picture. The term 'Salmonella' is derived from D.E. Salmon, who first isolated this organism (previously termed 'Eberth Gaffky' bacillus).

What is the incubation period of enteric fever?

A.1 (d) The incubation period varies from 3 to 21 days

Describe pathogenesis of enteric fever.

A.1 (e) It is not known as to why S.Typhi and Paratyphi A cause systemic disease and are host (human) restricted, whereas other Salmonella generally cause (restricted) gastroenteritis and have broad range hosts. The sequence of events are depicted in a flow diagram

Ingestion of infected food/water (infective dose 10^3-10^6 cfu)
↓
Reach the ileum and attach to epithelial cells of villi
↓
Enter mucosa by bacterial mediated endocytosis
↓
Penetrate lamina propria and submucosa
↓
Phagocytosed by polymorphs and macrophages (inside protected from antibodies and complement)
↓
Resist intracellular killing and multiply
↓
Disseminate in body via macrophages to RE system (Liver, spleen and lymph nodes)
↓
Enter mesenteric lymph nodes and multiply
↓
Via thoracic duct
↓
Primary transient bacteremia (till now little sign and symptoms)
↓
Bacilli seeded in various organs as liver, gallbladder, bone marrow etc and proliferate
↓
Secondary bacteremia (around 2nd week, bacteria again shed to small intestine)

It should be noted this bacillus proliferates profusely in bile and is discharged continuously into the small intestine (ileum) involving its Peyer's patches and lymphoid follicles. These can become inflammed undergo ulceration, bleeding and rarely perforation.

Generally anything that decreases stomach acidity; as achlorhydric disease and antacid ingestion, increases susceptibility to this disease.

What is the sensitivity of the blood culture technique in detecting enteric fever?

A.2 (a) The sensitivity of conventional blood culture is about 50%. This low sensitivity rate may be a reason that blood culture in this case was negative

Which sample could have increased the probability of isolating the incriminating pathogen from this case?

A.2 (b) Bone marrow is an excellent sample, as the culture positivity rate with it is approximately 90%. However, the sample has the limitation of being available only by invasive means.

Enumerate the aims to be considered, while performing laboratory diagnosis of enteric fever.

A.2 (c)
(i) Isolate the incriminating agent
(ii) Study the serological response, if required
(iii) Identify the carriers
(iv) Find the source of infection
(v) Epidemiological investigations
(vi) Antibiotic susceptibility pattern of the isolate

Outline the patient, carrier and epidemiological studies, performed in laboratory diagnosis of enteric fever.

A.2 (d) **Patient Studies**

Culture

Blood culture is the *gold standard,*

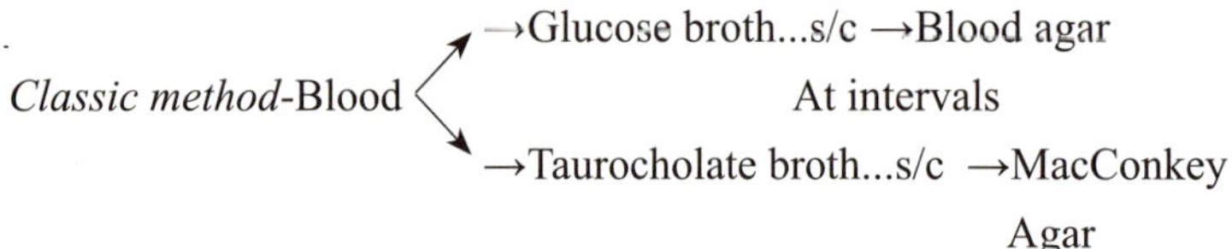

Critical factors: Skin disinfection, Amount of blood in blood culture bottle, Interval of subculture, Inactivation of antimicrobial taken by the patient.

Current methods: Automated systems-Sensors →Colorimetric
→Fluorometric

The advantage of this system is in the time saved in culture (isolation), so precious time is saved for appropriate intervention. In the antibiotic susceptibility testing of the S.Typhi isolate, one looks for chloramphenicol resistance, Nalidixic resistance (may indicate decreased susceptibilty to ciprofloxacin), ciprofloxacin resistance and multidrug resistance.

Other samples that are useful in culture include blood clot, bone marrow, bile, faeces and urine.

Serological: Widal test-The test has a number of limitations.

Typhidot test-This test is a more specific test, uses outer membrane protein antigen (o.m.p.) and is an immunochromatographic based (one hour assay).

Circulating antigen: Typhoidal antigen can be demonstrated in the first week of disease in blood and urine by ELISA and coagglutination studies.

Carrier Studies:

(i) Identify the site in the body harboring the bacteria; as Gallbladder or kidney.

(ii) Test to identify the structural abnormality in the organ, which is making the person a carrier; for example: gall bladder stone

(iii) Classify the carrier,whether is convalescent, chronic or other as paradoxical.

(iv) Diagnosis - Culture (isolation of organism) from bile (provides highest sensitivity), stool or urine.
- Serological-Vi antibody titer in serum ≥10 is significant.

There is no role of Blood culture or Widal test in the diagnosis of carriers.

Epidemiological studies
- Sewer swab→to find source of infection.
- Phage typing→Useful in outbreaks to identify strains.
- Pulse field gel electrophoresis→ – A genotypic based test to identify the strains, considered to be a gold standard

Describe the principle, procedure and limitations of the Widal test.

A.3 (a) **Status:** It is a common serological test performed to detect specific antibodies in enteric fever. However, the test has a number of limitations.

Principle: It is a tube agglutination test, which utilizes S. Typhi (T_O and T_H antigens) and S. Paratyphi A (A_H) antigens. Agglutination of O antigen, appears as; granular deposit at the bottom of the test tube, whereas agglutination of the H antigen, appears as; loose 'cotton wooly' clumps. Control tubes of H and O antigens are included in the test to demonstrate non-agglutination reactions, which appear as compact button formation. The antibodies in the patient start appearing in the patient, by the first week of infection.

Procedure: This test is conventionally carried out in tubes. Doubling dilutions of the serum are prepared in rows, to which different Salmonella antigens are added. The tubes are incubated at 37°C overnight.

Reporting: The report is given in titers for various antibodies. Significant (positive) titre varies from place to place.

Limitations:

(i) The test is negative in the first week of infection, as it takes about a week for antibodies to form

(ii) Baseline titre of local population varies from place to place, which should be known, to interpret results.

(iii) Vaccination and subclinical infections can affect the antibody titers.

(iv) 'H' antibodies persist for longer periods, hence relapse/reinfection may be difficult to diagnose.

(v) Anamnestic reaction can complicate the interpretation, as unrelated antigens can trigger similar antibody responses.

(vi) Administration of antimicrobial agents may hinder the antibody response.

(vii) Cases with liver disease; as cirrhosis and hepatitis, may give a false positive Widal test.

If a provisional diagnosis is possible with a Widal test (or some other serological test), what is the need of culturing clinical specimens and isolating the (Salmonella) pathogen from it?

A.3 (b) Isolating salmonella organism by performing blood culture is considered the 'gold standard' test. The isolate which becomes available after culture, makes it possible to perform antimicrobial susceptibility testing, which is not possible with a serological test. The molecular studies are also possible on the isolate, which provide information on various genes and also make it possible to conduct molecular epidemiologic studies, if required.

Discuss the role of the patient's visit to Jaipur in the development of this infection?

A.4 (a) Jaipur in India is an endemic area for enteric fever. The U.K. businessman could have acquired the infection during his meals at the local eatery.

Describe the epidemiology of enteric fever.

A.4 (b) **Agent:**

- S. Typhi along with S. Paratyphi A and S. Paratyphi B is responsible for the causation of enteric fever. Phage typing is a good phenotypic typing tool for tracing the source in typhoidal outbreaks An outbreak of MDR. S. Typhi E1 occurred in India in 1990, which peaked in 1992-93 in India and resulted in change of drug of choice from chloramphenicol to ciprofloxacin
- Pulse field get electrophoresis is on excellent genotypic typing tool used to type S. Typhi isolates.
  - *Reservoir of infection:* Man is the only reservoir of infection, namely cases and carriers.

    Carrier of infection: A chronic carrier is one, who excretes the bacilli through faeces and/or urine for a year or longer. Mary Mallon (Typhoid Mary) cook from USA (New York) is well known for having caused mortality and morbidity in few hundreds of people, who consumed food cooked by her.
  - *Source of infection:* These are faeces and urine of cases and carriers. The secondary sources are contaminated water, food and fingers

- **Host factors:** Enteric fever can occur at any age Carriage rate is higher in females than in males, on account of increased gall bladder disease in them. The infection is commonest in children. It is often symptomatic in children but sometimes asymptomatic in adults probably due to acquired immunity in them. Malnourished children have severe and recurrent infection often resulting in malnutrition.
  - *Immunity:* All ages are susceptible to infection. Natural infection and immunization provide temporary immunity.
  - *Gastric Acidity:* Acidity provides resistance to this organism by being detrimental to its survival. For this reason, antacids are recommended before intake of oral typhoid vaccine.
- **Environment:** Enteric fever occurs throughout the year. It has a worldwide distribution. The disease occurs wherever the sanitation is poor; as in poor colonies, slums, day care centers. Several localized outbreaks in India have been reported recently. Outbreaks do get reported in war; as occurred in the recent Rwandan civil war in 1994.

Is the picture of abnormal behavior of the case consistent with diagnosis of enteric fever?

A.4 (c) Currently, neuropsychiatric manifestations are common in enteric fever, which could be the reason for his odd/ abnormal behavior.

After the treatment of this case is over, what tests should be done to see that the case (Mr. Philip) is not an infectious threat to the society?

A.5 U.K. is a non-endemic zone, as far as enteric fever is considered. One has to monitor that this case does not become a chronic carrier for S. Typhi and is not a threat to the society. Approximately 1 to 3% of patients who have enteric fever, become chronic carriers for S. Typhi. Three stool cultures over a period of about 1 week should be performed, which should be all negative, to indicate eradication of this organism from the case.

What is the mechanism by which S. Typhi isolate becomes resistant to fluoroquinolones?

A.6 (a) By chromosomal mutations occurying in the gene coding for DNA gyrase (such strains are commonly designated as Nalidixic acid resistant S. Typhi strains-NARST.

Discuss general aspects of drug resistance in S. Typhi.

A.6 (b) See A.7b page. 42 Chapter 5, Section 1 (Clinical Vignette 2) and (Section 17, Chapter 6, Case-2, pg. 615

How could the businessman (in this case) have prevented the infection, he acquired?

A.7 The businessman should have been careful from, where he was consuming his food and water. If such a thing was not feasible, he should have taken about a few weeks, before his visit to this country, the Ty21a or Vi polysaccharide vaccine (pg. 631).

Integrated Clinical Based Study of Salmonella/Food Poisoning

Scenario 1: **An outbreak of food poisoning was reported due to *Salmonella enterica* serotype Weltevreden (S. Weltevreden) involving 34 students from Mangalore. The symptoms developed 8-10 hours, after consuming a non-vegetarian dish, probably fish. The identity of the implicated organism was confirmed at Central Research Institute, Kasauli.**

Scenario 2: **Five second professional students (Ramesh, Anil, Sandeep, Sarika and Tina) celebrate the passing of their second professional exam by eating special roasted chicken and 'Dal' preparation with extra helpings of fresh cream at dinner time. By early morning, two of the students are severely ill with vomiting, as a predominant symptom.**

Linkages: Pg. 255, 256, 260, 279

What is the provisional clinical diagnosis of the above two cases?

A.1 (a) Food poisoning.

What is the microbiological differential diagnosis?

A.1 (b) The entity could be caused by Salmonella sps. (except Typhi, Paratyphi A), *S. aureus, B.cereus* and others. List of Salmonella NT is at p. 260.

Classify food poisoning.

A.1 (c)

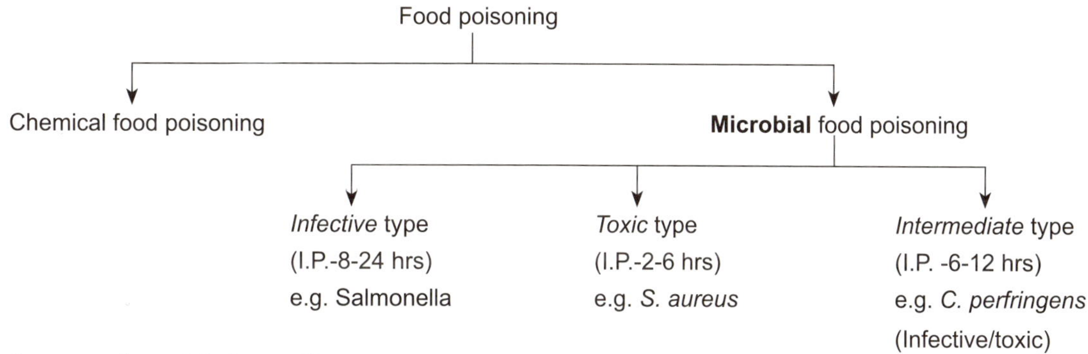

Enumerate the key species of Salmonella genus.

A.1 (d) *Salmonella enterica* and *Salmonella bongori.*

What are the key changes that have occurred recently in the nomenclature of Salmonellae?

A.1 (e) Previously the common Salmonella types; as S. Typhi, S. Paratyphi A, S. Typhimurium were given the status of species, but now these are given the status of serotypes. According to the current WHO recommendations, the serotype should be written with first alphabet in capitals; as S.Typhi (and not italicized).

What samples would be required to make a microbiological diagnosis in a food poisoning case?

A.2 (a) Faeces, vomitus and remnants of the food consumed; as fish, cream etc.

What are the ways the food can get contaminated with microbes?

A.2 (b)
- (i) Faeces of person may contaminate directly or indirectly through fomites (objects contaminated by hands of infected person or otherwise)
- (ii) Flies
- (iii) Water contaminated by faeces
- (iv) Contaminated dust–It may contaminate the exposed food kept outside

An Overview of the Antimicrobial options in the infections caused by Key Gram Negative Bacilli-Enterobacteriaceae

	Cell Wall Inhibitors	Cell-Membrane Inhibitors	Amino Acid Synthesis Inhibitors	Nucleic Acid Synthesis Inhibitors	Others
E. coli					
• Uncomplicated • Complicated (severe infections)	Ampicillin Cephalosporins (DOC) (3rd and 4th generation) Carbapenems As *E coli* strains are frequently multidrug resistant, treatment should be guided with antimicrobial susceptibility testing		Aminoglycosides	TM-SMZ (DOC) Nitrofurantoin (in UTI) Fluoroquinolones	
Klebsiella spp.	Cephalosporins (DOC) Piperacillin Aztreonam (esp. nosocomial infection) Ticarcillin-clavulanic acid Carbapenems as Meropenem As Klebsiella strains are frequently multi-drug resistant treatment should be guided with antimicrobial susceptibility testing		Aminoglycosides	TM-SMZ Fluoroquinolones	
Enterobacter species	Carbapenems (DOC) Cefepime (DOC) Aztreonam		Aminoglycosides	TM-SMZ Fluoroquinolone	
Proteus mirabilis	Ampicillin (DOC) Cephalosporins Carbapenems		Aminoglycosides	TM-SMZ Fluoroquinolones	
Proteus vulgaris	Cephalosporins (DOC) (3rd & 4th generation) Carbapenems				
Providencia stuartii	Is the most resistant of the Providencia spp. It is also resistant to disinfectants making it a key pathogen in burns ward				
Providencia alcalifaciens	Resistant to most antimicrobials				
Serratia marscescens	PnG Cephalosporins Carbapenems (DOC) Aztreonam Ticarcillin-clavulanic acid (Some strains are multi drug resistant)				
Salmonella Typhi (acute case)	Ceftriaxone, cefotaxime Ampicillin		Chloramphenicol (in non endemic areas, usually adminstered)	Fluoroquinolone (as ciprofloxacin) TM-SMZ Ciprofloxacin	

Contd.

Contd.

(Chronic case)	Ampicillin (high dosage, prolonged period)				
Salmonella Typhimurium, & other non-typhoidal salmonella					
Uncomplicated	Self limiting (fluid replacement)				
Complicated	Ampicillin In endemic areas, frequency of multidrug resistant strains is high, so antimicrobial susceptibility testing is recommended			Fluoroquinolones TM-SMZ	
Shigella spp.	Ampicillin Ceftriaxone			Fluoroquinolone (DOC) TM-SMZ	
Yersinia pestis			Doxycycline often combined with streptomycin (DOC) Chloramphenicol	TM-SMZ Ciprofloxacin	
Bacteriodes spp.	Cefoxitin Carbapenems Ticarcillin- clavulanic acid Piperacillin-tazobactam		Clindamycin	Metronidazole (DOC)	
Prevotella spp.	PnG Cefotetan Cefoxitin		Clindamycin (DOC)	Metronidazole	

NB:
- Treatment should be guided by antimicrobial susceptibility testing but empiric treatment can be initiated
- Strains of *P.vulgaris* are usually more resistant than of *P.mirabilis*
- DOC refers to drug of choice
- TM-SMZ is Trimethoprim-Sulfamethoxazole

10

Assessment/Examination Questions

1. What are the characteristics of the family enterobacteriaceae? A 3d., p. 262
2. What is the commonly used system in the lab, to classify the family enterobacteriaceae? A 3g., p. 262
3. Describe the morphological, cultural and antigenic characteristics of *E. coli.* p. 257
4. What is the habitat of *E. coli*? To which category most of the *E. coli* infections belong, i.e., endogenous or exogenous? A 7a,b., p. 263
5. What infections does *E. coli* cause, besides gastroenteritis? p. 259
6. Describe the tests used to categorize an isolate as one of enterotoxigenic *E. coli* (*ETEC*). A 4a., p. 262
7. Describe the mechanism by which ETEC causes diarrohea. A 4d., p. 262
8. Mention about the pathogenicity and diagnosis of infections, caused by enteroinvasive *E. coli.* A 7c., p. 263 and A 6., p. 263
9. Mention the epidemiology and diagnosis of infections caused by enterohaemmorhagic *E. coli* (EHEC).
10. Compare and contrast the pathogenicity of the different types of diarrheagenic *E. coli.* A 6., p. 263
11. Describe in detail the laboratory diagnosis of diarrohea caused by *E. coli.* P. 276, + p. 257 and chapter 4
12. Describe in detail the laboratory diagnosis of urinary tract infection caused by *E. coli.*
    chapter 4, p. 261 (section vi) and chapter p. 517 (section xvi)
13. Describe traveller's diarrohea. A 6 (see ETEC, p. 263)
14. Describe the following-*Klebsiella pneumoniae*, Citrobacter spp., Enterobacter spp., and *Serratia marscens.* p. 255-260
15. Classify the tribe Proteeae. Describe Dienes phenomenon. p. 257
16. Describe genera Morganella and Providencia. p. 255 and p. 257
17. What is the natural habitat of Shigella. p. 54-55
18. Describe selective and enrichment media used for isolation of Shigella. A 8b., p. 265-266
19. Describe the epidemiology of Shigellosis (include the classification of Shigella). A 8b., p. 265-266
20. Why do fomites become important in spread of this infection? A 8a., p. 265
21. Describe the pathogenesis of Shigellosis. A 9b., p. 266
22. Describe the laboratory diagnosis of dysentery caused by Shigella. A 276
23. Enumerate the two species of genus Salmonella. A 1d., p. 271
24. Describe the morphological and cultural characteristics (including media requirements) of S. Typhi. p. 258
25. Describe the Kaufmann-White scheme for Salmonella. A2e, A 2d, p. 272
26. Describe the Vi antigen. Enumerate the antigenic variation in Salmonella. A 2e., p. 272 and Vi vaccine
27. Describe the epidemiology of enteric fever. A4b., p. 269-270
28. Describe the pathogenesis of enteric fever. A 1e., p. 267-268
29. Enumerate the aims to be considered, while performing laboratory diagnosis of enteric fever. Describe in detail the laboratory diagnosis of enteric fever, including the patient, carrier and epidemiological studies to be performed. A 2c,d., p. 268-269
30. Describe the typhoid carriers including its diagnosis. p. 27
31. Describe the Widal test. A 3a., p. 269
32. Outline the treatment of enteric fever. Describe the mechanism of S. Typhi becoming resistant to fluoroquinolones.
    p. 278-279, A6a., p. 270
33. Describe typhoid vaccines. p. 631
34. Enumerate the causes of Food poisoning. p. 575
35. Describe the epidemiology of Salmonella gastroenteritis. A 4., p. 272
36. Describe Non–typhoidal Salmonella/Salmonella gastroenteritis/Salmonella septicaemia. p. 260 and chapter 7., p. 27
37. What are the indications of using antimicrobials in managing a case of Salmonella gastroenteritis? A 5., p. 272 and p. 279
38. How do you prevent Salmonella gastroenteritis? A 6., p. 272
39. How is plague defined? A 1b., p. 273
40. Describe the epidemiology of plague. A 4b., p. 274
41. Describe the virulent factors of *Y. pestis.* Outline the pathogenesis of plague A 4c, 275 and A3b., p. 274.
42. Describe laboratory diagnosis of plague. p. 277 and p. 257
43. Describe plague vaccine. p. 631 and A 4c., p. 275
44. Describe *Yersinia enterocolitica* and *Yersinia pseudotuberculosis.* p. 260, p. 255-257

Section VII: Gram Negative Bacilli–Non Fastidious, Oxidase +ve

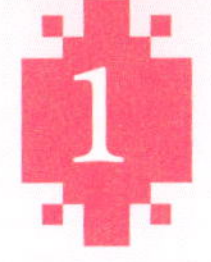

1 Classification, Metabolic Microscopic Features of Key Gram Negative Bacilli–Oxidase +ve

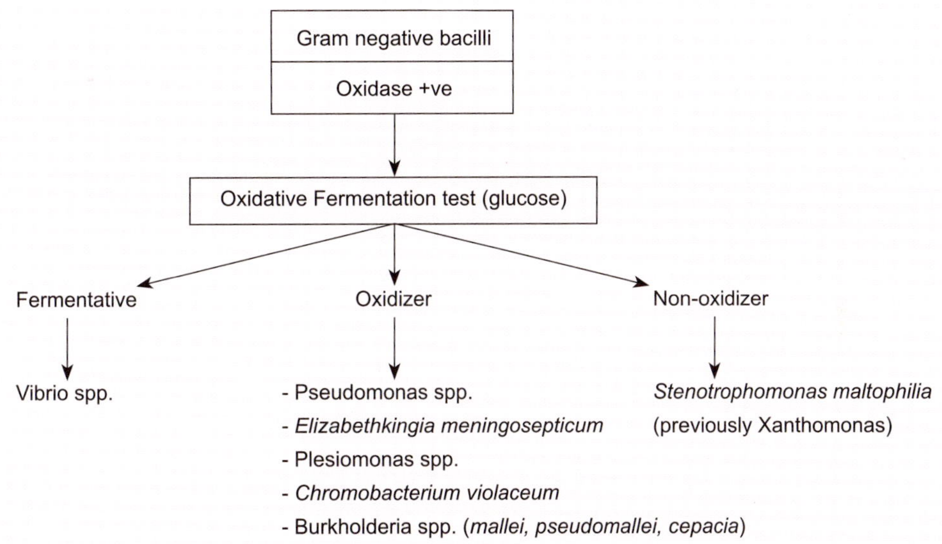

Fig. 7.1.1: Algorithm for identification of Gram Negative Bacilli - Oxidase +ve

NB: – Organism may fall into more than one group due to phenotypic variability of given trait.

– *H. pylori* and *C. jejuni* are oxidase +ve, but not categorized here, as are fastidious.

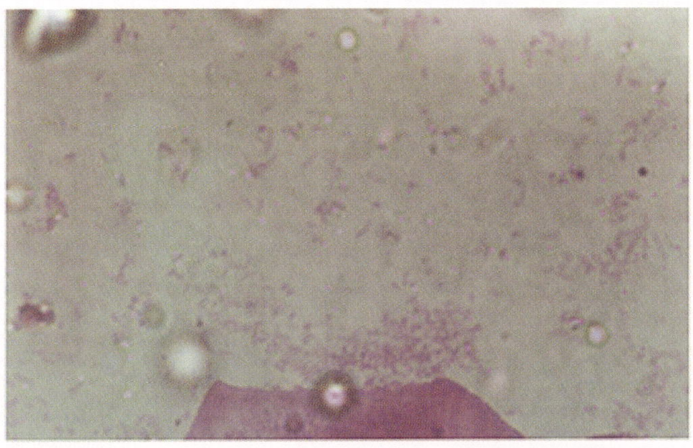

Fig. 7.1.1a: Cholera:Gram stained smear of faecal smear demonstrating comma shaped gram negative bacilli

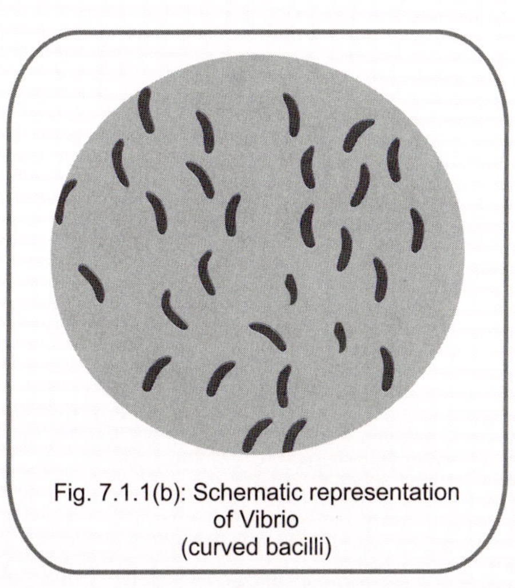

Fig. 7.1.1(b): Schematic representation of Vibrio (curved bacilli)

Metabolic and microscopic features of gram negative bacilli–oxidase +ve

Organism	Growth requirements						Cellular morphology and staining characteristics						
	O2 Requ.	Optimal Temp.	CO2 Requ..	Incubation Period Days	Weeks	Months	Shape	Gram	Arrangement	Capsule	Motility	Spore	Special Staining / microscopy / Special Features
Pseudomonas aeruginosa	Considered strictly aerobic (but can grow anaerobically	37°C	-	1	-	-	Bacilli	-ve	-	+ (some mucoid strains)	+	-	-
Stenotrophomonas maltophilia	Aerobic	37°C		1			Bacilli	-ve		-	+	-	-
Burkholderia mallei	Aerobic and facultative anaerobe	37°C		1			Bacilli	-ve	-	-	-	-	-
Burkholderia pseudomallei	Aerobic and facultative anaerobe	37°C		1			Bacilli	-ve	-	-	-	-	-
Pasterurella multocida	Aerobic and facultative anaerobic	37°C	-	1	-	-	Very small ovoid rods	-ve	In pairs/ small bundles	+(some strains)	-	-	Bipolar staining present
Elizabethkingia meningosepticum	Aerobic	37°C		1			Bacilli	-ve	-	-	-	-	-
Alcaligenes faecalis	Strict aerobe	37°C		1			Bacilli	-ve	-	-	-	-	-
Chromobacterium violaceum	Aerobe and facultative anaerobe	37°C		1			Bacilli	-ve	single or pairs	-	positive	-	-
**Kingella kingae*	Aerobic	37°C		-	+ weeks		Coccobacilli	-ve	-	+	_,twitch ing motility present	-	-
Vibrio cholerae	Aerobic (primarily) Slow growth anaerobically	37°C	-	1	-	-	Bacilli/ (curved/ comma shaped), S / spiral forms may occur} (Fig. 7.1.1a,b)	-ve	-	-	+	-	-
'El Tor' Vibrio	Aerobic	37°C		1	-		bacilli	-ve	-	-	+	-	-
Halophilic vibrios	Aerobic and facultative anaerobic	37°C		1			bacilli	-ve	-	-	+	-	-
Aeromonas hydrophila	aerobic and facultative anaerobe	37°C		1			bacilli	-ve	-	-	+	-	-
Plesiomonas shigelloides	aerobii and facultative anaerobe	37°C		1			bacilli	-ve	-	-	+	-	-

* Member of the fastidious bacteria, included in acronym HACEK.

2 An Overview of the Media Requirements, Colonial Characters and Diagnostic Characteristics of Key Gram Negative Bacilli–Oxidase +ve (Non Fastidious)

	Basal media	Enriched media	Selective/others	Characterization and confirmation of isolate
Vibrio cholerae	NA: + (oil drop appearance colony)	BA: + (El tor biotypes produce haemolytic colonies, classical biotype produces haemodigestion)	• MacConkey: initially NLF colony • Bile salt agar: oil drop appearance colony) • Monsur's GTTA medium: small translucent colonies with black centre & turbid halo because of gelatin liquefaction • Thiosulphate citrate bromothymol sucrose medium: yellow colonies because of sucrose metabolism, on continued incubation colonies may become greenish colonies • Alkaline peptone water (used as enrichment media) • VR medium as transport medium (Venkaraman Ramakrishnan) • Cary Blair (as transport medium)	• Microscopic features_ • Biochemical: Catalase +ve, Oxidase +, many sugars fermented producing acid (but not gas) excluding lactose,Indole +, reduces nitrate to nitrite, Cholera red reaction +ve • Suggestive colony is confirmed by slide agglutination with O group antisera • Biotyped into: Classical and eltor type • Serotyped into 3 serotypes by Ogawa & Inaba antisera (i) Agglutination (+) with Ogawa antiserum; serotype Ogawa (ii) Agglutination (+) with inaba antiserum; serotype inaba (iii) Agglutination with both of above antisera serotype Hikojima Phage typing (using 14 phages) (Mitra *et. al.* 1980)
V. parahaemolyticus (halophilic vibrio)	NA: +	BA: + (strains isolated from human sources are mostly haemolytic, Kanagawa phenomenon)	MacConkey: colorless colony (as NLF)	Resembles *V. cholerae*, except (i) doesn't ferment sucrose (ii) can grow only in media containing NaCl high concentration (iii) can tolerate sodium chloride concentration in media upto 8% (unlike 7% for *V. cholerae*)
V. alginolyticus (halophilic vibrio)	NA: + (swarms)	BA: + (swarming seen)	MacConkey: + TCBS: Yellow colony	Has higher salt concentration tolerance upto 10%
Aeromonas hydrophila	NA: +	BA: +	MacConkey: + (NLF) DCA: + TCBS: yellow colony	Differentiated from *V. cholerae* and Plesiomonas by utilization profile of amino acids (Lysine, arginine & ornithine
Plesiomonas shigelloides	NA: +	BA: +	MacConkey: + TCBS: no growth	• Doesn't ferment sucrose • Differentiated from *V. cholerae* and Aeromonas by utilization profile of amino acids

	Basal media	Enriched media	Selective/others	Characterization and confirmation of isolate
Pseudomonas aeruginosa	NA: + Large colonies often with bluish green pigment pyocyanin diffused into the medium. (Fig. 7.2.1) The color of the medium can vary depending on the predominant pigment being produced as pyorubin is a reddish brown pigments, fluorescein is a greenish yellow pigment and pyomelanin; a brown to blackish pigment	BA: + (beta haemolytic)	• MacConkey- colorless colonies (as non-lactose fermenting. • Cetrimide agar: + (grows because of ability of organism to resist cetrimide)	• Microscopic features • Fruity odor (because of production of 2-aminoacetophenone from tryptophan) • Motile (by polar flagella) • Catalase & oxidase +ve • Colonies fluoresce with u.v. light (because of fluorescent pigment) • Growth at 42°C (test used for organisms, which do not produce pigment) • Pyocin typing (type of Bacterocin typing) • Repeated isolation is recommended before significance attributed to isolate, as organism is saprophyte
Stenotrophomonas maltophilia	+	BA: +	-	• Acidifies maltose and glucose
Burkholderia mallei	NA: +	BA: +	MacConkey: ± (variable) colorless/pink colonies	• Microscopic characters • Biochemical characters
Burkholderia pseudomallei	Resembles *B. mallei*	BA: +	MacConkey: Pink/ colorless colonies	• Resembles *B. mallei*, but differs from if in liquefying gelatin, not forming acid from several sugars
Pasteurella multocida	NA: (–)	BA: +	MacConkey: No growth	• Resembles Yersinia but is oxidase +ve and indole +ve
Elizabethkingia meningosepticum	NA: + (produces yellow, non-diffusible pigment)	BA: +	MacConkey: slight growth or no growth	• Microscopic characters • Catalase +ve • Oxidase +ve
Alcaligenes faecalis	NA: +	BA: +	MacConkey: +	• Microscopic features • Catalase +ve • Oxidase +ve
Chromobacterium violaceum	NA: + (Violet pigment soluble in ethanol)	BA: +	MacConkey:+	• Microscopic features • Catalase +ve • Oxidase +ve
Kingella kingae	NA:(–)	Required prolonged incubation of weeks	Macconkey: (–)	• Microscopic features • Catalase –ve • Oxidase +ve • Ferments sugars

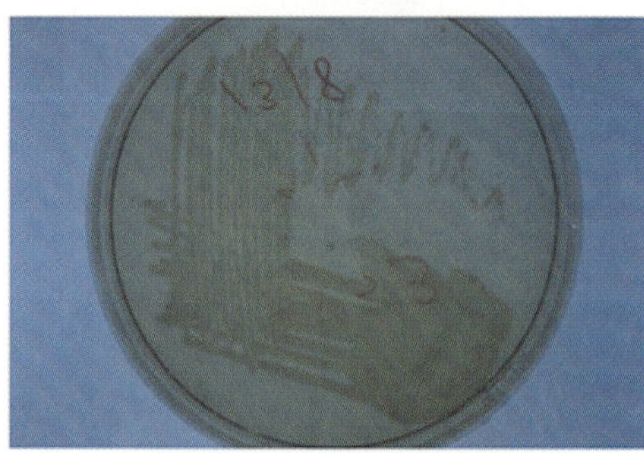

Fig. 7.2.1: *Pseudomonas aeruginosa*: Pigmented growth of *P. aeruginosa* on nutrient agar medium

3 Clinical (Pathogenicity) Profile of Infections Caused By Gram Negative Bacilli, Non Fastidious Oxidase +ve

Pseudomonas aeruginosa	Important nosocomial pathogen and causes opportunistic infections in burns cases, neutropaenic cases, cystic fibrosis and cases on ventilators The common presentations include skin infections, wound infections in the burns ward, UTIs following instrumentation, meningitis following injury or lumbar puncture, eye infections, otitis externa, otitis media, endoarditis in i/v drug users, ecthyma gangrenosum (acute necrotizing vasculitis in patients on respiratory ventilators) • Case: pg. 286-287
Other Pseudomonas species as *P. putida, P. fluorescens*	Opportunistic infections (getting increasedly involved)
Stenotrophomonas maltophilia	Opportunistic infections; as wound infections, UTIs
Burkholderia cepacia (previously P. cepacia)	Opportunistic infections and nosocomial infections especially in cystic fibrosis cases. Pulmonary infections
B. mallei (previously *P. mallei*)	• Acute fulminant febrile illness or chronic indolent infection, with abscesses in skin or respiratory tract. • Is an occupational disease seen in persons handling horses or laboratory professionals • In animals produce diseases; as Glanders and farcy involving the respiratory tract and skin, respectively.
B. pseudomallei (previously P. pseudomallei)	*Melioidosis:* (may present as asymptomatic, acute, chronic or even relapsing forms). In acute form; can present as 'typhoid' like illness, pneumonia or haemoptysis. In chronic form; can produce necrotic lesions.
Pasterurella multocida	• Cellulitis (at site of cat/dog bite/scratch) • Meningitis (following head injury) • Respiratory tract infections; as pneumonia • Other lesions; as appendicial abscess
Elizabethkingia meningosepticum	Opportunistic and nosocomial infections; as meningitis in infants and pneumonia especially in immunosuppressed
Alcaligenes faecalis	Opportunistic and nosocomial infections; as pneumonia, UTIs, wound infection
Chromobacterium violaceum	Skin lesions with pyaemia and multiple abscesses
Kingella kingae	Associated with bone & joint infections, endocarditis & septicaemia
Moraxella lacunata (previously included in genus Haemophilus)	Catarrahal (angular) conjunctivitis
Vibrio cholerae	Cholera (Acute diarrhoeal disease with extreme fluid loss, which can lead to extreme dehydration and even be fatal) Mild and asymptomatic infections, more common with el tor biotype Chronic carrier state also seen, more with 'El Tor' biotype • Case: pg 288-290
Non_O1 Vibrio cholerae (O2_0138)	Cholera like illness
Halophilic vibrios; as *V. parahaemolyticus,* *V. alginolyticus*	Food poisoning (especially with sea food)
Aeromonas hydrophila	Associated with diarrohea and opportunistic infections; as cellulitis, meningitis, UTI.
Plesiomonas shigelloides	• Gastroenteritis, septicaemia, neonatal meningitis and cellulitis

Section VII: Gram Negative Bacilli–Non Fastidious, Oxidase +ve

Integrated Clinical Based Study of *P.aeruginosa*/Pyogenic Lesions

A recently married woman, Srujana is admitted in the burns ward with 20% burns (dowry* related) in Safdarjung hospital, New Delhi. The surgeon examined the wound at the back of her body and noticed the oozing pus to be blue-green tinged and sweet smelling.

***property or money given to brides at their marriage time.**

Linkages: Pg. 281, 282, 284, 285, 291, 292

What is the most likely pathogen implicated in this case? Explain.

A.1 The case is most likely to be infected by *P. aeruginosa,* as it can produce a blush green pigment, due to production of pyocyanin and/or pyoverdin pigments. A. less likely cause of the pus having a green colour could be due to myeloperoxidase of neutrophils. Pus due to anaerobic infections is described as having a foul odour (sweet odor is associated with *P.aeruginosa*)

What are the characteristics P.aeruginosa possesses, that makes it an important nosocomical agent?

A.2 The numerous characteristics are:

(i) It is ubiquitous, probably as it has minimal nutrient requirements and tolerates wide range of temperature variations, which makes it easy to survive and multiply in diverse environmental conditions.

(ii) It has innate drug resistance to many antimicrobials; as pencillin, ampicillin, cephalothin, tetracycline, chloramphenicol, sulpha drugs, streptomycin etc. This is due to the organism's outer membrane porins, restricting entry of antimicrobials to periplasmic space, more than other gram negative bacilli. It is for this reason, these antimicrobials should not be tested in antimicrobial susceptibility testing and administered during management of cases infected with this pathogen.

(iii) It has acquired drug resistance to numerous antimicrobials; by plasmid mediated and mutational mechanisms.

(iv) It can grow in disinfectant solutions, like *dettol* and cetrimide.

(v) It has toxinogenicity and invasive abilities.

(vi) In hospitalized cases receiving broad spectrum antimicrobials, this organism colonizes various sites of the cases, suppressing the normal flora. This often results in wound and sputum getting secondarily contaminated by this organism.

What is the normal habitat of P. aeruginosa?

A.3 (a) It is a saprophyte and present in water and soil.

Why does ICUs forbid the use of flowers (bouquets) to cheer the patients and the staff?

A.3 (b) The flowers can be colonized with bacteria; as *P. aeruginosa* and other saprophytic bacteria, which can cause disease in patients admitted in ICU's, who have decreased immunity

What is the essential pathology of lesions caused by P. aeruginosa?

A.3 (c) The histologic picture is one of necrosis and haemorrhage.

Enumerate virulent factors caused by P. aeruginosa and describe the pathogenesis of lesions caused by this agent.

A.3 (d) (i) Extracellular products-Pyocyanin (disrupts many cellular functions)

(ii) Extracellular enzymes and haemolysins; as Proteases, lipases

(iii) Exotoxin A-It inhibits protein synthesis of host cells; just as *C. diphtheriae does*. A vaccine trial based on this toxin was carried out in a Delhi hospital.

(iv) Endotoxin

Pathogenesis: It is complex. The pathogen rarely causes disease in healthy individuals, despite presence of many virulent markers. It invades a case, when the cutaneous/mucosal barriers are breached and/or the immunological defenses are compromised. After colonizing a case, it can invade the blood stream and cause multiple organ dysfunction and death.

What does the term 'glucose non-fermenting gram negative rod' convey?

A.4 (a) Such an organism cannot ferment any sugars. These organisms are also designated as nil fermenting (fermenter) GNB. They utlize sugars oxidatively.

P. aeruginosa is an example of this category.

Mention the principle and procedure of oxidase test.

A.4 (b) See Section I, Page 67

Enumerate the common organisms that are oxidase positive.

A.4 (c) *V. cholerae*, Brucella sps, Neisseria sps, *C. jejuni*, *H. pylori*, *Pasteurella multocida*.

Describe pyocin typing.

A.4 (d) Chapter 9, Section 17, pg 623 (Bacteriocin typing)

With which clinical entity that has a respiratory pathology, is P. aeruginosa often associated with?

A.5 (a) Cystic fibrosis

What is the characteristic of P.aeruginosa, when it is isolated from such cases?

A.5 (b) The organism is responsible for causing chronic respiratory pathology in cases with this disease. Isolation of mucoid variant of *P. aeruginosa* from cystic fibrosis cases is the hallmark of the disease. The reasons for the expression of this characteristic are not known.

What is one complication that such cases (burns) often develop, that can be life threatening?

A.6 Sepsis is a common complication that develops in burns cases and is often precipitated by *P. aeruginosa* infection. It is for this reason that attempts were made to make a vaccine against this organism. A trial of a killed vaccine was conducted in burns ward of Safdarjung hospital, New Delhi.

Which antimicrobials should not be used (are not beneficial) in an infection caused by P. aeruginosa?

A.7 (a) See A 2 ii

Which classes of antimicrobials are useful in infections caused by P. aeruginosa?

A.7 (b)

- **Beta lactam group:** Carbenicillin, Ticarcillin, Mezlocillin, Piperacillin-Tazobactam
- **Newer Cephalosporins:** Ceftazidime, Cefoperazone, Cefpirome, Cefepime, Ceftobiprole
- **Quinolones:** Levofloxacin, Ciprofloxacin
- **Aminoglycosides:** Gentamicin, Amikacin, Tobramycin
- **Carbapenems:** Imipenem-Cilastin, Meropenem
- **Monobactams:** Aztreonam
- **Others:** Polymixin B, Colistin.

Describe the pathogenesis of cholera.

A.5 (c) For the *Vibrio cholerae* to produce the disease, it must be able to reach the small intestine in large numbers and be able to colonize it. To elude the effect of gastric acidity, large inoculum size of *V.cholerae* in the range of 10^4-10^5/ml is required to infect (compare in Shigella, lower number is sufficient) the GIT.

To be able to colonize, adhesion of the organism to intestinal epithelium is believed to be mediated by toxin co-regulated pilus (TCP). It is so named, as its synthesis is regulated in parallel with that of cholera toxin.

To traverse the small intestine, mucosal chemotaxis along with its motility and many proteases aid this process. ToxR gene products coordinate the regulation and expression of many other virulence factors.

The fluid loss in cholera can be extreme and reach life threatening levels. No pus cells or RBCs are present in the stool, as the organism does not invade the mucosa. However, the stool contains mucus flecks, giving it a classic appearance of 'rice–water' stool.

Aspects related to case theme and examination assessment

Mention the uniqueness of the seventh pandemic of cholera.

A.6 The seventh pandemic of cholera started in 1961 from Sulawesi (Celebes), Indonesia and by early 1970s had caused major epidemics in Africa and southern Europe. This pandemic was unique in many aspects

(i) It was the first pandemic to be caused by *V. cholerae* 'El Tor' *in contrast to the previous six pandemics, which were caused by *V. cholerae* biotype 'classical'.

(ii) It was the first pandemic to have arisen outside India

(iii) *V. cholera* biotype 'El Tor' displaced *V. cholerae* 'classical' strain in most regions, so the classical biotype strain are now infrequently encountered

(iv) Infection with the 'El Tor' biotype causes larger proportion of mild cases, higher carrier rate than 'classical' biotype but lower mortality rate.

*El Tor was first identified in 1905 at a quarantine camp on the Senai Peninsula El Tor, Egypt.

Describe epidemiology of Vibrio cholerae O139 infection.

A.7 This serogroup was first reported from an outbreak of cholera in Chennai in 1992. The new epidemic strain was designated O-139 (or O-139 Bengal). It is closely related to the O1 'El Tor' strain of the seventh pandemic strains and appears to have emerged from it, by horizontal gene transfer. Later on in 1992, this serogroup caused outbreaks in several parts of India. In 1993, it spread to Bangladesh, Pakistan, China and some parts of Europe. Some authorites believed this to be the beginning of the eighth global cholera pandemic. However by 1994, the 'El Tor' strain regained its prominence and the threat of O-139 pandemic diminished.

This serogroup is unique, as the first non cholera vibrio (i.e., non serogroup O1, *V.cholerae*) to have been associated with epidemics of cholera. This shattered the long-standing belief that only serogroup O1 *V.cholerae* could cause epidemic cholera. There was a fear of widespread outbreaks to be caused by this serogroup, as there was no immunity against this serogroup in man and the O1 strain vaccine would not be effective against it. Like other non-O1 *V. cholerae* strains, it produces a polysaccharide capsule. This may be responsible for these strains to be resistant to human serum and the occasional development of O-139 bacteremia.

Enumerate halophilic vibrios. Describe their pathogenicity and laboratory diagnosis.

A.8 Their natural habitat is sea water and marine life. They cannot grow in media lacking sodium chloride and grow only in their presence. Some of these are associated with human infection as depicted in table 7.5.3.

Table 7.5.3: Halophilic vibrios infective to man

	V. parahaemolyticus	***V. alginolyticus***	***V. vulnificus***
	Named 'parahaemolyticus' as causes haemolysis on blood agar		Previously designated L+ vibrio, as could ferment lactose
Pathogenicity	Food poisoning associated with consumption of sea food	Associated with marine wound infection (exposed to sea)	- Associated with marine wound infection - Consumption of undercooked sea food, at times associated with septicaemia
Diagnosis	- Morphology resembles *V. cholerae* - Optimal NaCl concentration in media is 2-4% and can tolerate NaCl concentration up to 8% - Does not ferment sucrose (so on TCBS, green colonies) appear - Kanagawa phenomenon#	- Resembles *V. parahaemolyticus* (higher salt tolerance of 10%) - Swarming growth on non selective media	Resembles *V. parahaemolyticus* (however ferments lactose and has salt tolerance of less than 8%)

Strains isolated from environmental sources as (water, fish) are mostly non haemolytic, when grown in blood agar with high salt concentration in comparison to strains, isolated from man, which are mostly haemolytic. This test has significance for pathogenicity.

Laboratory Diagnosis and Treatment (Overview)

An Overview of the comparative approach in Laboratory diagnostic of key Gram negative bacilli (non-fastidious)–Oxidase +ve

Organism/ Disease	Specimen	Stain Enhanced Microscopy	Detection of Microbial Antigen/ Metabolite/ Genome	Serological Tests	Culture of Organisms In Media/ Characterization and Confirmation of Isolate	Differential Diagnosis	Antimicrobial Susceptibility Tests
Vibrio cholerae	• Stool • Rectal swab • If delay in sample inoculaton ≥6 hrs, may inoculate sample in APW to prevent overgrowth of enteric bacteria • May use transport media as Cary Blair or Venkatraman & Ramakrishnan	• Gram staining • Methylene blue staining [Safety pin appearance, as (bipolar staining)] [Darting motility if gets inhibited by Vibrio antisera, is diagnostic]	–	Various serological techniques available as IHA, antitoxin assay, complement dependent vibriocidal assay. However little role in diagnosis, may be useful epidemiologically.	See chapter 2, page. 283	• Non 0-1 vibrio (138 different serogroup) • *Vibrio parahaemolyticus* • *Vibrio alginolyticus* • *Aeromonas hydrophila* • *Plesiomonas shigelloides* • Pseudomonas spp.	• Routinely method not required, as most cases do not require antimicrobials
Pseudomonas aeruginosa	Depends on site of lesion, can be: • Skin lesion (swabs) • Blood • C.S.F. • Urine • Pus	Gram stain can demonstrate the gram negative bacilli	–	Since this organism is often an contaminant, serologic response, can incriminate it as an etiological agent	• Nutrient agar (Large colonies often with Pyocyanin (blue-green), Pyoverdin (green fluorescent), pyomelanin (black) pigments • Nutrient broth (Growth with surface Pellicle because it is aerobic) • Details See Chapter 2, pg. 284	• *P.cepacia* • *P.pseudomallei* • *P.mallei* • *P.maltophilia*	• Routine tests (It is intrinsically resistant resistant to many antimicrobials. May be susceptible to sulphonamides, streptomycin, tetracycine 'in vitro' but resistant to them 'in vivo'. Following groups should be tested • Aminoglycosides-Gentamicin, Tobramycin, Polymyxin B • Quinolones-Ciprofloxacin • 3rd generation Cephalosporins-Ceftazadime- • 4th generation-Cefepime

An Overview of the antimicrobial options for infections caused by gram negative bacilli (non-fastidious)–Oxidase +ve

	Cell Wall Inhibitors	Cell-Membrane Inhibitors	Amino Acid Synthesis Inhibitors	Nucleic Acid Synthesis Inhibitors	Others
Pseudomonas aeruginosa	• Carbenicillin • Ticarcillin • Cephalosporins (as ceftazadime) • Carbapenems • Aztreonam	+	• Tobramycin • Other aminoglycosides DOC)	Fluoroquinolones as Ciprofloxacin	
Burkholderia mallei (previously *P. mallei*)			Streptomycin + Tetracycline Streptomycin + Chloramphenicol	(DOC)	
B. pseudomallei (previously *P. pseudomallei*)	• Ceftdazidime (DOC) • Amoxicillin-clavulanic acid • Carbapenems (DOC) as Imipenem		Chloramphenicol + Tetracycline	TM -SMZ	
Elizabethkingia meningosepticum	• Vancomycin (resistant to wide range of antimicrobials)		Clindamycin	• TM-SMZ • Rifampicin	
Chromobacterium violaceum	• Carbenicillin • Mezlocillin • Cefoxitin		• Erythromycin • Tetracycline	TM-SMZ	
Vibrio cholerae (acute case)			• Tetracycline (DOC) • Azithomycin	• TM-SMZ (DOC) • Fluoroquinolone	
Aeromonas hydrophila	• Cephalosporins • Aztreonam • Carbapenems (Uniformly resistant to ampicillin and penicillin. Often resistant to cefazolin & ticarcillin)		–	• Ciprofloxacin • TM-SMZ	
Plesiomonas shigelloides	Cephalosporins		Chloramphenicol	• TM-SMZ • Fluoroquinolones	

NB: –TM-SMZ is Trimethoprim Sulfamethoxazole
– DOC refers to drug of choice

7 Assessment/Examination Questions

1. What is the habitat of *P. aeruginosa*? — A 3a., p. 286.
2. Enumerate the virulent factors produced by *P. aeruginosa*. Describe the pathogenesis of lesions caused by this agent. — A 3d., p. 286
3. What are the characteristics *P. aeruginosa* possesses, that makes it an important nosocomial agent? — A 2., p. 286
4. Describe pigments produced by *P. aeruginosa*? — p. 284 and vignette., p. 286
5. Describe oxidase test. — pg. 67
6. Describe pyocin typing. — pg 623 Bacteriocin typing
7. What are the antimicrobials used to treat *P. aeruginosa* infections? Mention about drug resistance in *P. aeruginosa*. — A 7b., p. 287
8. Describe about Glanders and Melidiosis. — p. 285
9. Classify vibrios and describe its morphology. — Fig. 7.5.1., p. 288 and p. 282
10. Describe the differences between 'classical' and 'el tor' vibrios. — Table 7.5.1., p. 289
11. Describe Venkataraman Ramakrishna medium and selective media used for vibrios. — p. 283
12. Compare the pathogenicity of *V. cholerae* and non-agglutinating vibrios (non-O1). — p. 285 and A 2b., p. 287
13. Describe the epidemiology of cholera in India. Mention the uniqueness of the seventh pandemic of cholera. — A 3b., p. 288, A6., p. 290
14. Describe the role of O-139 strain in the epidemiology of cholera. — A 7., p. 290
15. Describe structure and mechanism of cholera toxin. Describe the pathogenesis of cholera. — A 6b., p. 289
16. Discuss the laboratory diagnosis of cholera. — p. 291 and chapter 5
17. Discuss prophylaxis against cholera. — pg. 632
18. Enumerate halophilic vibrios. Describe their pathogenicity and laborarory diagnosis. — A8., p. 290 and p. 291
19. Describe about Aeromonas and Pleisomonas spp. — p. 282, 283, 285

Section VIII: Gram Negative Bacilli–Curved/Spiral Shaped

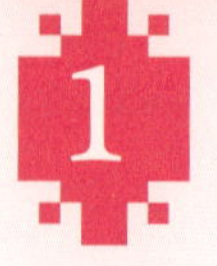

Classification, Metabolic and Microscopic Features of Key Gram Negative Bacilli–Curved/Spiral Shaped

General Species Listed in Category of Gram Negative Bacilli–Curved/Spiral Shaped

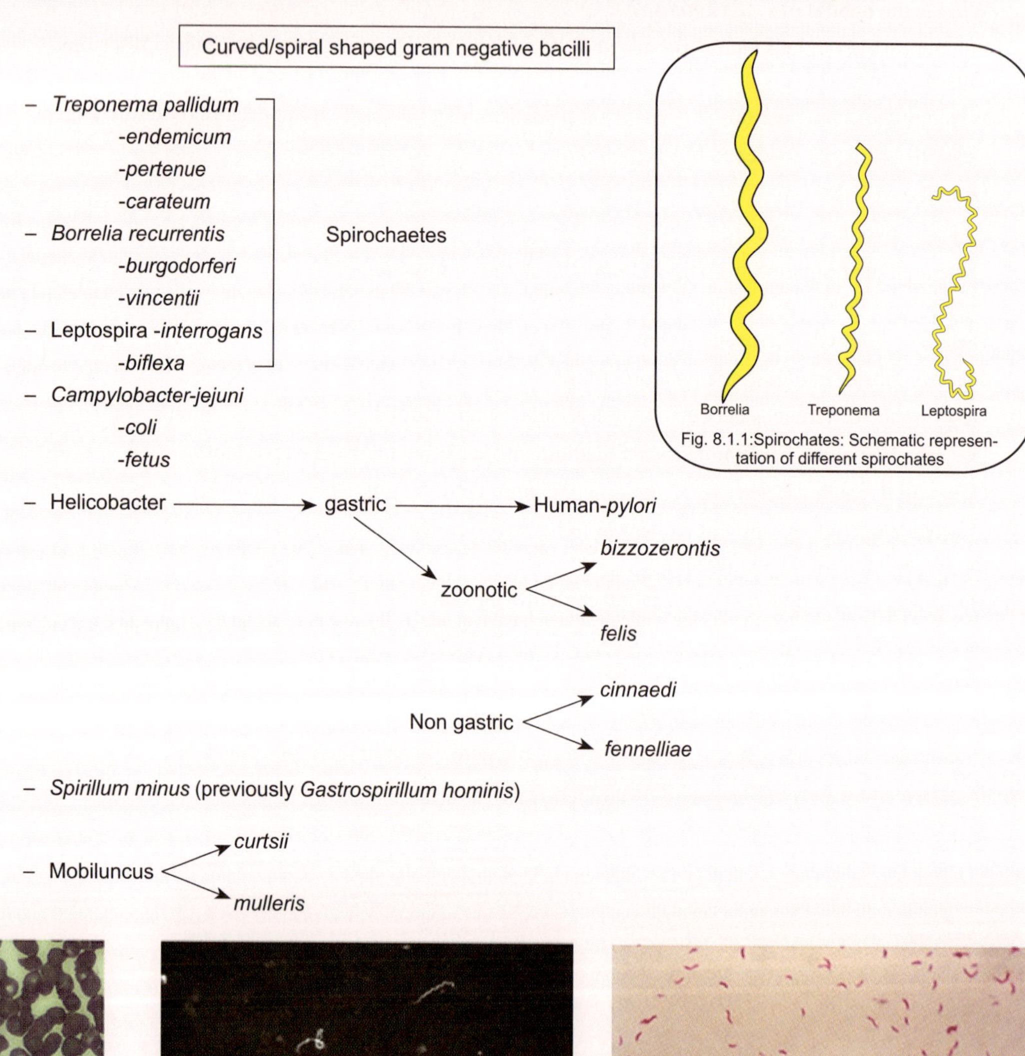

Fig. 8.1.1:Spirochates: Schematic representation of different spirochates

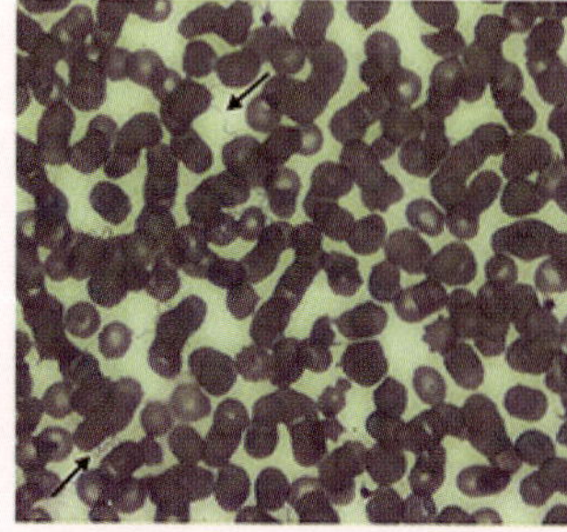

Fig.8.1.2: Borrelia: Peripheral blood smear demonstrating numerous borrelia (spirochates)

Courtesy: Port Collins, Colorado/CDC

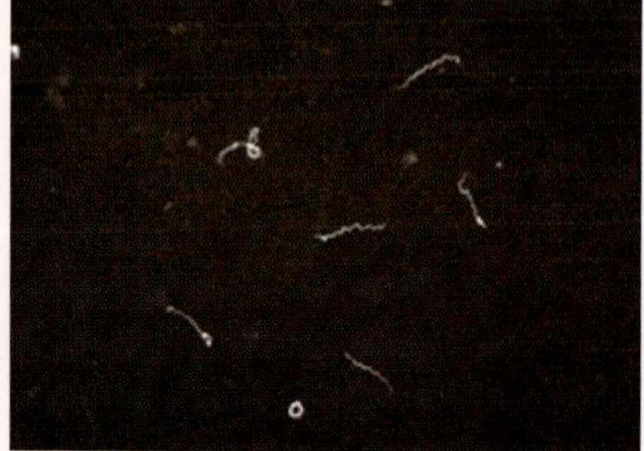

Fig.8.1.3: Syphilis: Dark ground microscopy demonstrating Treponema pallidum (400X)

Courtesy: Schwartz/CDC

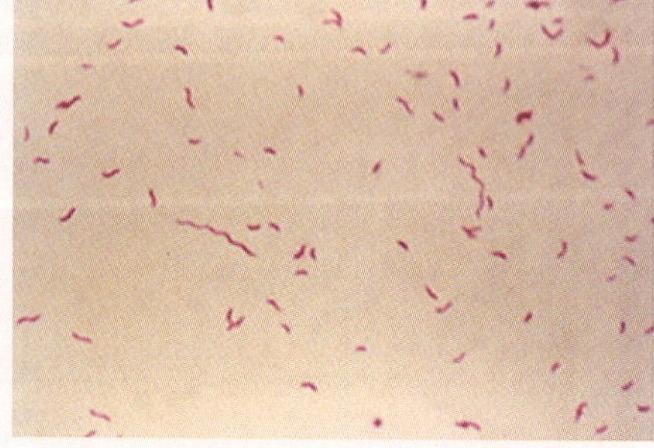

Fig.8.1.4: Campylobacter: Gram stained smear demonstrating spiral rods

Courtesy: Centers for Disease Control and Prevention, Atlanta, USA

Metabolic and microscopic features of gram negative bacilli - curved/spiral

Organism	*Growth requirements*						*Cellular morphology and staining characteristics*						
	O2 Requ.	*Optimal*	*CO2*	*Incubatior Period*			*Shape*	*Gram*	*Arrangement*	*Capsule*	*Motility*	*Spore*	*Special Staining / micros-copy / Special Features*
		Temp.	*Requ..*	*Days*	*Weeks*	*Months*							
Leptospira interrogans	Strictly aerobic	30°C	-	3 days to	3 weeks	-	Spirochaete, slim, numerous spirals (set very close) and ends are hooked (Fig. 8.1.1)	-ve (stains poorly with Gram stain)	-	-	-	-	Very thin difficult to see with conventional stains better with Giemsa, with silver impregnation & dark ground microscopy
Borrelia recurrentis	microaerophilic	28-30°C	-	Slow growing	-	-	Spirochaete (5-8 irregular spirals at intervals of about 2µm with pointed ends (Fig. 8.1.2)	-ve	-	-	+	-	-
Borrellia burgdorferi	microaerophile	33°C	–	–	≥2 weeks		spirochate	-ve	-	-	+	-	-
Borrelia vincentii	obligate anae-robe	37°C	-	Few			spirochate	-ve	-	-	+	-	Stained usually with Giemsa or Leishman Stain
Treponema pallidum	microaerophilic	Can not be cultivated on inanimate media					Spirochaete (6-12 evenly spaced coils / waves) -Slender (<0.15µm diameter) (Fig. 8.1.3)	Can not be stained by it	-	-	+	-	Giemsa and Fontana staining tech. used. Conventionally dark ground microscopy used
T. pallidum subsps endemicum, pertenue,carateum	similar features to T. pallidum							Can not be stained by it.					
Helicobacter pylori	microaerophilic	37°C	+(10%)	3-5	-	-	curved/spiral/ S shaped	-ve	-	-	Δ+	-	H&E,Warthin starry silver stain used in tissue samples
Campylobacter jejuni	microaerophilic	42°C	+(10%)	2	-	-	Curved (Fig. 8.1.4)	-ve	-	-	◊ + cork-screw type	-	tissue staining not required
Spirillum minus	microaerophilic	Can not be cultivated on inanimate media					spiral	-ve		-	+	-	Stained usually with Giemsa or Leishman Stain Also demonstrated with dark ground microscopy
Mobiluncus curtisii & mulieris	primarily an-aerobe	33-37°C	-	5			Curved	-ve	singly/pairs	variable/-	+		

Δ unipolar tuft of sheathed flagella

◊ single polar, flagellum at one or both ends

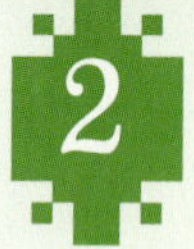

2 An Overview of the Media Requirements, Colonial Characters and Diagnostic Characterization of Key Gram Negative Bacilli–Curved/Spiral Shaped

	Basal media	Enriched media	Selective/ others	Characterization and confirmation of isolation
Leptospira interrogans	No growth	Culture technique is cumbersome and performed only in reference labs Media enriched with rabbit serum used as Stuart's, Fletcher's semi solid, EMJH (Ellinghausen's, McCullough, Johnson and Harris)	• Chorioallantoic membrane of chick embryo • Lab animals as guinea pig inoculated with material intraperitoneally	• In semi-solid media, growth occurs few mms below the surface • In guinea pig, heart blood is taken 10 mins. after i/p inoculation to obtain organism
Borrelia recurrentis	No growth	No growth on conventional enriched media	• Noguchi media containing ascitic fluid and rabbit kidney • Chorioallantoic membrane of chick embryo	• Classical colonial growth not obtained
Borrelia burgdorferi	No growth	Modified Kelley's medium: +	-	Not cultured routinely, as organism is slow growing and difficult to isolate
Borrelia vincentii	No growth	Media containing ascitic fluid and serum	-	Cultivation of organism is difficult
Treponema pallidum	No growth	No growth	• Not cultivable even in animate media as living membranes, specialized media • Nichol's strain has been maintained in rabbit testes by serial passage • *T. phagedenis* (Reiter's strain) grown in anaerobic conditions	Diagnosis essentially microscopic and serologic
Helicobacter pylori	No growth	Blood agar: + Chocolate agar: +	MacConkey: No growth	Culture requires microaerophilic conditions and incubation of few days up to 1 week • Colonies are circular, convex and translucent • Catalase +ve, urease +ve (biopsy urease test pg. 66), Oxidase +ve, biochemically inactive
Campylobacter jejuni	No growth	Blood agar: +	• MacConkey: NG • Camplylobacter selective media used, when samples as faeces are to be cultivated (medium has antimicrobials as Vancomycin, Trimethoprim, Polymyxin B, Cephalothin and Amphotericin B)	

3 Clinical (Pathogenicity) Profile of Infections Caused By Key Gram Negative Bacilli–Curved/Spiral Shaped

Leptospira interrogans	• Leptospirosis essentially a bacteremia, can present as aseptic meningitis (also as mild illness) • Weil's disease is a severe form of multiorgan Leptospirosis Details see A.2(a), (b), pg 306	
Borrelia recurrentis	Relapsing fever (epidemic and endemic form) (is bacteremia with relapses) Details see A3, pg 308	
Borrellia burgdorferi	Lyme disease [case see p. 309] I.P. _3-30 days • 1st Stage_Localized infection (erythema migrans) Fig. 8.3.1 • 2nd stage_few weeks later disseminated infection. Fever headache, myalgia, lymphadenopathy, meningeal and cardiac involvement may occur • 3rd stage_months to years later. Persistent infection, Chronic arthritis, polyneuropathy, encephalopathy.	
Borrelia vincentii	Vincent,s angina (ulcerative oropharyngitis or gingivostomatitis in association with fusiform bacilli (Fusobacterium fusiformis)	
Treponema pallidum	Syphilis	Primary (Fig. 8.3.2), secondary (Fig. 8.3.3, 8.3.4) Latent and tertiary stages. Details see A7, pg. 300
	Congenital syphilis	Details see p. 302-303.
T. pallidum subsps endemicum	Endemic syphilis (non venereal syphilis) • Details see A4, Pg. 305	
T. pallidum subsps pertenue	Yaws (non venereal syphilis) • Details see A4, Pg. 305.	
T. pallidum subsps carateum	Pinta (non venereal syphilis) • Details see A4, Pg. 305.	
Helicobacter pylori	Increased association with Duoednal ulcer, Gastric ulcer, gastric malignancies and non-ulcerative dyspepsias Decreased association with GERD and adenocarcinoma of oesophagus. nb: GERD_Gastro esophageal reflux disease	
H. cinaedi	Isolated from rectum of homosexual men with proctitis and cause of bacteremia in homosexual men, who are HIV positive	
H. fenelliae	Isolated from rectum of homosexual men with proctitis	
Campylobacter jejuni	Bloody diarrohea, abdominal pain and fever	
	Complcations_Reactive arthritis, Guillain-Barré syndrome (1 in every 100 to 2000 cases)	
	See details, p. 310	
C. coli	Similar to above except for the complications	
C. fetus	Commonly bacteremia, sepsis, endocarditis and meningitis Less common presentation is diarrohea	
C. sputorum	Associated with diarrohea and septicaemia	
Spirillum minus	Fever, skin rash and localized L.N. swelling (at bite site)	

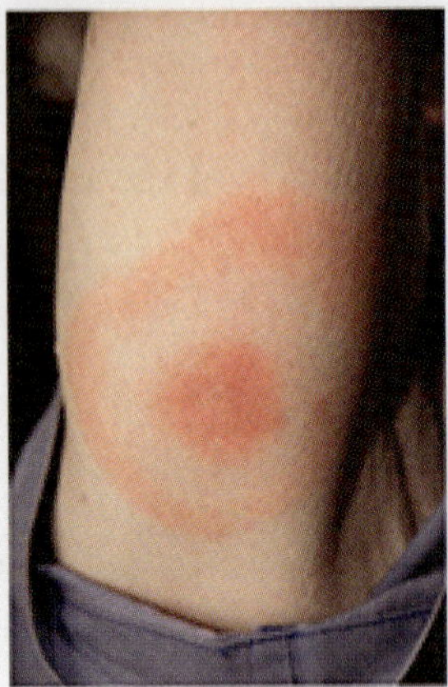

Fig.8.3.1: LYME DISEASE: Classic pattern of a "bull's eye" at site of tick bite

Courtesy: James Gathany/CDC

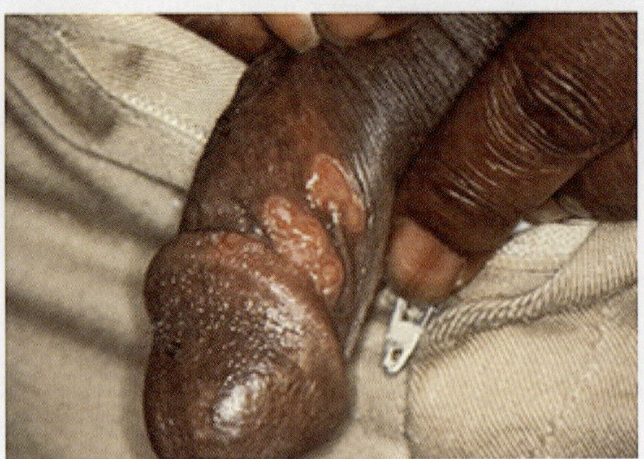

Fig.8.3.2: SYPHILIS: Chancre on the penile shaft caused by Treponema pallidum

Courtesy:M. Rein/CDC

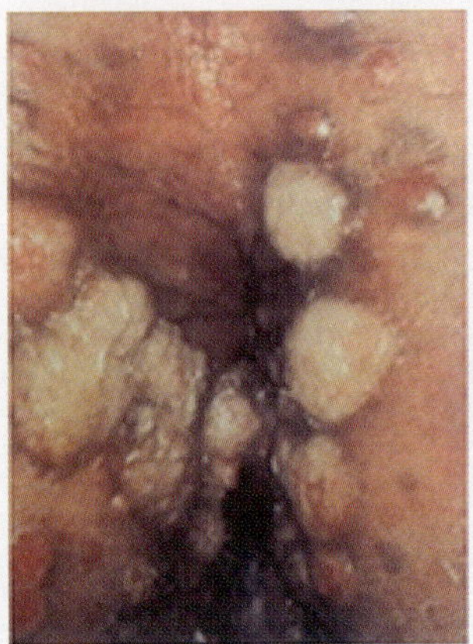

Fig.8.3.3: SYPHILIS: Condylomata lata, moist flat plaques on perianal areas

Courtesy: M. Rein/CDC

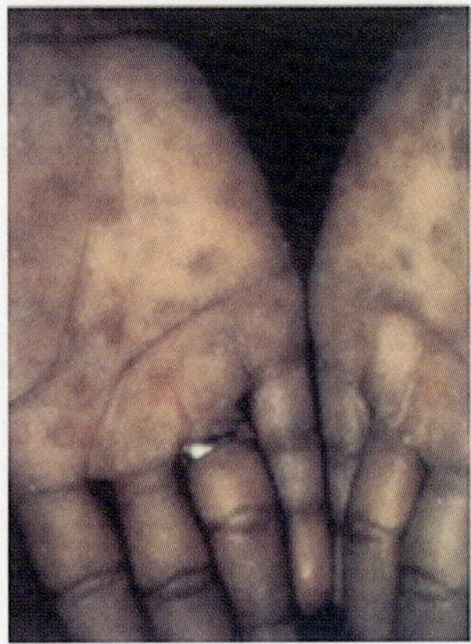

Fig.8.3.4: Secondary syphilis: Symmetrical macules on the palms

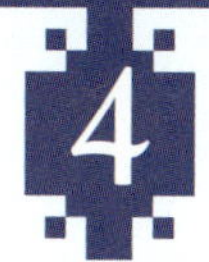

Integrated Clinical Based Study of *T.pallidum*/Syphilis-Chancre

A 35 year old truck driver, Satender reported to the O.P.D clinic with a painless, small ulcer on the glans penis (Fig. 8.3.2). Detailed history revealed, that he had an unprotected sexual intercourse with a commercial sexual worker of West Bengal, about two weeks back. Examination revealed enlarged, non tender lymph nodes in both groins.

Linkages: Pg. 294-298, Chapter 6, 314, 316

What is the clinical diagnosis the above case?

A.1 Syphilis

How should the specimen from the genital lesion be collected?

A.2 (a) Gloves should be worn to collect the specimen; as the lesions are highly infectious. If fresh exudate is present, it may be collected observing standard precautions. If the lesion appears dry, it may be cleaned with gauge soaked in warm saline and the margins gently scraped, so that the superficial epithelium is abraded. Gentle pressure may be applied to the base of the lesion to express fresh exudate.

What test can be done in the skin O.P.D setting, that may confirm the provisional diagnosis of syphilis?

A.2 (b) Dark ground microcopy for demonstration of spirochetes. However; expertise is required to differentiate *T. pallidum* form commensal spirochetes.

What is the role and mechanism of silver staining in the laboratory diagnosis of syphilis?

A.2 (c) *T. pallidum* is a slender, less* than 0.15 μm in diameter; which mandates the requirement of dark ground/phase contrast/electron microscopy for its visualization. The use of silver stain results in metallic silver (as reduction from silver nitrate) deposition on the organism, which increases its thickness to enable it to come in the range of resolution of a light microscope (Fontana's method used for films and Levaditi's for tissue sections).

* Is below the resolving power of light microscope and its refractive index is similar to that of the suspending media

What is unique about motility of T. pallidum? Mention; how it helps this organism to survive in its environment.

A.2 (d) It is an example of an organism, which is motile because of endoflagella and not due to exoflagella. In this organism, the flagella are not on the exterior but lie between the outer-membrane and the peptidoglycan. These flagella (3-4 in number) are anchored at each end and impart characteristic motility, which has corkscrew like character including flexion/extension and translatory movements. This type of motility helps the spirochaete to move easily through viscous environment and invade the host tissue.

If the genital lesion of the above case healed without giving treatment, is there still a need to treat this case?

A.3 (a) Yes. Complete treatment of the case must to done to prevent the case form progression to later stages of syphilis and to protect the sexual contacts of the truck driver from contracting the disease.

A towel being used by the commercial sex worker is used by another client. What is the probability of transmission of syphilis to that client?

A.3 (b) The probability is low, as the *T.pallidum* organism is very delicate and easily gets destroyed.

Describe the resistance characteristic of T.pallidium and its implications.

A.3 (c) Fortunately this organism is very delicate and is easily killed by drying and low heat, which accounts for this organism to be transmitted only by close contact. For the same reason, syphilis is unlikely to be transmitted by used towels (used by cases) at common facility places; as swimming pools. It is killed at 0-4°C in 1-3 days, so blood stored in refrigerator for 4 days, can't lead to transfusion syphilis, when used in transfusion. This organism is inactivated by soap, common antiseptics. Resistance of this organism to common antimicrobials; as penicillin, erythromycin and tetracycline has not developed.

Genome: Approx 1,138,000 (base pairs).

Unlike many pathogenic bacteria, the genome of it lacks transposable elements. This could be rendering the genome conserved and stable and possibly explain the susceptibility of this organism to penicillin for many decades.

What simple precaution, if taken by the truck worker, could have prevented this infection?

A.4 (a) Using condom, while having sex with a commercial sex worker.

What are the other important aspects in S.T.D. prophylaxis?

A.4 (b) Early treatment of the cases and follow up of cases and contacts.

Enumerate infectious genital diseases, which are transmitted non-sexually?

A.5 Folliculitis, Tuberculosis, Tularemia, Amoebiasis, Candidosis, and Histoplasmosis.

Describe the epidemiology of syphilis with special reference to men, who have sex with men (MSM).

A.6 **Agent:** *Treponema pallidum* subspecies pallidum.

Reservoir of infection: This organism is a strict human pathogen and resides in the genital tract of infected males and females.

Source of infection: Genital exudates/secretion and blood of cases.

Mode of transmission:

– Most cases by sexual contact, as during intercourse, kissing or other activities, involving with infectious lesions as (chancre/condylomata latum)
– Congenital route (transplacental to fetus)
– Blood transfusion
– Occupational (as on fingers of nurses)

Host:

– The disease has a worldwide distribution.
– Most cases occur in the sexually active age groups of 15 to 30 in women and 15-54 years in men.
– A recent increase in incidence of the disease has occurred because of change in sexual practices, despite initial control with penicillin therapy. These include oral sex and homosexuality including men who have sex with men, (MSM).

Approximately 30% of apparently uninfected individuals, who have sexual contact with infected persons, may develop disease, if not treated. The identification of these infected individuals by serologic means is an important part of the syphilis control programme. For this reason, pregnant women and military recruits are tested by serologic means.

– The disease is common in prostitutes and individuals, who have multiple sex partners.
– Co-infection of HIV and syphilis is common in many individuals.

Outline the clinical profile of syphilis.

A.7 I.P:10-90 days

Venereal	*Primary*	*Chancre (hard)*
	Fig. 8.3.2	*Men-heterosexual:* Penis *Homosexual:* Rectum, anal canal, oral cavity and external genitalia
		Women: Cervix and labia (often go unnoticed)
		Rarely on lips and nipple
	Secondary (Figs. 8.3.3 and 8.3.4)	- Macular to papular lesions on trunk and extremities (persist for few days to few weeks) - Condylomata lata on sites as lips, glans, vulva and anal canal (painless, erythematous, broad and moist plaques)
	Tertiary	As aneurysm, neurosyphilis and general paralysis of insane (stage is uncommon, due to treatment received in earlier stages). Disease is due to gummatous lesion of vessels, CNS and bones
Non-venereal	*Congenital*	- Presentation depends on number of factors - Stigmata in infant include Hutchinson teeth (notching), saddle nose, saber skin (anterior tibial bowing), frontal bossing etc
	Occupational	For instance in nurses and doctors on unprotected hand as fingers, due to contact with lesion during examination

Describe VDRL test and one of its modification, namely; Rapid plasma reagin test.

A.8
- **Historical:** The test has been developed at Venereal Disease Research laboratory, New York.
- **Principle:** VDRL test is a *slide flocculation test*, based on the presence of non-specific syphilitic antibodies (reaginic) in the syphilitic cases. Flocculation is a type of precipitation reaction, where the antigen and the antibody form a complex, which instead of sedimenting, remains suspended. The test uses cardiolipin (lipoidal antigen) as the non-specific antigen, which is an extract of beef heart. The lecithin plays the part of stabilization of the preparation. Cholestrol is added to the antigen preparation, to increase the reactive surface. The test detects the IgM antibodies, which appears after second week of infection.
- **Procedure:** The test is run on a VDRL slide. In the concavities of the slide, the dilutions of the inactivated serum and VDRL antigen are put. After mixture, the slide is rotated on the VDRL rotator for 180 revolutions/minute for 4 minutes.
- **Interpretation:** The reaction is broadly reported as reactive/positive or non reactive/negative. The presence of floccules is interpreted as positive. The reaction is reported as titer (in dilutions). A titer of more than eight is considered significant. The test gives false positive results in number of conditions namely: Tissue regeneration, severe trauma, intake of certain antihypertensives, heroin addiction, menstruation, vaccination, pregnancy, repeated blood loss, collagen disorders, rheumatoid arthritis, systemic lupus erythematosus, infective hepatitis, upper respiratory infection, infectious mononucleosis, HIV infection, malaria, tropical eosinophilia and lepromatous leprosy.
- The change in titer of the specimen on spaced repeat samples has diagnostic significance. Fall in titer of the test is reported, after successful treatment. For, interpretation in various stages of syphilis, see table 8.4.1.
- **Advantages of the test:** The test is simple, easy, inexpensive and rapid test. The test can become more specific, if rise in titer can be demonstrated in a follow up sample taken after few weeks.
- **Disadvantages of the test:** The sensitivity and specificity of the test is lower than many other treponemal antibody based tests.

Table 8.4.1: Sensitivity of key serological tests for syphilis

Test	Sensitivity (%)		
	Primary	*Secondary*	*Latent/late*
VDRL	70-80	100	60-70
TPHA	65	100	95-100
FTA-ABS	85-100	100	95-100

NB: all these tests have approximately a specificity of >97%

Modifications of the test:

(i) Rapid plasma reagin test (RPR)

(ii) VDRL–ELISA

(iii) Other related tests - see flow diagram at p. 315.

An comparison of the VDRL and RPR is depicted in table 8.4.2.

Table 8.4.2: Comparison between VDRL and RPR test

	VDRL	RPR
Equipment	Uses VDRL slide	Uses disposable cards
Specimen acceptable	Serum, CSF	Serum/plasma (but not CSF)
Antigen	To be prepared freshly daily	Readymade and longer stability
Interpretation	Requires microscope (low power) to observe floccules	Clumps can be read macroscopically (antigen is fine carbon particles)
Technique	Cumbersome	Easy
Sensitivity	Lower in primary syphilis	Higher in primary syphilis
Cost	Economical	Expensive than VDRL

Integrated Clinical Based Study of *T.pallidum*/Congenital Syphilis

A 6 week old male infant, Sunny was admitted to a paediatric ward with history of low grade fever, rhinitis, peeling rash on the hands and feet; with a TLC of 45,000/μL. Physical examination revealed hepatosplenomegaly. Radiographic study revealed extensive periostitis with osteolytic changes in metaphyseal regions of bones.

Linkages: Pg. 294-297, Chapter 6, 314, 316

What is the differential clinical diagnosis in this case?

A.1 (a) The differential diagnosis of this case includes congenital syphilis, Toxoplasmosis, CMV infection, Herpes simplex infection and Coxsackie virus infection.

What is the likely clinical diagnosis?

A.1 (b) The child is likely to have congenital syphilis, as the clinical profile includes peeling of skin in the hands and feet along with radiologic findings of periostitis and metaphyseal destruction, are indicative of congenital syphilis.

How did the infant likely acquire this infection?

A.2 (a) The infant is likely to have acquired the infection 'in utero' from the mother. The transmission has likely occurred transplacentally during pregnancy.

Why is it important to study the antigenic characteristics of T. pallidum? Describe its non-specific and specific antigens.

A.2 (b) It is important to study this characteristic, as serological diagnosis forms the mainstay of diagnosis in syphilis and the organism's structure needs to be characterized for development of diagnostic test. The treponemal antigens are poorly characterized. The outer membrane of the organism has LPS and is rich in phospholipids but contains few proteins. The antigens can be categorized into non-specific and specific antigen categories, on the basis of antitreponemal antibodies.

Non-specific antigen:

Antibodies formed against cardiolipin (wrongly termed 'reaginic', as is not related to IgE) is the basis of non-treponemal tests; as Venereal Disease Research Laboratory (VDRL) and Kahn. It is not clear, if this antigen is part of the spirochaete or is a modified component of the host cell. This difficulty in distinction arises, as the treponemes adsorb lipid from tissue, while multiplying.

The reagin antibodies react with a lipid haptene (disphosphatidyl glycerol) known as cardiolipin extracted from beef heart.

Specific antigens:

- *Group specific antigen:* This antigen is present in all pathogenic and non-pathogenic treponemes. The antibody to this antigen is detected using antigen derived from Reiter treponeme.
- *Species specific antigen:* It is probably a polysaccharide. The specific *T. pallidum* tests detect antibodies against this antigen.

How can you confirm the diagnosis of syphilis in this case?

A.2 (c) The lesion should be swabbed vigorously, so that cellular material is adequately collected. This specimen can be used to demonstrate the spirochaete, using dark ground microscopy.

What are the approaches and challenges in diagnosis of cases with suspected diagnosis of congenital syphilis?

A.2 (d) Two approaches can be utilized for diagnosing congenital syphilis. *One* is direct demonstration of spirochetes in mucous discharges, clinical lesions, placental and umbilical cord samples, using silver staining techniques or dark ground microscopy. These organisms can't be cultivated 'in vitro'. The *second* approach is serologic, i.e., demonstrating the antibodies to *T. pallidum*. The screening tests include RPR or VDRL, whereas the confirmatory tests; include FTA-ABS (fluorescent treponemal antibody absorption Test) and MHA-TP (microtitre haemagglutination *T. pallidum.* test).

The challenge in the diagnosis is that the sensitivity of tests demonstrating spirochetes in lesion is low. Secondly, the infant can be seropositive to serologic tests without having the disease. To counter this limitation, four fold rise of antibody titer between acute and convalescent serum needs to be demonstrated in tests as in VDRL. Demonstrating specific IgM for *T. pallidum* using Western blot assay or fluorescent antibody assay (IgM–FTA–ABS) is also diagnostic.

Compare and contrast the characteristics of Treponemal haemagglutination test (TPHA) and fluorescent treponemal antibody absorption tests (FTA-ABS).

A.2 (e)

	Treponemal pallidum haemagglutination test (TPHA)	**Fluorescent treponemal antibody absorption test (FTA-ABS)**
Category of test	*T.pallidum* serological test	*T.pallidum* serological test (fluorescent based)
Antigen used	Erythrocytes sensitized with extract of *T.pallidum* (Nichol's strain)	Killed *T.pallidum*
Principle of test	Haemagglutination test	Indirect immunofluorescent test
Procedure	• Patient's serum dilutions prepared • Reaction of the sensitized RBCs performed with various dilutions of serum	• Patient's serum first treated with extract of non-pathogenic treponemes (Reiter's) to remove reaginic and group reactive antibodies • Above serum reacted with smear of Nichol's strain • After incubation and washing, application of FITC conjugate (principle see pg. 130) • Incubate, wash and examine smear under UV light
Interpretation	Agglutination of RBCs is a positive reaction (+ve titer estimated)	Fluorescing treponemes is a positive reaction (+ve titer estimated)
Advantages	Simple, highly sensitive test, economical	Highly sensitive test, even in primary syphilis
Disadvantages	Lower sensitivity in primary syphilis	Requires expensive equipment and reagents
Status of the test	See table 8.4.1, pg. 301	See table 8.4.1, pg. 301

^TPHA test when performed in a microtitre plate is referred to as microlitre haemagglutination *T.pallidum* (MHA-TP) test

Can a case having syphilis infection remain asymptomatic?

A.3 Yes, many of the infected cases can remain asymptomatic for life.

What is the natural history of syphilis?

A.4 (a) The case may evolve through primary syphilis, secondary syphilis, latent syphilis and tertiary syphilis.

At what stage of infection, is this infant in?

A.4 (b) The case belongs to the stage of secondary syphilis, as it has a cutaneous lesion on the extremities. The clinician must wear gloves, while examining infectious lesions (likely to be teeming with spirochetes).

What is the drug of choice for the infant with syphilis?

A.5 (a) Penicillin G is the drug of choice for the case.

Disusss the treatment plan of parents of this child with syphilis?

A.5 (b) The mother must be treated, as she is the source of the infection for causing congenital infection of the infant. Sometimes the woman may be asymptomatic. Such a scenario is possible, as pregnancy can alter the course of syphilis. As this disease is sexually transmitted, all sexual partners of this woman should be screened and treated; if necessary to prevent the infection from developing in them.

8 Integrated Clinical Based Study of Leptospira/Leptospirosis

A thirty year farmer, Nileshwar from Port Blair*, who was involved in paddy (rice) plantation, presented with fever, jaundice and subconjunctival haemmorhage. After one day of admission in the medical ward, the patient presented with hemoptysis (bloody sputum).
***Is located in Bay of Bengal and is the capital of Andaman and Nicobar islands**

Linkages: Pg. 294-297, 315, 316

What is your clinical diagnosis of the case? Justify it.

A.1 Leptospirosis. The endemic area in which the patient is living, the occupation of the case (makes the case prone to leptospirosis) and the classic presentation in the case, makes this the likely clinical diagnosis.

Explain the occurrence of hemoptysis in this case.

A.2 (a) In the second stage of leptospirosis, numerous organs can get involved. In this case, the lung has got involved and has haemorrhagic pneumonitis. This clinical entity must be kept in mind, in cases from Andaman and Nicobar islands, Gujarat and Maharashtra, having hemoptysis. They are often misdiagnosed, with leptospirosis never being considered, as one of the differential diagnosis. Consequently; these cases never receive effective treatment.

Describe the clinical profile of Leptospirosis.

A.2 (b) **I.P.:** Usually 1-2 weeks (range 2-20 days)

Anicteric Leptospirosis: Most infections (90%) are mild, usually anicteric form (without jaundice) and may have meningitis (aseptic meningitis). A high degree of alertness on behalf of the clinician is required to clinch the diagnosis or the leptospirosis diagnosis would be missed out.The presentation is initiated by bacteremia.

Icteric Leptospirosis: About 10% of the cases present as icteric leptospirosis,a severe form of the disease, also known as the *Weil's syndrome*. The patient has jaundice and manifestations due to renal, pulmonary and haemmorhages. The case may present commonly as high fever, jaundice, renal failure, abdominal pain, chest pain and haemoptysis.

Mention the epidemiology of this disease with reference to the Indian subcontinent.

A.3
- **Agent:** *L. interrogans* is the pathogenic species (contrast with *L. biflexa,* which is a saprophytic species), is classified into 22 serogroups/serotypes, which are further subgrouped into serovars, according to their antigenic relatedness. As an example *L. interrogans* having Serovar Australis, is represented as *Leptospira interrogans* serovar Australis.

Reservoir/Source of infection: Leptospirosis is a *zoonoses* affecting rats, dogs cattle, pigs and other animals. The main source for the serogroup *icterohaemorrhagiae* and *canicola* are rat and dog, respectively. The leptospires multiply in the kidney and get shed in the urine in amounts that exceed several million leptospires per ml of urine.

- These organisms can survive for weeks, in the neutral or slightly alkaline water.
- Man gets secondarily the infection and is considered an *aberrant host*. There is no evidence of spread of infection from man to man.

Mode of Transmission: The organism can enter the body directly through skin abrasions by direct contact with infected urine or animal tissue. It can also occur indirectly by contact of the abraded skin with contaminated soil or water.

Host Factor: The disease has a worldwide distribution except Antarctica.

- In India, the disease is common in Andaman and Nicobar Islands, Tamil Nadu, and Gujarat, Kerala, Maharashtra and Orissa

- Agricultural workers; who work in rice (paddy) fields, miners or sewer workers who often come in contact with water contaminated with leptospires excreted by animals are more prone to this infection. Leptospirosis is a major cause of clinical syndromes; such as jaundice renal failure, myocarditis and atypical pneumonia.

Environment: Outbreaks usually follow natural calamities; as cyclones, floods and excessive rainfall (as in Mumbai). Outbreaks in Mumbai, a coastal city have been reported.

- Research on leptospirosis in India is carried out at Regional Medical Research Center (of ICMR), Port Blair. This center is also the National Leptospirosis Reference Center, which stocks the Leptospira strains.

What approach is commonly employed to confirm the clinical diagnosis of Leptospirosis?

A.4 (a) Demonstrating specific antileptospiral antibodies is a common approach used to confirm the diagnosis of leptospirosis.

Mention the serological test that is considered 'gold standard' in the diagnosis of Leptospirosis? Describe it.

A.4 (b) Microscopic agglutination test (MAT). It is a serotype specific test and helps to identify the infecting serovar by demonstrating specific antibodies. Essentially in the test, leptospires prevalent in the area are used. The test involves mixing of the live Leptospira with serial dilutions of patient's sera and examining microscopically in dark field for agglutination of the leptospira. Significant single serum titer or four fold rise in convalescent serum is considered positive. This test is highly sensitive and specific.

Mention the role of 'rapid dip stick' test in diagnosis of leptospirosis.

A.4 (c) The latter test helps to detect the Leptospiral specific IgM antibodies.

Mention the strategies to control leptospirosis.

A.5 (i) Disinfection of the water (as infection spreads by water)

(ii) Rodent control

(iii) Wearing of protective clothing

(iv) Vaccination has been attempted in dogs, cattle, pigs and individuals at high risk; as agricultural workers.

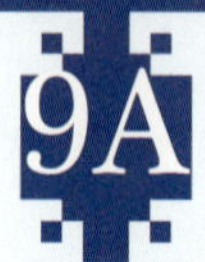

Integrated Clinical Based Study of *Borrelia recurrentis*/Relapsing Fever

An 23 year old college student Shailesh, who returned after visiting Sudan, complained of episodes of fever since the last few months. His current episode, i.e., the 3rd episode was less severe than the first two episodes and lasted only two days. His second episode of fever occurred about 10 days back and lasted for about 10 days. His first episode of fever occurred two months back and lasted for about 15 days. He gave history of exposure to lice. His physical examination was normal except for a palpable spleen, which was about 5 cm below the costal margin. The blood examination was within normal limits except for the presence of a spiral shaped organism in the peripheral blood smear, that were demonstrable with Giemsa staining.

Linkages: Pg. 294-297, 314 and 316

What is the provisional diagnosis in this case?

A.1 (a) Relapsing fever. *B. recurrentis* is present in the peripheral smear; as a spiral organism (Fig. 8.1.2.), pg., 294.

Compare and contrast the morphology of B. recurrentis and Leptospires.

A.1 (b) Leptospires possess numerous coils; set so close to each other that these can be distinguished only under the dark ground microscope.

B. reccurrentis has irregular,wide spirals and open coils (Fig. 8.1.1 and 8.1.2).

Which are the tick borne diseases, which can present as fever?

A.1 (c)
- Relapsing fever (is also louse borne)
- Colorado tick fever
- Rocky Mountain spotted fever
- Ehrlichiosis, Babesiosis.

What are the other diseases, which present with fever in episodic forms, having non-specific symptomatology?

A.1 (d) Malaria and Babesiosis

How is Borrelia able to evade the human immune response and cause recurrent fever?

A.2 Borrelia is able to undergo antigenic variation of their serotype specific outer proteins through gene rearrangement. The new antigens can evade the immune response, as the previous specific antibodies are not effective against the new strain. The variable major proteins (vmps) are encoded by the 'vmp' genes and the DNA rearrangement is responsible for the extreme variation in protein expression.

Compare and contrast the two types of relapsing fever.

A.3 Two distinct types of disease are known:

Epidemic: LBRF: Louse borne (epidemic) Relapsing fever	**Endemic: TBRF**=Tick borne-(endemic) Relapsing fever
Agent: *B. recurrentis*	*B. recurrentis, B. duttoni.*
Reservoir: Infected human	Rodent (infected), Ticks (infected)
Vector: *Pediculus humanus corporis* (Human body louse) **Transmission:** By crushing of lice into wound.	*Ornithodoros species [Soft ticks] By bite or through discharge
More severe Localized; as disease is controlled by improved socioeconomic conditions globally. Africa (especially eastern), China. Epidemics may occur **Environment:** Disease is associated with overcrowding, war and poverty.	Less Severe Worldwide Sporadic human case.

What is the treatment of choice for relapsing fever?

A.4 Tetracycline (including Doxycycline), Chloramphenicol and Erythromycin are effective drugs for treating this infection.

What is the prophylaxis of relapsing fever?

A.5
- Prevention of louse infestation/avoidance of tick infested places
- No vaccine is available

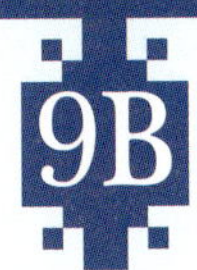

Integrated Clinical Based Study of *Borrelia burgdoferi*/Lyme Disease

A 14 year old boy, Vinod who recently returned from New York, U.S.A., reported fever of 6 days duration. Examination of the case revealed a rash on the back, which he reported to be increasing in size. He gave history of having trekked in a region with woods.

Linkages: Pg. 294-298, 315, 316

What is the likely clinical diagnosis of this case? Justify it.

A.1 Lyme disease (recognized in 1975). The rash with target like appearance having expanding borders is typical in this disease and has been described as 'erythema migrans' (Fig. 8.3.1, pg. 298). The history of having trekked in wooded areas made the boy prone to tick infestation.

Emphasize key epidemiological characteristics of Lyme disease?

A.2 The tick (*Ixodes scapularis*) is the vector responsible for transmission of *B. burgdorferi*(etiological agent for Lyme disease) to humans. The larval, nymph and adult stages of the tick can feed on a human host, but only the nymph and adult stages of the tick can transmit the disease. The organisms are transferred to humans during the blood meal of ticks, when they are likely to regurgitate the spirochetes into the wound. Transfer of spirochaetes to humans appear to require a long attachment period of about 2 days. For this reasons, deticking (removal of ticks), if performed before this period, mayn't result in the transmission of Lyme disease.

What complications can occur, if this disease isn't treated?

A.3 The boy in this case is in first stage of disease. He may go onto the second and third stages of disease, if not initially treated. In the latter stages, he could have arthritis and/or CNS complications.

How is the clinical diagnosis of Lyme disease confirmed in the laboratory?

A.4 Demonstration of specific antibodies in the serum of the case; using IFA or EIA technology, would be the technique of choice. Antibodies take 1-2 months to appear. Culture of this spirochete is difficult.

Mention measures that can be taken to prevent this disease.

A.5 Wearing appropriate clothing in endemic areas; as long pants, full-sleeved shirts and shoes would be helpful. Tick repellent chemical on skin and clothing; as diethyl toluamide (DEET) would be additionally helpful. Finally, the skin should be examined for any ticks, after coming out of the infested environment, which should be removed, before they can trasmit the disease.

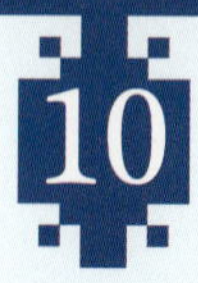

10 Integrated Clinical Based Study of *C. jejuni*/Campylobacteriosis

A 30 year man, Jefferson belonging to Shillong* complained of fever, abdominal pain and passing of stool mixed with blood, after consuming an undercooked chicken preparation. A faecal smear of this case, which was gram stained, revealed gram negative curved bacilli.

***is the capital of Meghalaya, a north eastern state of India**

Linkages: Pg. 294-297, 315, 316

What is the provisional diagnosis of this case?

A.1 *Campylobacter jejuni* infection of the gut.

What histopathological findings would be expected in such a case, in the small and large intestinal biopsy specimens?

A.2 (a) Acute non-specific inflammatory changes in jejunum, ileum and colon. The changes would include gland degeneration and crypt abscesses.

Describe the pathogenicity of Campylobacteriosis.

A.2 (b) The infection occurs orally with the incubation period being 1-7 days. The organism is an invasive one; with the jejunum and ileum, being the primary sites of colonization. The pathogenesis of the illness is not clear. The motility of the organism along with the enterotoxin (similar to cholera toxin) and cytotoxin (destroying mucosal cells), appear to play a part in the pathogenesis of this disease.

In the absence of findings suggestive of infective etiology in this case (i.e., microscopic findings), what could be the differential diagnosis of this case?

A.3 Crohn's disease/Ulcerative colitis. One should never give a diagnosis of Crohn's disease or ulcerative colitis, unless infective etiology has been ruled out.

Since; when has C. jejuni been a recognized as a human pathogen?

A.4 (a) This pathogen has been recognized after 1973, as an important human gut pathogen.

Why was this important gut pathogen missed for a long time?

A.4 (b) This pathogen was missed for a long time; as selective media with special conditions of high optimal temperature of 42°C and microaerophilic conditions, weren't provided to samples; possibly infected with this pathogen.

What complications can occur in this case (with C.jenuni infection)?

A.5 Reactive arthritis and Guillain Barré syndrome (one in every 100-2000 case)

Describe the epidemiology of Campylobacteriosis.

A.6 (a)

- **Agent:** *Campylobacter jejuni*
- **Reservoir of infection:** Campylobacter infections are usually zoonotic. This organism is found in the gasotrointestinal tract of many animals used for food (as poultry, cattle and pigs) and household pets (as birds, dogs and cats).
- **Source of infection:** Food and water contaminated with this organism.
- **Mode of transmission:** It is mostly transmitted to humans by ingestion of raw or undercooked food products; as poultry, meat. It is also transmitted by ingestion of contaminated raw milk or water and by oral–anal sexual contact.
- **Host:** The infections occur worldwide, but appear to be commoner in developed countries. This information may be incorrect, as selective isolation (culture) of *C. jejuni* isn't routinely performed in the developing countries. In fact this organism wasn't a pathogen before 1973, as specific conditions for its isolation were not being provided. The infection occur in all age groups, however the attack rates are highest amongst young children and adults.

How can Campylobacteriosis be prevented?

A.6 (b) Since Campylobacter infections are zoonotic, animal products should be thoroughly cooked and good personal hygiene should be kept.

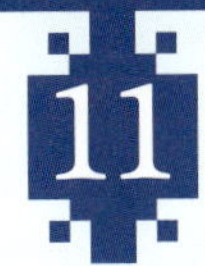

Integrated Clinical Based Study of *C. jejuni*/Guillain Barré Syndrome

A 30 year Indian male, Shailender presented with weakness of lower limbs, starting in lower legs and extending to thighs. His detailed history revealed three weeks back, an episode of febrile bloody diarrhea associated with vomiting.

Linkages: Pg. 297

What is the likely clinical diagnosis in this case?
(assuming a relationship between his past history of disease and presenting complaints)

A.1 Guillain-Barré syndrome.

What are the pathogens associated with Guillain-Barré syndrome?

A.2 *Campylobacter jejuni*, *Mycoplasma pneumoniae*, HHV-5 (Cytomegalovirus), Epstein Barr virus, and some vaccines (as swine influenza and older rabies type).

Section VIII: Gram Negative Bacilli–Curved/Spiral Shaped

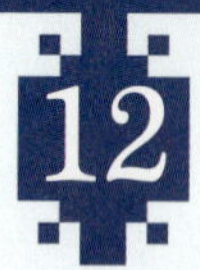

12 Integrated Clinical Based Study of *H.pylori*/Peptic Ulcer

An 45 year old male company executive, Anil complained of dyspepsia and long standing discomfort in upper abdominal areas that radiated above to the chest. An oesophagogastroduodenoscopy was performed, which revealed a gastric ulcer. A biopsy taken from the edge of the ulcer, revealed spiral shaped organisms.

Linkages: Pg. 294-297, 315, 316

Which bacterium is associated with peptic ulcer?

A.1 (a) *Helicobacter pylori.*

Why has the relationship between organism and G.U. described as an association and not as a causal relationship?

A.1 (b) The relationship between this organism and peptic ulcer, has been described as an association and not as causal relationship; as cases with gastric colonization with this organism exist, who don't have gastric ulcer.

Who is credited with the discovery of H.pylori?

A.2 (a) Robin Warren and J. Marshall in 1981 from Australia.

Why did it take a long period to discover an organism form upper gut lesions, which had been existing for many decades?

A.2 (b) *Helicobacter pylori* is an fastidious organism which requires specific environment for its growth, which include microaerophilic condition, high humidity and increased carbon dioxide concentration; besides prolonged incubation of many days for its growth. Such conditions wouldn't be routinely provided for cultivation of samples.

Student cartoon two

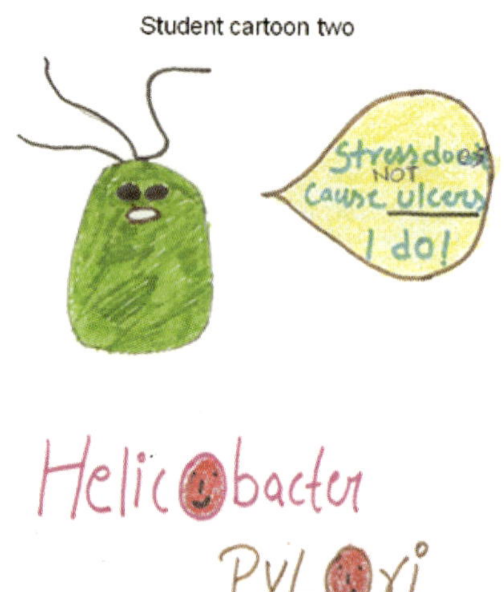

Rashmi meena

Highlight the importance of the discovery of H.pylori.

A.2 (c) For a long time, it was a firm belief with the medical fraternity, that etiology of peptic ulcer was related to the personality of the individual (usually type A) and required administration of antacids for its resolution. The work of Warren & Marshall challenged this concept. So; entrenched was this belief that Marshall had to infect himself with this organism (and then cure it by antimicrobials) and R. Warren had to face ridicule of his colleagues, for postulating this microbe-disease relationship. For their unique work, these two were awarded Nobel prize in 2005.

What is the gold standard for establishing infection with H. pylori from an ulcer site?

A.3 (a) Isolating (culturing) *H. pylori* in a culture from a gastric biopsy specimen would be the 'gold standard'

Describe breath test for H.pylori.

A.3 (b) **Principle:** Urea labeled with isotope of Carbon given orally to patient. If patient's stomach has *H.pylori*, then urea broken down and carbon-dioxide (with labelled isotope) appears in patient's breath.

Procedure: Isotope of carbon may be radioactive(14C) or a non-radioactive isotope(13C).

Commonly the non-radioactive isotope is used, as it is easy to handle. The labeled CO2 is detected in the breath by spectroscopic techniques.

Advantages: The test using the non-radioactive isotope is as simple, sensitive, specific, non-invasive and easy to perform technique, which is occasionally used for monitoring of treatment(test becomes negative with improvement)

What are the properties of H.pylori that allows it to exist in the inhospitable environment of the stomach?

A.4 (i) Production of enzyme urease; this enzyme is actively synthesized by this organism, even at low pH of gastric juice. This enzyme catalyzes the hydrolysis of urea, which is thought to raise the pH of the microenvironment, resulting in improved *H. pylori* survival.

(ii) The presence of multiple unipolar flagella, helps this organism to move in the thick mucous coat of the stomach.

(iii) Presence of 'cag' [cytotoxin associated gene] pathogenicity island, which codes for certain 'cag' proteins, associated with causing inflammation in stomach.

Describe the epidemiology of peptic ulcer associated with H.pylori.

A.5 The only reservoir of *H. pylori* is man. The transmission of the infection occurs from person to person, whether the route is oral-oral or fecal-oral isn't known. The seroprevalence rate of this infection in developing countries is approximately 80% in contrast to 30% in developed countries. Crowding appears to facilitate the spread of infection. The other risk factors for this infection are low socioeconomic status and poor hygiene. Many of the infected individuals are asymptomatic.

Does colonization with H.pylori offer any possible advantage to man?

A.6 Individuals infected with *H.pylori* are reported to have decreased association with gastroesophageal reflux disease (GERD) and adenocarcinoma of esophagus.

What is the treatment regimen for duodenal ulcer?

A.7 See chapter 13, pg. 316

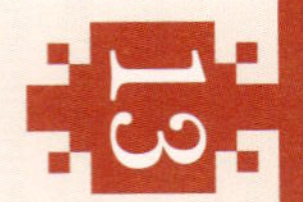

13 Laboratory Diagnosis and Treatment (Overview)

An Overview of the Comparative Approach in Laboratory Diagnosis of Key Gram Negative Bacilli-Curved/Spiral

Organism / Disease	Specimen	Direct Demonstration of Organism in Specimen Wet mount	Stain enhanced microscopy	Detection of Microbial Antigen/ Metabolite/ Genome	Serological Tests	Culture of Organisms In Media/Characteriza-tion and Confirmation of Isolate	Differential Diagnosis	Antimicrobial Susceptibility Tests
Treponema pallidum (Syphilis)	**Primary** • Exudate from ulcer etc • Aspirate from lymph node • Serum **Secondary** • Exudate/ secretion from lesions as on skin, Serum **Latent** • Serum **Tertiary** • Serum • CSF **Congenital** • Exudate/ secretion from lesion, • serum	Dark ground microscopy can demonstrate spirochaetes morphology & motility It has slow motility & has 10 spirals occurring regularly, sharply. Phase contrast microscopy can also demonstrate the organism's motility	With Gram staining, does not get stained. Silver impregnation techniques; as Fontana's method can demonstrate it Giemsa stain can also demonstrate it	-	Mainstay* of diagnosis, but the most specific test is direct demonstration of treponemes by Dark ground microscopy in exudate. 2 Forms **Non treponemal tests** • Screening test, lacks specificity • Monitor treatment (by titre estimation) • Can detect reinfection **Treponemal** • Confirm results of non-treponemal tests • Can detect latent syphilis & other cases, where non-treponemal tests are negative/ Details: A8, p. 301, A2e, p. 303	Not cultivable even in animate media, though virulent *T.pallidum* can be maintained by serial passage in rabbit testes	*T.pallidum* sub sps *pertenue* (causes Yaws) *T.carateum* (causes Pinta) *T.microdentium* *T.mucosum* [has lashing motility & lack uniform spirals at 1 µm]	- Cannot perform this, as can't be cultivated - Drug resistance reported
T.pallidum subsps endemicum, pertenue and T.carateum	Skin lesion, oral lesion and others	Dark ground microscopy		-	VDRL and RPR often employed. Consider in persons with symptoms in an endemic area or who as emigrated from endemic area	-	-	-
Borrelia recurrentis (Relapsing fever) Disease forms: • Tick borne • Louse borne	• Blood • Serum	Dark ground microscopy or phase contrast microscopy can demonstrate borrelia in blood (lashing motility)	Gram staining: Not stained by it Giemsa/ Leishman: can demonstrate it	-	C.F.T (earliest to become +ve) Indirect immunofluorescent test ELISA Immunoblot (proposed, as method for confirming diagnosis), specific IgM antibodies develop within 3-6 weeks	Primary isolation can be done by inoculating blood intraperitoneally into rat/mice and making smears from tail blood, after 2nd day, daily for about 2 weeks No role of even animate media in diagnosis as process difficult. Following available: Noguchi's medium (ascitic fluid containing rabbit kidney) Can support on Chorioallantoic membrane of chick embryo	Treponemes	-

Contd.

Contd.

Borrelia burgdorferi: • Early stage - Skin lesion • 2nd and 3rd stage (disseminated)	Rarely from skin lesion demonstrated	-	-	-	ELISA and IIF Specific antibodies appear after few months Serological diagnosis mainstay	Culture is difficult, as slow growing	-	-
Borrelia vincentii	Exudate from lesion	-	-	-	Not performed	Technique available, but difficult	-	-
Leptospira interrogans	In man - Blood - C.S.F - Urine - Body fluids - Serum In Animal: Kidney pieces (culture) Serum For water, shaved & scarified area of skin of a young guinea pig is immersed in water for 1hr	- Various fluids can be examined by dark-ground microscopy for Leptospires (urine may be alkalinized to prevent lysis of Leptospira by acidic urine) - In blood, leptospires can be demonstrated in 1st week, but sensitivity and specificity of technique is low - Gram staining not stained Giemsa/Silver impregnation technique can demonstrate the organism			Serological tests are essentially useful in diagnosis. The specific antibodies appear in the serum at end of first week, reach a peak and then decline after a month. Screening tests are genus specific and antigen based and includes ELISA, IFAT and rapid dip stick assay. Microscopic agglutination test: [(Live) Antigen mixed with serum & looked on card for agglutination Macroscopic agglutination: (formalinised) antigen mixed with serum & looked on card for agglutination C.F.T (not as sensitive) as agglutination **Note** : for these tests, antigens prevalent in area are tested. Serogroups & serotyping can be done using different types of antisera	Culture of specimens performed only in reference Labs Several liquid and semi solid media enriched with blood serum are available Commercially available are Korthof's, Stuart's, Fletcher's & E.M.J.H (growth occurs few mms below surface) Ellinghausen, McCullough, Johnson & Harrison (has bovine serum albumin fraction - V & polysorbate (Tween 80) - Chorioallantoic membrane of chick embryo can be used - Several laboratory animals as Guinea-pigs, hamster used - Identification of Leptospires isolates is done by agglutination with type specific (serotype specific) antisera	-	-
Helicobacter pylori	Biospy: duodenal : gastric Gastric aspirate Serum	Dark ground microscopy or phase contrast microscopy can demonstrate the organism	Gram staining can demonstrate organism	- Biopsy* urease test - Breath test (A 3b, 312)	Specific antibodies present in serum and gastric aspirate * Biopsy put in urea solution and urease activity detected	Blood agar (+) For isolation, selective media need to be cultured in microaerophilic conditions with high humidity and prolonged incubation (3-5 days)		
Campylobacter jejuni	• Stool • Serum	Dark ground or phase contrast microscopy can demonstrate organism	Gram staining can demonstrate organism	-	C.F.T E.L.I..S.A is currently used in aseptic arthritis & syndromes due to campylobacter	Blood agar + For isolation, selective media need to be cultured in microaerophilic conditions at high temperature (42°C) and prolonged incubation (up to 48 hrs.)	*C.fetus* *C.coli* *C.laridis*	

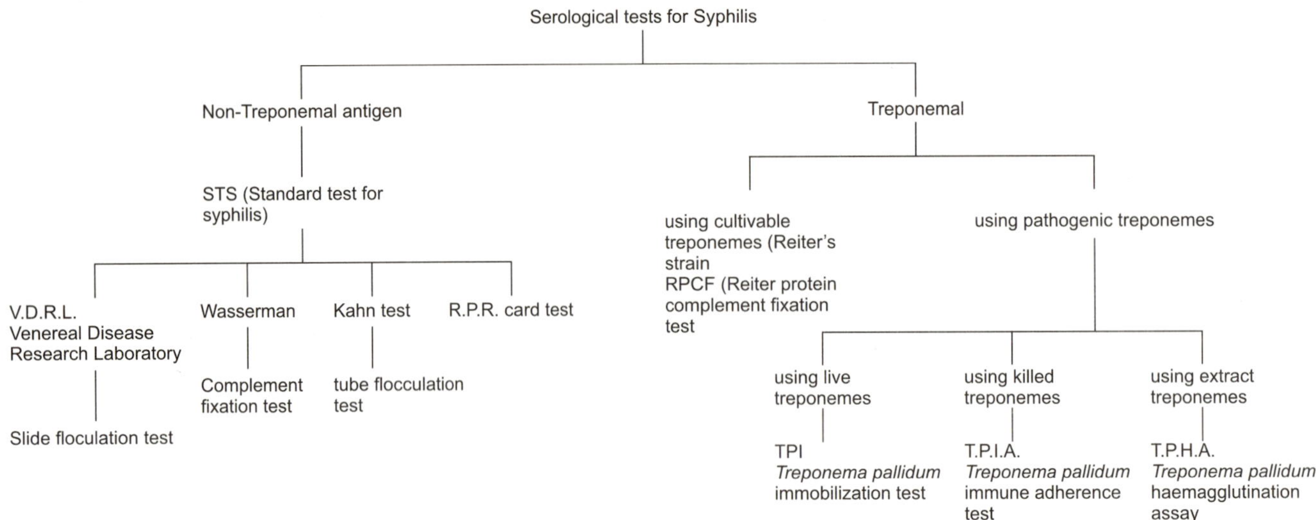

An Overview of the Antimicrobial Options for Infections Caused by Key Gram Negative Bacilli - Curved/Spiral

	Cell Wall Inhibitors	**Cell-Membrane Inhibitors**	**Amino Acid Synthesis Inhibitors**	**Nucleic Acid Synthesis Inhibitors**	**Others**
Leptospira interrogans	• PnG (DOC)		• Doxycycline		
Borrelia recurrentis	• PnG		• Doxycycline (DOC)		
B. burgdorferi	• Amoxycilin (DOC) • Cefuroxime (DOC) • Ceftriaxone • PnG		• Doxycycline (DOC) • Azithromycin • Clarithromycin		
Borrelia vincentii	• Pn G (oral hygiene)				
Treponema pallidum subspecies pallidum	• PnG (DOC) • Ceftriaxone		• Erythromycin (in penicillin allergic cases) • Doxycycline		
T. pallidum subsps endemicum	• PnG				
T. pallidum subsps pertenue	• PnG (DOC)				
Helicobacter pylori	• Triple combinations (including one proton pump inhibitor) [Amoxicillin+		Clarithromycin +	Omperazole](DOC)	
			[Tetracycline +	Metronidazole +	Bismuth subsalicylate]
			[Clarithromycin + Tetracycline		Bismuth subsalicylate]
Campylobacter jejuni	Resistant to penicllin and cephalosporins		• Erythromycin (DOC) • Azithromycin (DOC) • Tetracycline • Chloramphenicol		
C. fetus	• Ampicillin • Ceftriaxone		• Gentamicin • Ciprofloxacin		
S.minus	• PnG		• Tetracyline		

NB: DOC refers to drug of choice

14 Assessment/Examination Questions

1. Classify spirochaetes. Describe the morphology and cultural characteristics of *T. pallidum.* P. 294, 295, 297
2. Enumerate the sexually transmitted diseases and enumerate infectious diseases of genital tract that are transmitted non-sexually. P. 582 and A5., p. 300
3. Describe the epidemiology of syphilis with special reference to men who have sex with men (MSM). A 6., p. 300
4. Why it is important to study the antigenic characteristic of *T. pallidum*? Describe its non-specific and specific antigens. A 2b., p. 302
5. Describe the clinical profile of syphilis. A 7., p. 300
6. Describe laboratory diagnosis of primary syphilis. P. 314 and see chapter 5., p. 302-303
7. Describe Standard tests for syphilis (STS), VDRL test and Rapid plasma regain test (RPR). A 8., p. 301
8. Describe *T. pallidum* specific tests including TPHA and FTA-ABS test. A 2e., p. 303, p. 301
9. Describe congenital syphilis. P. 302-303
10. What are the approaches and challenges in the diagnosis of congenital syphilis? A 2d., p. 302-303
11. Describe the treatment of the infant with congenital syphilis (including parents). A 5b., p. 303 and p. 316
12. Describe Lyme disease. P. 297 and p. 309
13. Describe non-venereal treponematoses. P. 305
14. Compare and contrast the clinical profile of three forms of non-venereal treponematoses (i.e., Endemic syphilis, Yaws and Pinta). P. 305
15. Describe Leptospirosis (Weil's disease). A 3., p. 306
16. Describe the epidemiology of Leptospirosis with special reference to the Indian subcontinent. A3., p. 306
17. What approach is commonly used to diagnose cases of Leptospirosis? Describe the serological test considered 'gold standard' in the diagnosis of this entity? A4a., p. 307, A4b., p. 307
18. Describe Relapsing fever. P. 308
19. Compare the morphology of *B. recurrentis* and Leptospira A 1b., p. 308
20. How is Borrelia able to evade the human immune response and cause recurrent fever? A 2., p. 308
21. Compare and contrast the two types of relapsing fever. A3., p. 308
22. Describe *Campylobacter jejuni.* P. 294-297, 310-311
23. Describe laboratory diagnosis of diarrohea caused by *C. jejuni.* P. 315, 310-311
24. Describe *Helicobacter pylori.* P. 294-297, p. 312-313
25. What are the properties of *H. pylori* that allows it to exist in the inhospitable environment of the stomach? A4., p. 313
26. Describe the role of biopsy urease test and urea breath test in the diagnosis of *Helicobacter pylori* infection. P. 66, 315, p. 296, A 3b., p. 312

Section IX: Gram Negative Bacilli–Fastidious

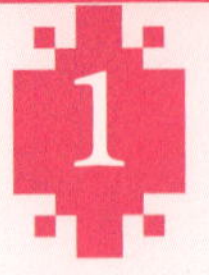

Classification, Metabolic and Microscopic Features of Key Gram Negative Bacilli–Fastidious

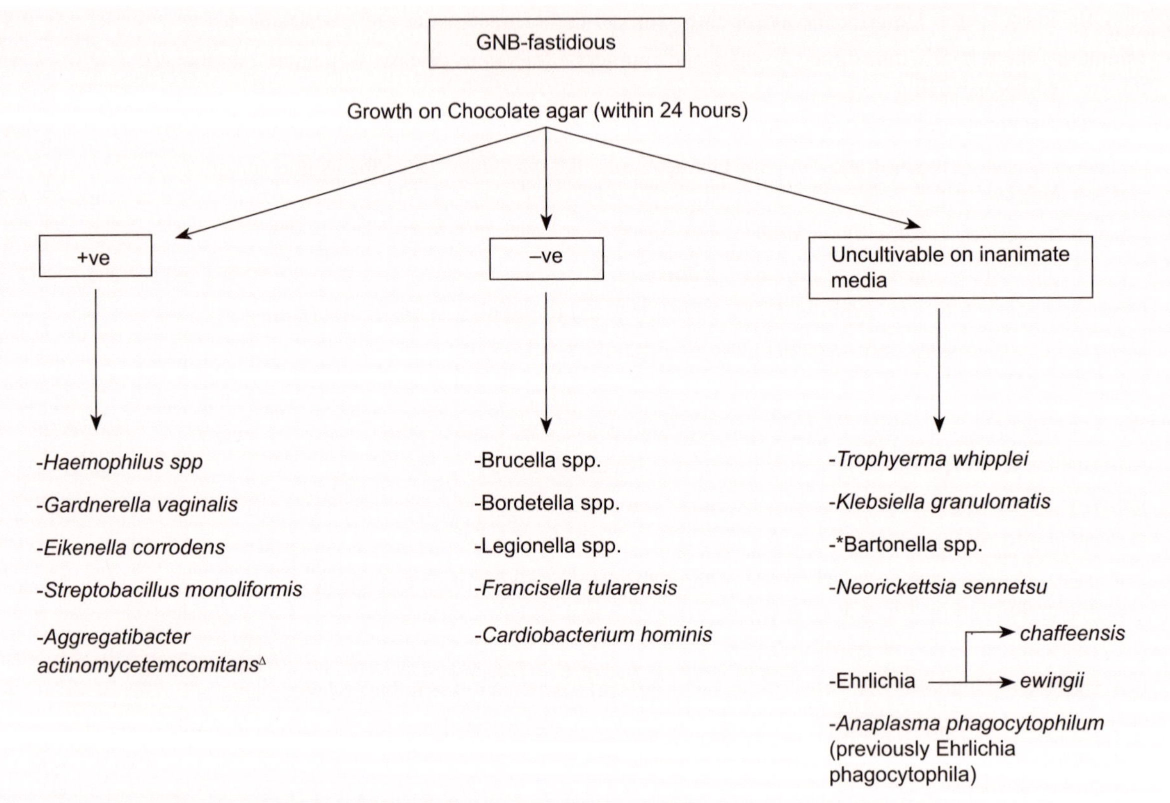

NB: *Three species of Bartonella can grow on Blood agar/Chocolate agar but takes many days to weeks for growth.
∆ Previously named as *Actinobacillus actinomycetemcomitans*

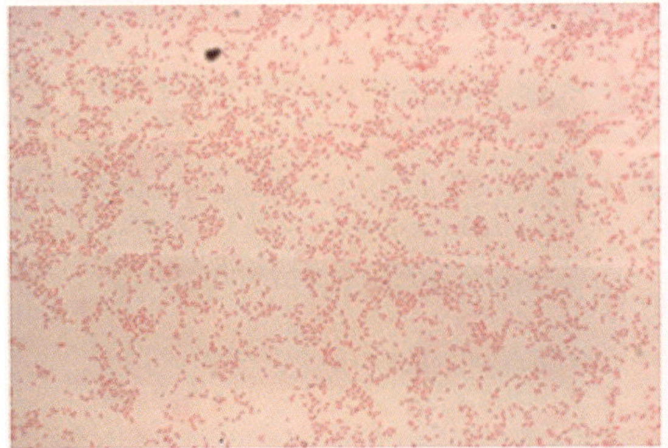

Fig. 9.1.1: Cocco-bacilli: Gram stained smear of Brucella spp.

Courtesy: Dr. W, A. Clark/CDC

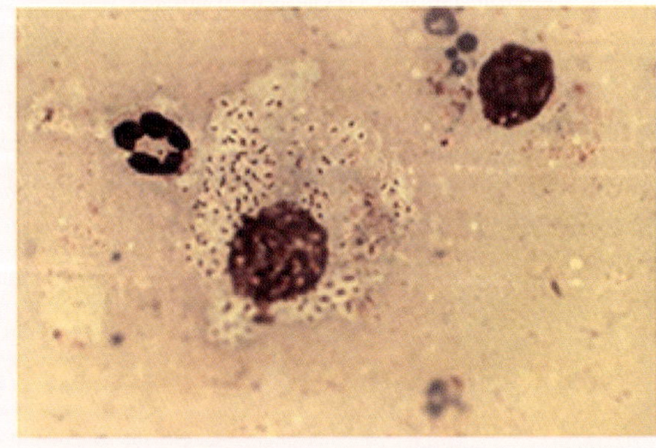

Fig. 9.1.2: DONOVAN BODIES: White blood cells containing pathognomic Donovan bodies (encapsulated gram-negative bodies; *Klebsiella granulomatis*, formerly designated *Calymmatobacterium granulomatis*)

Courtesy: Susan Lindsey/CDC

Metabolic and microscopic features of gram negative bacilli - fastidious

Organism	*GROWTH REQUIREMENTS*						*CELLULAR MORPHOLOGY AND STAINING CHARACTERISTICS*						
	O2 Requ.	*Optimal Temp.*	*CO2 Requ..*	*Incubation Period*			*Shape*	*Gram*	*Arrangement*	*Capsule*	*Motility*	*Spore*	*Special Staining / microscopy / Special Features*
				Days	*Weeks*	*Months*							
Haemophilus influenzae	Aerobic and Facultative anaerobic	37°C	+	1-2	-	-	Coccobacilli	-ve / stains with difficulty)	-	+ (some virulent strains)	-	-	-
H. ducreyi	Aerobic and Facultative anaerobic	37°C	+	1-3	-	-	Short ovoid bacillus	-ve	In pairs or short chains (smear may show `school of fish`apperance	-	-	-	Bipolar staining seen
Other Haemophilus species	Aerobic and Facultative anaerobic	37°C	-	1-2			Coccobacilli	-ve	-	-	-	-	-
Gardnerella vaginalis	Facultative anaerobic	37°C	+	2	-	-	Bacilli (pleomorphic)	Gram Variable to Gram –ve	Palisading may occur, bifurcating cells common	-	-	-	Albert's stain shows metachromatic granule
Bordetella pertusis	Aerobic	35°C	+	2-3	-	-	Coccobacilli / minute rods (Fig. 9.1.1)	-ve	Singly / in pairs, occasionally in filamentous forms	+ (young cultures)	-	-	Toludine Blue staining shows bipolar metachromatic granules
B. parapertusis	Aerobic	37°C	-	1-2	-	-	Coccobacilli/ minute rods	-ve	-	-	-	-	-
B. brochiseptica	Aerobic	37°C	-	1	-	-	Coccobacilli/ minute rods	-ve	-	-	+	-	-
Brucella sps.	Aerobic	37°C	+	1-3	-	-	Coccobacilli (small)	-ve	-	-	-	-	-
Francisella tularensis	Strictly aerobic	37°C	-	3-5	-	-	Coccobacilli	- ve	-	+	-	-	-
Legionella pneumophila	Strictly aerobic	35°C	-	3-5	-	-	Bacilli (Very pleomorphic)	- ve (stains poorly)	Filaments may be seen	-	+	-	Dieterle stain (silver impregnation tech.)
Eikenella corrodens	Facultative anaerobic	37°C	+	4-5	-	-	Bacilli (small)	- ve	-	-	+	-	-
Bartonella quintana	Strictly aerobic	35-37°C	+	-	Few	-	Rods slightly curved	-ve	-	-	-	-	-
Bartonella bacilliformis	Strictly aerobic	25°C	-	4-5	-	-	Rods (pleomorphic)	- ve	-	-	+	-	-
Bartonella henselae	Aerobic	35-37°C	+	5-15 days			bacilli		-	-	twitching motility	-	-
Ehrilchia chaffenesis	Obligate intra-cellular bacteria	Can not be cultivated in inanimate media											
Ehrichia ewingii	Obligate intra-cellular bacteria	Can not be cultivated in inanimate media											
Neorickettsia sennetsu	Obligate intra-cellular bacteria	Can not be cultivated in inanimate media											
Anaplasma phagocytophilum	Obligate intra-cellular bacteria	Can not be cultivated in inanimate media											
Streptobacillus moniliformis	Aerobic and Facultative anaerobic	37°C	+	2	-	-	Coccobacilli, (very Pleomorphic) (as chains & intertwining wavy filaments)	-ve	'String of beads' appearance, hence spp. name monoliformis	-	-	-	-
Cardiobacterium hominis	Aerobic and Facultative anaerobic	37°C	+	1-2			Coccobacilli (pleomorphic)	-	-	-	-	-	-
Aggregatibacter actinomycetemcomitans	Facultative anaerobic	37°C	-	Few days			coccobacilli	-ve	-	-	-	-	-
Klebsiella granulomatis (Donovania granulomatis)	Not cultivable easily on inanimate media, cultivable on animate media; as yolk sac						Cocobacilli (safety pin appearance) because of bipolar condensation of chromatin	- ve	-	+	-	-	Giemsa/Wright stain-pink capsule around blue bacillus,often as donovan bodies(when present in phagosome) (Fig. 9.1.2)
Tropheryma whipplei	Not cultivable on inanimate media						Characteristic not known, organism identified; following PCR amplification of 16S ribosomal RNA						Periodic acid Schiff stain of tissue reveal PAS +ve material in vacuole which are intracellular material

2 An Overview of the Media Requirements, Colonial Characters and Diagnostic Characteristics of Key Gram Negative Bacilli-Fastidious

	Basal media	Enriched media	Selective/others	Characterization and confirmation of isolate
Haemophilus influenzae	NA: NG	• BA plate with *S. aureus* streak: + • Chocolate agar: + (tiny transparent colonies) • Nutrient agar plate with X & V strips: + • Levinthal's, medium (prepared by boiling & filtering mixture of blood & NA): + (iridescent colonies) • Filde's agar: + (peptic digest of blood and NA)	MacConkey: NG	• Microscopic features: gram variable/ negative coccobacilli • Satellitism (Fig. 9.2.1) • Subculture of isolate to plate with X & V strip (Fig. 9.2.2) • Reduce nitrate to nitrite • Variable carbohydrate fermentation • Porphyrin test: tests the ability strain to convert-d-aminolevulinic acid to porphyrin • S-R transformation associated with loss of virulence • Serotypes a – f (depending on capsular antigen) • 8 biotypes I-VIII (on basis of urea, indole & ornithine decarboxylase activity) • 4 phages reported for *H. influenzae* types
Other Haemophilus sps (vary in their X and V requirement)				
Haemophilus ducreyi	NA: NG	• BA: + [10% CO2 and high humidity] • Chocolate agar with 1% isovitalex and vancomycin	• MacConkey: NG • Can be cultivated on chorioallantoic membrane	• Microscopic features; 'School of fish' appearance • Mostly biochemically inert
Gardnerella vaginalis (Clue cell, Fig. 9.2.3)	NA: NG	• BA: + (beta haemolytic colonies) • Chocolate agar: +	MacConkey: NG	• Microscopic features • Catalase test: –ve • Oxidase test: –ve • Hippurate hydrolysis test: +ve
Bordetella pertusis	• NA: NG *B. parapertusis* and *B. bronchiseptica* can grow	• BA: NG (usually) • B.G. glycerol potato blood agar: +ve [Fig. 9.2.4]	• MacConkey: NG (other Bordetella sps. can grow)	• Microscopic features • Toluidene blue staining- bipolar metachromatic granules • Catalase & oxidase +ve • Biochemically inactive, does not ferment sugars • Serotyping – based on capsular antigen has role in epidemiologic studies • Animal pathogenicity test- mice highly susceptible to intracerebral inoculation. Procedure used to test effectiveness of vaccine. Intranasal inoculation results in interstitial pneumonia

Contd.

Contd.

Brucella species	- NA: very slow grower	• BA: + • Trypticase soy agar and broth: +, Castaneda's medium (Fig. 9.2.5) • Liver infusion agar: + • Albimi agar:+	MacConkey: NG	• Microscopic features (gram negative cocco-bacilli) • Catalase, oxidase & urease +ve • Other biochemical characteristics • Utilize carbohydrates but produce acid not in sufficient amount for classification • Species differentiation done by antisera, phages, H_2S production and sensitivity to dyes
Francisella tularensis	NA: NG	• BA: ± (may grow) • Francis cystine Dextrose BA:+	MacConkey: NG	• Microscopic: gram negative cocco-bacilli
Legionella pneumophila	NA: NG	• BA: NG • CA: NG	• MacConkey: NG • BCYE: + (Buffered charcoal yeast extract agar)	• Stains poorly with Gram stain • Catalase +ve • Oxidase +ve • Hydrolyzes hippurate
Eikenella corrodens	NA: NG	• BA/CA: + (pitting colonies)	• MacConkey: NG	• Microscopic features • Catalase –ve • Oxidase +ve • Carbohydrates not fermented
Streptobacillus monoliformis	NA: NG	• BA: NG • Media supplemented with blood and serum:+ • Loeffler serum slope:+	MacConkey: NG	• Microscopic features • Catalase –ve • Oxidase –ve • Glucose fermented producing acid only • Generally biochemically inert
Cardiobacterium hominis	NA: NG	• BA: +	MacConkey: NG	• Catalase –ve • Oxidase +ve • Ferments sugars • Indole +ve • Nitrate reduction test +ve
Klebsiella granulomatis (Calymmatobacterium donovania)	NA: NG	• BA: NG • Egg - Yolk medium:+	• MacConkey: NG • Yolk sac of embryonated egg:+	• Microscopic features (not demonstrable with gram stain but with Giemsa stain)
Aggregatibacter actinomycetem-comitans	NA: NG	• BA: + (non-haemolytic)	• MacConkey: NG	• Microscopic features • Catalase +ve • Nitrate +ve • Glucose Fermented, but not lactose and sucrose
Tropheryma whipplei	Not cultivable			
Bartonella quintana	NA: NG	• BA: +ve (1-2 weeks incubation required)	• MacConkey: NG • Yolk sac of embryonated egg: poor growth • Xenodiagnosis -demonstrate in lice, after it is allowed to feed on patient's blood	• Microscopic features
Bartonella bacilliformis	NA: NG	• BA: NG • NA: +ve [containing rabbit serum and haemoglobin]	MacConkey: NG	-
Bartonella henselae	NA: NG	• BA: NG • CA: +ve	MacConkey: NG	-
Ehrlichia chaffeensis	NA: NG	-	Cultivable on macrophage cell lines, a research tool	-

NG-No growth, NA-Nutrient agar, BA-Blood agar, CA-Choclate agar

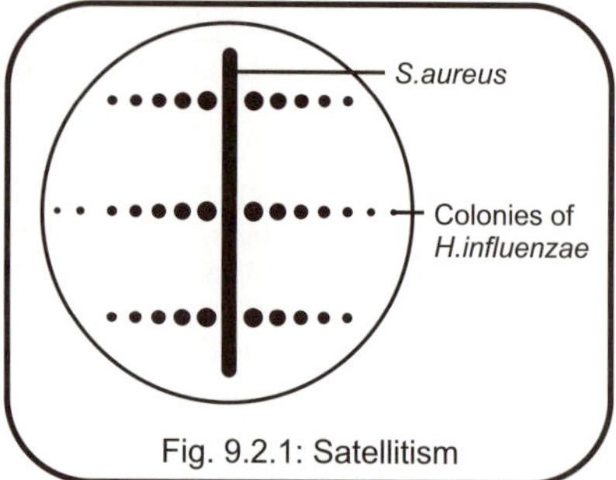

Fig. 9.2.1: Satellitism

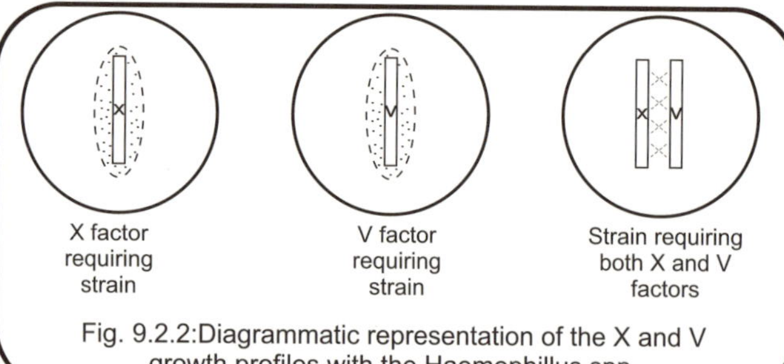

Fig. 9.2.2:Diagrammatic representation of the X and V growth profiles with the Haemophillus spp.

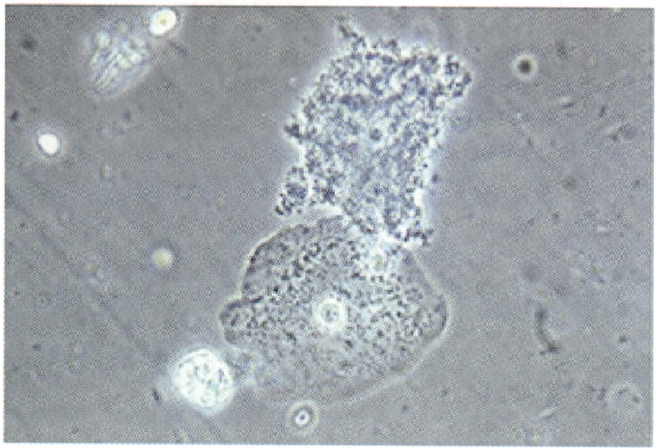

Fig. 9.2.3: CLUE CELL: Epithelial cell (here vaginal smear) with its external surface covered with bacteria, giving a stippled appearance. Finding suggestive of bacterial vaginosis.

Courtesy: M. Rein/CDC

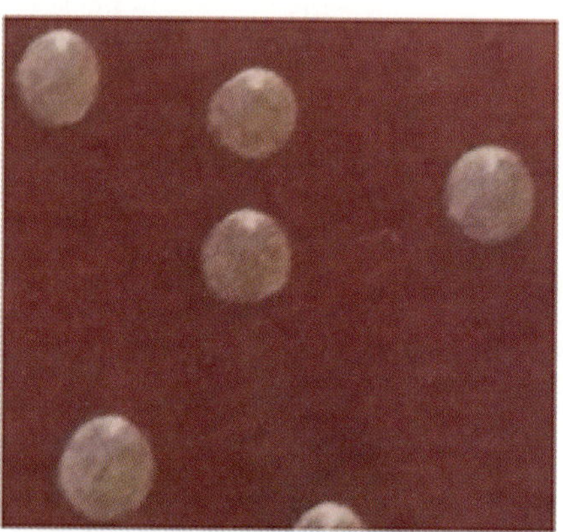

Fig. 9.2.4: Pertussis: Colonies of *B. pertussis* on Bordet gengou medium

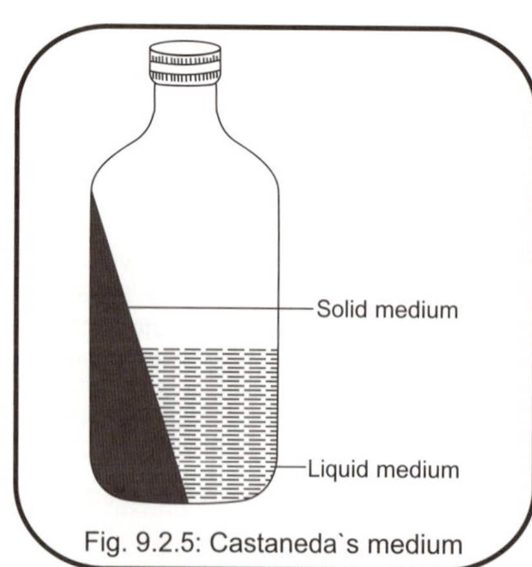

Fig. 9.2.5: Castaneda`s medium

Clinical (Pathogenicity) Profile of Infections Caused By Gram Negative Bacilli–Fastidious

Contd.

Haemophilus influenzae	In children, usually invasive infections (caused by capsulate strains); as meningitis, acute epiglottitis, cellulitis, arthritis and others • Details see pg. 325-326	
	In adults usually non invasive infections (caused by non capsulate strains) as otitis media, sinusitis, exacerbation of chronic bronchitis	
Other Haemophi lus species as parainfluenzae, haemolyticus, aprophilus	Associated with systemic infections; as endocarditis, meningitis, arthritis and pneumonia	
H. ducreyi	Chancroid (soft sore) (Fig. 9.3.1), Bubo.	
*H. aegyptius**	Conjunctivitis *also known as Koch-Weeks bacillus	
Gardnerella vaginalis	Associated with bacterial vaginosis (along with other bacteria)	
Bordetella pertusis	Whooping cough, 3 stages (Fig. 9.3.2) (i) Catarrahal (resembles common cold) (ii) Paroxysmal (paroxysms of cough)_this stage associated with complications; as secondary infections (pneumonia, otitis media), subconjunctival haemorrhage, etc. (iii) Convalescence (recovery) • Details see pg. 329-330	
B. parapertusis	Milder presentation (responsible for about 5% of whooping cough)	
B.brochiseptica	Responsible for about 0.1% of whooping cough	
Brucella sps.	Brucellosis (Undulant fever/Mediterranean fever/Malta fever) • Details see pg 327-328	
	- Acute brucellosis_fever sometimes associated with splenomegaly, hepatomegaly, and lymphadenopathy	
	- Subclinical (latent infection)_no symptoms, only serologically detectable	
	- Chronic brucellosis_when disease persists for more than 6 months	
Francisella tularensis	Tularemia,commonly presents as 3 types (i) Ulceroglandular form (following bite, most common) (ii) Typhoidal form (following ingestion) (iii) Pneumonia form (following inhalation)	
Legionella pneumophila	• Legionnaires disease (pneumonic illness) • Details pg 331-332 • Pontiac fever	
Eikenella corrodens	Opportunistic infections; as dental, peridontal, sinusitis, pneumonia, meningitis, wound infections (following human bite)	
Bartonella quintana	Trench fever	
Bartonella bacilliformis	• Oroya fever • Details A 6., p. 334 • Veruga peruana	
Bartonella henselae	Cat-scratch disease (details pg. 333-334)	
Neorickettsia sennetsu	Human monocytic ehrilichiosis	[- Senettsu ehrilichiosis, resembles glandular fever, seen in Japan and Malaysia, details page A.4, pg 335-336]
Ehrilchia chaffeensis	Human monocytic ehrichiosis (febrile illness with leucopaenia, thrombocytopaenia, lymphadenopathy, rash (40%), No eschar • Details A4, pg 335-336	
Ehrichia ewingll	Human monocytic ehrichiosis • Details see A4, 335-336	

Contd.

Contd.

Anaplasma phalgocytophilum	- Anaplasmosis (previously Human granulocytic ehrlichiosis)	[febrile illness with leucopenia, thrombocytopaenia, lymphadenopathy, no eschar or rash details. see A.4, pg. 335-336]
Streptobacillus moniliformis	Rat bite fever	
Cardiobacterium monoliformis	Rare cause of endocarditis, meningitis.	
Aggregatibacter actinomycetemc-omitans (Actinobacillus actinomycetemc-omitans)	Associated with SABE, periodontal disease, osteomyelitis and abscesses	
Klebsiella granulomatis (Donovania granulomatis)	Granuloma inguinale (Fig. 9.3.3)	
Tropheryma whipplei	Whipple's disease	

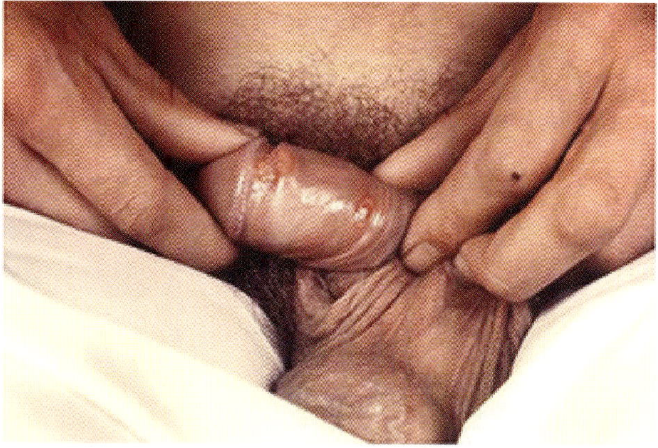

Fig.9.3.1: CHANCROID: Penile lesion caused by Haemophilus ducreyi

Courtesy: Dr. Pirozzi/CDC

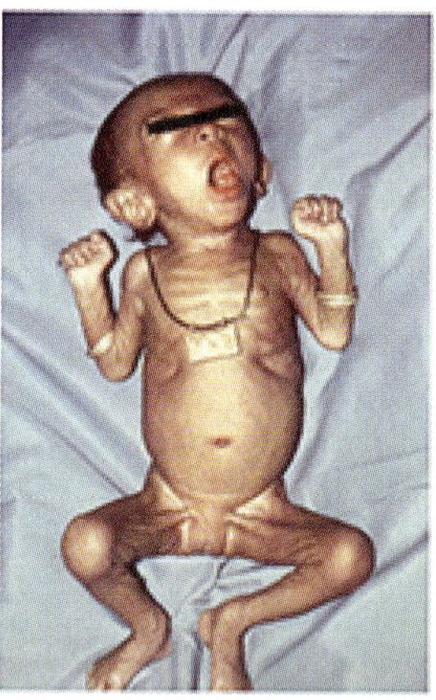

Fig.9.3.2: PERTUSIS: A female patient suffering from pertusis.

Courtesy: Centers for control and prevention, Atlanta, USA

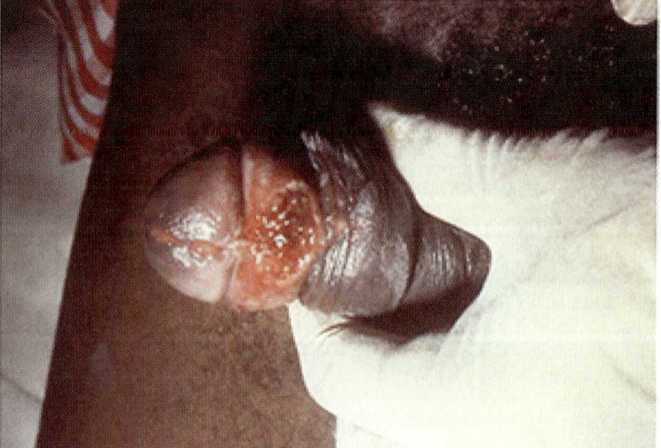

Fig.9.3.3: DONOVANOSIS: Case with granuloma (Donovanosis) of penis. These cases have Donovan bodies (intracellular bacteria) intracellularly.

Courtesy: Dr. Tabua, Joe Miller/CDC

Integrated Clinical Based Study of *H. influenzae*/Meningitis

A 14 month child, Shalu is brought to the paediatric emergency with complaints of fever and vomiting. Physical examination revealed neck rigidity. CSF examination revealed increased polymorph count, increased protein level and decreased glucose level. Gram stain of CSF demonstrated gram negative coccobacilli. On culture, no growth occurred on blood agar, however small colonies were demonstrated on chocolate agar.

Linkages: Pg. 318-321, 323, 337, 338

What is the clinical diagnosis in this case?

A.1 (a) Acute meningitis.

Which pathogen is likely to be the causative agent in this case?

A.1 (b) The pathogen is likely to be *H. influenzae*.

Enumerate other bacteria that have coccobacillary morphology.

A.1 (c) Bordetella spp., Brucella spp., Rickettsia spp. and Francisella spp.

Comment on the derivation of 'Haemophilus influenzae'.

A.1 (d) Haemo (blood) and philus (love) indicate that the organism is 'blood loving' or grows on enriched media; as choclate agar. 'Influenzae' term is associated with this organism; as in the 1892 Influenza pandemic, it was isolated from the sputum of cases and falsely thought to be the etiological agent of those cases.

What are the key factors required for growth of H. influenzae? Compare and contrast them.

A.1 (e) X and V factors

Table 9.4.1: Characteristics of X and V factors

	X	V
Composition	Hemin or other iron containing porphyrins	NAD/NADP
Effect of heat	Heat stable	Heat labile
Source	Factors in blood	*S.aureus*, certain fungi
Function	Synthesis of certain iron containing enzymes as catalase, peroxidase and cytochrome oxidase	Hydrogen receptor (involved in oxidation-reduction production)
Demonstration	Using X disc (Fig. 9.2.2)	• Using V disc (Fig. 9.2.2) • Satellitism (Fig. 9.2.1)

Which type of strain is liked to be responsible, for the clinical picture of this case?

A.2 The clinical picture in the case is an invasive *H. influenzae* infection. Invasive infections are caused by six major serotypes of *H. influenzae*, namely a through f, based on capsular polysaccharide composition. Out of these, *H. influenzae* type b is the most common serotype responsible for causing invasive infections.

What is the habitat for H. influenzae? Describe.

A.3 (a) *H. influenzae* is an exclusively human pathogen, which colonizes the upper respiratory tract (throat, nasopharynx). The colonization occurs shortly after birth. In majority of the children, the colonization is with the non-capsulated strains of *H. influenzae*. In contrast to colonization with capsulated strains, is seen in less than 5% of the children.

Describe the epidemiology of H. infuenzae infections.

A.4 (b) **Agent:** *H. influenzae*

This organism has been subdivided into eight biotypes, on the basis of three biochemical reactions; namely-indole production, unease activity and ornithine decarboxylase production. On basis of capsular composition, it has been divided into six serotypes; namely a to f; of which, serotype b is mostly involved in the invasive infections. Certain biotypes are associated with some clinical syndromes, as biotype 1 with meningitis. This organism has also been phage typed into four types.

Reservoir of infection:

- It is an exclusive human pathogen. Soon after birth, the upper respiratory tract respiratory tract (throat/ nasopharynx) gets colonized with non encapsulated strains, which are non-invasive. Colonization with invasive capsular strains in seen in a minority of children. Their characteristics are depicted in table 9.4.2.

Table 9.4.2: Comparison of *H.influenzae* types

	Type b strain	**Non Capsulated (untypeable)**
- Capsule	- Ribose p-ribitol Phosphate	- Unencapsulated
- Infection	- Invasive infections; as meningitis due to haemotogenous spread	- Mucosal Infections, due to contiguous spread; as otitis media
- Vaccine	- Conjugate type available	- None

- *Mode of transmission:* It is transmitted primarily by respiratory droplets. Direct transmission occurs with secretions and fomites also plays a part

Host: The disease occurs worldwide, but the incidence of invasive infections by this organism has fallen in the developed countries, after the introduction of conjugate vaccine. This vaccine has also been introduced in the Universal immunization programme in India. The disease occurs primarily in children.

The *H. influenzae* infections are usually sporadic in nature, although outbreaks in closed populations, as day care centers have been reported.

Describe the pathogenesis of H. influenzae infections.

A.3 (c) The transmission is essentially by inhalation of infective respiratory secretion. Following the colonization of nasopharynx, the infection of the entire respiratory tract occurs. This is followed by invasion of the blood stream, which can result in systemic disease (unlike *B. pertusis* infections which are localized).

The virulent factors include:

(i) Capsular polysaccharide (loss of it leads to, loss of virulence)

(ii) Pili and outer membrane protein (required for adherence to respiratory epithelial cells)

(iii) IgA protease (cleaves IgA1)

Describe clinical picture of infections caused by non typeable H. infuenzae.

A.4 The nontypable strains of *H. influenzae* are noncapsulated and cause mucosal infections, due to contiguous spread. The clinical menifestation seen with it include otitis media in infants and children, respiratory tract infections in adults; often presenting; as chronic bronchitis.

Which rapid laboratory test could have provided a bed side specific diagnosis in this case?

A.5 (a) Latex agglutination test of the C.S.F. would have detected the capsular type b polysaccharide of *H. influenzae*.

What fallacy by the medical personnel, after CSF collection, can result in false negative culture result for H. influenzae?

A.5 (b) As the organism is sensitive to low temperature, refrigeration (temporary) of the sample can result in culture negative result.

Which sign, if was to occur in this case, would indicate a poor prognosis?

A.6 Development of petechiae on the skin would be an ominous sign, though in *H influenzae* meningitis, petechial lesions are unusual.

How could this disease have been prevented in this child? Describe an advancement in vaccine manufacture that has been recently developed.

A.7 If this child had been vaccinated with a conjugated Hib vaccine,then the child was likely to have got protected from this infection.

Originally the Hib vaccine was a unconjugated polysaccharide vaccine, which comprised of polyribosyl ribitol phosphate (PRP) capsular polysaccharide. The disadvantage of this vaccine was that it was poorly immunogenic and wasn't effective in infants. To overcome this disadvantage conjugate vaccines have been synthesized, in which the PRP capsule is linked to a carrier protein. This carrier protein can be a diphtheria toxoid or a tetanus toxoid.

In USA, a substantial proportion of children population has been vaccinated with Hib vaccine. What change has been seen in the epidemiology of haemophilus infections caused by H.influenzae, as a result of this intervention?

A.8 (a) The other serotypes of *H. influenzae* (beside Hib) have taken over the ecological niche of the Hib in the body, resulting in rise of infections due to other serotypes of *H. influenzae*.

What is unique about the sequencing of H. influenzae?

A.8 (b) It was the first free living organism to be completely sequenced in 1996.

Integrated Clinical Based Study of Brucella/FUO

An army Jawan, Subedar Singh; presented to a tertiary care center with low grade fever, weakness and generalized lymphadenopathy of 4 weeks duration. Detailed history revealed visits to hilly region of Garhwal, where he consumed raw goat milk, during the period, he was in camp. Routine investigations; as Widal test, Rheumatoid factor, Paul Bunnel test, hepatitis markers, blood smear for parasities, chest X-ray, HIV serology, routine cultures and whole body CT scan have not yielded any clue. Liver biopsy showed non-caseating granulomas.

Linkages: Pg. 318, 319, 321, 323, 337, 338

What is the clinical diagnosis in the above case?

A.1 'Fever of unknown origin' (FUO), previously the term 'pyrexia of unknown origin' was used.

Mention one common classification for FUO?

A.2 One of the common classification used for this illness is of Durack and Street's. It categories this illness into four categories, namely Classic FUO, HIV associated FUO, nosocomial FUO and neutropaenic FUO.

What is the need of classifying FUO? Mention the features of classic FUO?

A.3 The number of conditions that have to be considered, while investigating FUO is very large, so it is easier to divide the cases into categories and focus on specific causes.

The key features of 'classic' FUO are:

(i) An illness of more than 3 weeks duration

(ii) A temperature of greater than 38.3°C(101°C) on several occasions

(iii) No specific diagnosis after 3 days of investigations.

Which pathogen is likely to be incriminated in this case?

A.4 (a) Brucella species (David Bruce isolated this organism in 1886)

Describe the epidemiology of brucellosis.

A.4 (b)

- **Agent:** *B. melitensis* (Isolated from sheep), *B. abortus* (isolated from cattle), *B. suis* (isolated from pig) *B. canis.*
- **Reservoir/Source of infection:** Brucellosis in an important zoonotic disease. The organisms are part of normal flora of genital and urinary tract of many domestic animals. So; these organism are excreted in the urine, milk, placenta, uterine and vaginal secretions, especially during birth or abortion.
- **Modes of transmission:** The transmission occurs usually from animal to man.

  Rarely; transmission can occur from man to man. The routes are as follows:

  (a) *Contact infection:* This is the commonest mode in which professionals; as butchers, and veterinarians contract the infection, when they come is direct contact with infected tissues; as placenta, blood and urine. The infection takes place through abraded skin.

  (b) *Food borne infection:* This occurs by ingestion of infected food items; as dairy products and meat.

  (c) *Air borne route:* This can occur by inhalation of infected dried animal material; as dust from wool or aerosol from wool or aerosol from heavily infected cowshed. By this route, the laboratory personnel in the lab can also get infected.
- **Host:** The disease is worldwide is distribution and has certain endemic foci. In U.K. and India, *B. abortus* and *B.melitensis* are the predominant species responsible for human infection in comparison to *B. suis* being the predominant species in U.S.A. Predominantly male adults are affected. They are often farmers, shepherds, butchers, abattoir workers, veterinarians and laboratory workers.
- **Environment:** An environment which has predominant domestication of animals, lacking of hygiene, favours the propagation of this infection.

day' fever. The name 'trench fever' derives from the trenches of the first world war, where this disease was very common. The disease is *transmitted* by the faeces of the infected lice, while it is taking the meal from the host. The louse becomes infected after about 5-10 days of its infectious meal. It remains infected throughout its life but there is no transovarial transmission. However; it does not have any morbidity due to the infection.

The trench fever is an exclusively human disease. The disease is *mild* with no mortality. However the disease may become chronic and recrudescences are reported to occur after many decades of the primary infection. *B. quintana* can be cultured on blood agar but the procedure is time consuming and difficult. *Xenodiagnosis* is possible by allowing non infected lice to feed upon the infected case and culturing the organism from the gut of the lice after a week. PCR tests are not warranted due to the mild clinical nature of the cases.

Describe Bartonellosis.

A.6 Bartonellosis is caused by *B.bacilliformis*. The disease has clinically two forms; namely the acute form called the Oroya fever and the subsequent cutaneous form called the *Verruga peruana*. The name 'Oroya' is derived from one of the two places, i.e., Lima and Oroya, between which the epidemic of this disease had occurred in 1870, while building the railway line. The disease Bartonellosis is also called *Carrion's disease*, after the medical student named Daniel Carrion. He in 1885 established the bacterial etiology of the two forms of the disease, by developing Oroya fever; after inoculating himself with the blood from a patient's skin lesion. The term 'peruana' of the skin lesion is likely to have derived from Peru in South America, where the disease is prevalent.

Bartonella bacilliformis, the etilogical agent of this disease is a small gram negative, pleomorphic and motile organism. It stains poorly with gram stain and stains reddish purple with Giemsa stain. It is often seen in clusters and is a strict aerobe. It has optimal growth, when grown at 28-30ºC in a semisolid nutrient agar, containing fresh rabbit serum and haemoglobin.Growth is slow and may take 10 days or longer. This disease is prevalent in S. American countries; as Peru, Ecuador and Colombia. This limited regional occurrence is likely related to the limited habitat of its sandfly (Phelbotomus) vector.The organism has an affinity for the erythrocytes and it invades endothelial cells. The *incubation period* of bartonellosis is approximately 3 weeks. In *Oroya fever*, the presentation is of fever and headache, which is followed by severe anaemia.After resolution of the Oroya fever, the patient may present with nodules over exposed parts of the body; over a period of few months, which may persist for years. The organism can be demonstrated in blood smear by Giemsa stain. Culture is time consuming. The acute stage of the disease responds well to penicillin and chloramphenicol. *Prevention* of the infection requires control of the sandfly.

9 Integrated Clinical Based Study of Ehrlichia/Ehrlichiosis

A colonel, Jung Bahadur reported to the base hospital; with fever, headache, myalgia, and respiratory distress (respiratory rate of 55-60/min). He had served recently in a forested area, infested with ticks. A blood smear of the case, stained with Giemsa revealed cytoplasmic inclusions (morula) in monocytes.

Linkages: Pg. 318, 319, 321, 323, 324, 338

What is the presumptive diagnosis of this case?

A.1 (a) The case is likely having an infection with *Ehrlichia chaffeensis*. Pneumonitis in this case, an entity currently reported with Ehrlichia infection is responsible for the respiratory distress in this case.

What are the characteristics of organisms that belong to Ehrichia genus?

A.1 (b) The Ehrlichiae are small, obligate intracellular gram-negative bacteria that grow in cytoplasmic vacuoles of blood cells; as monocyte, granulocyte and neutrophils but not RBCs.

In whose honour has genus Ehrlichia been named?

A.1 (c) The genus Ehrlichia was established in 1945 and named in honor of German Nobel laureate; *Paul Ehrlich*.

Describe the epidemiology of human Ehrlichiosis.

A.1 (d) Most of the human ehrlichiosis appear to be a tick-borne zoonoses. The infection is propagated by a horizontal transmission that depends on a tick-mammal-tick cycle. Human gets accidentally infected, when they enter natural habitats of ticks and mammals.

What is the limitation in basing the diagnosis of Ehrlichiosis, on demonstration of morulae in peripheral smear of blood?

A.2 (a) In HGA, morula can be demonstrated in about two third of cases, whereas; in HME it can be demonstrated in less than 10% of cases (also see A4)

What diagnostic approach is often used in diagnosis of Ehrilichiosis?

A.2 (b) Serological diagnosis (i.e., demonstration of specific antibodies) using IFA technique.

Why is culture technique not resorted to in diagnosis of Ehrlichiosis?

A.2 (c) This organism cannot be cultivated on inanimate media and culture on macrophage derived cell lines is possible only in a few references laboratories.

What are the reasons for Ehrlichiosis to be reported more frequently currently?

A.3 (i) Better diagnostic techniques for demonstrating Ehrlichia spp. are currently available.

(ii) Current life style including increased outdoor activities in forests may increase exposure to ticks.

Tabulate the characteristics of diseases associated with Ehrichia group (including A.phagocytophilum and N.sennetsu).

A.4

	Human monocytic ehrlichiosis (HME)	**Human granulocytic anaplasmosis (HGA)**	**Human granulocytic ehrlichiosis (HGE)**	**Sennetsu neorickettsiosis**
Etiological agent	*E. chaffeensis*	*Anaplasma phagocytophilum*	*E. ewingii*	*Neorickettsia sennetsu*
Geographical range	USA, Europe, Africa, Thailand	USA, Europe	USA	Far east (Japan, Malaysia)

Contd.

Contd.

Transmission	Tick bite (*Amblyomma americanum*)	Tick bite	Tick bite (*Amblyomma americanum*)	Ingestion
Vector	Tick (*Amblyomma americanum*-lone star tick)	Tick (*Ixodes scapularis*)	Tick (*A. americanum*-lone star Tick)	Trematode in Fish
Reservoir	white tailed deer, domestic Dog	Mice, squirrels, white-tailed deer	Dog and white-tailed deer	Raw fish infected with flukes
Target cell	Macrophage/monocyte	Granulocytes	Granulocytes	Macrophage/Monocyte
Distinctive features	Rash(20%), Fever, headache, systemic involvement including CNS, leucopenia, thrombocytopenia	Granulocytopenia	Fever, headache, myalgia, predominant in immunocompromised Individuals	Fever, headache, resembles mononucleosis like illness
Seasonality	April through September	Year around	April Through September	-
Mortality	2-3%	<1%	None Reported	-
Direct demonstration of organism	Giemsa stain-morulae (cytoplasmic inclusions) <10%	Morulae (frequently seen) in cytoplasm of WBCs	Morulae (rarely seen)	-
Culture on animate media	Few reference labs can grow in macrophage derived cell lines	In research laboratories	In research laboratories	-
Serological Diagnosis	IFA>1:128	IFA>1:80	IFA is gold standard	-
Drug of choice	Doxycycline	Doxycycline	Doxycycline	Doxycycline

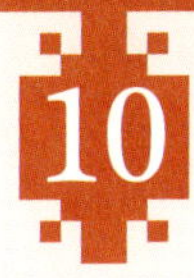

10 Laboratory Diagnosis and Treatment (Overview)

An overview of the comparative approach in laboratory diagnosis of key Gram negative bacilli-fastidious

Organism / Disease	Specimen	Stain enhanced microscopy	Detection of Microbial antigen/ metabolite/genome	Serological Tests	Culture of Organisms in Media/ Characterization and Confirmation of isolate	Differential Diagnosis	Antimicrobial Susceptibility Tests
Brucella sps. commonly: • *abortus* • *melitensis* • *suls* [Undulant fever/ Mediterranean fever/ Malta fever]	*In Man:* • Blood • Fluid/Secretions • Urine • CSF • Abscesses • Vaginal/Seminal fluid - Tissues (*) • Lymph node • Bone marrow • Liver biopsy • Brucellosis* is a disease of reticuloendothelial system and organisms are present in macrophages. *In animals and animal* products: as milk.	- Gram stain: Gram negative coccobacilli	- - - **For animal infection:** *Milk ring test* detects infection in animals by demonstration of antibodies in milk. A group of concentrated suspension of killed *B.abortus* stained with *haematoxylin* is added to 1ml of milk in narrow tube. It is incubated at 70C for 40-60 mins, if agglutinins are present in milk, bacteria are agglutinated and rise with cream to form blue ring at top. If no antibodies are present, milk remains uniformly blue and no blue ring is formed *Brucellin test* - skin test to detect hypersensitivity to Brucella antigen	1. Tube agglutination test: Standard test - indicates acute infection, sufficient dilutions to be put to exclude prozone phenomenon 2. Mercaptoethanol test: indicates chronic infection (this reagent destroys IgM and leaves IgG for agglutination 3. Coomb's test: uses antihuman globulin, if tube agglutination test is negative, but clinical picture otherwise, one should test for blocking antibodies (a) C.F.T. (b) ELISA	N.A.: (very slow growth) Details see pg. 321	- Other brucella sps. as • *B.ovis* • *B.canis* • *B.neotomae* Other non fermenters of carbohydrates, which are gram negative coccobacilli - Bordetella sps. - Acinetobacter sps. - Moraxella sps. - Kingella sps.	
Bordetella pertusis (whooping cough)	(a) Nasopharyngeal secretions - cough plate method: Plate of B.G medium held about 4° in front of patient during coughing episode (b) Postnasal swab: Calcium alginate/ Dacron swab passed through mouth to collect secretion (c) Pernasal swab: Swab passed through anterior nare to collect secretion	- Gram stain: Gram negative coccobacilli - Direct fluorescent antibody test available	- - PCR available for *B.pertusis* and *B. parapertusis*	- Antibodies appear 2-3 weeks after infection, so role limited Tests available C.F.T. I.H.A. ELISA	N.A: other Bordetella sps. can grow on Bordet gengou glycerine potato blood agar (has high % of blood approx 20-50% to neutralize inhibitors Colony: Mercury drop/Bisected pearl appearance Details see pg. 320	- *Bordetella parapertusis* - *B.bronchiseptica* - *B.avium*	
Haemophilus influenzae	- C.S.F. - Blood - Sputum (in pneumonia) - Pus (in arthritis, otitis media) - Muscosal swab (in epiglottitis)	- Gram stain (Gram negative coccobacilli) - Immunofluorescent test - Quellung test to demonstrate capsular swelling, using type b antisera	Capsular antigen can be demonstrated by - Precipitation roaction - C.I.E.P. - Latex/coagglutination test	-	NA: NG Details see chapter 2, pg. 320	- *H. parainfluenzae* - *H. haemolyticus* - *H. parainfluenzae* - *H.suis* - *H.ducreyi* - *H.aphrophilus*	- Special protocol to be followed, as organism is fastidious and high prevalence of drug resistance in organism

An overview of the antimicrobial options for infections caused by gram negative bacilli-fastidious

	Cell Wall Inhibitors	Cell-Membrane Inhibitors	Amino Acid Synthesis Inhibitors	Nucleic Acid Synthesis Inhibitors	Others
Haemophilus influenzae (respiratory infections)	• Ampicillin • Amoxicillin • Cephalosporins • Amoxicillin-clavulanic acid (DOC)		• Azithromycin • Clarithromycin	• TM-SMZ • Fluoroquinolone	
(Meningitis & other serious infections)	• Cephalosporins (DOC) • Meropenem		• Chloramphenicol		
H. ducreyi	• Ceftriaxone		• Erythromycin • Doxycycline	• TM-SMZ • Sulfonamide • Ciprofloxacin	
Gardnerella vaginalis			• Clindamycin	• Metronidazole	
Bordetella pertusis	• Ampicillin		• Erythromycin • Chloramphenicol	• TM-SMZ	
Brucella sps.			• (Tetracycline + Rifampin) (DOC) • [Doxycycline + Gentamicin]		
			• Gentamicin +	TM-SMZ • Ciprofloxacin + Rifampin	
Francisella tularensis			• Streptomycin • Gentamicin • Doxycycline		
Legionella pneumophila			• Azithromycin (DOC) • Erythromycin • [Doxycycline ± Rifampicin]	• Levofloxacin (DOC) • TM-SMZ	
Eikenella corrodens	• PnG • Ampicillin • Cephalosporins • Ticarcillin				
Bartonella quintana			• Tetracycline • Chloramphenicol		
Bartonella bacilliformis	• PnG		• Tetracycline • Chloramphenicol		
Bartonella henselae	(usually self limiting)		• Erythromycin • Gentamicin		
Streptobacillus moniliformis	• PnG		• Doxycycline • Erythromycin • Clindamycin		
Cardiobacterium hominis	• PnG		• Gentamicin • Chloramphenicol • Erthromycin		
Klebsiella granulomatis (Donovania granulomatis)			• Doxycycline • Erythromycin		

NB: DOC refers to drug of choice

Section IX: Gram Negative Bacilli–Fastidious

11 Assessment/Examination Questions

1. Enumerate organisms that have coccobacillary appearance. A1c., p. 324
2. Describe the origin of the name *H. influenzae*. Describe the morphology of *H. influenzae*. Describe satellitism A1d., p. 324, pg 319, pg 320 and 322
3. What are the key factors required by *H. influenzae* (for its growth). Compare and contrast them. Describe the cultural characteristics of this organism.
4. What is the habitat of *H. influenzae*? Describe the epidemiology of *H. influenzae* infections. A1c., p. 325, p. 325-32
5. Describe the pathogenesis of *H. influenzae* infections.
6. Describe the laboratory diagnosis of infections caused by *H. influenzae* with special reference to meningitis. A 3c., p. 326
7. Describe Hib vaccine. pg. 632
8. Describe *H. ducreyi, H. aegyptius* and *Gardnerella vaginalis*. pg. 318-320, 323
9. Classify FUO. Define FUO and enumerate the causes of it. Discuss the laboratory diagnosis of FUO. A1-A3., p. 327+see p. 567
10. What special media and condition need to be met for culturing Brucella? A 6b., p. 328
11. Describe the epidemiology of brucellosis. A 4b., p. 327
12. Mention the role of serological tests used in diagnosis of brucellosis. A 5a., p. 328
13. Describe Castaneda's medium. A 4b., p. 327
14. Describe laboratory diagnosis of brucellosis including in animals. A 5a., p. 328, p. 337
15. Mention the principles in managing a case of brucellosis. A5c., p. 328
16. What is the habitat of *B. pertusis*? Describe the epidemiology of whooping cough. A3d., p. 330, A3c., p. 330
17. Discuss the antigenic structure of *B. pertusis*. Describe Bordet–Gengou medium. Describe the acellular pertusis vaccines. A3b., p. 329, pg 55, pg 632
18. Describe the laboratory diagnosis of whooping cough. p 337 and chapter 6., p. 329-330
19. What is the likely habitat of *Legionella pneumophila*? Describe the epidemiology of Legionellosis? A3., p. 339
20. Describe the laboratory diagnosis of Legionellosis. p. 321, chapter 7., p. 331-332
21. What is the treatment of choice of Legionnaires disease? A 7b., p. 332, p. 338
22. Describe Cat scratch disease. Chapter 8., p. 333
23. Describe Trench fever. A5., p. 333-334
24. Describe *Bartonella bacilliformis*. A 6., p. 334
25. Describe *Ehrlichiosis* Chapter 9., p. 335-336
26. Describe *Francisella tularensis*. p. 318, 319, 321, 323 and 338

Section X: Atypical/Unconventional/ Obligate Intracellular Bacteria

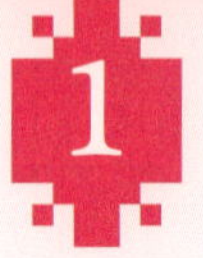

Classification, Metabolic and Microscopic Features of Key Atypical/Obligate Intracellular Bacteria

Algorithm for Identification of Atypical Bacteria/Obligate Intracellular Bacteria

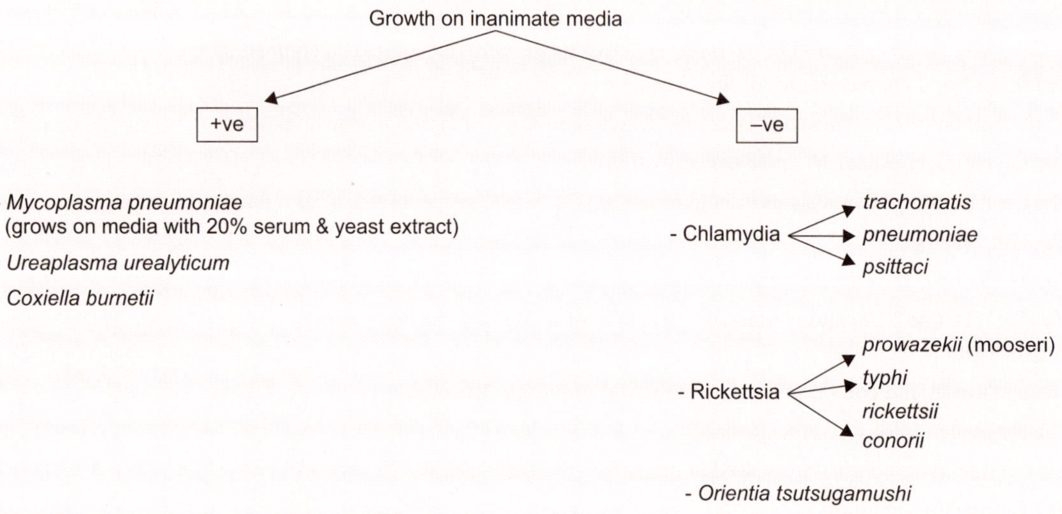

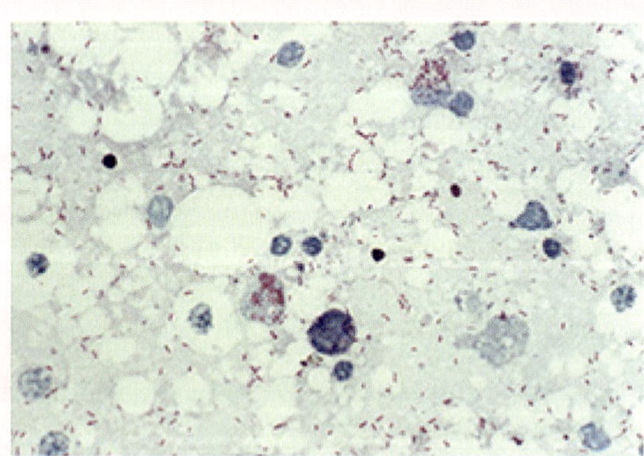

Fig.10.1.1: GRAM NEGATIVE COCCOBACILLI: Yolk sac smear demonstrating Rickettsia ricketsii, appearing as gram negative cocco-bacilli, stained by routine histologic stain, as Gimenez stain (in this case)

Courtesy: Billie Ruth Bird/CDC

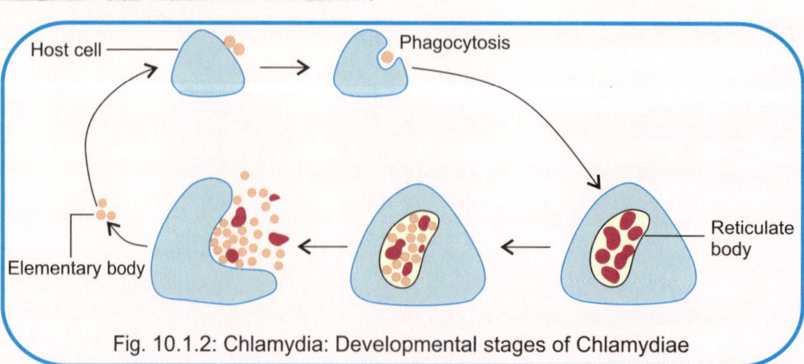

Fig. 10.1.2: Chlamydia: Developmental stages of Chlamydiae

Metabolic and microscopic features of atypical bacteria/obligate intracellular bacteria

Organism	*Growth Requirements*						*Cellular Morphology And Staining Characteristics*						
	O2 Requ.	*Optimal Temp.*	*CO2 Requ..*	*Incubation Period: Days*	*Weeks*	*Months*	*Shape*	*Gram*	*Arrangement*	*Capsule*	*Motility*	*Spore*	*Special Staining / microscopy / Special Features*
Mycoplasma pneumoniae (considered by some as L form)	Facultative anaerobic	37°C	+	2-3	-	-	Very pleomorphic varing from small spherical shape (125-250nm diameter) to long branching filaments (500-1000nm)	-ve (better stained with Giemsa)	-	-	- (in some gliding motility)	-	Difficult to stain by Gram stain as lack cell wall, better stained with Giemsa
M. hominis	Facultative anaerobe	35°C	+	2-3				-ve					
M. genitalium	Facultative anaerobe			isolation difficult may require few weeks				-ve					
Ureaplasma urealyticum	Facultative anaerobe, placed in separate genus because of unique urease activity							-ve					
Rickettsia prowazekii,	Obligate intra-cellular bacteria (Fig. 10.1.1)	Can not be cultivated in inanimate media					Coccobacilli	-ve (do not take stain well) as usually inside host cell	-	-	-	-	Giemsa & Giminez stains bacteria bright red and purple respectively
R.mooseri	do	Can not be cultivated in inanimate media					Coccobacilli	-ve	-	-	-	-	do
R. rickettsia	do	Can not be cultivated in inanimate media					Coccobacilli	-ve	-	-	-	-	do
R. akari,	do	Can not be cultivated in inanimate media					Coccobacilli	-ve	-	-	-	-	do
Orientia tsutsugamushi	do	Can not be cultivated in inanimate media					Coccobacilli	-ve	-	-	-	-	do
Coxiella burnetti	do	Can not be cultivated in inanimate media					Coccobacilli	-ve	-	-	-	+	do
Chlamydia sps. (as trachomatis, pneumoniae, psittaci)	Obligate intracellular bacteria	Can not be cultivated in inanimate media					Exists in two forms (i) Elementary body (EB) (spherical particle 200-300nm in diameter) (ii) Reticulate body (RB) (500-1000 nm). (Fig. 10.1.2)	-ve	-	-	-	-	Giemsa, Giminez and immuno-fluoroscent staining tech. often used. Inclusion bodies (multiple EBs within a vacuole seen in clinical material. (Fig. 10.1.3)

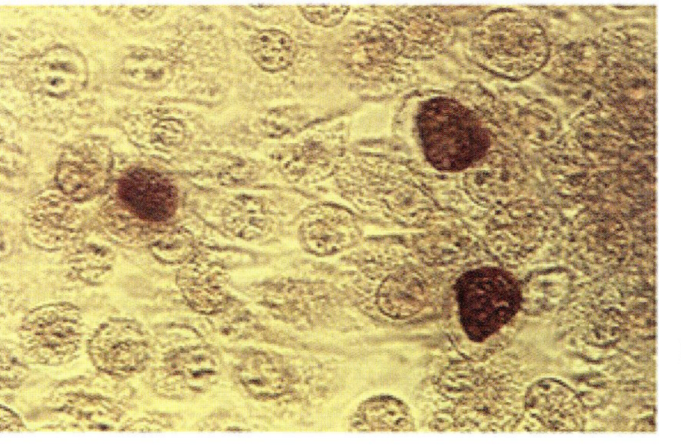

Fig. 10.1.3: CHLAMYDIA TRACHOMATIS: Inclusion bodies of *C. trachomatis* in McCoy cell monolayer (200X)

Courtesy: Dr. E. Arum; Dr. N. Jacobs/CDC

2 An Overview of the Media Requirements, Colonial Characters and Laboratory Diagnostic Characteristics of Atypical/Obligate Intracellular Bacteria

	Basal media	Enriched media	Selective/ others	Characterization and confirmation of isolate
Mycoplasma pneumoniae	NA: NG	- BA: NG - PPLO: Used for broth isolation (contains serum yeast extract, glucose and phenol red as indicator) Once growth occurs, subculture done in medium containing selective agents Subculture done using small agar (medium) and not conventionally using platinum straight wire Fried egg colonies appear after a week of incubation (β haemolytic) (Fig. 10.2.1)	- MacConkey: NG - Penicillin, Thallium acetate and amphotericin B added to make medium selective (Mycoplasma are resistant to penicillin and thallium acetate, as lack cell wall)	- Colonies stained with Diene's method or by Giemsa stain - Colonies adsorb guinea pig erythrocytes - Ferment glucose producing acid - Reduce tetrazolium (colorless) to red color
M. hominis	NA: NG	- BA: NG	- MacConkey: NG	- On mycoplasma medium, inhibiton of growth with specific antisera used to differentiate from other genital mycoplasmas - The organism can break down arginine with production of potentially cytotoxic amounts of ammonia
Ureaplasma urealyticum	NA: NG	- BA: NG - Mycoplasma medium with urea used (this organism can split urea and is a useful growth factor for the organism)	- MacConkey: NG	- As colonies produced are tiny (15-50 μm), these were earlier termed T-strain mycoplasma (T- for tiny)
Chlamydia sps (pneumoniae, trachomatis, psittaci)	Cannot be cultured on inanimate media	(–)	Cultivated on a) mice inoculated by various routes; as i/p, i/c b) yolk sac of embryonated chick c) McCoy cell line treated with cycloheximide, mouse fibroblast cell line, HEP-2	Growth detected by presence of incluson bodies (by Giemsa staining)

Contd.

Contd.

	Basal media	Enriched media	Selective/ others	Characterization and confirmation of isolate
Rickettsia sps (including Orientia)	Cannot be cultivated on inanimate media Isolation should be attempted only in reference laboratories with adequate protection level (as BSL-3/4) as without them, fatal infections can occur in laboratory workers	–	- Can be cultivated in yolk sac of embryonated chick egg (5-6 day old) - Guinea pig and mice (intraperitoneal route), as lab animals can be used - Cell lines used for maintenance of this organism, but not for primary isolation – arthropod cell lines, HeLa, HEp	The organism grows in cytoplasm of the cell (except for Rickettsia causing spotted fever, which grows in nucleus) - Weil Felix test (see A.2b, chapter 5)
Anaplasma phagocytophilum	Cannot be cultivated on inanimate media	–	Culture on myelocyte cell lines, a research tool	

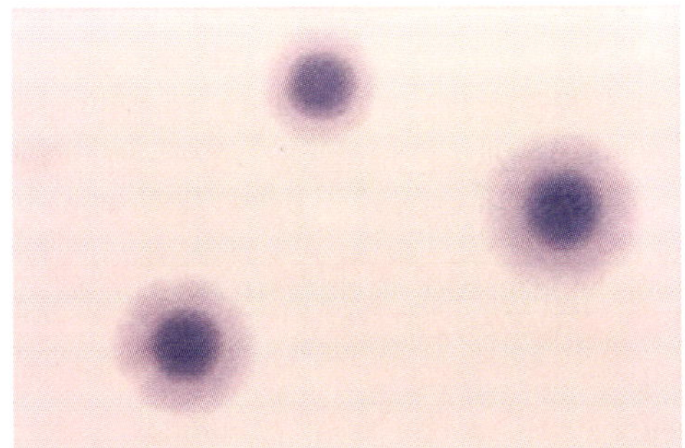

Fig.10.2.1: MYCOPLASMA COLONY: `Fried egg` appearance of Mycoplasma spp., cultivated on solid medium

Courtesy: Dr. E. Arum; Dr. N. Jacobs/CDC

3 Clinical (Pathogenicity) Profile of Infections Caused By Atypical/Obligate Intracellular Bacteria

<table>
<tr><td rowspan="2">Mycoplasma pneumoniae</td><td colspan="3">Primary atypical pneumonia ('Walking pneumonia')</td></tr>
<tr><td colspan="3">Tracheobronchitis, pharyngitis, acute haemorrhagic bullous myringitis, Otitis media</td></tr>
<tr><td>M. hominis</td><td colspan="3">Incriminated in Postpartum (post abortal) sepsis, pelvic inflammatory disease (in women), vaginitis, cervicitis, salpingitis, proctitis</td></tr>
<tr><td>M. genitalium</td><td colspan="3">Urogenital tract disease (Difficulty in identifying it, makes it difficult to estimate cases caused by it)</td></tr>
<tr><td>M. fermentans</td><td colspan="3">Not associated with any disease
Colonizes respiratory and genital tract in 20% of adults</td></tr>
<tr><td>Ureaplasma urealyticum</td><td colspan="3">• In men associated with urethritis, proctitis & Reiter's syndrome
• In women, associated with pelvic inlammatory disease, post abortal fever, chorioamnionitis</td></tr>
<tr><td>Rickettsia prowazekii</td><td colspan="3">• Epidemic typhus (fever, headache, centrifugal rash (no eschar), severe illness if not treated, Details pg. 348-349)
• Brill-Zinsser disease (reactivation form, similar to epidemic typhus, but milder)</td></tr>
<tr><td>R. typhi (mooseri)</td><td colspan="3">Endemic typhus (Clinically similar to epidemic typhus, but milder)</td></tr>
<tr><td>R. rickettsii</td><td colspan="3">Rocky mountain spotted fever [Fig. 10.3.1] (fever, headache, centripretal, rash (no eschar), systemic complications, details pg. 350-351)</td></tr>
<tr><td>R. akari</td><td colspan="3">Rickettsial pox (Fever, headache, vesicular rash (eschar)</td></tr>
<tr><td>Orientia tsutsugamuchi</td><td colspan="3">Scrub typhus [Fever, headache, rash (approx. 50% have eschar), systemic complications, details pg. 352-353]</td></tr>
<tr><td>Coxiella burnetii</td><td colspan="3">Q fever: Acute or chronic. [Headache, fever, pneumonia, systemic complications details pg. 352-353]</td></tr>
<tr><td rowspan="3">C. trachomatis</td><td rowspan="2">Genital</td><td>• Male
• Female
• Both sexes (adults)</td><td>Urethritis*, epididymitis*
Urethritis*, cervicitis*, salpingitis*
Lymphogranuloma inguinale (LGV, by serotypes L1, L2a, L2b and L3), proctitis, Reiter's syndrome</td></tr>
<tr><td>Infants</td><td>Pneumonia</td></tr>
<tr><td>Non genital</td><td></td><td>Endemic trachoma (by serotypes A,B,Ba and C), Inclusion conjunctivitis*, Opthalmia neonatorum*</td></tr>
<tr><td>C.pneumoniae</td><td colspan="3">Pharyngitis, sinusitis, bronchitis, pneumonia (adults), chronic vascular infection</td></tr>
<tr><td>C.psittaci</td><td colspan="3">Psittacosis, (systemic infections).</td></tr>
</table>

* are by serotypes D to K

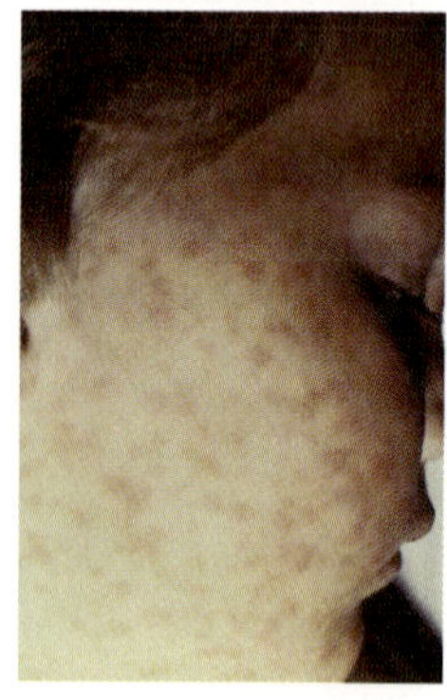

Fig. 10.3.1: ROCKY MOUNTAIN SPOTTED FEVER: A female child face with characteristic rash of RMSF

Courtesy: CDC, Atlanta

4 Integrated Clinical Based Study of *M.pneumoniae*/ Community Acquired Pneumonia

A 19 year first year college student, Shalini presented to the Medical O.P.D with history of two weeks; non-productive cough and fever. Her detailed history and examination revealed, diffuse painful rash over her extremities for the last three days. She gave no history of contact with any sick persons and examination of the respiratory system revealed no significant findings. However, her chest radiograph revealed bilateral diffuse interstitial infiltrates.

Linkages: Pg. 340-342, 344, 360, 362

What is the clinical diagnosis in this case?

A.1 **(a)** The case appears to be one of a community acquired (atypical) pneumonia.

What are the microbes that are associated with community acquired pneumonia?

A.1 **(b)** The microorganisms that could be responsible for this entity include *M. pneumoniae*, *S. pneumoniae, M pneumoniae*, *Legionella pneumophila*, *Coxiella burnetii*, viruses and some fungi as *H.capsulatum* and *C. immitis*.

What is the most likely pathogen involved in the above case?

A.2 **(a)** The respiratory pathology is most likely to be caused by *M. pneumoniae*, as the age group of the case is between 5-20 years and X-ray chest findings are suggestive of a *M pneumoniae* chest infection. The manifestation of a skin rash; as erythema multiforme is likely to be extrapulmonary Mycoplasma manifestation. This agent was first isolated by Nocard and Roux in 1898. These were initially called 'pleuropneumonia like organisms' because of their resemblance to organism causing bovine pneumonia.

What extrapulmonary manifestations, sometimes a case of Mycoplasma pneumoniae can present with? Mention its importance.

A.2 **(b)**

System	Manifestation
Neurological	Meningoencephalitis, meningitis, Cranial nerve palsy and others
Cardiovascular	Pericarditis, Myocarditis
Gastrointestinal	Nausea, vomiting and diarrhea
Dermatological (Skin)	Erythema multiforme, Steven-Johnson syndrome and others
Musculoskeletal	Arthalgia, Myalgia
Haematological	Haemolytic anaemia, Cold haemagglutinin synthesis

Mycoplasma cases often have paucity of symptoms, despite marked radiological changes. Because of this, the entity is also called 'Walking pneumonia'. Sometimes the extrapulmonary presentations can complicate the respiratory presentation and at times is the only clue, that a case could be having an unremarkable mycoplasmal respiratory infection.

Outline the taxonomical status of M. pneumoniae.

A.2 **(c)** *Mycoplasma pneumoniae* belong to family Mycoplasmataceae, which has 2 genera; namely Mycoplama and Ureaplasma, which have around 100 species.

Most of the species in these genera are commensals. Only two are established human pathogens; namely *M.pneumoniae and Ureaplasma urealyticum*. *M. hominis* and *M. genitalium* are associated with some diseases.

Enumerate unique characteristics of Mycoplasma.

A.2 **(d)** (i) Smallest free living microorganism (it is for this reason; these pass through bacterial filters, as have a diameter of about 0.2-0.3 μm)

(ii) have the smallest genome (amongst free living bacteria, *M. genitalium* has 580,073 base pairs)

(iii) Filamentous forms with true branching (explains resemblance to fungi at times)
(iv) Lack cell wall
(v) Trilaminar cell membrane is unique in containing cholesterol (unlike other bacteria)
(vi) Are gram negative, but stain with difficulty with this stain. Better stained with Giemsa or Dienes stain.
(vii) Growth media requires sterol; as a constitutent (for synthesis of unique plasma membrane component). During binary fission, cytoplasm division, may lag behind DNA (genome) replication. This may result in the formation of various shapes.
(viii) Resistant to antimicrobials that act on cell wall

Why is Mycoplasma sometimes confused with viruses?

A.2 (e) (i) Many pass through *bacterial filters because of their small size

*The size of pore size is such that it should have retained classical bacteria

(ii) Not easily stained by classic gram stain, as lack cell wall
(iii) Often contaminate cell lines used to cultivate viruses and mistakenly reported as viruses.
(iv) Do not get inhibited by many antibiotics, used in cell lines to inhibit viruses, as these organism lack cell wall (the site; at which many antibiotics act).

Why are Mycoplasma not categorized as viruses?

A.2 (f) (i) Have trilaminar cell membrane
(ii) Have both DNA and RNA
(iii) Can multiply in cell free media
(iv) Also show extracellular parasitism 'in vivo' (besides intracellular existence)
(v) Inhibited by antibiotics acting at sites other than cell wall

How are Mycoplasmas different from L forms?

A.2 (g) (i) Have sterols in the cell membrane (ii) Remain stable and donot revert to any other form
(iii) Have unique genome, which is one of the smallest for the free living bacteria (L forms resemble parent bacterium)

Why do Mycopalsma pneumoniae have limited biosynthetic capabilities (as require cholesterol and other sterols for their growth)?

A.2 (h) It is one of the smallest free living organisms with its genome having only 8.16×10^5 base pairs and about 679 putative protein coding sequences (ORFs). This limited DNA coding capacity limits its biosynthetic capabilities, making it dependent on readymade molecules.

Describe the epidemiology of M.pneumoniae infections.

A.2 (i) **Agent:** *Mycoplasma pneumoniae*

Reservoir of infection: Upper respiratory tract of man.

Source of infection: Respiratory secretions of infected persons.

Mode of transmission: Nasal secretion in the form of aerosols; which if inhaled lead to transmission of the infection. Direct close contact between individuals facilitate transmission.

Host: The infection is present worldwide with increased incidence in temperate zones.

It causes upper and lower respiratory tract infection in all age groups. Symptomatic *M. pneumoniae* infection is commonest between 5-15 years of age. Asymptomatic infections do occur.

Mostly causes sporadic cases, though outbreaks at intervals of 4-6 year intervals have been reported especially in closed population; as schools and military installation. Because of relatively long incubation period of 2-3 weeks and prolonged shedding of organisms in nasal secretions, infections tend to spread over time.

Which approach can be used to confirm the diagnosis in this setting?

A.3 (a) In this setting, where a respiratory specimen is not clinically available, serologic approach involving demonstrating specific antibodies against common respiratory pathogens, as Mycoplasma is a rational approach.

What is the consequence of the small colony size of Mycoplama, in reference to culturing it?

A.3 (b) The small colony size (0.2-0.5 mm) makes it difficult for the unaided eye to pick it up (an isolated colony). Hence a small size of the agar is blindly taken and subcultured onto fresh medium for isolation (by rubbing)

Describe cold agglutination test.

A.3 (c)
- **Type of test:** Non specific antibody detection type (based on antigenic similarity between Mycoplasma membrane and antigen of RBCs).
- **Principle:** Agglutinins (macroglobulin) appear in the blood of more than half of the patients with *M.pneumoniae* infection, when present to the health care provider.
- **Characteristic of the antibodies:**

  These are antibodies that agglutinate human 'O' blood group RBCs at low temperature, hence called cold agglutinins.
- **Procedure:**
  - Prepare serial dilution of patient's serum
  - Add washed suspension of the human 'O' erythrocytes to all dilutions
  - Incubate at 4°C (overnight) and observe for red cell agglutination
- **Interpretation:**
  - A titer of ≥ 1:32 is suggestive of *M.pneumoniae* infection (note this agglutination gets dissociated at 37°C)
- **Disadvantage of test:**

  Such antibodies are also demonstrated in sera of cases, who have infections by Rubella, adenovirus and in conditions; as cirrhosis of liver and haemolytic anaemia. This test is not in vogue.

nb: these agglutinins (antibodies) can cause anaemia and other complications.

Describe Streptococcus MG agglutination test.

A.3 (d)
- **Principle of the test:** It is a type of non-specific antibody detection test, based on antigenic similarity (cross-reactivity) between mycoplasma membrane and carbohydrate antigen of Streptococcus MG.
- **Procedure:** Serial dilutions of patient's serum are prepared. Heat inactivated suspension of Streptococcus MG is added to it. The test is incubated at 37°C overnight.
- **Interpretation:** A titer of 20 or more is considered suggestive of *M. pneumoniae* infection. The reaction that is observed, as the name indicates is an agglutination reaction.
- **Status of the test:** The test is not commonly used.

Aspects related to case theme/examination assessment

Which molecular biology test facilitates a syndromic surveillance, in case with respiratory infections (where a panel of pathogens is incriminated)?

A.4 (a) Multiplex PCR, which utilizes multiple primer sets designed for amplification of multiple targets.

Can some bacteria mimic Mycoplasma, in certain conditions?

A.4 (b) Yes. Many bacteria (with cell walls), when grown in presence of antibiotics acting on cell wall, start appearing morphologically (microscopically); as Mycoplasmas. These forms are called 'L' forms. However; on removal of the stimulus i.e., the presence of antimicrobial, the bacteria may revert to their original form.

How are Mycoplasmas similar to L forms?

A.4 (c) (i) Microscopically both appear similar (ii) Both macroscopically form 'fried egg' colonies

(iii) Agglutinins to Streptococcus MG are frequently formed, following infections with *M.pneumoniae.*

How are L forms different from Mycoplamas, i.e., unique characteristics of L-forms?

A.4 (d) L forms have

(i) remnants of cell wall

(ii) L-forms are not filterable

(iii) Do not require sterol for growth

(iv) resemble antigenically, biochemically, and genetically the parent bacterium

(v) Play role in chronic infections during antibiotic therapy

(vi) Unstable L forms can revert to their original morphology, on removal of precipitating stimulus

What are the antimicrobials of choice to treat a case of atypical pneumonia caused by M. pneumoniae?

A.5 Tetracycline/Erythromycin.

Integrated Clinical Based Study of *R.prowazekii*/Epidemic Typhus

A 40 year old man, Brijesh presented with chills, weakness, high temperature, severe headache and a rash on the trunk. History of louse bite about two weeks ago was elicited. The rash developed 5 days, after the onset of symptoms. Four days after his admission to the medical ward, the rashes became haemorrhagic and the patient progressed to coma.

Linkages: Pg. 340-344, 361, 362

What is the presumptive clinical diagnosis in this case?

A.1 (a) Epidemic typhus, caused by *R.prowazekii.*

What does the progression of this case to coma indicate?

A.1 (b) It indicates severe involvement of the central nervous system in the disease process.

To which the family, does the etiological agent for this disease belong?

A.1 (c) It belongs to family Rickettsiaceae, which consists of three genera, namely Rickettsia, Orientia and Ehrlichia. The name Rickettsia is given in honour of Howard Taylor Rickets, who did pioneering work on spotted fever and typhus, contracted the latter disease.

Enumerate features of Rickettsia, which resemble those of viruses.

A.1 (d) (i) Obligate intracellular existence (ii) Inability to grow in cell free media

(iii) Some of them can pass through bacterial filter

Enumerate features of Rickettsia, which resemble those of bacteria.

A.1 (e)
- (i) Have cell wall resembling gram negative organism and contains LPS and muramic acid
- (ii) Have trilaminar cell membrane
- (iii) Have both DNA and RNA (single unbounded chromosome of DNA and also ribosome)
- (iv) Multiply by binary fission
- (v) Susceptible to antibacterial antibiotics

Which infectious diseases are transmitted by louse?

A.2 Epidemic typhus,Trench fever and Epidemic relapsing fever (also see chapter 2 of Section XVI, p. 599).

What serological test can confirm the clinical diagnosis of Epidemic typhus?

A.3 (a) Weil-Felix test or complement fixation test (using specific rickettsial antigen) can be performed or IFAT.

Describe Weil Felix test.

A.3 (b) History:

In the early 1900s; an interesting observation of serum from typhus patients agglutinating certain Proteus strains, led to the development of this test.

Principle:

Non motile (Proteus is usually motile) strains of Proteus, namely *P. vulgaris* OX-19, OX-2, and *P. mirabilis* OX-K cross react (or share some antigens) with certain Rickettsial organisms. This forms the basis of the heterophile agglutination test, in which antibodies of rickettsial fever cases get detected by the strains of Proteus species that share alkali stable carbohydrate with the rickettsia.

It is to be appreciated that Rickettsial antigen itself is not used in rickettsial diagnostic tests because rickettsial antigen are difficult to obtain.

Procedure:

- Inactivate the patient serum

- Make serum dilutions in triplicate (in tubes)
- Add three antigens, namely OX-19, OX-2, and OX-K to three series of serum samples
- Incubate the preparation
- Observe for agglutination

Interpretation:

Disease	OX-19	OX-2	OX-K
Epidemic typhus	+++	±	-
Brill Zinsser disease	±	-	-
Endemic typhus	+++	±	-
Tick borne spotted fever group	++	++	-
Rickettsial pox	-	-	-
Scrub typhus	-	-	++

+++ = strong agglutination, ++ = moderate agglutination, + weak agglutination, (-) negative, +/- positive or negative

The agglutinins appear as early as 5-7 days after infection and reach peak by end of 2nd week and decline thereafter. A single titre of $\geq$ 160 is considered diagnostically significant.

Limitation of the test:

(i) Test has poor specificity, false positive reactions also occur in certain Proteus and Salmonella infections

(ii) Test has poor sensitivity

(iii) Test can't differentiate amongst many rickettsial clinical entities.

Recommendation:

A positive test should be confirmed by a specific test; as indirect fluorescent antibody test, which is considered a serological test of choice. The sensitivity and specificity of the Weil-Felix test is low

Describe Neil Mooser test.

A.3 **(c)** Neil–Mooser reaction (Tunica reaction)

- **Principle:** The diagnosis of rickettsial infection is a challenge. This was a biological test used in the past to differentiate between *R. prowazekii* and *R. mooseri;* which are similar.
- **Procedure:** Inject male guinea pig intraperitoneally with blood from a case of endemic typhus or *R. mooseri*.
- **Interpretation:** If the male guinea pig develops fever and typical scrotal inflammation, the test is considered positive for *R. mooseri*. In such a case, the testes of the guinea pig cannot be pushed back into the abdomen due to inflammatory adhesions between the layers of tunica vaginalis. Final confirmation of the infection is with the demonstration of intracytoplasmic rickettsia in the stained smear of scrapings from the tunica.
- **Limitation:** This test is currently of limited use because of the development of better diagnostic tests and other concerns in infecting the animal for diagnostic use.

Can epidemic typhus manifest decades after its first manifestation, despite initially having been adequately treated?

A.4 Yes. The latent infection, when reactivated, leads to recrudescent typhus and this is named as 'Brill-Zinsser' disease.

Outline the two groups of the genus Rickettsia.

A.5 i) Typhus fever group: It consists of epidemic typhus, recrudescent infection (Brill-Zinsser disease) and endemic typhus.

ii) Spotted Fever group: It consists of Rocky mountain spotted fever, Rickettsial pox and other tick borne diseases.

Integrated Clinical Based Study of *R.ricketsii*/Rocky Mountain Spotted Fever

A 30 year adult, Shailesh who recently returned, after trekking in the Himalayan region, presented with fever, headache (frontal and retro-orbital, i.e., behind the eyes) and myalgia. He gave history of ticks being removed from his scalp about 9 days back. Two days after his admission to the hospital, he developed a macular rash, which started initially on both upper and lower extremities and then gradually spread to the trunk. The significant findings of his blood examination were low platelet count of 20,000/micro-lit and significantly increased coagulation time. Four days later, he developed *paraplegia and clouded consciousness.

***Decreased/loss of function in lower limbs**

Linkages: Pg. 340, 341, 343, 344, 361, 362

What is the likely diagnosis of this case?

A.1 Rocky mountain spotted fever (RMSF)/India Tick typhus.

What are the diseases transmitted by ticks?

A.2 (a) Bacterial: Tularemia (*Francisella tularensis*)

Lyme disease *(B. burgdorferi)*

Relapsing fever (also by lice)

Rocky mountain Spotted fever (*R. rickettsii*)

Human Ehrlichiosis

Viral: Colorado tick fever

Powassan encephalitis

Parasitic: Babesiosis (*Babesia microti*)

Discuss the role of ticks in the pathogenesis of RMSF.

A.2 (b) Most of the cases of RMSF occurs between the months of April and September, which is a period, when ticks actively feed. The tick infected with *R. rickettsi* must attach to the human host for a minimum period of five hours for a possible transmission of the infection to human host. For this reason, a frequent deticking of the individual in the tick infested areas is critical in minimizing the occurrence of this disease.

How are rickettsia cultivated?

A.2 (c) They are obligate intracellular bacteria, so can grow only in living cells of eukaryotic origin

They are cultivated on cell lines as of Arthropod lineage, HeLa, HEp2

(useful in maintenance of Rickettsia, not for primary isolation of Rickettsia)

They can also be cultivated on yolk sac of 5-6 day old chick embryo (incubated at 33-35°C), this route is useful for preparation of rickettsial antigens and vaccines. Cultivation also occurs in Laboratory animals; as mice and guinea-pig

Discuss the implications of the blood findings present in this case.

A.3 (a) Vasculitis (in many organs) can occur, following infection with *R. rickettsi*. The vascular injury along with some immune-mediated mechanisms, can result in disseminated intravascular coagulation (DIC). The findings of low platelet count and increased coagulation time are indications that the process of DIC has begun. Purpura in a setting of sepsis indicates that the patient is suffering from DIC.

Describe the pathology of Rickettsial infections.

A.3 (b) The basic changes are vascular with resultant widespread lesions in adjacent parenchymal organs; as skin muscle, heart, lung and brain. Nodules can form in the latter, which are essentially perivascular aggregation of PMNs, lymphocytes and macrophages associated with blood vessels of grey matter. Rickettsia essentially causes systemic infections(not localized).

Explain the pathogeneses of paraplegia in this case.

A.4 (a) Vasculitis (vascular injury) in *R. rickettsii* infection leads to leakiness of blood-vessels that can lead to edema and petechial hemorrhage. The vasculitis may also result in occlusion of the blood vessel. The CNS is a commonly involved site, besides skin involvement in the pathology. In this case, occlusion of some blood vessels supplying motor neurons (to lower limbs) has possible occurred, resulting in paraplegia.

Outline the pathogenesis of Rickettsial infections.

A.4 (b) The disease is transmitted by the bite of the infected arthropod

↓

Rickettsia multiply at the inoculated site, producing a dark swollen crusted lesion (called eschar, not produced by all Rickettsia)

↓

Infect the vascular endothelium (special predilection for these cells)

↓ ↓

Enters blood and spreads via the bloodstream | Damages vascular endothelium

↓

Swelling and spotting destruction of endothelial cells results in

↓ ↓

Bleeding, thrombosis and purpuric skin lesions

Nb-vascular manifestations are more severe in RMSF

Integrated Clinical Based Study of *C.trachomatis*/Pelvic Inflammatory Disease

A 20 year female, Dimple presented to the emergency room of a hospital with severe abdominal pain. She gave no history of UTI. Her examination revealed her to be having temperature of 38.5°C and no masses could be palpated on abdominal examination. However, tenderness was elicited in left lower quadrant. Pelvic examination revealed cervical motion to be reduced and presence of right and left adnexal tenderness.

Linkages: Pg. 340-342, 344, 361, 362

What is the clinical diagnosis in the above case?

A.1 (a) This case is likely to have pelvic inflammatory disease-P.I.D. (acute cervicitis and salpingitis)

What do you understand by 'urogenital' chlamydiasis?

A.1 (b) 'Urogenital chlamydiasis' are infections of urogenital tract caused by *C.trachomatis* (D-K).

The profile of these infections and their laboratory diagnosis is depicted at page 344 and 361. The importance of these infections can be gauged by the fact, that these are more prevalent than the ocular trachoma and cause major complications; as acute pelvic inflammatory disease, infertility and infantile pneumonia. Reliable data on prevalence is not available due to scarce testing for this entity.

C. trachomatis genital infections represent one of the commonest sexually transmitted diseases. The clinical spectrum resembles that of gonococcal infections. Majority of the infected females are asymptomatic (asymptomatic rate lower in males). The age of peak prevalence of this infection is late teens and early twenties.

What are PLT or TRIC agents?

A.1 (c) Chlamydia organisms (parasites) were also known by as Psittacosis-lymphogranuloma trachoma (PLT) or Trachoma - inclusion conjunctivitis (TRIC) organisms.

What microorganisms are responsible for causing P.I.D.?

A.2 (a) *C. trachomatis* (b) *N. gonorrhoeae*
(c) *Bacteroides fragilis* (d) Anaerobes other than *B. fragilis*

How can cervical specimen be collected?

A.3 (a) A sterile swab is inserted 1cm into the cervical canal and rotated for about 5 seconds; before withdrawing.

What is the best approach to isolate C. trachomatis?

A.3 (b) Tissue culture is regarded as the 'gold standard' for diagnosing *C. trachomatis* infection. McCoy cells are often used for it. The inanimate media including enriched agar media can't be used, as this organism is an obligate intracellular pathogen.

Can C. trachomatis cause asymptomatic infection of the genital tract in the females?

A.4 (a) Yes, majority of infected females are asymptomatic.

If so, is there any need to treat such infections?

A.4 (b) Treating the asymptomatic infected woman is essential to prevent these women from developing serious sequelae; as infertility and to prevent the spread of this infection to their sexual male (and female) partners.

What population should be screened for in an attempt to prevent P.I.D. in women?

A.5 (a) Sexually active women should be screened.

What samples are commonly taken for demonstrating Chlamydia infection?

A.5 (b) Uretheral swab and cervical swab can be taken for doing antigen detection studies.

What is the role of genome and antigen detection techniques in diagnosis of 'Urogenital chlamydiasis'?

A.5 (c) Antigen detection techniques and genome detection using molecular biology techniques are licensed in USA (F.D.A. approved) for only *C. trachomatis*. The specificity level for the two techniques is high and comparable, although higher for the genome detection techniques than the antigen detection kits. The genome detection (NAAT), nucleic acid amplification tests, techniques are expensive but have a significant role in diagnosis of *C.trachomatis* genital infections. It provides early diagnosis, treatment and prevent further transmission of genital infections. This also gets important, as a large proportion of women may have asymptomatic infections and untreated can lead to serious complication and spread of infection.

Screening programmes may be conducted for high risk women for presumptive chlamydial infection.However a positive result in *single NAAT* should be considered as a presumptive evidence of infection, as false positive result can have adverse social impact on the patient. So; an additional test should be performed before reporting a case as positive. A word of caution is to be kept in mind, that clinical sample may contain amplification inhibitors, as nitrites; that may result in false negative report.

Mention empiric therapy strategy for treating sexually active women in whom P.I.D. is suspected (in situations where laboratory support isn't available).

A.6 Beta–lactam antimicrobials can be effective against *N. gonorrhoeae* and anaerobes. Addition of doxycycline would cover *C.trachomatis* infections, as beta lactam antibiotic have poor intracellular penetration.Instead of the combination of beta lactam antibiotic and doxycycline, newer fluoroquinolones; as Ofloxacin can be used, however strains of *N. gonorrhoeae* with resistance to fluoroquinolones have been reported. It should be noted that co-infection with *C. trachomatis* and *N. gonorrhoeae* is possible. It is also essential to treat sexual partners of cases who have PID.

Aspect related to case theme/examination assessment

Describe Lymphogranuloma venerum with special reference to Frei test.

A.7 As the name indicates, it is a distinct venereal disease characterized histopathologically by granuloma in late stages. This disease is caused by three distinct serotypes (L_1-L_3) that aren't associated with other genital chlamydial infections. The disease is still endemic and occurs primarily in S. America, Africa, Asia (including India) and the Caribbean.

The disease is essentially sexually transmitted, though other routes have been documented. The peak incidence of disease is the second and third decades of life, which correspond to increased sexual activity. A recent trend in the disease has been the involvement of homosexual men with the disease, who develop disease after receptive anorectal intercourse. These individuals present as haemorrhagic proctitis/proctocolitis with regional lymphadenitis. The incubation period of disease varies from three days to thirty days. The *primary stage* of the disease involves a small painless papule or ulcer on the external genitalia or in the vagina. The lesion usually heals without scarring and the lesion may go unnoticed by the individual. The organism may gain entry into the lesion through minute ulcerations or lacerations. The primary lesion may also be urethral, anal or rectal in orgin, with the organism spreading via the regional lymphatics.

The *secondary stage* occurs days to weeks after the primary lesion heals and is characterized by localized lymphadenopathy and systemic symptoms. In heterosexual men, the inguinal syndrome is the most common presentation, characterized by painful inguinal lymphadenopathy. Metastatic complications involving meninges, eyes and joints may occur. The last stage or the *tertiary stage* of the disease may present as 'esthiomene' (Greek 'eating away'), which implies hypertrophic chronic granulomatous enlargement (sometimes with ulceration) of penis, scrotum or vulva. Elephantiasis of the male and female genitalia may occur. These occur as a consequence of scarring and lymphatic blockage.

The outline of its lab diagnosis is depicted at page 361. A test that needs more explanation is the **Frei test.**

- **Status:** Used in the past, now not currently used, due to availability of other tests with increased sensitivity and less turnaround time (Time to positivity)
- **Principle:** delayed hypersensitivity reaction.
- **Procedure:** 'Lygranum', commercially available antigen, (prepared from infected yolk sac) used. Specific heat inactivated specific antigen and control antigen (non-infected yolk sac) injected on left and right arms; respectively.
- **Interpretation:** A nodule appearing after 48-72 hours of administration and reaching a maximum size after 4-5 days is interpreted, as a positive test (for infection). This test becomes positive 2-6 weeks after infection and remains positive for several years.

What are the general approaches in laboratory diagnosis of Chlamydial infections?

A.8 The simplest and effective technique for diagnosis of infection would be demonstration of inclusion bodies in the smear sample, but however its sensitivity is low for *C. pneumoniae* and *C. psittaci*. Culture techniques for isolation of organism is cumbersome and time consuming. It has poor sensitivity for *C. pneumoniae* and *C. trachomatis* (LGV serotypes). However, it has the status of being a reference method for diagnosis of chlamydial infections. Nucleic acid amplification tests (NAAT), especially PCR give promising results. The sensitivity, specificity and predictive values of serologic methods (antibody demonstration) are not high to make it clinically useful for diagnosis of active infections except in cases of LGV, psittacosis and infant pneumonia. The approaches to the serologic diagnosis are based on:

(i) Complement fixing genus specific antigen-lipopolysaccharide (present in EBs and RBs).

(ii) Species specific antigen present on envelope surface.

(iii) Serotype specific antigens present in the major outer membrane proteins (demonstrated by microimmunofluorescence).

Integrated Clinical Based Study of C.trachomatis/Trachoma

A seven year boy, Satender belonging to lower socioeconomic status from a village, presented to the Primary health center with swelling of right upper lid. The examination of the eye revealed conjunctival inflammation, papillary hypertrophy and inflammation of the cornea.

Linkages: Pg. 340-342, 344, 361, 362

What is the likely diagnosis in the above case?

A.1 (a) Trachoma, stage 2 (stage 1, is relatively asymptomatic).

How is conjuntival swab collected?

A.1 (b) A fine, flexible swab pre-moistened with sterile saline is introduced into lower conjunctiva swabbed and transported to the laboratory.

How was the name 'Chlamydia' derived?

A.1 (c) The name 'Chlamydia' is derived from the typical inclusion bodies produced by these bacteria, which are seen as enclosing the nuclei of the infected cells; as a mantle (Chlamys, meaning mantle).

Describe the life cycle of Chlamydia.

A.1 (d) The Chlamydia species exist in two forms, namely Elementary body (EB) and Reticulate body (RB)-pg. 340-341. The elementary body is the extracellular, infectious, metabolically inactive forms, sized 0.2-0.3 μm/200-300 nm in contrast to the reticulate body, which is intracellular, replicating, metabolically active form and sized 0.5-1.0 μm/500-1000 nm (see Fig. 10.1.2).

The elementary bodies attach to the specific receptors on the host cells and are subsequently endocytosed. Inside by about 12 hours; the elementary bodies transform to the reticulate body, which has a diffuse nucleoid. The reticulate body is metabolically active and by about 24 hours reorganize to form elementary bodies. The vacuoles containing EBs enlarge in size to form the inclusion body, which has a diagnostic significance, as is demonstrable by histologic and fluorescent stains. The mature inclusion body ruptures to release the numerous EBs by 48 hours. The EBs can infect new host cells.

Compare the morphological characteristics of the three species of Chlamydia.

A.1 (e) Morphological characteristics of Chlamydiae

	C.trachomatis	*C.pneumoniae*	*C. psittaci*
Inclusion body Morphology (approx. 1000 nm)	Round, vacuolar^	Round, dense	Large, irregular, dense*
Glycogen in Inclusion body	Yes (as organism gets stained with iodine)	No	No
Plasmid presence	Yes	No	Yes
Natural host	Man	Man	Birds (including parrots)

*Levinthal Cole Lillie bodies (LCL)

^Halbaerstaedter-Prowazek bodies (H.P.)

What are the epidemiological factors that could have led to the boy acquiring this infection?

A.2 (a) The likely poor hygiene kept by the child and the dusty conditions in the village, may be the likely factors in the causation of this disease.

Describe the epidemiology of trachoma.

A.2 **(b)** **Agent:** *C. trachomatis* (Serotypes A, B, Ba, C).

Reservoir of infection: Chronically infected eye of older children and adults.

Source of infection: Ocular discharges of infected persons and contaminated fomites.

Mode of Transmission – Eye to eye transmission occurs, which may occur by direct contact with ocular discharges of infected person by infected fingers or indirectly by fomites; such as towels.

Host: – The infections occur worldwide. It is endemic in Africa, Middle East, India and the Far East. It is responsible for visual impairment of blindness in 1.8 million people.

Age: – Children from the age of two to five years are the most infected.

– Poverty, poor hygiene and illiteracy favour this infection.

Environment: – Sunlight, dust and smoke predispose to this infection.

In India, the incidence of active infection is found during April-May and from July-September.

How can you provisionally differentiate Inclusion conjunctivitis from Trachoma?

A.3 In *Inclusion conjunctivitis*, the lower lid conjunctiva is most often involved, unlike the *trachoma* which often involves the upper tarsal conjunctiva.

Describe Chlamydia trachomatis (including endemic trachoma).

A.4 *C. trachomatis* is an obligate intracellular bacterium and strict human pathogen. It causes disease primarily by direct destruction of infected host cells during multiplication and by eliciting inflammatory responses in the host. The organism multiplies intracellularly and probably escapes destruction, by prevention of lysosomal fusion with the phagocytic vacuole having the organism. Natural infection with *C. trachomatis* appears to confers little protection against reinfection. Multiple or persistent infections are often caused by this organism.

Endemic trachoma:

It is a *chronic keratoconjunctivitis* and forms typical inclusion bodies named after Halberstaedter Prowazek, who in 1907 transmitted this infection to organutans and demonstrated these inclusion bodies in the organutans experimentally infected. It forms an important public health problem in the developing countries in Africa, Middle East and Asia. It is responsible for 20 million cases of blindness, which can be prevented.

It is usually contracted in early childhood from close contacts by *fingers or fomites*. It may also be transmitted by dust. The first exposure results in acute conjunctivitis, which usually resolves without sequelae; unlike the subsequent exposures. Reinfection usually occur and their persistence is associated with associated inflammatory reaction responsible for the pathology in the eye. Blindness results from conjunctival deformities and severe corneal scarring that may ensue.

The *treatment* is usually difficult, as reinfections continue to occur, due to poor hygiene; in which most patients live and the colonization of extraocular sites; as nasopharynx, rectum, and vagina, which reduce the effectivity of topical antibiotics. For the latter reason, the systemic antibiotics have a role. In public health programs, mass application of eyes of all children with erythromycin or tetracycline ointment is instituted for 3 weeks to two months.

Aspects related to case theme/examination assessment

Describe Inclusion conjunctivitis and Opthalmia neonatorum.

A.5 **Inclusion conjunctivitis:**

It is an acute conjunctivitis (unlike chronic in trachoma) disease of the adults, caused by D-K serotypes (unlike A-C in trachoma) of *C. trachomatis*. The disease is *usually benign*, as there is no chronicity or permanent eye damage. It is sexually transmitted with exposure to infected genital secretions. The *diagnosis* is similar to that; as performed for trachoma. *Topical antimicrobials* are effective in most cases but they may fail in some cases due to extracellular colonization of *C. trachomatis*, which may cause reinfection.

Ophthalmia neonatorum:

It is the *neonatal form* of inclusion conjunctivitis, acquired from the infected birth canal, 6-18 days post-delivery. The organism apparently gains entry through the conjunctival mucosa. The condition develops in about 35% infants of mothers infected with *C. trachomatis*. This can be *prevented* by local adminstration of doxycline. The acute conjunctivitis in this population can also be caused by number of other agents; as gonococcus, herpes or chemicals.

If the child is not properly treated, what serious sequelae could develop in the case?

A.6 Conjunctival scarring, trichiasis, lid abnormalities; as entropion, secondary eye infections; as corneal ulcer and sequelae; as corneal opacities and blindness.

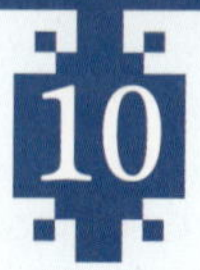

Integrated Clinical Based Study of C.psittaci/Psittacosis

A 40 year old widow, Mrs Sudershan was admitted to the medical emergency with history of abrupt onset of non-productive cough, high fever and prostration. Her home attendant gave history of parrot (her pet) having died 5 days before the onset of her illness. During her admission in the hospital, her consciousness got clouded.

Linkages: Pg. 340-342, 344, 361, 362

What is the most likely diagnosis of this case?

A.1 (a) The case is most likely to be having psittacosis.

Outline the taxonomical status related of the organism; implicated in this case.

A.1 (b) *C. psittaci* belongs to the family Chlamydiaceae. The latter has single genus; namely Chlamydia and four species psittaci, pneumoniae, trachomatis and pecorum). *C. trachomatis* has two biovars; namely TRIC (D to K) causing trachoma, PID, inclusion conjunctivitis and LGV (L1-L3) causing lymphogranuloma venerum.

Why was Chlamydia initially confused with viruses?

A.1 (c) Earlier they were thought to be viruses and were known by the name 'PLT' viruses (Psittacosis, lymphogranuloma venereum, trachoma). The confusion with viruses occurred because of their filterability through filters (0.45 μm pore size), obligate intracellular existence (inability to synthesize their own ATP and dependence on host's metabolism) and inability to be cultured on inanimate media.

What are the characteristics that have made Chlamydia being classified as bacteria?

A.1 (d) The workers agreed to classify them as bacteria (adapted to obligate intracellular existence) due to numerous features, as having a cell wall resembling gram negative bacteria, possessing both DNA and RNA (like bacteria), possessing numerous bacterial enzymes, possessing ribosomes and synthesizing own proteins, growth in cytoplasmic vacuoles, division by binary fission (with no eclipse phase) and susceptibility to antibacterial antimicrobials. The characteristic feature of these organisms is the unique biphasic life cycle.

Do all patients of psittacosis, give history of exposure to birds?

A.2 No.

How do you explain the development of clouded consciousness in the case?

A.3 In the case, the disease could have spread to the C.N.S. and caused meningoencephalitis, which could be responsible for this presentation.

Describe human psittacosis.

A.4 Human psittacosis is a zoonoses, contracted through inhalation of infected aerosol. The term psittacosis (in Latin, 'psittacus' a parrot) was applied by Morange in 1892, after studying the association of human cases with sick parrots. The infected parrot with this disease may be asymptomatic or clearly sick. This infection is seen in many other birds; as turkey, chicken and is likely in all birds, as all are susceptible. As a result, the term *ornithosis* (in Greek, 'ornith' means bird) was used to describe infections contracted from birds other than parrots or parakeets, but for unknown reasons the term psittacosis has persisted for all human infection, acquired from infected birds including parrots. The disease is usually latent in the birds but may become manifest with stress of capturing or transporting the birds. The prevalence or incidence of disease has decreased recently due to the malpractice of antimicrobial addition in bird feeds and the policy of many countries to quarantine imported birds. Man essentially *acquires* the disease by inhalation of infected aerosol. The I.P. is 5-15 days. The disease onset can be both insidious or abrupt. The disease can present both ^sporadically or as outbreaks. The disease is essentially seen in individuals, who remain in contact with birds such; as pet-shop owners, taxidermist, veterinarians, and individual pet owners. The disease usually present as *fever* and a *lower respiratory tract infection* in humans. However the disease can spread systemically and present; as meningoencephalitis, endocarditis, pericarditis, arthritis or as septicaemia. Case to case transmission is rare. The diagnosis is essentially suggested in individuals by history of exposure to birds. The *diagnosis* is essentially serologic, as culture of samples as blood or sputum can be hazardous, in absence of BSL-3 facilities. The *treatment* of choice is Doxycycline or azithromycin, which should be given for at least 1-2 weeks after defervescence (abatement of fever). The disease can be *prevented* by treating all infected birds with doxycycline for at least 45 consecutive days. All imported birds may be treated prophylactically or be quarantined adequately.

^occurying occasionally/irregularly

How could the infection have been prevented in this case?

A.5 (i) minimal contact with the infected bird.

(ii) Prophylactic antibiotics; as chloramphenicol or tetracycline, in this case at the time of the death of the parrot.

Aspects related to case theme/examination assessment

Describe C.pneumoniae.

A.6 It is the third species of Chlamydia being described in the past quarter century. It was called *TWAR*, after the first conjunctival isolates of the species (TW-183 and AR-39). The organism can be distinguished from the other species on basis of DNA hybridization and elementary body morphology; as seen electron microscopically.

The infections occur throughout the year and are *spread by* the respiratory droplets (aerosol). The infection begins in early childhood and reaches a peak in young adulthood. It is an important cause of pharyngitis, bronchitis and pneumonia ('walking' pneumonia); with serological studies showing seroprevalence exceeding 40% in many parts of the world. However in most cases, the infection is subclinical/asymptomatic. The *clinical spectrum* is similar to *Mycoplasma pneumoniae* infections. Seroepidemiological studies studying antibody to *C. pneumoniae*, immunocytochemical and PCR studies of atheroma (for genome in atheroma) have implicated this organism to atherosclerosis and coronary artery disease. The *diagnosis* of *C. pneumoniae* infection is difficult, as it is difficult to culture and commercial antigen and genome detection tests are not available. The antibody tests can't differentiate the antibodies formed against *C. pneumoniae,* from those formed against the other species. The *treatment* of choice is erythromycin or tetracycline administered for 10-14 days.

Section X: Atypical/Unconventional/Obligate Intracellular Bacteria

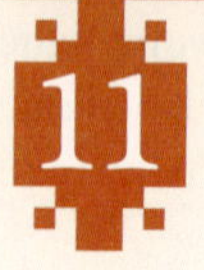

Laboratory Diagnosis and Treatment (Overview)

An overview of the comparative approach in laboratory diagnosis of key atypical/obligate intracellular bacteria

Organism / Disease	Specimen	Stain enhanced Microscopy	Detection of Microbial antigen/ metabolite/genome	Serological/ Hypersensitivity Tests	Culture of Inanimate Organism In Media / Characterization of Isolate	Differential Diagnosis	Antimicrobial Susceptibility Tests
Mycoplasma pneumoniae	- Throat swab - sputum - Nasopharyngeal aspirate, - tracheal aspirate, - BAL, - Pleural fluid For *M. hominis* and *Ureaplasma urealyticum* Uretheral, prostatic secretions, cervical swab, urine etc. No need to look for *M. genitalium* in routine specimens; as lower genital tract because are commonly found in healthy individuals, so make results uninterpretable. However may consider in sterile specimens; as joint fluid with evidence of inflammation; which are culture negative for conventional microbes	Gram stain: stains poorly, is gram negative	Antigen can be demonstrated by direct immunofluor-escence test and ELISA PCR available for respiratory sample –	- *Non-specific* - : 'cold agglutination test' - agglutination of O'RBC at 4°C, titre > 1:32 (dissociation at 37°C), details pg. 347. - *specific*: C.F.T. and others	- Diagnosis requires reference labs - Media enriched with serum & yeast extract used (colonies can take a few days to appear) - Penicillium & Thallium acetate used to make selective media (this organism is resistant to thallium & Penicillin, as organism lacks cell wall) - colonies confirmed on media by staining with Giemsa stain (violet) or Diene's-stain (red purple), observed with hand lens - Fluorescent conjugated antimycoplasmal antibody can also be used for staining Subculturing growth on media containing antimycoplasma serum (sub-culture not done by platinum loop, but cutting agar with growth & spreading - For characterization & confirmation of isolate pg. 342	- *Mycoplasma hominis* (can breakdown arginine) - *Ureaplasma urealyticum* (produces urease) - *M. genitalium*	

Contd.

Contd.

Chlamydia psittaci	Sputum, blood	In smear, inclusion bodies can be demonstrated by giemsa stain	- NAAT (Nucleic acid amplification test)	- C.F.T test - Micro-immunofluorescence (MIF, most sensitive and specific)	specimen inoculated into 6-8 day yolk sac of chick egg intraperitoneally or intracerebrally into mice. McCoy and Hela cell lines useful After 1-2 weeks elementary body L.C.L (Levinthal Cole Lillie) can be demonstrated For characterization & confirmation of isolate see p. 342		
Chlamydia pneumoniae	Throat swab, sputum, serum	Giemsa stain and fluorescent stain can detect EBs [Low sensitivity]	ELISA helpful in detecting genus specific antigen - NAAT	- MIF (most sensitive and specific) - Single sample IgG titre ≥ 512 and IgM titre ≥ 16	- Cell culture difficult, HEp-2-used For characterization & confirmation of isolate see. p 342		
Chlamydia trachomatis							
(i) A→C sero-types [Hyperendem-ric trachoma]	Conjunctival smear & scraping (for trachoma)	- Gram stain: poor staining - Giemsa stain - Fluorescent stain demonstrate inclusion body (Halberstaedter Prowazek body)	- NAAT; as PCR, LCR, SDA, TMA	C.F. antibodies also appear (not usually helpful in diagnosis of trachoma - MIF	NA: NG Material after t/t with streptomycin or polymyxin B is inoculated into Yolk-sac. Idoxuridine/ Cycloheximide t/ted McCoy cells (McCoy cells rendered non-replicating by irradiation/ antimetabolite often used. Inclusion bodies in it, detected by staining with fluorescent antibody - Isolation also possible by mice inoculation		
(ii) D→K serotypes (numerous syndromes)	- Exudates (as from Inclusion conjuctivitis, opthalmia neonatorum, genital infections. The lesions could be conjunctivitis urethritis, cervicitis, salpingitis, PID etc. - Cervical swab, blood	Inclusion bodies of *C. trachomatis* contain glycogen, so can also be stained with Iodine. DNA probes helpful in diagnosing *C. trachomatis*			-		
(iii) L1-L3 (Lympho-granuloma venereum)	- Smear from bubo - Scraping from different sites	-	- DNA probe useful	- MIF, ELISA, CFT - Frei test	- NG, NA: details see pg. 342, 355		
Rickettsiae	skin/biopsy specimen, serum	- Poorly stained with Gram stain, stains bluish purple with Giemsa	- Bacterial genome detection in samples; as eschar attempted with PCR	- Serological tests- C.F.T,ELISA,I.F.A.T - Weil-Felix test- Agglutination pattern (See pg. 348-349)	Not cultivable on inanimate medium / ISOLATION performed ONLY IN REFERENCE LABS, as can cause fatal infection in lab personnel		
					Cultured in yolk sac/ chorioallantoic membrane (limited growth): arthropod cell lines : Vero, Lab animals Details see pg. 343.		

An overview of the antimicrobial options for infections caused by atypical/Unconventional/Obligate Intracellular Bacteria

	Cell Wall Inhibitors	**Cell-Membrane Inhibitors**	**Amino Acid Synthesis Inhibitors**	**Nucleic Acid Synthesis Inhibitors**	**Others**
ORGANISM					
Mycoplasma pneumoniae	No role of these, as organisms, lack cell wall		• Tetracycline • Erythromycin (DOC) • Azithromycin (DOC) • Clarithromycin	• Fluoroquinolones	
Ureaplasma urealyticum	-do-		• Erythromycin		
Rickettsial species insluding Coxiella			• Doxycline (DOC) • Chloramphenicol	• Fluoroquinolones	
Chlamydia trachomatis			• Doxycycline (DOC) • Azithromycin (DOC)	• Ofloxacin • Sulfonamide	
Chlamydia pneumoniae			• Doxycycline (DOC) • Azithromycin (DOC)	• Fluoroquinolones	
Chlamydia psittaci			• Chloramphenicol • Tetracyline (DOC)		

NB: Sulfonamides may enhance the disease process in rickettsial infections, hence contraindicated..

DOC refers to drug of choice.

12 Assessment/Examination Questions

1. Outline the taxonomical status of Mycoplasma. Can some bacteria mimick Mycoplasma under certain conditions? A2c., p. 345, A 4b., p. 347
2. (a) Enumerate unique characteristics of Mycoplasma. A 2d., p. 345-346
   (b) Why are Mycoplasmas sometimes confused with viruses? A 2., p. 346
   (c) Why are mycoplasma not categorized as viruses? A 2e., p. 346
3. (a) How are Mycoplasma similar and different from L forms? A 2g., p. 346
   (b) How are L forms different from Mycoplasma? A 4d., p. 347
4. Describe laboratory diagnosis of Mycoplasma infections. p. 360 and chapter 4., p. 345
5. Describe *Mycoplasma pneumoniae* and *Ureaplasma urealyticum*. p. 340-342, 344, chapter 5., p. 345
6. Describe cold agglutination test and Streptococcus MG agglutination test. A 3c,d., p. 347
7. Classify Rickettsial infections. p. 340, A3., p. 353
8. Describe laboratory diagnosis of Rickettsial infections. A 3b., p. 352, p. 361
9. Describe Epidemic typhus, Brill-Zinsser disease, Scrub typhus, Rocky mountain spotted fever, Typhus fevers, Trench fever and Q fever. A 3., p. 353, chapter 5-7., section 10
10. Describe Weil-Felix reaction and Neil-Mooser reaction. A 3b., p. 348-349, A3c., p. 349
11. Classify Chlamydiae. Enumerate general characteristics of Chlamydiae. A1e., p. 356, A 1c, d., p. 356, p. 341, 343
12. Describe morphology of Chlamydiae emphasizing the relationship of elementary body and reticulate body. A1d, p. 356
13. Describe laboratory diagnosis of chlamydial infection with special reference to 'Urogenital chlamydiasis'. A 5a,b., p. 354, p. 361, A7, 8., p. 355
14. Describe Lymphogranuloma venereum with special reference to Frei test. A 7., p. 355
15. Compare the morphological characteristics of three species of Chlamydiae. A 1e., p. 356
16. Describe Trachoma, Psittacosis and Ornithosis. A 2b, 3,4., p. 357, A4., p. 358
17. Describe TRIC agents and NGU. A1c., p. 354, A 1b, A8., p. 208

Section XI: General Virology

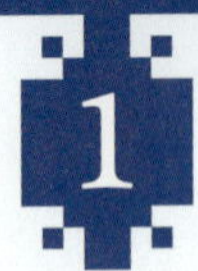

General Properties of Viruses

If Charles Darwin reappeared today, he might be surprised to know that humans have descended from viruses as well as from apes. — *Robin A. Weiss*

It appears that the viruses exist in the twilight zone that separates the 'living entities' from the 'non-living entities'. However their importance, cannot be underemphasized, as the viruses are both the commonest 'entities' found in the environment and the commonest cause of human infections. Let's study these agents.

Mention how the concept of viruses developed; as agents of disease during the last 100 years.

A.1 (a) For many centuries the causes of diseases as small pox, chicken pox and polio remained unclear, although it was clear that these diseases were transmitted from person to person. It was Louis Pasteur, who proposed the term 'virus' (Latin for poison) for this group of infectious agents. He postulated that this group of infectious agents were smaller than bacteria, hence could not be observed under the light microscope. It is for this reason that these were also termed as 'ultramicroscopic'. Pasteur also proposed a viral etiology for rabies and was able to develop a vaccine (1884) for it, even before the etiological agent could be isolated and identified!

The key historical development in virology are given in a tabular form (Table 11.1.1)

Table 11.1.1: Historical developments in virology

Year	Development
1892	• D. Ivanovsky, a Russian biologist, was the first to isolate a virus, named tobacco mosaic virus. Showed it to be ultramicroscopic (beyond resolution of light microscope) and demonstrated its transmissibility.
1898	• Loeffler and Frosch isolated a filterable agent (i.e., devoid of particles equal to or smaller than size of bacteria) and discovered it to be cause of foot and mouth disease of cattle
1900-1901	• Walter Reed and his colleagues from Cuba identified the virus that caused yellow fever. The epidemiology and role of mosquito in the transmission of disease was worked out. This was the first human disease in which viral aetiology was worked out.
1903	• Remlinger and Riffat Bay identified the virus that caused rabies
1907	• Asburn and Craig identified the virus that caused dengue
1909	• Landsteiner and Popper and Flexner and Lewis identified the virus that caused poliomyelitis and successfully transmitted this disease to monkeys
1910	• Francis Rous, an American pathologist discovered viruses causing cancer
1915-1917 1930	• F. Twort; a British biologist and F.D. Herelle; a French biologist discovered bacteriophages (bacterial viruses) • Goodpasteur developed the chick embryo technique for cultivation of viruses
1933? 1934 1935	• Smith isolated/discovered influenza virus • Hyashi Isolated/discovered Japanese encephalitis virus • Wendell Stanley successfully crystallized tobacco mosaic virus and demonstrated that it retained its ability to cause infection.
1933-38	• German Ernst Ruska invented the electron microscope, which made feasible the study of small virus particles
1940	• Tissue culture techniques developed for cultivation of viruses
1953	• Row isolated/discovered the adenovirus
1957	• D. Carleton Gajdusek discovered causes of slow viral diseases
1983	• Luc Montagnier discovered/isolated the HIV virus (for which he shared the Nobel prize in 2008)

Enumerate the scientists who got Nobel prize for contribution in the field of virology.

A.1 (b) **Table 11.1.2:** Scientists awarded Nobel prize for contribution in virology

Year	Scientists	Work
1966	Peyton Roux	Viral carcinogenesis
1975	Dubecco, Temin & Baltimore	Reverse transcriptase and Cancer
1976	Carlton Gajdusek	Kuru
1977	Stanley Pruisner	Prions
2008	• Harald Zur Hausen • Luc Montagnier	• Human Papilloma virus • Human Immunodeficiency virus

Enumerate the characteristics of viruses that resemble those of 'non living' agents?

A.2 (i) Do not have any cellular organelles or cellular organization

(ii) Some viruses; as Tobacco mosaic virus can be crystallized, just as chemicals

(iii) Viruses cannot exist independently of the host cells

Enumerate the characteristics of viruses that resemble those of 'living agents'?

A.3 (i) Viruses that are crystallized retain their infectivity

(ii) They reproduce and have a growth curve just like 'living entities'

(iii) Can spread from one cell to another cell

(iv) Their reproduction can be interrupted by drugs

What are the differences between bacteria and viruses?

A.4 (a) **Table 11.1.3:** Differences between bacteria and viruses

Bacteria	Viruses
• Larger (seen with light microscope)	• Smaller (ultramicroscopic, not seen with light microscope)
• Contain *both* DNA and RNA	• Contain *either* DNA or RNA
• Have cellular organelles & organization	• Lack both of them
• Enzymes present for synthesis of important molecules	• Lack the enzymes for synthesis of important molecules
• Retained (not filtered) on routine bacterial filters	• Filterable through these filters due to their small size
• Replicate intracellularly and extracellularly	• Replicate only intracellularly
• Antibacterial antimicrobials usually effective	• Antiviral drugs sometimes effective

Mention about the origin of viruses.

A.4 (b) The origin of viruses is not clear. There are various hypotheses to suggest their origin. According to one hypothesis, viruses evolved from self replicating molecules in the precellular world.

Another hypothesis suggests that viruses were once cells, that lost all cellular organization and function. A third theory suggests viruses to have extraterrestrial planetary origin!

Describe the challenges in classification of viruses.

A.4 (c) The function of the taxonomy is not just categorization, its knowledge helps in predicting organisms in related taxa and plays key role in understanding the epidemiology and pathogenesis of newly isolated viruses.

Initially; when viruses were discovered, little was known about their structure and they were classified by the type of host and host structure infected, e.g., bacterial viruses (bacteriophages), plant viruses and animal viruses. The latter could be further grouped, as dermatropic (if; infecting skin) or neurotropic (if; infecting CNS).

As more viruses started getting discovered, conflicts starting arising. This led to the establishment in 1966 of International committee on taxonomy of viruses (ICTV), which led to a uniform and universal taxonomical system for viral classification.

As viruses differ tremendously at the cellular organization from living organisms, it is difficult to classify them by the typical taxonomic structure; as Kingdom, Phylum etc.

The highest taxonomic category by the ICTV for the viruses is the family (ending; for the name of the virus family as 'viridae', e.g., Herpesviridae. The next level may be subfamily, which ends in 'virinae', for example beta-herpes virinae. The next level is the genus to be further followed by species level. However despite advances in classification, the issue of defining species has not been resolved. Species of the same virus that may differ from each other in nucleotide sequence are referred to as strains of the same species.

The main criteria for virus classification is the structural and chemical composition in genetic makeup. Currently English common names rather than Latinized binomial term are used to designate a viral species, e.g., Human immunodeficiency virus.

How large are the viruses?

A.5 (a) Size

Viruses are approximately 100-1000 fold smaller than the cells they infect.

Most of them are so small* that it requires the help of an electron microscope to view them (except poxviruses). It is for this reason, they are described as ultramicroscopic (not visible by light microscope). The animal viruses range in size from the smallest parvoviruses (approximately 20 nm (0.02 µm) in diameter) to the poxviruses 300 nm (0.30 µm) in length), which are as large as small bacteria.

Nb: Some cylindrical viruses; as Tobacco mosaic virus may be relatively long (300 nm/0.3 µm) but so narrow in diameter (15nm/0.015 µm) that their visibility is limited without the high resolution and magnification of an electron microscope.

*The extremely small size of these particles makes them able to pass filters, that would retain most bacteria.

Can the viruses be detected by light microscope?

A.5 (b) Most viruses are beyond the limit of resolution of light microscope, i.e., 20 nm, except poxviruses (size is 300 nm or 0.30 µm)

Describe the structure of the virus?

A.6 (a) Viral Structure

The whole structure of viral particle/virion is sometimes described as nucleocapsid ±envelope.

The organization of its structure can be represented as below: (Fig. 11.1.1)

- **Covering**
  - Envelope/membrane (presence is +-)
  - Capsid
- **Central core**
  - DNA or RNA molecule (but never both)
  - Enzymes (sometimes, only few enzymes are present)

The detailed study of structure of the mature viral particle, (i.e., the virion) has been possible by electron micrographs (images) of negatively stained preparation of the clinical material and by X-ray crystallography studies (reveal arrangement of polypeptide chains) of the virions.

The basic structure of a virion is a protein capsid, which covers the nucleic acid strand. The outermost covering of a virion is an envelope, which is present in some virions (many of the animal virus families). This layer is external to the capsid and is derived from the nuclear or cytoplasmic membrane of the host cell during release of the nucleocapsid/virion from the infected cell (by process of budding). Enveloped viruses have a space between the envelope and the capsid of the virion, which is filled with matrix or *tegument* proteins, which help to stabilize the viral particle. Viruses that lack the envelope are known as *naked (non-enveloped)* viruses. The entry (and exit) of the naked virions differs from those of the enveloped virions. The *envelope* is composed of combination of carbohydrates, lipid and proteins. Sometimes the envelope has glycoprotein spikes projecting to the outside, which help to attach the virions to specific receptor sites on susceptible host surfaces. What other *benefit* this structure gives to the virion is not clear? The covering of the virion with the host cell molecules can prevent the attack from the host immune system and help in the spread of the viruses by fusion of the envelope with the host cell membrane. However, enveloped viruses are more susceptible than naked viruses to environmental conditions. The environmental conditions that can damage the membrane include lipid solvents; as ether, increased temperature, drying, extreme pH, cycles of freezing and thawing and chemical disinfectants; as phenol.

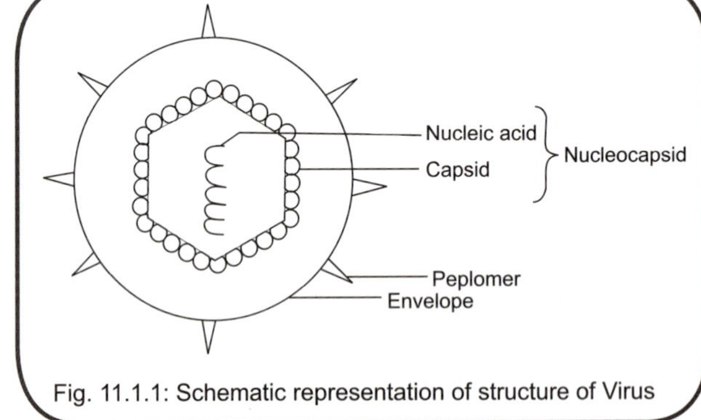

Fig. 11.1.1: Schematic representation of structure of Virus

The envelope remains maintained only in aqueous solutions. Hence to remain viable, these viruses have to remain wet and are consequently spread usually by blood, fluids and respiratory droplets. These viruses need not kill the cell to spread.

Capsid

The nucleic acid of most virions is covered by a capsid, which is composed of protein. The capsid performs many functions including attachment of the virion to host cell, giving the virus a shape, organization of the viral genome and protecting the viral genome from enzymes; as nucleases in the environment may destroy it.

Each capsid is made of smaller building blocks called capsomeres. They are usually *identical but there can be a variety in it. Each capsomere is made of polypeptides of a configuration that permits it to interlock with other capsomeres. These are tightly packed and often gives a crystalline appearance. X-ray crystallography reveals the symmetry of arrangement of these molecules. These capsomeres are usually held together by noncovalent bonds, which are usually demonstrable by electron microscopy. The capsid makes the virus withstand harsh environmental conditions, as it is a tough structure. Hence, these viruses can withstand acid and bile of GIT including sewage and consequently do get transmitted by faecal-oral route.

NB: capsomeres are morphological units, whereas protomers (one or more polypeptide) are structural units.

* because of limited genetic complexity of viruses.

The capsomeres assemble into capsids with icosahedral, helical or complex symmetry.

Icosahedral symmetry (Fig. 11.1.2a)

Capsids with icosahedral symmetry are more complex than those with helical symmetry, as the capsomeres in it consist of several different polypeptide groupings. Icosahedral structures approximate sphere. They should be economically constructed, so as to create maximal internal volume. A icosahedron is a rigid structure and in its simplest case will be a polygon with 20 triangular faces with characteristic two fold, threefold and fivefold rotational symmetries.

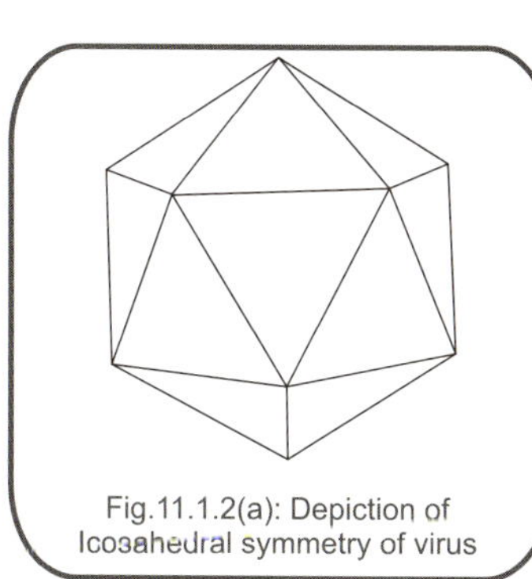

Fig.11.1.2(a): Depiction of Icosahedral symmetry of virus

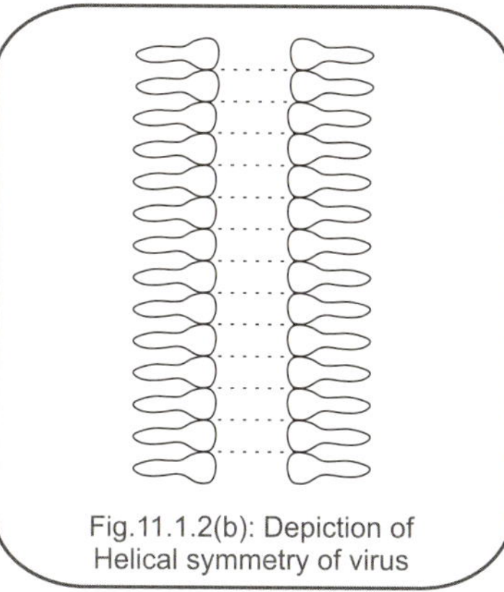

Fig.11.1.2(b): Depiction of Helical symmetry of virus

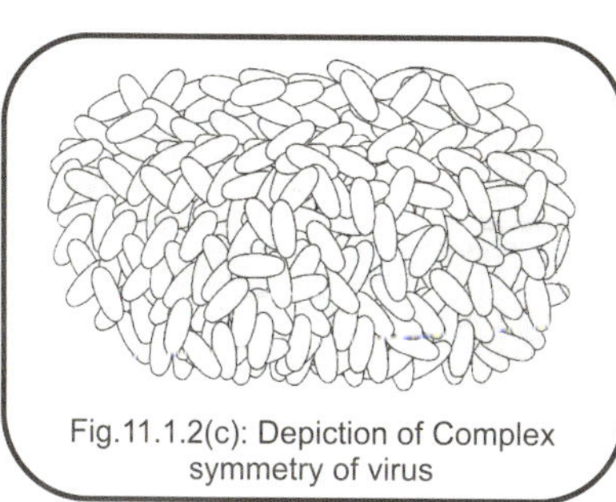

Fig.11.1.2(c): Depiction of Complex symmetry of virus

Helical symmetry (Fig. 11.1.2b)

This is seen in RNA viruses, most of which are enveloped viruses. This type of symmetry is unsuitable for DNA viruses. Here the capsomeres and nucleic acid are wound together in a helical or spiral structure. One can visualize this helical structure by rolling a two-dimensional lattice into a cylindrical structure that can accommodate a nucleic acid inside.

Complex symmetry (Fig. 11.1.2c)

Some viruses capsids don't get categorized into helical or icosahedral symmetry, form complex capsids and are categorized into complex category eg some animal viruses of family Poxviridae and Retroviridae.

Shape of viruses

- Most of the enveloped viruses are round or pleomorphic
- Some animal viruses with unique shapes are:
  - Bullet-shaped (Rhabdovirus)
  - Brick-shaped (Poxvirus)
  - Rod-shaped (Tobacco mosaic virus)

Nucleic acids

The genes in viruses vary from few in the smallest viruses to several hundred in the largest viruses, which may exist as DNA genome or as a RNA genome but genome never exists as both DNA and RNA.

Arenaviridae/Spherical	Arenavirus/Lymphochoriomeningitis virus, Lassa virus, Machupo virus, Junin virus, Sabia virus & others	Lymphocytic choriomeningitis, Lassa fever and others
Caliciviridae/Icosahedral	Calicivirus/Human Calciviruses, Hepatitis E virus, Norwalk virus	Diarrhoeal disease, Jaundice
Picornaviridae/Icosahedral	Human enterovirus A-D & others see below*	* see below
Coronaviridae/Petal shaped spikes project (peplomer) project from surface	Coronavirus/Human Coronaviruses	Respiratory infection
Flaviviridae/spherical	• Flavivirus (Flavi=yellow)/Yellow fever virus, Dengue virus, Japanese encephalitis virus, St. Louis encephalitis virus • Hepacivirus/Hepatitis C virus & others	• Yellow fever, Dengue, Encephalitis • Hepatitis C infection
Togaviridae/Icosahedral (Toga, Greek for "Mantle")	• Alphavirus/Chickengunya virus, Sindbis virus, Eastern, Western and Venezuelan equine encephalitis viruses (EEE., WEE and VEE) • Rubivirus	• Chickengunya, • Encephalitis • Rubella
Retroviridae (positive strand/positive sense)/spherical	• Delta retrovirus/Human T lymphotropic virus 1, Human T lymphotropic virus 2 • Lentivirus/HIV- 1,HIV- 2	• Adult T cell leukemia/Lymphoma (Associated with HTLV-1) • AIDS

* Viruses in family Picornaviridae

Genus	Species	Disease
Human enterovirus A	Human Coxsackie A (types 2, 3, 5, 7, 8, 10, 12, 14 & 26), enterovirus 71	Aseptic meningitis, Herpangia, Hand-foot and mouth disease by Group A viruses
Human enterovirus B	Human Coxsackievirus A (type 9), Human Coxsackie-virus B (types 1 to 6)	Epidemic myalgia (Bornholm disease), Myocarditis, Pericarditis, Aseptic meningitis by Group B viruses
Human enterovirus C	Human Coxsackie A (types 1, 11, 13, 15, 17-22 & 24)	
Human enterovirus D	Human enterovirus (types 68 & 70)	• Pneumonia and bronchitis (type 68) • Acute haemorrhage conjunctivitis (type 70)
Poliovirus	Human poliovirus (types 1to 3)	Poliomyelitis
Human rhinovirus A, B and C	>100 serotypes	Common cold
Aphthovirus	Foot and mouth disease virus	Foot and mouth Disease
Hepatovirus	Human Hepatitis A virus	Hepatitis A
Parechovirus	Parechovirus (previously classified as Echovirus)	

Provide a detailed account of viral multiplication.

A.8 It is important to understand this, as it helps to appreciate the pathogenesis of viral diseases, find the role of viruses in cancer, understand antiviral chemotherapy and devise newer strategies for antiviral drugs and vaccines.

These are number of steps involved in the virus multiplication, but the overall production of viruses can be studied in the one-step growth curve. It is a representation of the overall change with time, in the amount of infectious virus in a single cell that has been infected by a single virus particle. The curve begins with the eclipse period to be followed by the exponential growth period and the plateau phase. The eclipse period represents the time elapsed from initial viral entry, disassembly of the parental virus to the assembly of the first progeny virion. This period for most viruses of human viruses varies from one to twenty hours. The exponential growth period is characterized by exponential increase in the number of progeny virus produced within an infected cell. The maximum yield per cell is characteristic for each virus cell system and the yield can vary from 100 to several thousands virions per cell.

The viral multiplication can be divided into 6 phases, though there may be overlapping in some phases (Fig. 11.1.3).

1. **Adsorption:** A pre-requisite for this step is a collision between the *virion and the host cell.

   This is the first step in the infection of host cell. Ideally, to prevent the viral infections, the antiviral drugs and vaccines, should be targeting this step. During this step, viral attachment protein (VAP); as the surface capsid/ envelope attach to receptors on host cell (Table 11.1.7). Damage to VAPs can inactivate the virus. Production of antibodies against these structures can also prevent viral infection.

This step involves the interaction of specific viral structure; as glycoprotein spikes in rabies virus or gp 120 in HIV, with receptor (specific) on target cells of the host. If the receptors are lacking from a target cell, then the natural viral infection is not possible. Lack of acetylcholine receptors in the rodents, explains their resistance to the rabies disease. If this phase of adsorption is bypassed and the nucleic acid of rabies virus is introduced directly into the rodent cells, they become susceptible to this disease.

NB: *Virion –A mature, extracellular particle that is virulent (which can establish infection in a host) is called virion.

Table 11.1.7: Target cell and Receptors of some viruses

Virus	Viral attachment protein	Target cell	Receptors
Rhinovirus	VP1-VP-2-VP3 complex	Epithelial cell	Intercellular adhesion molecule-1 (ICAM I)
Influenza A	HAgp	Epithelial cells	Sialic acid▲
Rabies	G protein gp	Neuron	Acetylcholine receptor, NCAM
HIV	gp 120	Helper T cell	♦CD4 molecule and chemokine receptors.

▲ Sialic acid is a sugar found widely on different human cells, which explains the ability of influenza to infect many different cells.

♦ CD4 molecule is found on a limited number of cell types, which explains the restricted range of cells, HIV can infect.

NB: A thousands of receptors can be present on a cell surface to which hundreds of virions can adsorb, once the cell is infected by a specific virion, it is resistant to infection by other virions.

2. **Penetration:** This step can occur by two processes, namely endocytosis (viropexis) and fusogenic pathway. *Endocytosis* is a normal path used by mammalian cells to ingest nutrients. Here the cell subverts this pathway to facilitate entry of virions, e.g., in non-enveloped viruses.

   Fusogenic pathway, as the name indicates involves fusion of the viral envelope with the plasma membrane of the host cell releasing the nucleocapsid into the cell. This pathway obviously occurs in enveloped viruses.

3. **Uncoating:** For most of the viruses the lysosomal enzymes of the host cell can carry out this step, but for some, new enzymes (proteins) may be required to be synthesized to complete the process.

   This process involves removal of the outer layer (if present) and capsid of the virus, so that the nucleic acid of the virus is released into the host cell. This could make the viral genes ready for expression to initiate the viral replication.

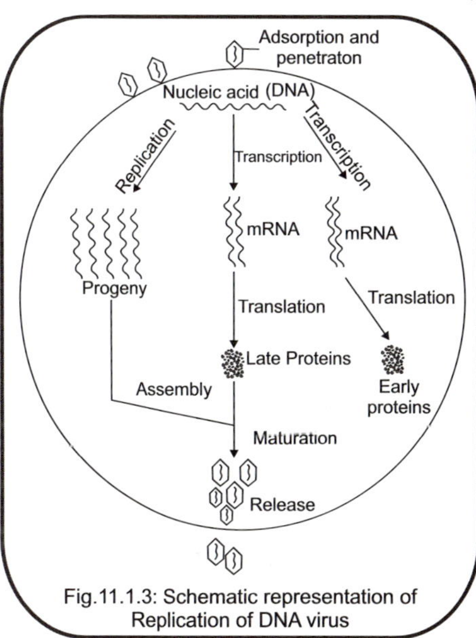

Fig.11.1.3: Schematic representation of Replication of DNA virus

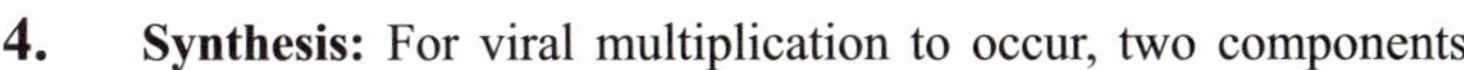

4. **Synthesis:** For viral multiplication to occur, two components need to be synthesized; namely viral protein and viral nucleic acid. *Viral protein* (required for capsid) is always synthesized in the host cell cytoplasm. The *nucleic acid* of most DNA viruses is synthesized in the nucleus of the host cell nucleus; except the poxvirus, for which the synthesis occurs in the cell cytoplasm. The nucleic acid of most RNA viruses occurs in the cytoplasm of the host cell excepting some orthomyxoviruses, paramyxoviruses and retroviruses, which are synthesized partly in the host cell nucleus.

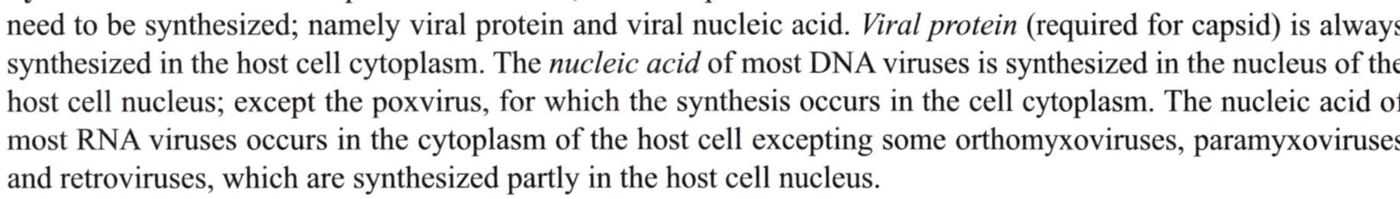

   DNA viruses vary tremendously in their genome size, which may make them vary in their dependence on host cell enzymes; from total dependence to no dependence, e.g., Parvovirus is totally dependent on host cell enzymes while poxviruses (one of the largest viruses) is totally independent of host cell enzymes, i.e., generally smaller the viral genome, more it has to depend on the host cell to provide the functions for viral replication.

   The *translation* of the first viral mRNAs into enzymes (protein) has a very important function to perform, i.e., takeover the host cell processes and divert them to those of viral replication. The genes of the viral nucleic acid can be categorized into early genes and late genes. The transcription products of *early genes* are referred to as early mRNAs and their translation products; as early protein, which are involved in viral genome replication. The *late proteins* of the late mRNA (of late genes) are involved in protein synthesis required for capsid synthesis. They are also involved in coordination of viral maturation and viral release processes.

The mechanism of nucleic acid synthesis varies in the different classes of viruses. Most viruses contain double stranded (ds) DNA or single stranded (ss) RNA. One must appreciate that the *central theme* in them is the transcription of specific mRNAs from viral nucleic acid (except for positive sense RNA viruses, which can directly act as mRNAs). Following are the various mechanisms:

1. *ss DNA viruses:* Here the cellular DNA polymerase (not viral) is used to make a complementary strand of DNA. The double stranded DNA form (also called replicative form) acts as a template for it replication and also for its transcription into mRNA for translation into viral proteins, e.g., Parvovirus.
2. *ds DNA viruses:* Here the process starts with a part of the viral DNA getting transcribed and translated into early proteins.
3. *ss RNA virus (with positive polarity):* Here the RNA molecular can serve directly as mRNA, so this category there is no dependence on cellular RNA dependent RNA polymerase. So, the parental RNA molecule serves both as mRNA for translation of polypeptide and in the later stage as a template for the synthesis of complementary (-ve) strand, from which multiple (+ve) RNA strands are synthesized.
4. *ss RNA virus (with negative polarity)*: The negative stranded RNA of the virus cannot be translated until it is converted into a positive stranded RNA and the host cell has no RNA - dependent RNA polymerase

   So the infecting virus particle must contain (viral) RNA - dependent RNA polymerase, as the host cell has no means of replicating viral RNA. The virus must bring this enzyme with its genome into the host cell. The positive stranded RNA (single stranded) virus strand, once synthesized is able to synthesize viral proteins and numerous negative RNA strands, required for synthesis of numerous virions.
5. *ds RNA virus:* The virus in such a category indicates that each consists of nucleic acid; as one positive and one negative strand RNA (intertwined) in a segmented form, each segment coding for one polypeptide.
6. *ss RNA (positive polarity*, replicated via a DNA intermediate): e.g., retroviruses

   Here the key enzyme present is the RNA dependent DNA polymerase (reverse transcriptase), which converts the ss RNA first into DNA-RNA hybrid and then into DNA-DNA molecule, which gets integrated into the host DNA. From the latter, viral ss RNA and other viral proteins get synthesized for virion multiplication.

5. **Maturation:** When the concentration of the virion components; as capsomeres, nucleic acid reach a high concentration, then the self assembly of this components into virion starts occurring. For most viruses the assembly of nucleocapsids takes place in the compartment of the host cell, where the nucleic acid replication occurs, i.e., cytoplasm for most RNA viruses and nucleus for most DNA viruses. This implies that for DNA viruses, the capsid proteins have to be transported, from the cytoplasm (site of synthesis of proteins) to the nucleus. As far as the naked viruses are concerned, the virion maturation is complete at this stage. For enveloped viruses, however the envelope is to be acquired from the nuclear membrane (e.g., herpes virus) or from the plasma membrane of the host cell (as orthomyxoviruses and paramyxoviruses). This implies that for most enveloped viruses, infectious progeny is extracellular.
6. **Release of virions:** Many of the non-enveloped viruses are released from the host cell, as a result of the death of host cell, which leads to lysis of the cell. No specific enzymes are required for causing the death of the host cell, which usually occurs as a result of the host cell functions not getting carried out.

   The *enveloped viruses* are released by a process of *budding*. This process is actually a part of the maturation process. First the virus specific glycoprotein is synthesized and transported to the host cell membrane. Then the cytoplasmic domains of these proteins binds. The nucleocapsid is enveloped by the host cell membrane and finally released from the cell. In some cases, host cell damage does not lead to cell death, as the plasma membrane can be repaired following budding.

   The period from the adsorption of the virus to appearance of first infections virus progeny inside cell takes about 15-30 hours for most animal viruses (15-30 mins for bacteriophages). This period is known as eclipse phase.

Abnormal replicative cycle

Many types of abnormal replicative cycles can occur as follows:

- *Abortive infection:* As the name indicates, in this case either premature or unviable non-infectious virions gets produced. This occurs due to a defect in the host cell type, e.g., infection of the virus into an inappropriate host.

- *Incomplete viruses:* Here the defect is in the incomplete assembly of the virions, which may lead to the formation of incomplete daughter viruses that may not be infective, e.g., in replication of influenza virus, assembly of haemagglutinins may be normal but defect could be in other components. This may lead to a situation, where the haemagglutination titre of the virus sample may be high but has low infectivity. This phenomenon is called *'Von magnus' phenomenon.*
- *Pseudovirions* (pseudo=false): here the false virions gets produced by; host cell nucleic acid getting enclosed in a capsid, instead of the viral nucleic acid. So, this leads to production of virions, which are nonreplicative and non-infective.
- *Defective viruses:* Some viruses cannot replicate independently in a host cell but can do so only in presence of a helper virus.

  e.g., adeno-associated viruses can replicate only in a host cell, if it is already infected with an adenovirus.

  e.g., hepatitis D virus can only replicate in a hepatic cell, if it is already infected by a hepatitis B virus.

Describe the effect of viral infection on the host cell.

A.9

The effects can vary from little or no detectable effect to cell death (*cytocidal*) with or without cell lysis (*cytolysis*). The effects can be:

1. **Little or no detectable effect:** This can occur, when the virus has had a genetic change in itself and cannot replicate or is infecting cells, that are semi permissive or non-permissive to the virus. A *semi permissive cell* is defined; as a cell that supports some but not all stages of viral infection, whereas *non-permissive cell* is defined; as one which does not support any stage of viral infection. A non-permissive cell may lack a receptor, key enzyme pathway or express a metabolic pathway that does not support the viral replication.
2. **Antigenic alteration of host cell *but* no host cell death** (viral persistence).

   The alteration of host cell can occur; as acquiring some viral glycoproteins on cell membrane surface. The viral replication and release from the host cell does not interfere with the functions of the host cell, so it can survive. This infection is so said to be persistent; as neither the host cell can destroy the virus, nor the virus can destroy the host cell.

   e.g., Togaviruses can persist in arthropod cells but not kill them (however the same Togaviruses can kill some human mammalian cells.
3. **Latent viral infection of the host cell**

   As the name of the condition indicates, in this condition the viral genome persists in the host cell but no production of progeny virus occurs. This condition differs from the *persistent* viral conditions, where in the virus keeps producing continuously.

   However, the viruses that cause latent viral infection, can get reactivated after a period; varying from months to years and then again go in a state of latency, e.g., Herpes viruses.

   In some cases, these viruses can get stably integrated with the host cell chromosome and alter the cellular metabolic functions and replicative patterns. Some of such viruses can cause malignancies in the host cells and the cells infected such are said to be *transformed*. e.g., Hepatitis B virus.
4. **Host cell death with or without cell lysis.**

   The replication of many viruses leads to death of the host cell (*cytocidal*) with or without lysis of the host cell (*cytolysis*).

   In reality one can have many combinations of these effects: for instance; a cell having a latent virus infection can undergo cell death with lysis.

Mention the effect the viral infection can have on the host?

A.10 One can study the effect of interaction of viruses with host cells in cell cultures ('in vitro'). However in humans ('in vivo'), the outcome of such interactions; as measured by symptoms of disease depend on numerous factors that may be independent of the effect, the virus would have had on the host cell.

Inapparent acute infections:

As the term indicates, in this there are no symptoms or disease. This occurs; as the quantity of virions produced is below the threshold required to elicit symptoms in the infected individual. This entity must be differentiated from unsuccessful viral infections, where the virus is not able to multiply and produce virions. The latter outcome is designated as failed infection (abortive infection).

This type of pattern is often seen in well adapted viruses (to hosts), as has been seen in poliovirus infections in man, where greater than 90% of infections are inapparent.

Apparent (clinical/overt) Infection: See Table 11.1.8

Table 11.1.8: Apparent (Clinical/Overt) infections

	Disease	Characteristic
Acute infection	e.g., Rota virus diarrhoea	Short, self-limiting infection (usually)
Latent infection	e.g., Herpes group of viruses	Infectious virus is only demonstrable during reactivation. Disease usually manifest, only during recurrences
Chronic infection	e.g., Hepatitis infection	Virus is always demonstrable and disease may be absent, develop late or be chronic and may have neoplastic character.
Slow virus infection	e.g., AIDS, CJD, Kuru	Infections have a long incubation period and usually a slowly progressive and often lethal course (details see case 2, pg. 506-507 section 14)

Δ An aspect that needs clarification in virology, is that original Koch's postulates cannot be applied to viruses. Criteria were developed by Rivers and Huebner to include viruses. Viruses have been implicated in causation of many psychiatric, neurological and malignant diseases but it is very difficult to have a proof of the causation in many of them! Even if the viral genome can be demonstrated in the pathologic tissue, it may not be proof of its causative role. This occurs as many viruses are ubiquitous and can cause lifelong chronic infections; as herpes group of infections. Certain criteria that may be helpful in establishing causation include presence of disease to be significantly higher in the exposed than in controls not exposed, spectrum of host responses following exposure to putative viral agent and significant immunological response.

How are viruses cultivated?

A.11 Cultivation of Viruses

As viruses are obligate intracellular pathogens, they cannot be cultivated in any cell-free (inanimate) medium, no matter how complex it is (Fig. 11.1.4). Media containing living cells is essential for cultivating viruses.

Viruses need to be cultivated, so that the virion can be characterized, its mode of replication studied and gets identified preferably by a classical diagnostic technique, which is considered to be a 'gold standard'.

Three systems are available for cultivating viruses namely laboratory animals, embryonated eggs and tissue culture.

1. **Laboratory animals:** This was the first method used to cultivate viruses, but now this technique is hardly used in the laboratory diagnosis of viruses for numerous reasons. Currently suckling mice is used for isolating coxsackie viruses and other mice have also been used for isolating rabies and arboviruses.

   The other animals that have been used in cultivation; include rabbits, guinea pigs, monkey and hamsters. Numerous inoculation routes; as intracerebral, intraperitoneal, subcutaneous and intranasal have been utilized. The reason of their becoming redundant, is that better system for cultivation of viruses is available now. The laboratory animals have the disadvantage of being difficult to handle/maintain, show genetic diversity, may have latent viruses and their immune system can interfere with the cultivation of viruses.

2. **Embryonated egg:** In the 1930s, this approach was used to cultivate some viruses. However, only embryonated and intact eggs can be used, as they have membranes and embryos, which have living cells (Fig. 11.1.5). Chick and duck eggs available in market cannot be used for this purpose as they are non-fertile, i.e., have no embryo, so no living cells. One advantage of this approach in contrast to the laboratory animals, is that the egg does not have an immunological system to interfere with the viral growth, but this system can support limited number of viruses and the embryo is prone to bacterial contamination.

   To cultivate a virus, first the route of administration is to be decided; for instance; for sample containing suspected herpes virus, the sample is to be inoculated into the chorioallantoic membrane. After inoculation, the egg is incubated at appropriate temperature and period; for the replication of virus (usually 35°C for 3 days). After the incubation period is over, the egg is harvested, i.e., the necessary portion of the egg is isolated. The presence of virus in the isolated portion can be detected by numerous techniques; as electron microscopy examination or performing a haemagglutination assay or a haemagglutination inhibition assay of the suspected virus, when it has the ability of haemadsorption. The isolation of herpes viruses or pox viruses on chorioallantoic membrane can also be assessed by gross examination of the membrane. It can have opaque spots called *pocks* (may contrast them with plaques seen in viral cell culture), which represent localized area of damage in the membrane, which occur from multiplication of single virion. The different viruses can produce pocks with varying morphology (Fig. 11.1.6a,b).

   The other routes of inoculation are depicted in figure 11.1.5. The embryonated egg is commonly used to cultivate influenza virus and manufacture of vaccine; as yellow fever and Rabies ('Flury', in yolk sac).

   NB: Generally, duck egg is larger than chicks egg, so give greater yield of viruses.

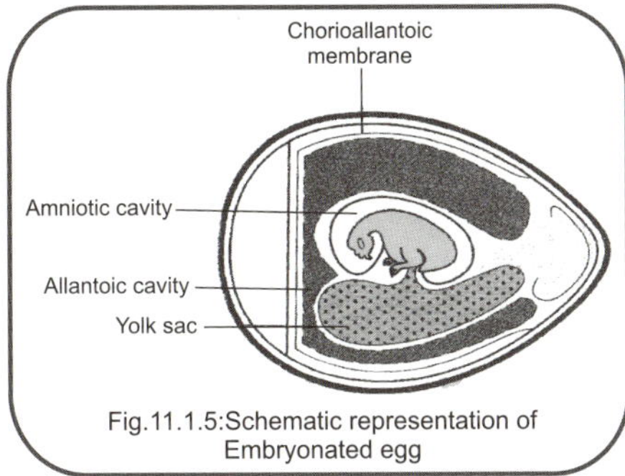

Fig.11.1.5:Schematic representation of Embryonated egg

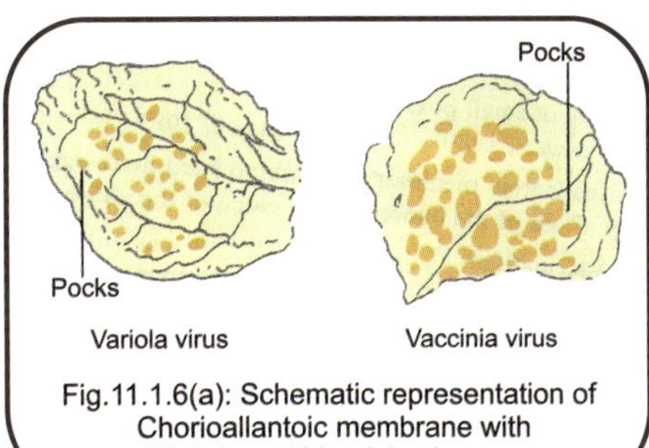

Fig.11.1.6(a): Schematic representation of Chorioallantoic membrane with Variola and Vaccinia viruses

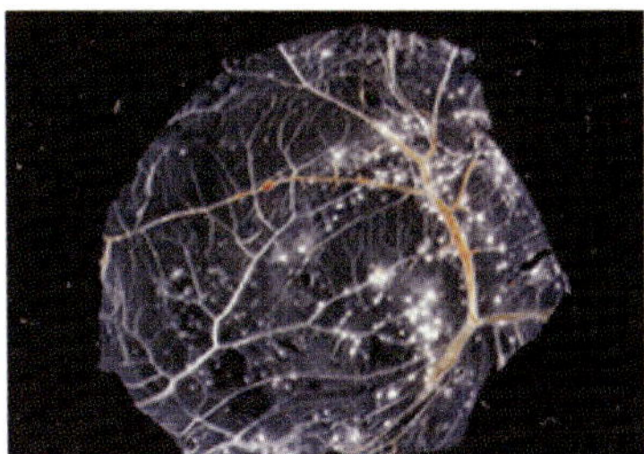
Fig.11.1.6 (b): Photomicrograph of CAM with pocks of Variola (capillaries with red blood cells are visible)

3. **Tissue Culture:** It is categorized into three types, namely:
   (a) **Organ culture:** In it, a small bit of organ is maintained in tissue culture medium, e.g., tracheal ring culture; as a form of organ culture is utilized for isolation of corona viruses.
   (b) **Explant culture:** It is rarely performed currently. Here, small tissue is grown as 'explant' embedded in plasma clot, e.g., adenoid tissue explants for isolation of adenoviruses.
   (c) **Cell culture:** The term tissue culture is often used for this technique but the term, cell culture is more appropriate. Virus isolation by cell culture remains the 'gold standard' for diagnosis against which newer techniques for viral diagnosis must be compared. This technique remained unutilized for many decades till *antibiotics* and *trypsin* could be used in the cell culture medium. The antibiotics minimized the contamination of cell lines with bacteria, fungi and mycoplasmas, whereas trypsin helped the cells to be free from surrounding tissues without damaging the freed cells. This technique led to the isolation and characterization of hundreds of viruses in the period between 1950 to 1970s.

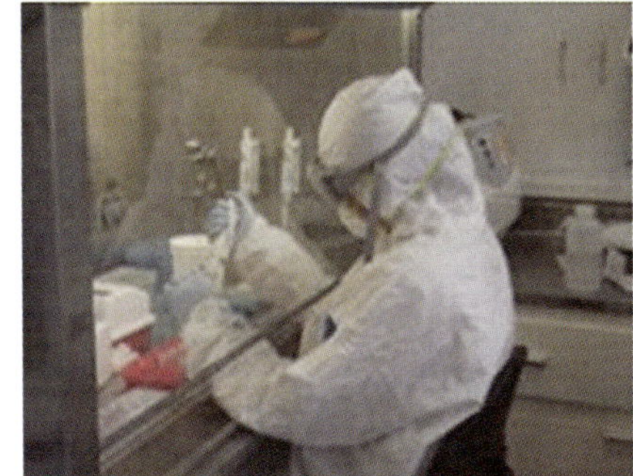
11.1.4: A Virologist at work (eye mask, head cover and other protective gear are in use in the biological safety cabinet)

The bacterial viruses grow rapidly than animal viruses one reason that the study of bacterial viruses has been more rapid. The viruses can be cultivated in sterile plastic tubes, petri dishes and flasks (Fig 11.1.7a,b). The nutrients in the cell culture container easily support the growth of bacteria and fungi, so strict aseptic procedures have to be used during the viral culture work. The cells which are bathed in the nutrients, *attach* to the plastic surface on the bottom part of the container, multiply and eventually form a complete sheet of one cell thickness, which is termed a *monolayer*. One can propagate these cells by removing them from one container and transferring them to a new container, the process is called *subculturing*.

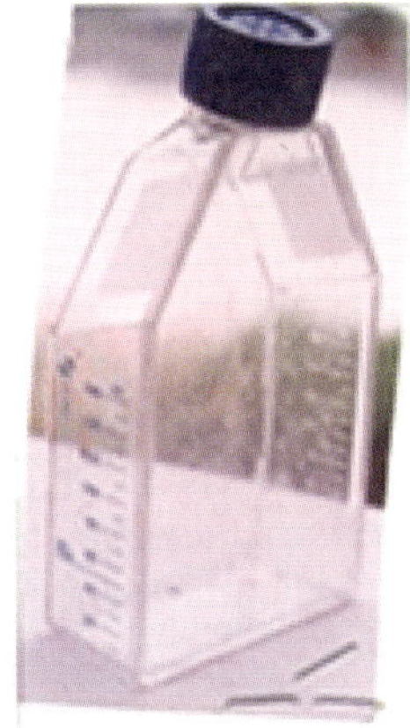
Fig.11.1.7 (a): Tissue culture bottle (uninoculated)

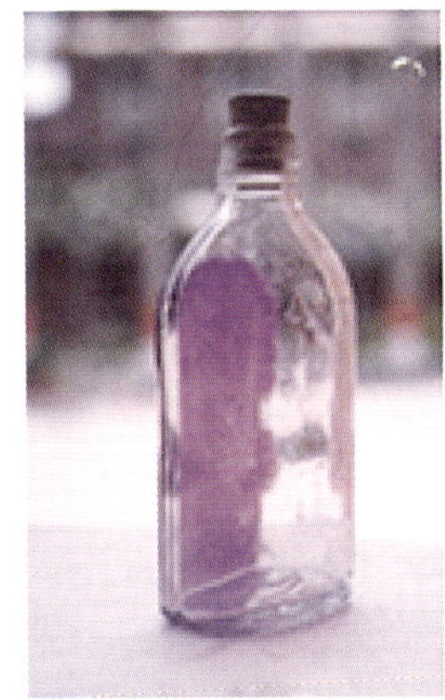
Fig.11.1.7 (b): Tissue culture bottle with cell line

Fig.11.1.8: Schematic representation of normal monkey tissue culture line, 400X

One of the best known medium to cultivate viruses is known as Eagle's medium, which has been developed by Eagle. It is an isotonic solution of simple salts, glucose, amino acids (thirteen), vitamins, phenol red (as indicator), antibiotics and serum (often fetal calf buffered at pH 7.4). The purpose of the serum is to provide some growth factors; without which the cell lines, cannot multiply. In recent years, the growth factors for some cell lines have got chemically defined.

Three basic types of cell cultures are used in diagnostic and research virology, namely, primary cell culture, diploid cell, cultures, and continuous cell culture. Their characteristics are given in table 11.1.9.

Table 11.1.9: Characteristics of cell culture lines

	Primary cell culture	Diploid cell culture	Continuous (heteroploid) cell culture
Source	Obtained from fresh tissue of organs of animals	Derived from foetal tissues	From immortalised cell lines (cancer cells)
Chromosomal character	Same as that of the cell of origin	Diploid	Haploid, heteroploid (have different number of chromosomes, so are genetically diverse)
Growth	• Limited growth (5-10 division) • Cannot undergo subculture	• Rapid • Can undergo 50-100 serial passages	• Rapid • Can undergo infinite passages (as derived from cancer cells)
Cell character	• Initially consist of mixture of cells; for example: epithelial and muscle cell. On subculture, one cell type becomes predominant, such a culture is called cell strain • Support growth of a wide range of viruses	• Immature cells (as derived from foetus) • Support growth of a wide range of viruses	• Cells are ^'dedifferentiated' (have undergone numerous sequential mutations^ in their long history in culture) and have simple growth requirements • Support growth of a limited range of viruses
Examples	• Primary money kidney (PMK)	• Human embryonic fibroblast (HEF) • WI 38 (human embryonic lung cell strain)	• Hela (human carcinoma cervix cell line) • HEp 2 (human) epithelioma of larynx cell line • Vero (vervet monkey kidney cell line) • McCoy (human synovial carcinoma cell line) • BHK-21 (Baby hamster kidney cell line)
Uses	• Isolation of viruses(sensitivity is good) • May harbour latent viruses, so can cause diagnostic confusion	• Isolation of viruses • Used in vaccine production (as usually free of latent viruses)	• Limited use in isolation of viruses • Use in research
	• May be avoided in vaccine production		• Avoided for vaccines (as malignancy in a line could have arisen because of virus, although vero cells line are used in rabies vaccine).

^ Cells have lost the specialized morphology and biochemical abilities, that they possesed; as differentiated cells in vivo.

NB: *'Hela'* cell line has been usage since 1951, has been derived from a woman with cervical cancer and is named after the first letters of her name.

For virus cultivation, the sample containing suspected virus is mixed with cell lines in an tissue culture container and incubated at appropriate temperature for appropriate time. The infected cells may get lysed and the unlysed cells and cell debris are removed by centrifugation. The light small virions remain in the liquid (the supernatant). The fluid containing the virions is termed as '*lysate*'.

How is viral growth detected in cell cultures?

A.12 (a) Detection of viral growth in cell cultures

Gross examination of the cellular monolayer for a *plaque* (in CAM, one can look for pocks) can be helpful in eliciting viral growth (Fig. 11.1.8). Plaques represent macroscopic appearance of roundish, clear spaces that correspond to areas of dead cells. It develops, when virus infect a host cell and forms multiple progeny, which are released to the neighbouring host cells in the medium. This way new cells become infected and the process can lead to cell death and lysis.

Following are the different phenomena employed to detect viral growth in cell lines:

(i) **Cytopathic effect:**

Commonly morphological changes at microscopic level occur in the cellular monolayer caused by viral proliferation, which is best observed by an inverted phase contrast microscope, and these are known as 'cytopathic effects' (CPE). An experienced virologist can make provisional identification observing the distinctive changes (Fig. 11.9.a,b,c). The cell cultures may be observed thrice a week to see the development of CPE. However some viruses grow slowly and do not cause a CPE in the classical cell lines used in clinical virology. Following are the CPE changes that may be observed:

- Discrete, focal change; indicate Herpes virus infection
- Cell necrosis and lysis; indicate Enterovirus infection
- Cellular clumping (grape like cluster); indicate Adenovirus infection
- Syncytium formation (multinucleate giant cell) indicate Measles infection.

Viral infection of cell may induce apoptosis of the infected cell, which is defined as a preset cascade of events that when trigerred, lead to cellular suicide!

(ii) **Inclusion bodies:** These are viral specific structures that develop during the course of virus multiplication within cells and get demonstrable because of shape, large size about 20-25 μm (visible under light microscope), altered staining character in the cytoplasm and/or nucleus. These could represent developmental sites of virus development; as masses of virus particles or scars remnant of virus multiplication. These can be classified according to stain and site in the cell; as depicted in table 11.1.10.

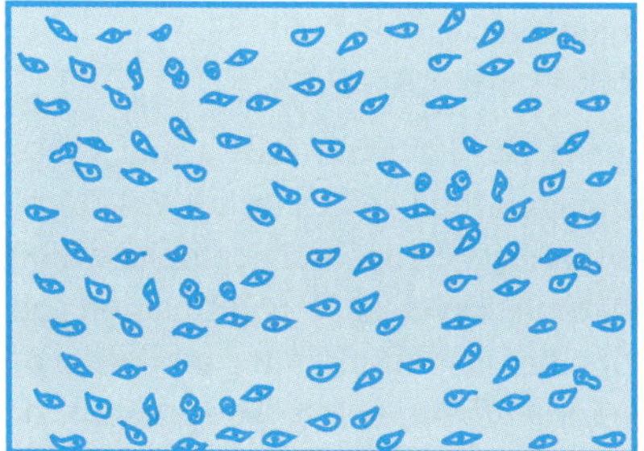

Fig. 11.1.9a: Cell necrosis/lysis

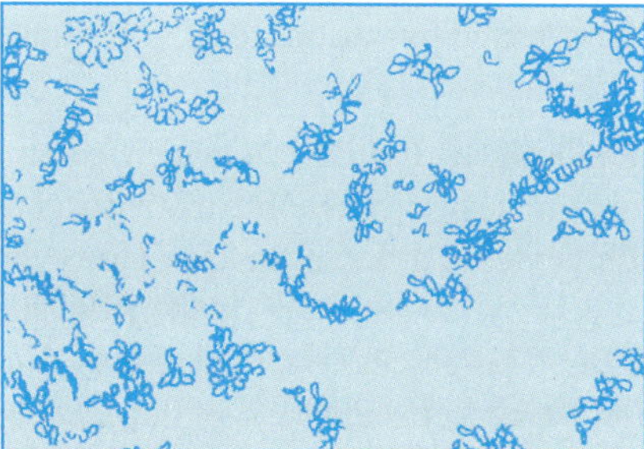

Fig. 11.1.9b: Cellular clumping

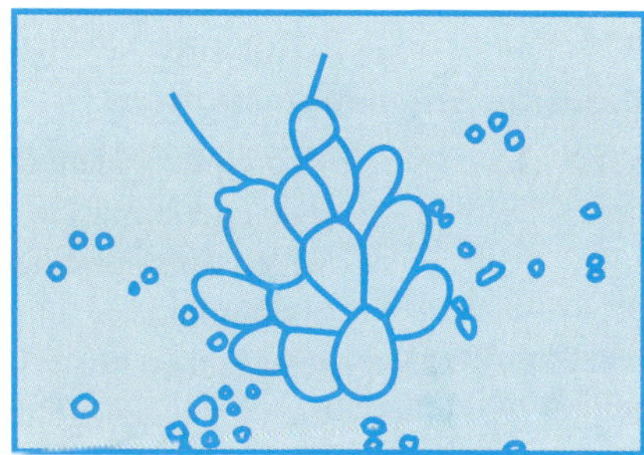

Fig. 11.1.9c: Syncytium formation

Table 11.1.10: Classification and Characteristics of Inclusion bodies

According to staining [by Giemsa stain or H & E stain] • Basophilic (blue) – Adenovirus • Acidophilic (Pink) – others **According to site** • *Cytoplasmic* – Poxviridae o Small pox Guarnieri body o Fowlpox (Bollinger body) o Molluscum contagiosum – Rhabdoviridae – Rabies virus (Negri body) – Paramyxoviridae	• *Nuclear* – Papovaviridae – Adenovirus (Cowdry type B) – Herpes viruses (Cowdry type A) – Yellow fever (Cowdry type A)	• At both sites – Measles – Cytomegalovirus

NB: Some authorities consider inclusion bodies to be also a type of CPE.

(iii) **Monoclonal antibodies (Immunofluorescence/ELISA)**

The classical technique for detecting viral growth by observing CPE may take days to weeks. So currently emphasis is on detection of viral antigen, which is *expressed earlier* in cell lines and can be detected much earlier. Specific monoclonal antibodies, which are fluorescent or enzyme labelled are used for this purpose.

So, fluorescent antibody assays or ELISA, technology is used for this purpose. Similar principle is used in *'shell vial' technique*.

(iv) **Electron microscopy or immune electron microscopy** is also helpful (IEP) (Fig. 11.1.10) in differentiating viruses, which are morphologically resembling; for instance members of Herpesviridae.

(v) **Haemadsorption:** Certain members of the orthomyxoviridae and paramyxoviridae acquire certain glycoprotein, (haemagglutnins) on their envelope, which gives them the property of adsorbing RBCs of some species on their surface, resulting in haemadsorption and visible as haemagglutination (Fig. 11.1.11a,b).

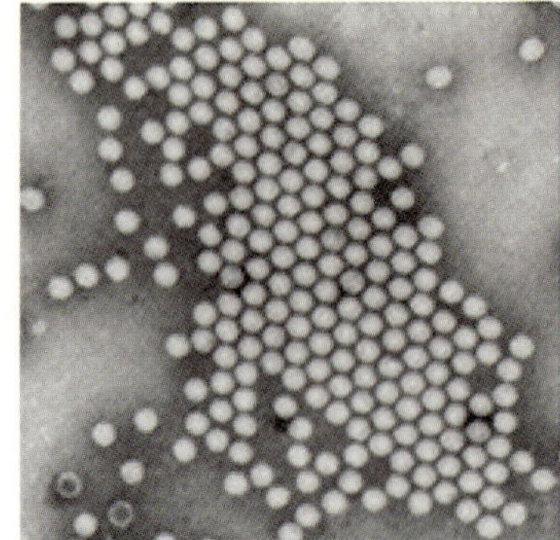

Fig.11.1.10: Poliovirus: Transmission electron micrograph of poliovirus

Courtesy: Dr. Joseph J. Esposito; F. A. Murphy/CDC

Specific antibodies against the virus receptors can block this haemadsorption. This is the basis of the *haemagglutination inhibition (H.I.) test*.

(vi) **Inteference:** The growth of a *non-cytopathogenic virus* in a cell culture can be tested by subsequent *challenge* with a known cytopathogenic virus (which can usually produce CPE). The growth of the first virus (if it occurs) will inhibit the infection by the second virus by interference. For example; measles virus does not produce any CPE in a cell line (primary African green monkey kidney) in which it can replicate. When this cell line is subsequently challenged with a virus that can cause CPE in this line, no CPE can be seen).

(vii) **Detection of antigen** (in cell culture supernatants): when the virus is replicating in the cell line, it is producing a whole range of antigens (as complement fixing) or enzymes (as reverse transcriptase in retroviruses), which can be detected by various tests; including serological tests.

Describe Haemagglutination.

A.12 (b)

- **Principle:** Haemagglutination is a reaction, in which certain antigens can act with RBCs and cause *haemagglutination*. Certain viruses; such as influenza virus, have haemagglutinin spikes on the envelope, which can agglutinate erythrocytes of different species. However, this virus also has another peplomer called neuraminidase, which can destroy the receptors on the RBC and result in the reversal of agglutination and release the viruses from RBC. This process is called *elution*. Viral antibodies also result in the inhibition of the viral haemagglutination which forms the basis of the *haemagglutination inhibition test*. The principle of haemagglutination is also used in Rose-Waaler test used for detection of RA factor in case of Rheumatoid arthritis.
- **Procedure:** In the viral haemagglutination assay, double dilutions of virus are used. The test is performed in plastic trays or test tubes. Red cells which are not agglutinated settle at the bottom and form a 'button'. This is confirmed by tilting the wall of the tray and looking for free flow of RBCs, which indicates absence of agglutination. (Fig. 11.1.11a,b). The last well which shows haemagglutination has *one unit of haemagglutination*. The well which is previous to it (in twofold dilution series) has double the units of haemagglutination. Similarly, the one previous to it has 4 HA units.

Controls: – *RBC control:* Shows button formation – *Virus control:* Shows haemagglutination

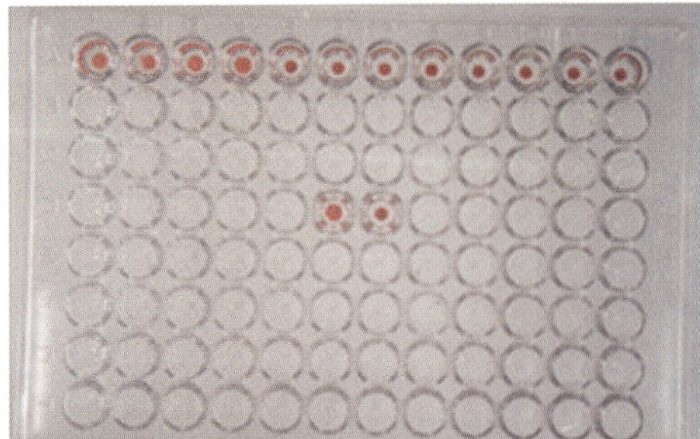

Fig.11.1.11 (a): Viral haemagglutination test in a microtitre plate with agglutination and cell control (Hawmagglutination visible uptil 4th well)

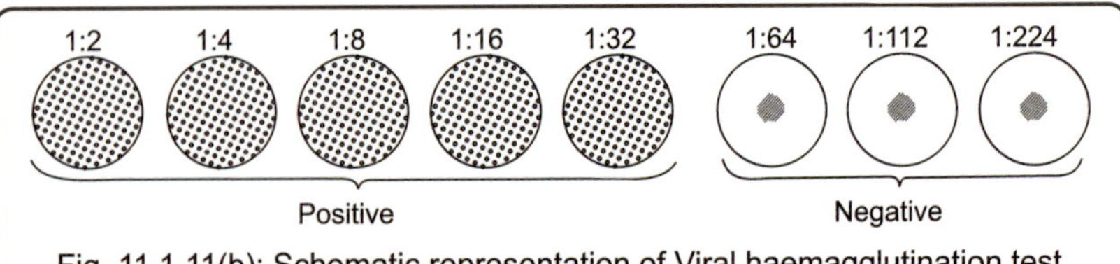

Fig. 11.1.11(b): Schematic representation of Viral haemagglutination test

- **Uses:** The principle of haemagglutination is used in purification of viruses, identification of viruses and estimation of antibody by haemagglutination inhibition test (HAI)

Describe the transmission of viruses emphasizing the routes of transmission?

A.13 Transmission of Viral Infections

It is important to study transmission of viral infections, as it helps to explain the role of various factors that determine the frequency and distribution of viral diseases in a community. Transmission of viruses is important for the viruses to survive in nature, for they can do so only; if they pass from one animal to another of the same or another species. It involves specific routes of entry of viruses into the body and their exit from body; which involve skin, mucosal surfaces of gastrointestinal tract, respiratory tract and genitourinary tract (Table 11.1.11). One thing must be realized that man can shed virus, when there are no symptoms or signs of disease. This is possible in three conditions. One; virus being shed significantly; in latter part of the incubation period. Two, the individual is having subclinical/asymptomatic infection or thirdly; infection has become chronic, i.e., the infection has persisted beyond the evidence of the original disease. It must be realized that presence or absence of envelope plays a key role in determining the mode of transmission (see A6a,p. 366).

Table 11.1.11: Routes of transmission for common human viruses

Viral Family	ROUTES
Parvoviridae	Respiratory, contact
Papovaviridae (includes papilloma viruses)	Contact♦
Adenoviridae	Respiratory, enteric, contact; as causes of conjunctivitis
Herpesviridae	• Salivary contact (HHV-1 (HSV), HHV 4 (EBV), HHV 5 (CMV) • Venereal contact (HHV-2) • Respiratory- HHV-3 (varicella)
Poxviridae	• Respiratory, contact (small pox, now eradicated) • Arthropod (tanapox) • Contact (mollusum contagiosum, orf, cow pox)
Hepadnaviridae	Injection, contact (perinatal and venereal)
Calciviridae	Enteric, contact
Picornaviridae	• Respiratory, contact (Rhinovirus) • Enteric, respiratory (Enterovirus)
Coronaviridae	Respiratory, contact
Flaviviridae	• Arthropod (yellow fever virus, dengue virus) • Blood injection, venereal, perinatal (hepatitis C)
Togaviridae	Arthropod (alpha viruses-arboviruses) Respiratory, congenital (rubella)
Orthomyxoviridae	Respiratory, (direct contact with secretion)
Paramyxoviridae	Respiratory, (direct contact with secretion)
Rhabdoviridae	Animal bite (In India, dog bite-rabies)
Filoviridae	Contact, injection
Retroviridae	Contact, injection, blood, ▲congenital, perinatal (HIV)
Reoviridae	• Enteric (Rotavirus) • Arthropod (orbivirus)

♦ 'Contact route' can imply different meanings, here it implies transmission by physical contact by salivary exchange (as kissing) and transfer of respiratory secretions (including saliva) via hands and fomites (as tissue papers and towels)

▲ Congenital refers to transmission across the placenta, in the egg or in the sperm/as part of the germplasm.

Pathogenesis of Viral Infections

Viral pathogenesis deals with the entire process with which viruses cause disease. There is no easy answer to this apparently straight forward process. Let's study it.

What is the goal of the virus?

A.1 The goal of the virus is to be able to achieve maximal multiplication. To achieve this, viruses must endure and infect new, susceptible hosts. Most viral population survive in nature due to serial infections (a chain of transmission among hosts).

Why do we say that 'there is no clear cut answer to the apparently straight forward process of viral pathogenesis'?

A.2 The ideal scenario would be to study natural human infections in outbred populations but this approach has limitations especially of studying the initial part of pathogenesis; when the individual is not aware of infection. It is also not ethical to infect humans with viruses; even if they are avirulent.

What are the sources, from where we gather information about human viral pathogenesis?

A.3 Our understanding occurs essentially from the epidemiological, clinical, diagnostic and research studies on the clinical viral cases that occur, including some of the accidental natural infections.

Experimenting with animal models is not easy, as many animal rights groups oppose such work. However, though work has progressed along these times, the findings cannot be totally extrapolated to man for instance, mice is not susceptible to poliovirus through the oral route.

Advancement has occurred in the field of experimental animal work. Transgenic and knockout mice have been created, which have added valuable information in this field. Introduction of a gene in the germline (using genetic engineering technology) of the animal results in the production of a transgenic animal, e.g., transgenic mice expressing the hepatitis B genome has been used to study the HBV-immune response interactions. New mouse models for poliomyelitis and measles have been established by producing transgenic mice that synthesize the human viral receptors.

- Knockout animals (as mice) are genetically modified animal, in which specific gene have been inactivated 'or knocked out'.

Mention two examples of accidental natural viral infections that have added to our understanding of the pathogenesis of human viral infections.

A.4 *One classic example* is of during the World War II, when approximately 45,000 U.S. soldiers were administered yellow fever vaccine. Yellow fever was a serious problem then and military personnel were frequently vaccinated then. By mistake, this lot of vaccine had been contaminated with hepatitis B virus. The results of this disaster were astonishing, as fortunately only 900 soldiers (2%) developed clinical hepatitis and less than 36 developed severe hepatitis.

Another incident is the *'Cutter' incident* of 1955, when more than one lakh school children were administered improperly inactivated Salk poliovirus vaccine. Vaccine prepared by Cutter laboratories, was not properly inactivated and contained live polio (virulent) virus. About 10-25% of this population got infected by the vaccine virus; as detected by appearance of symptoms, shedding of virus in faeces, and appearance of antibodies. Most of these cases escaped this disease, excepting approximately 60 cases; who developed paralytic poliomyelitis.

Describe the four possible categories of the host virus interactions to explain patterns of human viral disease.

A.5 *Mathematical* models are being developed to describe patterns of disease transmission in population; especially human. Such models can help to determine the critical population size necessary for effective transmission of viruses and help understand the emergence factors for viral diseases. The spectrum of possible interactions between hosts and viruses is complex. To understand the dynamic host virus interactions and their outcomes, *four categories* of interactions can be defined, namely stable, evolving, dead-end and resistant.

The *stable host virus interactions* are those in which both members (i.e., host and virus) survive and multiply. This often occurs, when the virus population becomes solely dependent on one host. For instance; humans are believed to be the sole natural host for measles, herpes simplex and small pox viruses. This situation can constrain the further evolution of the virus. However, this stable relationship, may not remain permanent.

The *evolving host virus interactions* imply that stability is unlikely to be achieved instantly. For instance, some host subpopulations may experience high infection rates, while others may be minimally affected. This occurred in the past, when the English invaded the Americas and caused high rate of measles and small pox in the native population. Currently, HIV causes high morbidity in the humans, but individuals who harbour mutations in chemokine or chemokine receptor genes are resistant.

The *dead end interactions* are characterized by the host often getting killed with minimal or no subsequent transmission of virus to others. For instance arboviruses causes yellow fever and dengue have maintained a stable relationship with their natural host and insect vectors. However; when human ventures into such zones and gets infected, it manifests with high morbidity and mortality. Another example of this category the Marburg and Ebola infections.

The *resistant host-virus interactions* are characterized by the host not getting infected by the virus. It must be appreciated that all organisms are exposed virtually continuously to numerous viruses, but majority of these interactions are uneventful. This category may be the largest amongst the four discussed.

Outline the three stages involved in the pathogenesis of viral infections.

A.6 I. Entry of virus into the body via various routes

- Respiratory tract
- Alimentary tract
- Genitourinary tract or genital
- Skin, conjunctiva
- Congenital (horizontal transmission)

II. Interaction of the virus with the target tissue and ability to cause cytopathology (including viral spread)

- Stability of the virus in body (during varying temperature and environment exposure; as acid and bile of the gut)
- Capacity to establish viremia
- Capacity to spread through the reticuloendothelial system
- Target cell – presence of viral receptors
- Efficiency of viral replication in the host cell
- Altered cell metabolism, which includes inhibition of cellular macromolecule synthesis
- Cytopathology; which could exist as apoptosis, presence of viral proteins and/or structures (inclusion bodies in the host cell)

Nb: The term virulence is synonymous with pathogenicity. It deals with the capacity of the virus to cause disease.

III. Host immune response to infection (may lead to resolution or persistent infection): It depends on

- Viral immune escape mechanisms
- Innate immune responses
- Acquired immune responses
- Antibody-dependent cellular cytotoxicity-ADCC (including processes dependent on complement, immune complexes)
- T-cell mediated (includes DTH) responses

Factors on which severity of viral disease may depend

- Age of host
- Host genotype
- Overall health of the host (including nutritional status)
- Body temperature
- Usage of any hormones including steroids by the host
- Quantity of the virus inoculated
- Virulence of the virus
- Quality of immune response by the host

Describe the first stage of the pathogenesis process, i.e., the entry of the virus into the body via various routes.

A.7 The various routes utilized by the viruses are depicted in Table 11.2.1

Respiratory tract

The respiratory tract offers probably the commonest way of spread of viruses, from one individual to other, by means of droplets released from the nose or mouth of infected persons; during activities; as talking, laughing, 'coughing' or sneezing. The particles of 10 micrometer diameter, usually get deposited on the nasal mucosa in the nasal cavity. The smaller particles (5 μm or less) may get inhaled directly into alveoli of the lungs, where the virions may get destroyed by the alveolar macrophages. The mucociliary blanket in the nasal cavity, acts as a protective mechanism. The mucus traps the foreign particles and may have inhibitors that prevents the viruses from interacting with the specific receptors on the cells of respiratory tract. If the virions can pass through the mucus layer, they can multiply in the ciliated cell or pass between them to reach the basement membrane. The latter is another physical barrier, which if the virus crosses, can then reach into lymphatic capillaries and reach blood. Many of the viruses; such as influenza and rhinovirus remain restricted to the respiratory tract, where they multiply and cause localized disease but some others that enter via the respiratory tract produce their key effects, elsewhere in the body following *systemic spread; as human herpesvirus 3 (V.Z. virus), human herpes virus 5 (CMV), Rubella and measles virus.

(*Utilizing haematogenous and/or lymphatic path).

Alimentary tract

Human herpes virus 1 (HSV 1) and human herpes virus 4 (EBV) initiate infection via the mouth or oropharynx. The oesophagus is usually spared of direct infection, probably, as it has stratified squamous epithelium and the material containing virions has a rapid passage over the surface. The viruses that initiate infection of the intestinal tract are acid and bile resistant; as adenovirus, calcivirus, enterovirus and rotavirus. Some of these viruses multiply locally and produce localized infection; as rotaviruses, however some of these also spread systemically and affect other body organs; as hepatitis A virus and polioviruses. The sIgA and mucus provide protection to the intestinal tract, however viral particles may lodge in sequestered places; as in the crypts and cause infection on the availability of specific receptors in that place.

Skin

It is the largest organ of the body, which provides a tough and impermeable barrier to the entry of viruses. The few viruses that enter the skin through minute abrasions and produce localized lesions are depicted in the Table 11.2.1. It must be emphasized that more viruses are introduced into the skin by bites of arthropods or animals than through localized trauma. The other aspect that needs emphasis is that most of the viruses that enter skin by bites or blood do not cause skin lesions. Skin lesions are more often caused by viruses that have entered the body through routes other than skin; as measles and rubella that enter the body through respiratory tract and cause skin lesions.

Conjunctiva

It is much less resistant to viral invasion than the skin. The flow of secretions (tear) and the presence of sIgA in it, act as protective defense mechanisms. The viruses that gain entry through this route are depicted in Table 11.2.1.

Genitourinary tract

This route is also called the venereal. It must be emphasized that of the viruses spread by this route; only Papillomaviruses and human herpes virus 2 (HSV 2) cause localized lesions on the genitalia and perineum, whereas the others produce lesions in other organs of the body.

Placenta

It refers to the congenital transfer of virus from mother to foetus, which occurs through placenta. This type of transmission is also known as *vertical transmission*. It should also be noted that transmission of HHV-2 (HSV-2) from mother to foetus can also occur during passage of it, from the infected genital tract during delivery. In the current HIV pandemic, this virus is also known to spread during lactation from the lactating mother to the infant.

Table 11.2.1: Various routes of transmission of viral infections

Respiratory tract	
• *Both upper and lower tract*	• **Skin**
– Influenza A and B viruses	– *Minor trauma of skin*
– Parainfluenza virus types 1-3	o Human papilloma virus
– Respiratory syncytial virus	o Human herpes virus 1 (HSV 1)
– Adenovirus types 1-7, 14, 21	o Human herpes virus 2 (HSV 2)
• *Localized upper tract*	o Molluscum contagiosum
– Rhinovirus (common)	o Cowpox
– Coxsackie virus	o Orf
– Coronavirus	o Milker's node
– Arenavirus	– *Arthropod/animal bite*
– Hantavirus	o Arboviruses – insect bite
– Others	o Rabies virus – animal bite
• *Localized lower tract*	o Herpes B virus – monkey bite
– Respiratory syncytial virus	– *Needle pucture/sexual contact*
– Others	o Hepatitis B virus
• *Systemic spread (entry via respiratory tract)*	o Hepatitis C virus
– Poxviruses	o Ebola virus▲
– Human herpesvirus-3 (VZV)	o HTLV and HIV (by various routes)
– Foot and mouth disease virus	▲Two major epidemics of African haemorrhage fever caused by it occurred in Sudan and Zaire.
– Rubella virus	
– Measles virus	• ***Conjunctiva***
– Mumps virus	– Adenovirus
– Hantavirus	– Enterovirus 70
– Arenavirus	– Human herpes virus-8
• **Alimentary tract**	• ***Urogenital tract*** *(venereal)*
– *Localized*	– Human Papilloma viruses (genital type)
o Calcivius	– Human Herpes virus 2 (HSV 2)
o Norwalk	– #Hepatitis B virus
o Coronavirus	– #Hepatitis C virus
o Rotavirus	– #HIV
– *Systemic*	• ***Placenta*** *(congenital)*
o Adenovirus	– *Rubella
o Coxsackie	– Cytomegalovirus (also called vertical transmission, which refers to transmission of viruses between parent and offspring)
o Enterovirus	
o Reovirus	– #HIV
o HHV-4 (EBV)	– #HBV
o HHV-5 (CMV)	– HHV-5 (CMV)

NB: Horizontal transmission (is the transmission from person to person via various routes), includes all forms of transmission of viruses excepting vertical
#Indicates transmission by multiple routes

*The risk of rubella fetal infection from mother, who has been infected with rubella virus during first trimester is approximately 80%.

How does the virus spread in the body?

A.8 The following stages are involved:

– **Multiplication at the site of entry:** Most viruses after their entry into the body, multiply near the site of entry, which could be respiratory epithelium, intestinal mucosa or a breached skin. The viruses that cause localized infections, as Papilloma virus (on skin), Rhinovirus (upper respiratory tract) or Rotavirus (intestine); multiply locally and cause localized pathology. These viruses may minimally invade the underlying tissue and enter the lymphatics with a potential to spread. However, due to unknown reasons these viruses do not spread. The possible reasons could include absence of specific viral receptors on other host cells. These viral infections have *short incubation* of few days, as the portal of entry of the virus and the site of the lesions are the same; as in Influenza (Table 11.2.2). This is unlike the other viruses, which produce a pathology; at a site distant from the site of entry of the virus, as the polio virus enters the body through the alimentary tract, but causes the classic lesions in the spinal cord. Some viruses can have incubation period extending from months to years; as rabies virus and slow viruses.

– **Subepithelial invasion and lymphatic spread:** Some viruses cause systemic infections after entry and localized multiplication, spread to subepithelial tissue and reach the lymphatics that lie beneath all the surface epithelia. The virions from the lymphatic capillaries reach the local lymph nodes. Here the antigen presenting cells (APCs) may ingest the virions and present their antigens to lymphocytes, K cells and NK cells, to initiate the immune response. Some viruses can multiply within the macrophages itself; as HIV, measles virus, some adenovirus and some herpesviruses, however some viruses pass from the lymph node into the blood.

Table 11.2.2: Incubation period of common human viral infections

Viral Infection	Incubation period	Viral Infection	Incubation period
Warts (by HPV)	50-150 days (approx 2-6 months)	*Poliomyelitis*	5-20 days
Herpes simplex type 1	5-8 days	*Common cold (by Rhinovirus)*	2-4 days
Chicken pox (HHV 3)	13-17 days	*Influenza*	1-3 days
Infectious mononucleosis (HHV 4)	30-50 days	*Rubella*	17-20 days
Small pox (now eradicated)	12-14 days	*Measles*	9-12 days
Hepatitis B	50-150 days (approx 2-6 months)	*Mumps*	16-20 days
Hepatitis A	15-40 days	*Rabies*	30-100 days (approx 1-3 months)
Hepatitis C	15-60 days	*AIDS (by HIV)*	1 year – 10 ^years

^Hoping that new vaccines can prolong it very long.

– **Haematogenous spread:** The viruses that escape the local defense; ultimately enter the blood stream, and can then spread to any organ. The term viremia refers to the presence of infectious virus particles in the blood. This stage of viremia that is produced, after the multiplication of the virus in the lymph nodes is called *primary viraemia*. The virions can be circulating 'free' in the plasma or be cell-associated; as depicted in Table 11.2.3.

The concentration of viruses in the primary viraemia stage is low. After this, the viruses reach the replication sites; as liver, spleen, muscle and blood vessels, which act as the 'central foci' for viral multiplication. In these sites, extensive multiplication of the virus, occurs and the concentration of virions reaches a high level in the blood. This stage is called *secondary viremia*. The leucocytes can pass through the small blood vessels by diapedesis and initiate infection in the various parts of the body.

NB:

(i) Cells of voluntary muscle may be important site of multiplication of some enteroviruses and togaviruses.

(ii) Reticuloendothelial system (RE) system is a site for virus multiplication, but virions circulating in the blood are also continuously removed by cells of the RE system. Viraemia can only be maintained, if there is continuous release of virus into the blood, from cells in contact with it or if the clearance system is grossly impaired.

Table 11.2.3: Cells associated with plasma viremia

Cell type	Virus
Erythrocyte	• Colorado tick fever virus
Neutrophil	• Influenza virus
B lymphocyte	• HHV-4 (EBV)
T. lymphocyte	• HIV • Human T lymphotropic virus type I • HHV- 6 (human B cell lymphotropic virus) • HHV 7 (RK virus)
Monocyte- macrophage	• HHV 5 (CMV), • Dengue virus • Measles virus, • Rubella virus • Lymphocytic choriomeningitis virus • HIV
Free in plasma	• Hepatitis B virus • Poliovirus • Yellow fever virus

– **Invasion of target organs**

A host cell may be susceptible to infection, if the viral receptor(s) is present and functional. If the appropriate form of viral receptor is not available, the tissue cannot become infected. Viruses have selective affinity for one or more target organs in the body. This property is known as tropism. The specific viral receptors on host cells are necessary for infection, but are not sufficient to explain viral *tropism*. Based on tropism, viruses may be classified as *neurotropic* (affinity for neurons), *dermatropic* (affinity for skin), *hepatotropic* (affinity for liver) or *pneumotropic* (affinity for lungs).

The common target organs (sites) include CNS (brain), skin, liver, kidney and mucous membranes. Viruses can reach the brain via the blood stream or via the peripheral nerves, causing encephalitis. Viruses that cause meningitis; often traverse the blood-CSF junction in the meninges. Viruses reach the CNS also via peripheral nerves, as seen in HHV-1, HHV-3 (VZV) and rabies virus. In herpes virus infection, when virions move from the skin to ganglia (nerve body), they are said to move in a *retrograde* fashion (as are moving in opposite direction of nerve impulse). When the virions move during reactivation, from the ganglia to the skin, they are said to move in *antegrade* fashion (as move in direction of nerve impulse). Cytocidal infections of the neurons by herpes virus, poliovirus flavivirus and togavirus are characterized by three hallmarks of encephalitis; namely cell necrosis, phagocytosis by glial cells (neuronophagia) and perivascular infiltration of inflammatory cells. The slow viruses cause slow neuronal degeneration, vacuolization and changes in cell membrane leading to demyelination. Post infectious encephalitis seen commonly, after measles is characterized predominantly by demyelination without neuronal degeneration.

When the skin is the target organ, the lesions may manifest; as macules, papules, vesicles or pustules. It must be appreciated that in measles and chickenpox, the virus enters via the respiratory tract and the skin gets affected only, after the viruses have caused secondary viraemia in the body (Table 11.2.4).

Rubella virus which can cause congenital abnormalities, causes relatively noncytocidal, minimal inflammatory or necrotic changes in the infected foetus.

Table 11.2.4: Systemic viral diseases with skin rashes

Characteristic of rash	Virus
Maculopapular	• Echovirus • Coxsackie • Rubella • Measles
Vesicular	• HHV-1, HHV-3 Coxsackie
Haemorrhagic	• Small pox (now eradicated) • Arbovirus • Measles

– **Viral shedding**

This is the last stage in the pathogenesis of many viruses. However; some viruses can persist in the body for a life time; as herpes group of viruses, HIV, HBV (chronic cases) HCV and slow viruses. Persistent infections can be chronic (productive), latent (no virus synthesis), recurrent (periods of production and no synthesis interpersing) or transforming (immortalizing).

The shedding of the virus is essential for the virus to survive within a species. It should, however be noted that virus release to the environment also occurs in the initial stages of viruses in many viral diseases. In some diseases, where man is the dead end; as rabies, arboviruses; shedding does not occur. In localized viral infections; as some gastrointestinal infection, the shedding route is the same as entry point.

In systemic viral infections, various routes act as focus for viral shedding. Skin lesions are formed in many systemic viral infections, however in only a few of them; the shedding is of a level, that can be significant for transmission of these viruses. The vesicular lesions of small pox (now eradicated) and herpesvivus infections have profuse virions to play a part in the transmission of these infections. Viruses; as HHV-3 (chicken pox), HHV – 4 (EBV), HHV 5 (CMV), Rubella and measles are shed in significant level from the respiratory tract to play a part in their transmission. Many viruses of the respiratory tract get swallowed and are shed in the feces, but only a few of them remain in an active state to be effective for transmission. Rhinoviruses and many enveloped viruses get inactivated by the hostile acidic pH in the stomach and bile salts in the small intestine (including duodenum).

The presence of viruses in the urine is called *viruria*. Many viruses; as polyoma viruses (as BK, JC), HHV-5 (CMV), measles and mumps are shed in the urine. This aspect is of public health importance. Some viruses replicate in the kidney, e.g., Hantaviruses and arenaviruses, infect rodents and cause persistent viruria. This infected urine can contaminate the dust and infect humans.

Other fluids that can participate in viral shedding are milk and semen. From milk HIV, HHV-5 (CMV) and some tick borne flaviviruses get shed. From semen, HIV-1 gets shed.

The viral diseases that can be transmitted by blood include:

• HHV-5 (CMV), • HBV, • HDV, • HCV, • Some arboviruses, • HIV

Describe the third stage of the pathogenesis process, i.e., Host immune response to infection, on which the severity of the viral disease depends.

A.9 Man is literally clouded by viruses of countless types. Defense mechanism in it are imperfect, despite million of years of evolution, as the virus can evade the response by numerous mechanisms including modifying its genome by antigenic shift and drift. There is also existence of viral immune escape mechanisms.

The intrinsic cellular defences must be differentiated from the immune defense mechanisms, which are dependent on white blood cells and cytokines. Apoptosis (programmed cell death) is a process of cell destruction, in which the infected cell dies quickly after infection, when it can detect biochemical alterations induced by the infection. The function of this process is to eliminate particular cells during development.

- **Innate immune response:** Natural killer cells plays a key role in the first line of defense against the viral infections. The NK cell cytotoxic activity peaks within 1-2 day, earlier than most of the other responses (excepting interferon synthesis). It may be noted that interferon is a key inducer of NK cell activation.

The interferons which were described by Issac and Lindemann in 1957, play a crucial role in the antiviral defense. Interferons; especially α and β can inhibit many steps in viral life cycle, as viral penetration and uncoating, synthesis of viral mRNAs, viral peptide replication and virion assembly and its release. These actions are mediated by the various proteins translated, after the hundreds of genes are transcribed. Macrophages and complement (alternate pathways) also play an important part in the innate immune responses.

Acquired immune responses

- At the outset it must be clarified that the immune response acts as a double edged sword. At occasions, it is responsible for immunopathology, whereas in many other cases it helps in providing the immunity to viral diseases. Antibody (humoral) mediated immunity and cell mediated immunity are two components of this category.
- Specific IgG, IgM and IgA antibodies are produced in response to viral infection about 7-10 days after infection. They play a key role in infections against extracellular viruses. sIgA is effective against viruses acting at respiratory, gastrointestinal and genitourinary tracts. This also provides protection to infants, who take breast fed milk, as sIgA is also secreted into milk. The humoral immunity plays a key role in recovery from papovavirus, picornavirus and togavirus infections. Parenteral administration of readymade antibodies (passive immunization) gives man satisfactory protection against challenge with hepatitis A and B, polio, measles and rabies viruses .

The antibody acts by the following mechanisms namely (i) neutralization of the virus, which prevents it's attachment and penetration to the host cell, (ii) opsonisation of the virus, facilitating its destruction by the various cells (iii) antibody and complement mediated cytotoxicity, (of viral infected cells).

In the following instances, antibody response has been seen to participate in the immunopathology of viral diseases.

(i) Respiratory syncytial virus infections are more severe in young infants with increased maternal antibody levels, which suggest that bronchiolitis (in RSV) may have an immunological basis.

(ii) Infection of a case with a serotype of dengue other than with which it had been previously infected, produces severe morbidity rather than protection.

(iii) Periarteritis nodosa manifested in some cases of hepatitis B infection, is attributed to immune complex formation and its deposition in small arteries.

The cell mediated immune response occurs about 7-10 days of infection. These chiefly comprise of HLA class II restricted CD4+ helper T lymphocyte responses and virus specific HLA class I restricted CD8+ cytotoxic T lymphocyte responses. The latter are involved in the direct killing of virus infected cells. Antibody dependent cell mediated cytotoxicity (ADCC) is another mechanism, in which the antibody helps cells like killer cells, and neutrophils to lyse viral infected cells. This immunity play a key role in diseases; as caused by herpes group, measles virus, poxivirus and HIV. It must be noted that some viral infections can suppress especially cell mediated responses; as measles and HIV. This information about the role of measles came, when it was seen in some studies that tuberculin positive individuals, when acquired measles, become tuberculin negative. Studies of Eskimos is Greenland have shown that measles exacerbates pre-existing tuberculosis. The role of HIV as an immunosuppressant is dramatic and clear cut.

- CMI also participates in the pathologic manifestation and symptoms of viral disease. This response is involved in the inflammatory manifestations at the site of infection, which may manifest as erythema, edema and lymphadenopathy. The characteristic rash of measles, is absent in children with a congenital absence of T cells.

Factors on which severity of viral disease may depend

1. **Age:** Generally speaking at the two extremes of life, man is more susceptible and the severity of viral disease is greater than at other periods. The exceptions are chicken pox, hepatitis A and infectious mononucleosis; if contracted in adulthood cause severe disease. Mumps, if contracted in adolescent period is likely to be complicated with orchitis. The most grim scenario is of poliovirus infection, likely to be inapparent in childhood, but contracted in adulthood is likely to be complicated with motor neuron disease.
2. **Host genotype:** There is sufficient circumstantial evidence available to support that the human genotype predisposes to certain viral infections, however this is an area, which requires case controlled studies for definitive evidence. For instance, West Africans appear to be more resistant to yellow fever than Europeans. This could be explained on the basis of genetic difference in MHC (including immune response gene), which could alter the immune response to a viral antigen, which could affect the control of that viral infection.
3 **Overall health of host including nutritional status:** This is clearly a factor, that the health implementing authorities can take to curtail the incidence and severity of viral infections. For instance, children in many developing countries with malnutrition have severe viral infections, which unfortunately exacerbate their malnutrition, as such children have been seen to have significantly reduced body weight. Emphasis can be also placed on the nutrition of lactating mothers, so that the milk the infants receive is rich in nutrients and maternal antibodies. Malnutrition acts by interfering with the humoral and cell-mediated immunity of the individual, thus increasing susceptibility.
4. **Body temperature:** Fever accompanies most viral infections. It occurs chiefly due to production of interleukin-I, which is produced mainly by macrophages. Fever acts as a natural defense mechanism against many viral infection, as the activity of many viruses is inhibited at body temperature of above than 39°C. The exact mechanism of fever in inducing antiviral effect is not known.
5. **Usage of hormones including steroids by man:** Administration of corticosteroids enhances most viral infection. This may be related to the ability of the steroids to suppress interferon synthesis and reduce inflammatory and immune responses. In fact, injudicious use of these drugs, in a case of HSV keratoconjunctivitis; may lead to blindness. Benign viral infection; as varicella can be fatal in case the patient is on cortisone.

   Pregnancy significantly increases the likelihood of severe disease following infection with herpes or polioviruses. Latent viral infection; as HHV-2 (HSV-2), Papovaviruses and HHV-5 (CMV) often get reactivated during pregnancy. The presence of herpes viruses in the birth canal may lead to infection of infant, while it is passing through it during delivery.
6. **Quantity of virus inoculated:** Exact data is not available on; what quantum of virus would be required for infection to occur or cause a severe infection? But is appears logical that this factor could play a part in the pathogenesis of viral infections.
7. **Virulence of the viruses:** e.g., HIV clades
8. **Quality of immune response:** This aspect has just been discussed.

Mention the emerging viruses in the recent past

A.10

Table 11.2.5: Emerging viruses in the recent past

Viruses	**Family**	**Possible emergence factors**
Norwalk	Calciviridae	Newer methods for detecting viruses
Dengue	Flaviviridae	Increase in urban population, increased usage of open water storage (which favours Aedes breeding), e.g., water coolers, used tyres
West Nile	Flaviviridae	Not known
Influenza	Orthomyxoviridae	Integrated pig/duck agriculture, increased mobile population
Marburg	Filoviridae	Unknown, possibly importation of monkeys in Europe
Ebola	Filoviridae	Contact with unknown natural host in Africa, importation of monkey
Machupo and Junin	Arenaviridae	Agriculture techniques, which favour human contact with rodents
Rift valley	Bunyaviridae	Dams, Irrigation
Human T lymphotropic (virus)	Retroviridae	Transfusion of blood products, contaminated needles
HIV	Retroviridae	Change in sexual practice (as homosexuality), transfusion of blood products

NB: Xenotransplantation is a dangerous proposition, as animal viruses can invade host tisue bypassing innate defences, when host is immunosuppressed, as having received steroids.

3 Bacteriophage

One of the virus types is an excellent cloning vector, besides playing a significant part in the pathogenicity of many bacterial diseases. Let's study it.

What is the name of this agent? Describe it.

A.1 Bacteriophage. Bacteriophage (in Greek 'phagein' means to eat) literally means a bacteria-eater or destroyer. Initially there was considerable excitement on their discovery, as it was thought that their use could lead to control and treatment of bacterial diseases. But subsequent trials belied such hopes. The phages are filterable through filters, which can hold back bacteria. They are inactivated by boiling. They have high host specificity. The phages may be transferring DNA from one bacterium to another in nature. The studies of water, soil and intestinal contents of man and animals by electron microscopy, have revealed that phages are common in nature.

Mention the historical events leading to its discovery.

A.2 Such concept was first suggested by Twort (1915), who observed degenerative changes in a culture of Staphylococcus. Subsequently D'Herelle (1917) reported lytic properties of a faecal filtrate on broth culture of Shigella.

Describe the structure of phage and the stages in the life cycle of the lytic phage.

A.3 Structure:

The virulent phage which has been studied most intensively is denoted as the T-even phage (T2, T4, T6).

Fig. 11.3.1 and 11.3.2

nb: Understanding of animal viruses and mammalian host cells is much less in comparison with understanding of phage bacteria (as former is complex). Animal cell genome contain 10,000 times more DNA than bacterium and the time it takes for animal cell to divide is about 100 times longer than what *E. coli* takes.

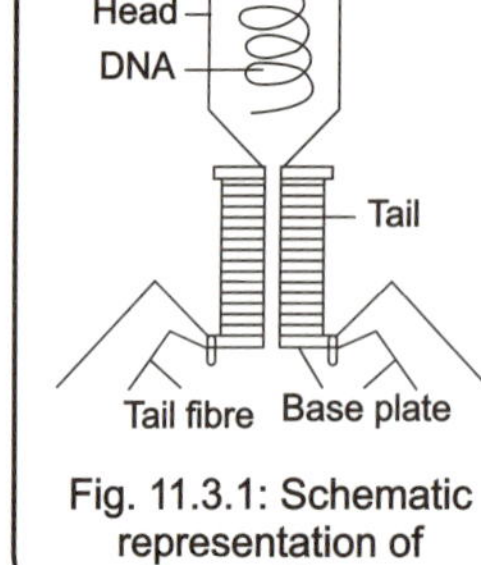

Fig. 11.3.1: Schematic representation of T even Phage

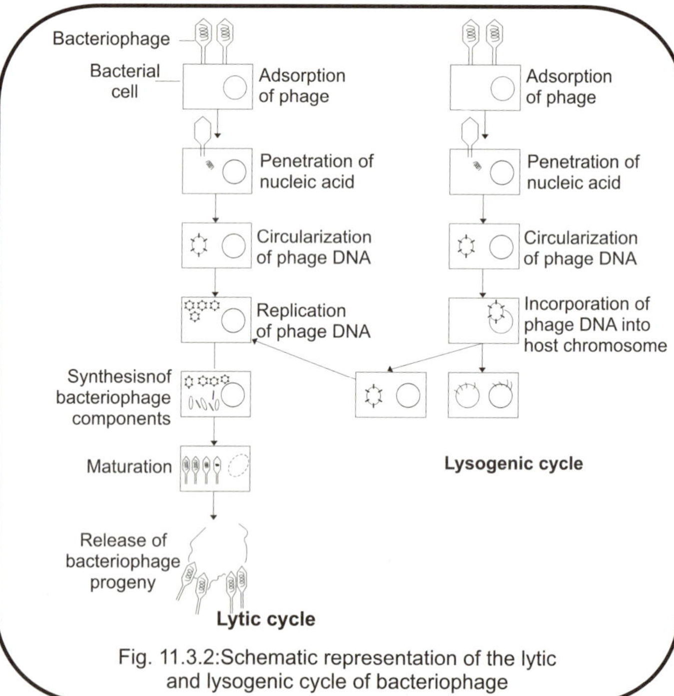

Fig. 11.3.2:Schematic representation of the lytic and lysogenic cycle of bacteriophage

Stages (steps) in life cycles of lytic phage.

Stage 1: Attachment of phage to host (bacterial) cell receptors.

The protein fibers at the end of phage tail attach to specific receptors on the bacterial cell wall. This stage can be bypassed, as experimental infection of the host cell directly with phage DNA is possible. The infection of the bacterium with naked phage nucleic acid is called *transfection*.

Stage 2: Entry of the viral nucleic acid into the host cell.

At the site of phage attachment to the bacterial cell wall, a degradation of the site is carried out by lysozyme at the tip of the phage tail. By an unknown mechanism (just like an injection), the nucleic acid (DNA) present in the head of the phage enters the bacteria, after the opening by the tail tip.

Stage 3: Transcription of phage DNA leads to production of specific protein.

Firstly; the phage DNA is transcribed into mRNA, which is then translated into proteins. The first proteins to be synthesized are the enzymes that are essential for replication of phage DNA and synthesis for phage coat protein. The synthesis of these enzymes is carried out on bacterial ribosomes. There is also degradation of bacterial chromosome into numerous pieces, as a result of synthesis of enzyme deoxyribonuclease by phage DNA.

Stage 4: Synthesis of phage structural protein.

The phage DNA *replicates to form many copies of itself, so that each copy can go into each of the phage particle that would be synthesized. There is synthesis of the phage components as phage head, tail etc.

*this function is beside the function of phage DNA to transcribe into mRNA

Stage 5: Assembly of phage DNA and phage components (proteins) to form mature phage (particles) virions.

This is a self-assembly process; initiated by the late-induced enzymes (from the phage DNA).

Stage 6: Release of phage virions from the host cell.

This stage is initiated, by a lysozyme coded by the phage DNA. The number of phages released per cell is termed the *burst size,* which varies from phage to phage. For T-4 phages, the burst size is about 200.

The replication study of bacteriophage can be done, by measuring the number of phages inside and outside the bacteria at different times, after the phage have adsorbed to the bacterium. The results of the release of phages released over a period of time are plotted serially over a period of time, on a graph known as *one step growth curve.*

Latent period: It is the length of time between entry of nucleic acid into the cell and phage release.This period could be about 40 minutes.

Eclipse period: It is the period in the bacterium shortly after infection, when no intact phage can be detected in the cell. It is a reflection of the separation of protein coat and DNA from each other.

Describe the life cycle of the temperate phage (lysogenic).

A.4 The most extensively studied temperate phage is the *phage lambda (λ),* which infects *E. coli.* It is similar in structure to the T-4 phage.

The first two steps/stages are the same; as with the lytic phage. At this stage, *two possibilities* exists, i.e., either the phage DNA replicates and goes into the lytic cycle or gets integrated with host cell DNA and goes into the lysogenic cycle. On entry into the cell, the phage DNA integrates with the bacterial chromosome at a specific site(s) (Fig. 11.3.2). This occurs, where the phage and the bacterial chromosome DNA is homologous, this allows the two to synapse, following which the phage DNA to become integrated into the bacterial chromosome. This integration can continue for numerous cell cycles (may be hundreds), but ultimately the prophage gets released from the bacterial chromosome, phage reverts to the lytic mode and eventually lyses the cell. The integration of the phage DNA with the host cell chromosome requires, that a group of genes synthesise a *repressor protein;* that helps to maintain this state. If this protein is not synthesized for any reason, as inactivation of this gene, then the enzyme that *excises the prophage* from the bacterial chromosome gets synthesized and the lytic cycle of the phage gets started. The repressor protein also makes the host cell immune (resistant) to infection from the same type of phage, but not to infection by other phages, as the repressor can't bind to their DNA.

Nb: One characteristic of a λ phage, that makes it useful as cloning agent, is the presence of at either end of the molecule, a short 12 nucleotide stretch of single-stranded DNA, which can base pair with other (as complementary) to form circular, double-stranded molecule. Complementary single strands are also referred to as 'sticky' ends or 'cos' sites (cohesive sites).

Describe about the significance of the Lysogenic conversion.

A.5 Lysogenic conversion: The lysogenic cells (i.e., which have prophage) sometimes acquires new properties, that can play a key part in their structural and functional organization, this phenomenon is called *lysogenic conversion* egs.

- *Presence of prophage beta is responsible for toxigenicity (pathogenicity) of *C. diphtheriae.*
- ^Presence of phage CEβ and DEβ in *C. botulinum* type C and D; respectively, are responsible for their toxin production.
- Lysogenic strain in *S.pyogenes* is responsible for scarlet fever (due to erythrogenic toxin)
- *V. cholerae* (cholera toxin).
- Modification of the somatic antigen (lipopolysaccharide layer of cell wall) of Salmonella can occur due to presence of specific phages (*S. Anatum* can get converted to S. Newington)
- Possible origin of viral origin of cancer (if prophage can excise and alter regulation of some genes)
- Toxin of EHEC (O157:H7)
- Use of genetic engineering studies (including gene mapping)

- Plasmid mediated drug resistance in *Staphylococcus aureus* can spreads from one strain to other by transduction.

  *Can these pathogenic strains lose their toxigenicity/pathogenicity?

  Yes, if the phage is excised (lost from the bacterial chromosome).

  ^Δ Can nontoxigenic (non-pathogenic) *C. diphtheriae* and *C. botulinum* (type C and D) acquire toxigenicity (pathogenicity)?

  Yes, if they get lysogenized by the relevant phages.

Describe the types of transduction.

A.6 Types of transduction:

1. **Generalized** (when involves *any* segment of the donor DNA; at random)
2. **Specialized/Restricted** (involves only *limited* segments of donor DNA)

Generalized: This occurs in the setting of a host cell, in which lytic cycle is undergoing and the host cell contains numerous bacterial chromosome pieces (produced by the replicating phage, which can lyse it). In the frenzy to assemble new phage virions; due to a packaging error, a piece of fragmented bacterial chromosome may be packed into the phage head instead of the phage DNA. This process is termed *generalized transduction*, as any bacterial gene stands an equal chance of getting transduced to a recipient cell, in contrast to specialized transduction in which only a few gene can be transduced. This process occurs at a frequency of about 1 in 10^6 phage assemblies. Once the newly synthesized phage particle (with new DNA) leaves the host cell, it may infect the new host cell transferring the new genes (bacterial) to the recipient cell.

[Before advanced molecular techniques became available, researchers used generalized phage induction in the lab oratory to transfer DNA segment from one bacterial strain to another]

Specialized: This occurs in the setting of a prophage, which can integrate at a few specific sites (not randomly) in the host chromosome. When activated, the prophage separates entirely from the host chromosome. In few cases, (about 1 in 10^5 or 10^6 assemblies), the prophage excision is imprecise and it carries with it bacterial genes adjacent to the sites of attachment. As these possible sites are few and specific, this is called *specialized* transduction. The transducing phage usually contains both phage and bacterial DNA, which is joined together.

Outline the significance of phages.

A.7 The *virulent* phages are used in phage typing (see A8 of this chapter)

The *temperate* phages have a role in:

(i) As a cloning vector, e.g., Phage M13. Cosmid is a cross of a lambda phage and plasmid.

(ii) In transfer of drug resistance as in *S. aureus*.

Other role see A.5, pg 389-390

Describe bacteriophage typing.

A.8 *Phage (Bacteriophage) assay:* Phages are characterized by causing areas of clearing or lysis, after adequate incubation period, when applied on lawn cultures of a susceptible. bacterium. These zones are called *plaques*. Each plaque represents a lesion, which has been produced, after a single phage proliferated to form millions of phages at that site. The plaques are analogous to bacterial colonies, the latter being produced after proliferation of bacteria. Like bacterial colonies are characterized by features; as size and shape etc.; plaques are also *characterized* by similar features. Plaque assay can be used for titrating the number of viable phages in a test preparation, as under optimal conditions, a single phage particle is capable of producing one plaque.

The specificity of the phage (virulent)-host cell (bacterium) interaction is exploited in identifying and typing bacteria, e.g., Tigley species specific phage for *B. anthracis*, Mukerjee phage IV (biotype specific) phage for classical *V. cholerae*. Intraspecies (strain) typing is performed for *S. aureus*, *S. Typhi*, *S. Typhimurium* and S. *Paratyphi A*. The importance of such typing, is in study of epidemiology of these infections, as locating the source of an outbreak in a neonatal unit or in a field study.

To obtain/synthesize specific phages, principle of serial passage of the phage in a strain of bacterium is used, which makes them specific for that and related strains, a phenomenon known as *adaptation of host range*. To do strain typing, a lawn culture of the test strain is obtained on a nutrient agar plate. Subsequently, the set of phages are applied at *routine test dose*▲. After appropriate incubation, period, the plate is read for the pattern of lysis and interpretation is done.

▲*Routine test* dose is defined as the highest dilution of phage preparation that just produces *confluent lysis.

**Confluent lysis mean total absence of any growth at site of application of phage. When lower concentration of phages are used, it produces a picture, in which plaques are produced, which can be counted.*

Section XI: General Virology

4 Laboratory Diagnosis of Viral Diseases (General Principles and Techniques)

A few decades back, many physicians used to question the utility of the making a viral diagnosis, as the viral culture techniques used to take a long time and specific antiviral drugs were mostly lacking. But now the scenario has changed drastically with viral diagnosis possible in a few hours and the increased availability of specific antiviral drugs for many diseases. The increased number of immunocompromised patients with opportunistic infections has contributed to making viruses, as the most frequent cause of human infectious diseases. Let's study the role of laboratory diagnosis in controling viral diseases.

Enumerate the conditions, where making laboratory diagnosis of viral infections is of key importance.

A.1 I. *Where specific antiviral drugs are available:*

1. Herpetic encephalitis
2. HIV disease

II. *Where making the viral diagnosis affects the patient's management*

1. Diagnosis of rubella in the first trimester of pregnancy, calls for *abortion of the foetus

   *as the probability of the baby being borne with congenital abnormalities is high
2. A baby borne of an HBsAg (especially with HBeAg) positive mother calls for active/passive immunization
3. If the pregnant women has genital herpes of the time of delivery, caesarean section may be indicated

III. *Where suspected viral exposure calls for PEP*

1. Health care personnel getting exposed to HIV positive patient, while caring for the patient
2. A person getting a dog bite from a dog, whose rabies status is not clear.

IV. *Where making a viral diagnosis can avoid unnecessary treatment and diagnostic testing*

1. Many times, while working up vague syndromes; as lower respiratory tract infection or aseptic meningitis, presumptive antibacterial treatment is started, which won't be useful and sophisticate expensive tests get carried out. Such a situation can be avoided, if early in the work up, it becomes clear that the patient is suffering from a viral disease.

V. *Where the diagnosis is of public health importance*

1. Blood banks have to test the donated blood for HBV, HCV and HIV, so that these diseases are not transmitted to the recipients
2. Diagnosis of diseases; as arboviruses, can alert the authorities to initiate control measures.

VI. *Where diagnosis mandates measures to prevent nosocomial spread*

e.g., Diagnosis of diseases; as rotavirus, respiratory syncytial virus in the inmates of hospital, calls for specific measure to prevent the disease spread within the hospital.

VII. *When new outbreak occurs in a community or a country.*

e.g., the outbreak of avian influenza (H5N1), which occurred in 2008 in India.

e.g., the outbreak of Crimean Congo haemorrhagic fever (CCHF) in Ahmedabad in 2011.

These are signals to the civic and other authorities to go into action.

VIII. *To make current (new) vaccines and antiviral drugs*

- Many viruses as Influenza frequently undergo genetic change, which makes the available vaccine stock, useless for the infection; with a new strain, when it evolves. In such a situation, the virologists have to be ready to quickly make a vaccine stock ready for the new virus strain.

- HIV frequently undergoes mutation, making it resistant to current antiviral drugs. It is important to manufacture (design) new drugs.

IX. *Epidemiologic monitoring*

- Gathering data about viral infections; as arboviruses and enteroviruses is important and valuable.
- Detecting antigenic variation (is important).
- Detecting and predicting epidemics

Enumerate the common specimens to be taken in the diagnosis of various categories of viral infections.

A.2 Specimen Collection

Collecting an appropriate sample from the site of active infection and other sites, depending on the disease stage (especially when viral shedding is maximum), is vital to make a correct diagnosis. Following are the recommended samples; for the various categories of infection.

Category of infection	Usual specimens	Appropriate invasive one
CNS infection	CSF, throat swab, saliva, stool, paired sera	Brain biopsy
Conjunctivitis	Tears, *conjunctival swab	Scraping from conjunctiva and cornea
Upper respiratory tract	*Throat swab, nasal swab, nasal washing, nasopharyngeal aspirate, sputum, stool	None
Lower respiratory tract	-do-	Bronchoalveolar lavage, lung biopsy
Cardiovascular system	CSF, *throat swab, faeces	None
Gastrointestinal tract	*Rectal swab *Stool (Faeces)	None
Urinary tract	Urine	None
Cutaneous	Vesicle fluid, ulcer, scrapping, throat swab, faeces	None
Blood (for HIV, HBV, HCV, HTLV)	Blood	Lymph node biopsy

* Specimens from conjunctiva and vesicle require presence of epithelial cells in the specimen for specimen quality validation. Similarly nasopharyngeal/throat swab and bronchoalveolar lavage/sputum requires columnar cells and alveolar macrophages for these specimens validation, respectively.

Mention the considerations, while transporting specimens likely to contain viral agents.

A.3 Transport of Specimen

- The specimen should be transported as early as possible, so that virus remains intact and viable and has a chance to grow; if required. Attempt should also be made to prevent overgrowth of bacterial and fungal contaminants.
- If there is likelihood of a delay in transport, the specimen may be kept at 4°C.
- If the delay is likely to be longer, the samples may be frozen at -20° except for whole blood (serum, however may be frozen) and tissue of organs should only be kept at 4°C.
- Viral transport medium (VTM), which contains a buffered salt solution, protein stabilizer, pH indicator and antibiotics (to prevent bacterial and fungal contamination) may be used for sample transportation.
- A multipurpose viral, chlamydial and mycoplasma transport medium is also available

Mention the special considerations in diagnosis of viral diseases.

A.4

1. *Choosing a test:* If the patient belongs to early stage illness, rely essentially on tests that depend on direct identification of virus, viral antigen or viral nucleic acid in the clinical specimen.
2. *Isolation (culture)* of a virus from a clinical specimen is *not necessarily* equivalent to establish it as a cause of the infection under investigation (as in many diseases carrier state are known; as adenoviral infection and CMV, can which cause life long infection).
3. *Dual infection* of viruses are possible. Serology also may be useful; if two viruses are 'isolated' to find, which one or if both; are clinically active.

Mention the three broad category of methods employed in diagnosis of viral infection and the indications for the same.

A.5 I. Direct demonstration of virus, viral antigen or nucleic acid in clinical sample or in cell line used for isolation.

Techniques: To demonstrate *virus*, particle, electron microscopy* and immune electron microscopy. Detecting viral *antigen* using monoclonal antibodies; which are fluorescent labelled (fluorescent microscopy) or enzyme labelled (enzyme immunoassay), other serological tests to demonstrate viral antigen. *Staining technique*; as Giemsa to detect inclusion bodies or Tzanck preparation to detect multinucleated giant cells of HSV etc. Nucleic acid probes; as DNA and RNA, to detect viral nucleic acid. *Nucleic acid amplification techniques*; as PCR, multiplex PCR (as for respiratory viruses) real time PCR, NASBA (for mRNA).

Indications:

1. When rapid diagnosis is to be established in early or initial period of disease
2. In immunodeficient cases, as serological response is poor
3. For diagnosis of new diseases, as Rota virus was discovered by electron microscopy technique
4. To diagnose uncultivable viruses

* Is not a standard clinical laboratory method.

II. Cell culture or its newly developed modifications; as shell vial technique.

Indications:

1. It is considered the gold standard for detecting viruses, against which other techniques are evaluated.
2. Detecting unexpected and new viruses.
3. Detection of antigenic change of viruses, as influenza virus in epidemics. These changes are utilized to make better diagnostic kits and effective vaccines (old vaccines can be rendered ineffective by antigenic change).
4. Confirms serological diagnosis.
5. Resolve any controversy, that is clinical or laboratory oriented.

- *Preparation of inocula* (from clinical sample) is a specialized technique; which requires mincing of the tissue (using scissors) in trypsin (for separation of cells). For making sample bacteria free, antimicrobials are used or millipore filter is used.
- *Techniques to detect* viral growth in cell culture, see A.12a, P 376-378. The culture results need to be carefully interpreted. Viral isolation for sterile sites is usually significant. However isolation from some other sites, as faeces, can occur intermittently for long periods, without any role in the pathology of the concerned case.

III. Measurement of serum antibodies

Principle: Rising (classically four fold rise) titers of antibodies to virus specific antigen (in acute vs convalescent phase sera) and shift from IgM to IgG antibodies are taken, as diagnostic criteria for acute viral disease. Presence of antibodies in single sample are considered significant, if infection is exotic and one is determining susceptibility to infection; as CMV.

Indications:

(i) Conditions; where good serological test is available. (ii) Epidemiologic studies to find prevalence of infection.

(iii) Test effectiveness of vaccine as, titer in serum of anti HBs of more than 10 IU/ml is considered protective against Hepatitis B virus.

Techniques:

- ELISAs (being sensitive and automated, they are replacing haemagglutination assays, immunofluorescence tests) latex agglutination, CFT, immune electron microscopy, virus neutralization (in cell cultures).
- HAI, reverse passive agglutination, immunodiffusion.

Limitation in serology:

- Lack of specificity: This is being take care these days with availability of specific monoclonal antibodies.
- Rheumatoid factor (RF) – Screen for it. If serum is positive for it, false positive in IgM immunoassays can occur. This problem can be avoided by making assay in which anti-human IgM is used as a capture antibody.

Nb: RF is antibody, mainly of the IgM class, directed against the constant region domains of normal IgG. This RF is present in many infectious diseases including of TORCH agents. In neonate, antibodies may be made against mother's IgG allotype.

5 Assessment/Examination Questions

Chapter 1

1. Discuss general properties of viruses. A 2-A4., p. 365, A1a., p. 364
2. Depict diagrammatically the structure (morphology) of virus and describe it. A 6a, b., p. 366-367
3. Describe viral inclusion bodies. A 12a ii., p. 377
4. Describe nomenclature of viruses. Enumerate DNA viruses and list the diseases caused by them. A4c., p. 365, A7a., p. 368, A7bi, 369
5. Enumerate the RNA viruses and list the diseases caused by them. A7bii., p. 369-370
6. Describe viral multiplication. A. 8., p. 370-373
7. Enumerate the effects of viral infection on the host cell and describe in detail the cytopathic effects on the host cell., A 9, 10., p. 373-374.
8. Describe cultivation of viruses with special emphasis on cell culture. A 11., p. 374-376
9. Describe techniques to detect viral growth in cultures with emphasis on using principle of cytopathogenic effect (CPE) of viruses. A 12a,b., p. 376-379
10. Describe haemagglutination. A 126., p. 378-379
11. Describe viral latent infections. A9; (3)., p. 373
12. Discuss challenges in ascribing viruses as causative agents in diseases. p. 374Δ

Chapter 2

1. Describe two accidental natural infections that have added to our understanding of viral pathogenesis. A 4., p. 380
2. Discuss pathogenesis of viral infections. A 6., p. 381-387
3. Describe the various routes, by which viruses enter the human body and cause infection. A6, p. 381-383
4. Describe emerging viral infections in the recent past and mention the possible emergence factors. A 10, p. 387

Chapter 3

1. Describe morphology of T even phage and life cycle of bacteriophage. A 3., p. 388-389
2. Describe lysogenic conversion. A4, 5., p. 389, 390
3. Discuss significance of phages with a special mention on phage typing. A 7, A 8., p. 390

Chapter 4

1. Discuss the indications of performing laboratory diagnosis of viral infections. A 1., p. 391, 392
2. Describe the considerations in transporting specimens for making viral diagnosis. A 3., p. 392
3. Discuss the special considerations in diagnosis of viral disease. A 4., p. 392
4. Classify the three major categories of techniques used to make diagnosis of viral infection and mention their indications. A5., p. 393

Section XII: DNA Viruses

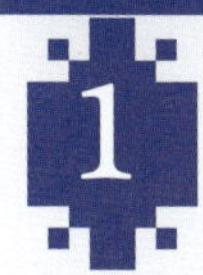

Overview of Clinical Profile (Pathogenicity) of DNA Viral Infections

Erythrovirus (Parvovirus B19)-Details see. pg 398

Disease	Host target
Erythema infectiosum (fifth disease)	Children
Arthralgia and arthritis	Adults
Transient aplastic crisis	Chronic haemolytic anaemia cases
Chronic anaemia	Immunodeficient individuals
Hydrops fetalis and fetal death	Fetus

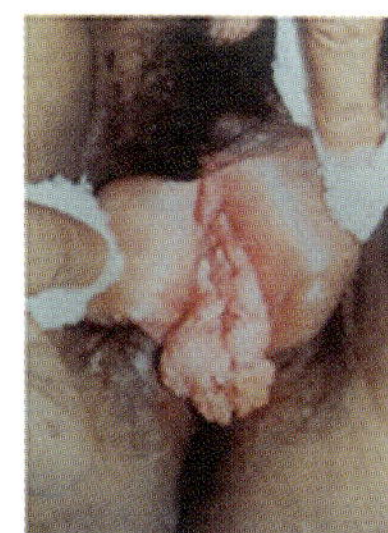

Fig.12.1.1: Condylomata acuminata,warts in the vulvar region caused by Human Papilloma viruses

Papilloma virus-Details see pg 400-401

	Disease	*Site*	*Predominant Human Papilloma Virus (HPV) types*
Skin warts	Common warts (Verrucae vulgaris)	Skin (esp. hands)	2, 1
	Plantar warts (Verrucae plantaris)	Heel, sole foot (weight bearing areas)	1, 2
	Flat warts (Verrucae plana)	Face, heel	3, 10
	Epidermodysplasia verruciformis	Skin (esp. sun exposed areas)	5, 8, 9
Benign tumours of head and neck (Papilloma)	Oral papilloma	Oral cavity (buccal)	6, 11
	Congenital papilloma	Conjunctiva	11
	Laryngeal papillomatosis (Recurrent respiratory papillomatosis)	Larynx	6, 11
Anogenital warts	Condylomata acuminantum (Fig. 12.1.1)	Vagina and cervix in females	6, 11
		Shaft of penis, perianal region in males	
	Premalignant intraepithelial neoplasia	Cervix, Penis	6, 11, 16
	Cervical carcinoma	Cervix	16, 18 (strong association)

Polyoma viruses	
BK polyoma virus	Asymptomatic viruria in pregnant women and immunocompromised individuals (including renal transplant cases)
JC polyoma virus	Progressive multifocal leucoencephalopathy–PML, (rare, fatal, sub-acute demyelinating disease, may occur on reactivation)
Adeno Associated Viruses (defective in human cells, for growth require to be complemented by adenoviruses	So far not been found to cause any illness in human beings

		Associated serotypes	Those at risk
Adenoviruses (details pg 402-404)	**Respiratory**		
	Acute febrile pharyngitis	1-7	Infants, young children
	Pharyngoconjunctival fever	1-7	Infants, young children
	Acute respiratory disease	4, 7, 14, 21	Adults
	Pneumonia	1, 2, 3, 7	Infants, young children
	Ocular		
	Follicular conjunctivitis	3, 4, 11	Any age
	Epidemic keratoconjunctivitis	8, 9, 37	Adults
	Others (associations)		
	Haemmorhagic cystitis	11, 21	Infant and young children
	Diarrhoea and vomitting	40, 41	Infant and young children
	Intussusception	1, 2, 5	Infant
	Disseminated infection	5, 3, 4, 35-47	Immuno-compromised
	C.N.S.	3, 7	
	S.T.D.	2, 19, 37	

POX VIRUSES

Genus	Virus	Primary host	Diseases
Orthopoxvirus	**Variola major** (details pg. 405-407) **Variola minor**	Man	*Small pox* (Variola major and minor) Details see. pg 405
	Vaccinia	Man	*Vaccinia* *Vaccine complications*
	Monkeypox	Monkeys	*Monkeypox*
	Cowpox	Cow	*Cowpox*
Parapoxvirus	**Orf**	Sheep	*Orf*
	Milker's node	Cow	*Milker's node*
Yatapoxvirus	**Tanapox**	Monkey	*Tanapox*
	Yabapox	Monkey	*Yabapox*
Molluscipox virus	**Molluscum contagiosum**	Man	*Molluscum contagiosum* (Benign skin lesions)

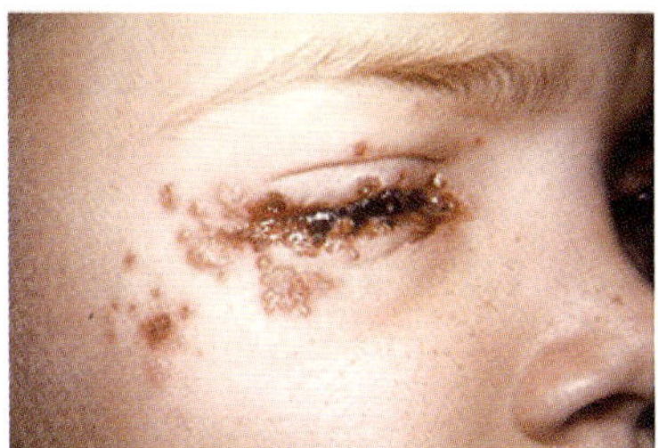

Fig.12.1.2: Herpetic lesions: A young child with periocular herpes simplex vesicular lesion
Courtesy:Dr K.I. Hermann/CDC

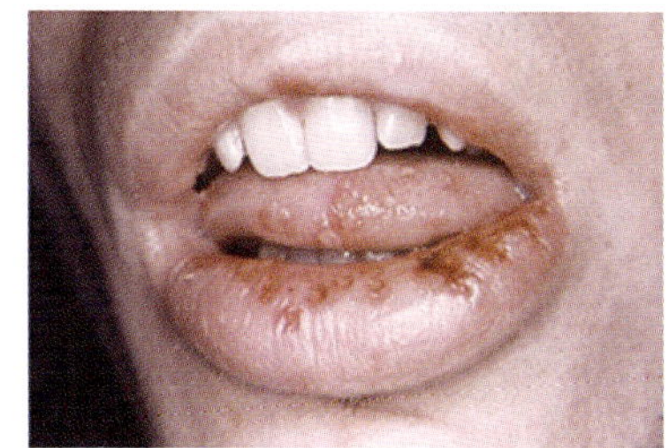

Fig.12.1.3: Herpes Simplex Virus: Lesion on a young male patient`s lips and tongue by this virus
Courtesy: Robert E. Sumpter/CDC

HERPES Viruses **Human herpesvirus 1 (HHV-1)**	
	• Gingivostomatitis (lesions in perioral region) (Fig. 12.1.2) • Herpes labialis (lesion on lip) (Fig. 12.1.3) • Keratitis/keratoconjunctivitis (involvement of cornea, conjunctiva or both) • Encephalitis (pathogenesis unclear, high morbidity and mortality; if untreated) • Eczema herpeticum (occurs in children with eczema lesions) • Herpetic whitlow (infection of finger) • Herpetic *gladiatorum (infection of body, which occurs through abrasions of skin, often seen in *wrestlers)
Human herpesvirus 2 (HHV-2)	
	• Genital herpes (on sites; as penis, urethra, cervix, vulva etc.). Detail see. p. 408-417 • Neonatal herpes (acquired by neonate, during birth)
Human herpesvirus 3 (V-Z virus)	
Primary infection in normal children	Varicella (chicken pox) Maculopapular lesions, centripretal in distribution. Details see pg., 413-416
Reactivation in elderly	Zoster (painful vesicular lesion)
Human herpesvirus 4 (E.B. Virus) Details-pg., 417-419.	• Infectious mononucleosis (Kissing disease in adolescents) • Fever, lymphadenopathy and pharyngitis • Burkitt's lymphoma (in children of Sub-Saharan, Africa) • Nasopharyngeal carcinoma (in adults of Southern China) • B cell lymphoma (seen in immunodeficient children and adults) • Oral hairy leucoplakia (in HIV infected patients)
Human herpevirus 5 (CMV)	• Congenital (Prenatal transplacental spread) • (Congental cytomegalic inclusion disease) Only 1% of all babies have this infection at birth. Out of this only 5% are symptomatic at birth. • The syndrome is characterized by small infants with growth retardation, hepatosplenomegaly, jaundice, thrombocytopenia, pneumonitis (not always seen in entirety) • Details of presentation, See table 12.8.1, pg. 420.
Human herpesvirus 6	Associated with roseola infantum or exanthem subitum
Human herpesvirus 7	Associated with roseola infantum or exanthem subitum
Human herpesvirus 8	Associated with Kaposi's sarcoma (in HIV patients)
Hepatitis B Details-p.424-430	Serum hepatitis Three phases namely; preicteric, icteric and Convalescent. See table 14.4.5, pg 513-514 of Section 14 for comparison of the hepatitis viruses Carrier state may also occur. Details A 5b, pg. 526., Hepatocellular carcinoma may develop

*'gladiator' means an armed man, who fought against men or wild animals in a public place.

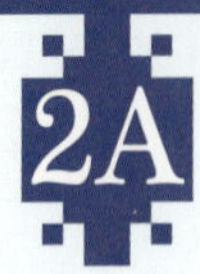

Integrated Clinical Based Study of Parvovirus B-19

Paulina, a nine year girl presented to the paediatric OPD in Birmingham (U.K.) with fever and a facial rash (slapped cheek appearance).

Linkages: Pg. 368, 395, 431

What is the provisional diagnosis of the case?

A.1 Human Parvovirus B19 infection. The virus belongs to family Parvoviridae.

What approach is to be followed to laboratory diagnose Human Parovirus B19 infection?

A.2 The diagnosis essentially relies on demonstration of B19 specific serum IgM and IgG antibodies by ELISA kits (see pg. 431, Chapter 10). Specific viral DNA can be demonstrated in bone-marrow, RBC and foetal liver (in hydrops fetalis) samples, where facilities for molecular biology exists. The virus can be cultured only at labs, where advanced research facilities exist. Electron microscopy of the serum can demonstrate B19 virion.

Mention the historical aspects and morphological characteristics of Human B19 virus.

A.3 It is one of the smallest DNA animal viruses. It is the only parvovirus, presently known to be a human pathogen. The name B19 is derived from the code number of the human serum, in which the virus was discovered. It was discovered unexpectedly in 1974, when parvovirus like particles were found in asymptomatic blood donors, undergoing routine testing for pathogens.

The virus has an outer capsid; formed by two structural protein (other details see table 11.1.4, pg. 368). Its genome has been sequenced and is 5.5 kb large. It has failed to grow in classical cell culture lines but can replicate 'in vitro' in erythroid progenitor cells, derived from human bone marrow and other sites (as umbilical cord, peripheral blood, foetal liver).

Describe the clinical profile of Human B19 viral infection.

A.4 B19 infections occurs worldwide, year-round and can occur at any age. B19 virus is highly contagious and numerous outbreaks have been reported. The infection is presumed to be transmitted via respiratory droplets. Vertical transmission of B19 (from mother to fetus) and parenteral transmission with contaminated blood products is documented. The role of oral route secretions in the transmission is not clear. There is no evidence of suggest that B19 infection of fetus increases the risk of congenital malformations in live-born infants.

The major clinical manifestations of B19 infection are depicted at pg. 395.

The transient aplastic crisis in chronic haemolytic anaemia patient was the first clinical manifestation of B19 infection to be noticed in the early 1980s. Subsequently by 1985, it was recognized as the cause of the characteristic childhood exanthematous illness, *erythema infectiosum (fifth disease)*. This entity is also called fifth disease because it was classified fifth in a series of six exanthems of childhood. This disease is characterized with a facial rash (slapped cheek appearance) that may subsequently spread to the arms, legs and other sites. The severe manifestations of B19 viremia relate to its propensity to infect and lyse erythroid blood precursors in the bone marrow.

No specific antivirals or vaccine is available. Handwashing is recommended to reduce transmission, although this has not been specifically studied before eating or after contact with respiratory/other secretions.

Aspects related to case theme/examination assessment

Mention the clinical importance of Simian virus 40.

A.5 Polyomaviruses include several animal viruses; especially simian virus 40 (SV 40) and two human viruses; namely JC polyomavirus and BK polyoma virus. The polyomavirus of mouse, which is a prototype of this genus can produce a wide variety of tumors under some conditions, hence the name 'polyoma' (poly, many; oma tumor). They belong to polyomaviridae.

Simian virus 40 infects monkey subclinically but can induce tumors, when inoculated into baby rodents. This virus became the model in the 1970s for the molecular investigation of the virus induced malignancy. It also has medical importance, as live viral vaccines produced from monkey kidney tissue, must be free from this virus because of the oncogenic potential it possesses. It may be pertinent to point out here that declaring animal cell lines being used in vaccine production; free from various viruses is a key activity, which requires tremendous expertise. The animal cell lines may be infected with viruses, whose existence, we may not be knowing at the moment. Inoculation of vaccines produced by cell lines infected with unknown viruses could be disastrous.

Describe BK polyoma virus.

A.6 This virus was isolated in 1970 (like JCV), from urine specimen obtained, from a renal patient with the initals BK, who developed ureteral stenosis postoperatively. The structural details of the virus is given in table 11.1.4, pg. 368. In comparison to the papillomaviruses, it has a smaller virion (45 vs 55 nm diameter). Its genome size is approximately 5000 base pairs long.

BK virus infections are ubiquitous. This virus infects children early in life and by the age of 10 years, almost all children have antibodies to this virus. It spreads likely by the respiratory route. The virus establishes latent infection primarily in the kidney and persists for life. Reactivation may occur; whenever the immune system is impaired, as after any disease or administration of immunosuppressant drugs. The asymptomatic BK viruria is seen in 3 percent of pregnant women. The virus excretion occurs primarily during the third trimester of pregnancy and usually ceases in the postpartum period. This virus besides being associated with ureteral stenosis in renal transplant patients is also associated with hemorrhagic cystitis in bone marrow transplant patients.

Laboratory diagnosis

The examination of the urine is the commonest method to detect BK viruria. The cytologic examination reveals characteristic infected cells to have an enlarged nucleus with a single large basophilic intranuclear inclusion. The electron microscopic examination of the urine can also reveal the BK virions. PCR technique can also detect specific BK sequences in the urine. The virus is slow growing and difficult to culture on traditional cell lines, hence viral isolation is not a routine method.

Treatment

The majority of patients with BK virus are asymptomatic and don't require treatment.

Describe JC polyoma virus.

A.7 This virus like BKV was isolated in 1971, but was isolated from brain tissue of a patient with progressive multifocal leukoencephalopathy. JC was the initial of the patient. The basic gross structural details resemble that of BK virus. The JCV and BKV share 75 percent homology at the level of the nucleotide sequence.

The epidemiology and pathogenesis of this infection has many similarities with the BK infection. Both infections are ubiquitous and asymptomatic viruria is seen in both infections, in the pregnant women and immunocompromised individuals. Adults have a 75% seropositivity to the viral antigen. This virus also establishes a latent infection in the kidney but also infects the B cells and the monocyte lineage cells. In some cases, the infection results in the progressive muitifocal leukoencephalopathy disease. It is a rare subacute demyelinating disease, that results from direct infection of the oligodendrocytes with JCV and results in decreased myelin production and demyelination. These patients present with rapidly progressive focal neurologic deficits, without signs of intracranial pressure. The neurologic findings commonly include hemiparesis, visual field defects, aphasia, ataxia and cognitive impairment.

The AIDS epidemic has significantly altered the epidemiology of PML. In the pre-HIV era, PML was seen primarily in the older patients with haematologic malignancies; as Hodgkin's disease or chronic lymphocytic leukemia. Now PML is common and may be seen in approximately 1-4 percent of patients with HIV. Now PML is an AIDs defining disease, according to the CDC case definition and may be the initial presentation of HIV infection.

Laboratory diagnosis

The PML can be diagnosed with the histological examination of the brain tissue. The picture would be one of demyelination of the neurons; accompanied by proliferation of bizarre astrocytes. The nucleus of the oligodendrocytes is enlarged with presence of intranuclear deeply basophilic homogenous staining material. The electron microscopy, if performed of this material can reveal the JC virions. Immunofluorescent techniques can reveal the specific viral antigen in the brain lesions. Viral isolation is not performed, as a routine because the virus grows slowly and requires uncommon cell lines and human fetal brain cells. CT scans in patients with PML can reveal hypodense nonenhancing lesions of the cerebral white matter. MRI scan may be more sensitive than CT scan in detecting PML lesions.

Treatment

The majority of patients with JCV infection are asymptomatic and do not require treatment.

Integrated Clinical Based Study of Adenovirus/Diarrhoea

A diarrhoeal outbreak occured in a military camp in Dehradun, India. No bacterial pathogens were isolated. Viral cultures were ordered from the stool specimen.

The stool specimens were inoculated into cell cultures. The pattern of cytopathogenic effect (CPE) observed on the Hela cell line was of cells: becoming swollen, rounded, refractile and getting clustered together as a 'bunch of grapes'.

Linkages: Pg. 368, 396, 431

What is the likely diagnosis the above case?

A.1 Adenoviral infection

How can the provisional diagnosis be confirmed?

A.2 (a) The viral isolate can be confirmed, as one of adenovirus by; performing direct immunofluorescence test on the cell monolayer showing CPE.

How can the viral isolate be typed?

A.2 (b) Appropriate type specific antisera can be chosen to type, the isolate by haemagglutination inhibition and/or neutralization tests.

What is the need of typing the viral isolates?

A.2 (c) The typing of the isolate can help in epidemiologic studies and could help in finding the source of the infection and detect the routes of spread of the infection.

Comment on the derivation of the term 'adenovirus'.

A.3 (a) The virus was first observed in a culture of adenoid tissue, maintained in tissue culture in 1953, by Rowe and colleagues. Hence; the derivation of the name.

Mention about the morphological characteristics and classification of adenoviruses.

A.3 (b) The basic structure of it is depicted in table 11.1.4, pg. 368 The icosahedral shell (capsid) is composed of 20 equilateral triangles (sides) and 12 vertices. It is composed of 240 capsomeres; as hexons. (each have six neighbour, which make up the 20 triangular faces of icosahedron) and 12 penton (each has 5 neighbours) capsomeres at the vertices. From each vertex, emerges a rodlike structure with knob, so the resemblance of this virion to a space vehicle. (Fig. 12.3.1)

The human adenoviruses belong to the genus Mastadenovrus, which has 51 serotypes. The genetic maps of few of these types (as types 2, 5 and 7) have been constructed and functions assigned to most of the regions of the DNA viral genome. The human adenoviruses have been divided into six subgenera (A through F), on the basis of the homology of DNA genomes and other properties; as haemaglutination of RBCs and oncogenicity potential in hamsters. These viruses have been divided, on the basis of antigenicity into subgenera and serotypes, that bear a letter 'h' (for human) and a number for serotype; for instance mastadenovirus h9.

Can we ascribe the isolation of the adenovirus (from the cases) definitely to them, being the etiological agents of the diarrhoeal outbreak in the military camp?

A.4 (a) No, the adenoviruses are often shed intermittently, for long periods from asymptomatic cases also. Adenovirus serotypes 40 and 41 are associated with diarrhoea.

If not, then what additional test may be required to ascribe etiological significance to the isolation of adenoviruses?

A.4 (b) Serologic testing of the acute and convalescent sera from the cases to demonstrate a fourfold rise of adenoviral antibodies may be necessary.

From which samples, the isolation of adenoviruses, would be considered definitely significant?

A.4 (c) From samples; as brain biopsy and lower respiratory tract.

Outline the laboratory diagnosis of adenoviral infections.

A.4 (d) A diagnosis of adenoviral infection should be made frequently in the proper setting of a clinical criteria; for instance an outbreak of acute respiratory disease in military recruits or an outbreak of pharyngoconjunctival fever. In most cases, however the disease caused by adenoviruses, cannot be differentiated from other viral agents and/or *Mycoplasma pneumoniae*. A definitive diagnosis of adenovirus infection depends on various tests as depicted at pg. 431. Isolation of adenovirus from oropharynx and faeces should be interpreted cautiously because of the common asymptomatic long intermittent shedding of the virus from these sites. If significance of an isolate is doubtful (questionable), serologic testing of acute and convalescent sera may be necessary. Isolation of the adenovirus from lungs, eyes or brain sample is significant.

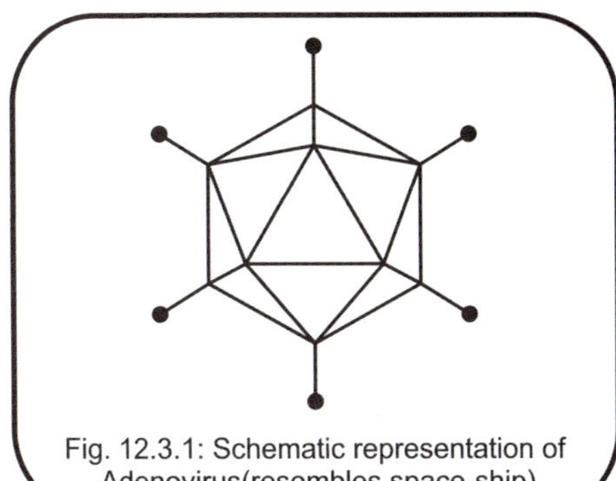

Fig. 12.3.1: Schematic representation of Adenovirus(resembles space-ship)

What are the diseases besides diarrohea, adenovirus infection is associated with?

A.5 (a)

Age group	Syndrome	Associated serotype
Neonates	Fatal disseminated infection	3, 7
Infants	Pharyngitis, Coryza	1, 2
Children	Upper respiratory disease	1, 2
	Pharyngoconjunctival fever	3, 7
	Pneumonia	1, 2
	Meningoencephalitis	2, 6
	Diarrohea	2, 3
	Intussusception	1, 2
	Haemorrhagic cystitis	11, 21
Young adults	Acute respiratory disease	3, 4
	Epidemic keratoconjunctivitis	8, 19
Immmunocompromised	Disseminated infection	5, 13, 34
	CNS disease; as encephalitis	7, 12

Mention about the pathogenesis of adenoviral infections.

A.5 (b) These viruses are *transmitted* by inhalation of aerosolized virus, by inoculation of virus into conjunctival sac and likely by the faecal-oral route also. The adenoviruses multiply initially in the pharynx, conjunctiva or small intestine and rarely spread beyond the draining cervical, preauricular or mesenteric lymph nodes. As the disease remains localized and does not spread further, the disease is often mild/asymptomatic/self limiting and has a short incubation period (5-10 days). The immunity is *serotype specific* and long lasting. Second, attacks from the same serotype are usually rare. Adenoviruses can interact with the cells in three ways. Firstly, it can cause a lytic infection of the cell, which results in the lysis of the cell, producing thousands of progeny viruses per cell. This interaction produces the typical adenoid type of CPE (enlarged round, grape like clusters). The other two type of interactions are latent/chronic infection of the lymphoid cell and oncogenic potential of the infected cell.

What could be the target population for usage of a potential good adenoviral vaccine?

A.6 (a) Military recruits or other critical population that are frequently prone to such infections.

Why is the development of adenovirus vaccine not seriously considered for general population?

A.6 (b) The reasons include:

(i) many of the infections are self-limited.

(ii) numerous serotypes exist currently the number is 52 serotypes of human adenoviruses. They are divided into seven species (namely; A to G).

(iii) ability to adenovirus to cause tumors in animals; as baby hamsters, but no such evidence exists in man.

Describe the adenovirus vaccine in current usage.

A.6 (c) Considering the critical job of military personnel, live vaccines against adenovirus types 4 and 7 have been used to counter the acute respiratory disease in the military recruits. This vaccine is not !! attenuated and given as enteric coated capsule. The basis of the vaccine is that inoculation of the adenovirus into the gastrointestinal tract does not result in illness, in contrast to the inoculation into the respiratory tract.

What are the uses of adenoviruses?

A.7 **(a)** (i) As vectors for gene delivery of human CFTR cDNA in individuals with cystic fibrosis.

(ii) As model to study carcinogenesis.

(iii) As novel anti-cancer therapy (using attenuated strain to directly kill tumor cells, by viral 'lytic' replication)

Describe Human adenovirus–associated viruses.

A.7 **(b)** These are small icosahedral viral particles, which belong to the *genus 'Dependovirus'*. They have been named so, as these often contaminate adenovirus preparations. These are defective and need a helper virus as adenovirus or herpesvirus for their proliferation, hence also the name *dependoviruses*. These are detected in several adenovirus preparations by *electron microscopy*. Very little is known about their life cycle. They commonly infect humans but have *not been* associated with any disease. They persist in the human cells by integrating with the human cell genome and establishing latent infection. Their ability to persist and lack of pathogenicity have created interest in their being used, as *potential vectors* (tools) for gene therapy.

What measures could have been successful in preventing the above outbreak?

A.8 Chlorination (disinfection/sterilization) of water being consumed and proper management of waste water.

Integrated Clinical Based Study of Smallpox (Variola Major/Accidental Outbreak)

The last natural case of small pox (Variola major) occurred in Assam (India) in May, 1975. An laboratory (accidental) outbreak of this virus occurred, in August, 1978 in a laboratory in Birmingham, U.K., in which one fatality occurred, for which Dr. Henry Bedson Professor of the Lab took responsibility and ended his life.

Linkages: Pg. 368, 396, 432

Is it necessary to maintain stocks of small pox virus in laboratory? Explain.

A.1 (a) It is important to maintain the smallpox virus for many reasons, namely

(i) For academic (study) reasons

(ii) Any time this disease reemerges, the medical community should be able to tackle it; including vaccine manufacture.

(iii) Any time the terrorists use this agent as a bioweapon, the microbiologists should be in a position to diagnose the syndrome effectively.

Classify poxviruses causing human infection.

A.1 (b) Classification of poxviruses causing human infections: see pg. 396.

Describe Molluscum contagiosum.

A.1 (c) Molluscum contagiosum is a benign epidermal tumor-like lesion (also see pg. 396).

Pathology: The lesion is small (few mms in size) and umbilicated. They involve the whole of the body excepting the soles and palms. The cut section of the lesion, when stained with histopathologic stains, reveal hyaline inclusion bodies (molluscum bodies) within the proliferated epidermal cells.

Pathogenicity: The disease is transmitted by direct and indirect contact; including sexual transmission in adults. The disease is self limiting and usually disappears within few months.

Laboratory diagnosis:

(i) Characteristic histopathological appearance

(ii) The virus is non-cultivable

Treatment: The lesions are surgically removed by ablation

Describe the morphology of poxviruses with special reference to their large size.

A.1 (d) The poxviruses are the *largest* viruses that infect vertebrates. The virions are just large enough to be seen under a light microscope (using critical illumination), but details of its structure come only from electron microscopic studies. The large virion size is *accounted* partly by the large DNA molecules that include all genes for all proteins needed for DNA synthesis and production of viral mRNAs. These viruses are unique from the other DNA viruses in having several specific enzymes, replicating in the cytoplasm rather than nucleus and being minimally dependent on the host cell. With in the cytoplasm, they produce eosinophilic, inclusion bodies called *Guarnieri bodies*.

The structure of poxviruses is complex as can be evident from table 11.1.4, pg. 368 and Fig. 12.4.1 and 12.4.2 The nucleocapsid symmetry does not conform to either of the two common types of symmetry, i.e., icosahedral or helical. So; it is sometimes called a *'complex' virion*. The virus particles are brick shaped and asymmetric and very resistant to chemical and physical inactivation.

Which year was the immunization programme for small pox stopped throughout the world?

A.2 (a) In U.S.A., the vaccination programme was stopped in 1972 and throughout the world in 1980.

What is the significance of the above data, as far as the usage of Variola virus, as a bioweapon is considered?

A.2 (b) Any time this disease reemerges naturally or as a bioterrorism event, the individuals borne after this date would be prone to this infection. In case the structure of the virus is significantly different from the one before 1980s, then all the population may be prone to the new virus.

What is the incubation period of smallpox?

A.3 (a) The incubation period of smallpox is 8-17 days.

What is the route of transmission of small pox?

A.3 (b) The disease spreads by *respiratory route.*

Outline the pathogenesis of small pox.

A.3 (c) Virus enters humans by inhalation into the respiratory tract

↓

Local multiplication in lymphoid tissue

↓

Enters blood and multiplies (primary viraemia)

↓

Reaches systemic organs and multiplication

↓

Re-enters blood and multiplication (secondary viraemia)

↓

Reaches skin and causes classical lesions

One of the striking feature in the pathogenesis of the smallpox, is that the virus enters the body through respiratory tract, follows a long path, before finally causing lesions on the skin (entry point is not skin). The incubation period on an average is 12 days with a prodromal period of 2-4 days during, which the virus can be isolated from the blood.

What were the factors that made it possible for the smallpox to be eradicated from the world?

A.4 The factors include

(i) no known animal reservoir
(ii) existence of only single serotype
(iii) No subclinical infections or carriers
(iv) Transmission of the disease is low with a long incubation period
(v) Disease identification easy
(vi) Availability of potent vaccine, which provides lifelong immunity
(vii) Aggressive surveillance and containment measures
(viii) International coordination

Mention briefly about the origin of the Vaccinia virus.

A.5 (a) Little is known about the origins of this virus. It has probably evolved from the cowpox. This virus has no natural host of itself. It causes localized skin infection, when introduced into hosts of broad range.

Describe vaccinia virus.

A.5 (b) The basic structure of the Vaccinia virus is *similar* to that of Variola virus (Figs. 12.4.1 and 12.4.2). The dumbbell shaped core contains the viral DNA. On either side of the concavities of the core are two *lateral bodies* of unknown nature. Outer to it, is a double layered *membrane* (consists of irregularly arranged tubules visible on surface view). Outermost some virions are seen to have an *envelope*, which originates from altered Golgi membranes. Little is known about the origins of the Vaccinia virus. It has possibly evolved from cowpox. It was Edward Jenner in 1798, who first observed that pustular material from the lesions of cowpox, when inoculated into humans protected them from small pox. The Vaccinia virus has no natural host of itself. It causes *vaccinia*, which is a localized skin infection, when introduced into hosts of broad range. It caused numerous complications, when it was used as a smallpox vaccine ranging from generalized vaccinia to central nervous system complications; as encephalitis. It plays an important role in development of recombinant vaccines.

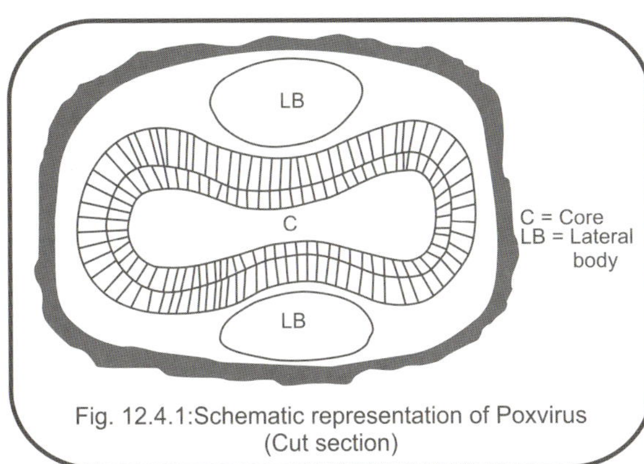

Fig. 12.4.1:Schematic representation of Poxvirus (Cut section)

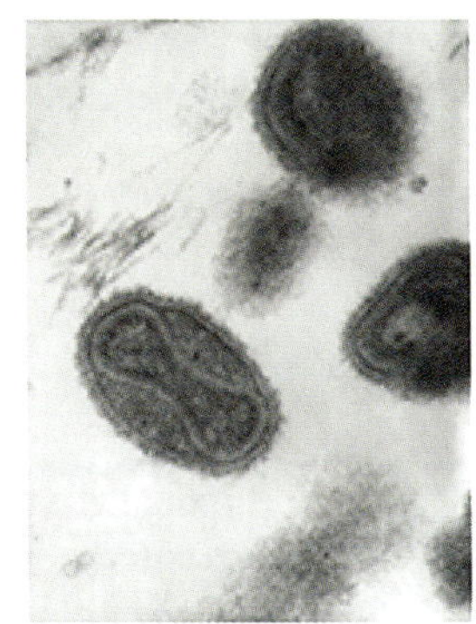

Fig.12.4.2: SMALL POX VIRION: Transmission electron micrograph(TEM) depicting "dumbbell shaped' structure of smallpox virion(370,000X)

Courtesy: Dr. Fred Murphy: Sylvia Whitfield/CDC

Outline the laboratory diagnosis of small pox.

A.6 Since the eradication of the small pox in 1977 from the world, the laboratory diagnosis of it is more of an academic interest. However, one should be prepared to diagnose it, should variola virus be used any time in the future as a biological warfare agent or the disease reappears in a modified form.

The outline of the laboratory diagnosis is depicted at pg. 432. Chapter 10. This virus can be easily grown on chorioallantoic membrane of chick embryo, producing typical *pocks* (Figure 11.1.6a, 11.1.6b, pg. 375). The pocks produced by variola are small, shiny, white, convex, non-necrotic and non-haemorrhagic in contrast to larger, flat, greyish, irregular and haemorrhagic lesions, produced by the vaccinia virus. The phenomenon of *'ceiling temperature'* also aids in the differentiating the various poxviruses. It is defined as the highest temperature, above which the pocks are not produced. The ceiling temperature for Vaccinia is 41°C and for Variola major is 38.5°C.

Mention about the composition of smallpox vaccine, its side effects and the contraindications.

A.7 In 1798 Edward Jenner observed that pustular lesions of cowpox, when inoculated into humans protected them from smallpox. The currently available smallpox vaccine is a live form of Vaccinia virus, which can result in adverse effects; as eczema vaccinatum,generalized vaccinia and rarely post vaccinial encephalitis. Details see pg. 633, Section 17.

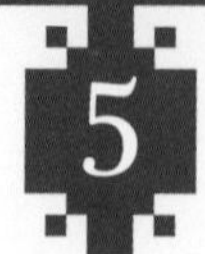

Integrated Clinical Based Study of HHV-2/Genital Lesion

A 24 year old woman, Savita presented with painful genital lesions, which were preceded 3 days back with fever and myalgias. Pelvic examination revealed a few vesicular and ulcerative lesions on the right labia majora.

Linkages: Pg. 368, 397, 431

What is the differential diagnosis of the case?

A.1 The genital infection in her could be due to viruses; as human herpes virus 2 and bacterial agents, as *C. trachomatis, N. gonorrhoeae* and *T. pallidum.*

So; specimens may be taken for culturing the viruses and the bacterial agents.

What is the most likely diagnosis of this case?

A.2 (a) As the lesions are vesicular, the most likely diagnosis is genital herpes, caused by Human herpes virus 2 (Human Herpes simplex virus 2)

Enumerate the diseases caused by HHV-1and HHV-2. Mention their clinical features.

A.2 (b) One must realize that primary HHV infections may often be inapparent. HHV-1 and 2 have been isolated from all mucocutaneous and visceral sites. The incubation period ranges from 1 to 26 days (median 6-8 days). The clinical profile and course of HHV infection depends on the age, anatomical site involved, immunity status of the host and the antigenic type of the virus. The diseases caused by HHV 1 and 2 are depicted at pg. 397. Broadly HHV-1 causes lesions above the waist, whilst HHV-2 causes lesions below the waist.

Immunocompromised cases may present; as disseminated herpes, where the gastrointestinal and respiratory system are commonly involved presenting; as esophagitis, hepatitis, tracheobronchitis or pneumonia.

What test can help to make the microbiological diagnosis?

A.2 (c) A Tzanck preparation can be prepared from the edge of the lesion and (Fig. 12.5.1) giemsa stained. It could demonstrate characteristic pathological changes; including presence of multinucleate giant cells and Cowdry type A intranuclear inclusion bodies.

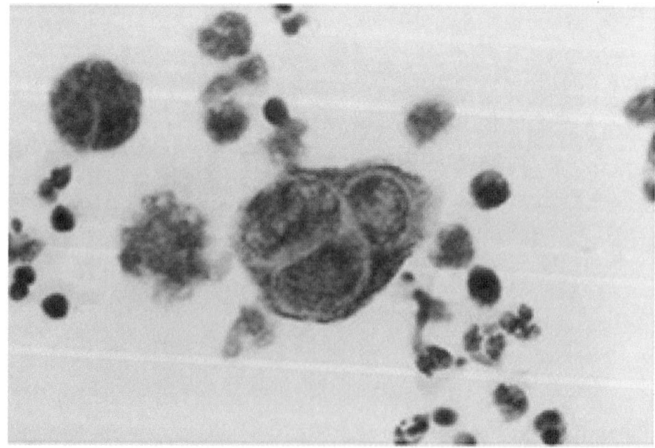

Fig.12.5.1: Tzanck Test: Photomicrograph depicting multinucleated giant cell (Tzanck cell) in a penile ulcer of a case of herpes progenitalis

Courtesy: Centers for Disease Control, Atlanta, USA

Classify Herpes viruses based on their biological properties.

A.3 (a) Classification of Herpes viruses based on biological properties

Sub gamily	Growth cycle	Cytopathology	Primary target cell	Site of latency	Official name	Common name
Alpha herpes virinae	Short (i.e., replicate fast (12-18 hr)	Cytolytic	Mucoepithelial cell	Neuron	Human herpes virus-1	Herpes simplex virus type 1
			Mucoepithelial cell	Neuron	Human herpes virus-2	Herpes simplex virus type 2
			Mucoepithelial cell	Neuron	Human herpes virus-3	Varicella zoster virus
Beta herpes virinae	Long (i.e., replicate slowly > 24 hours)	Cytomegalic	Monocyte, lymphocyte and epithelial cell	Glands, kidney (Fig. 12.5.2)	Human herpes virus-5	Cytomegalovirus
		Lymphotropic	Lymphocytes, Epithelial cell	Lymph node	Human herpes virus-6	Human β-lymphotropic virus
			Lymphocytes	T cell	Human herpes virus-7	RK virus
Gamma herpes virinae	Variable	Lymphoproliferative	B cells	Lymphoid tissue	Human herpes virus-4	Epstein Barr virus
			Epithelial cells, Endothelial cells	Vascular endothelium	Human herpes virus-8	Kaposi sarcoma associated virus (Fig. 12.5.3)

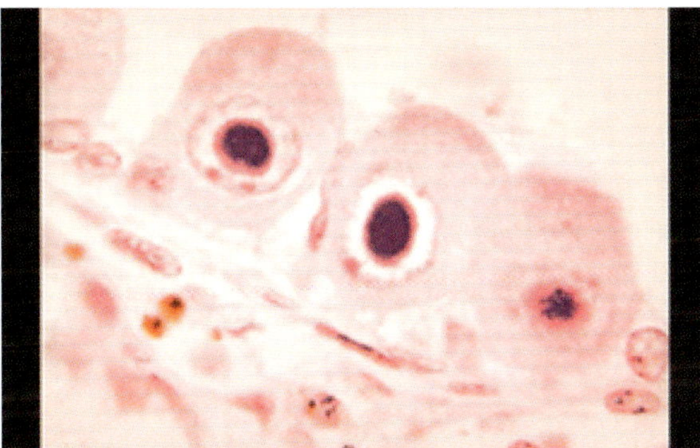

Fig.12.5.2: Cytomegalovirus: Photomicrograph depicting histopathologic changes in kidney infected with CMV

Courtesy: Dr Harasgh/CDC

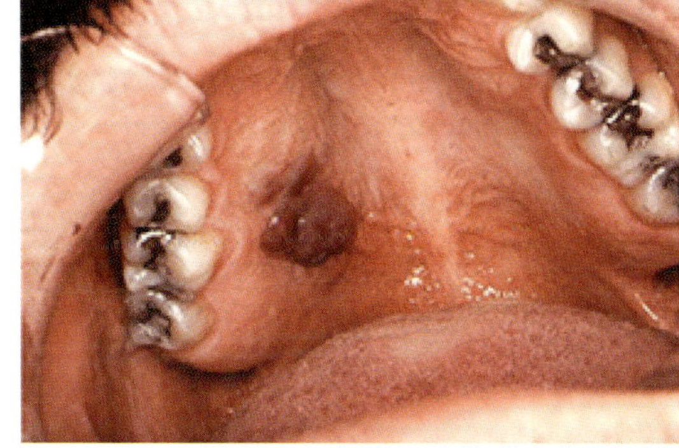

Fig.12.5.3: Kaposi's Sarcoma:HIV patient presented intraoral Kaposi`s sarcoma of the hard palate(secondary to the AIDS infection)

Courtesy: Sol Silverman/CDC

Comment on latency, reactivation, and explantation with reference to herpes viruses.

A.3 (b) Latency

HSV infection of some neuronal cells is unique, in that it does not result in their death. Instead; viral genome is maintained by the cell in a repressed state, which is compatible with the normal activities of the cell. How normal transcription of viral DNA is blocked is unknown? Perhaps low level or sporadic transcription of immediate and early genes occur, is not enough to initiate viral replication. This state is called latency.

Reactivation

It is the process of activation of viral genome, which is earlier in a state of latency and can result in replication of the virus. This process in some cases can result in re-development of herpetic lesions.

Explantation

The process of maintenance and growth of infected neuronal cells, when can result in production of infectious virions.

What are the general characteristics of Herpes virus infections?

A.3 (c) (i) Herpesviruses are DNA virus, enveloped with icosahedral symmetry and sized 150-250 nm. A space exists between the envelope and the capsid, which is called *tegument*.

(ii) The envelope is formed from the nuclear membrane. The nucleic acid replicates in the nucleus and characteristic *Cowdry type A* intranuclear inclusion bodies are present in all the infected cells.

(iii) Infections are life long

(iv) Many of the herpes virus infections are *associated* with malignancies.

(v) Many of the herpes virus infections are *amenable* to antiviral drugs.

Describe the structure of herpes viruses 1 and 2.

A.3 (d) An outline of the structure of herpes viruses is given in table 11.1.4 (pg. 368). The herpes virion has a complicated structure. The diameter of the herpes virus capsid is 100nm but because of the presence of additional layer of tegument and envelope, the complete virus is a large particle, varying in diameter from 150-250 nm.

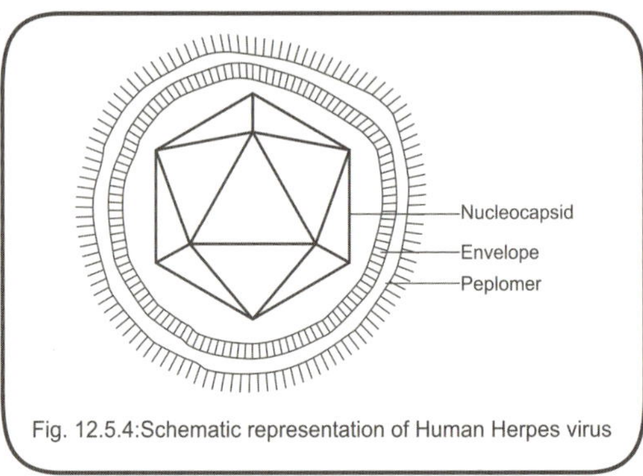

Fig. 12.5.4:Schematic representation of Human Herpes virus

The outermost element of the herpes virus is the *envelope*, which is derived from the portions of the nuclear and cytoplasmic membrane, that are acquired, as the developing particle traverses the nucleus into the cytoplasm and finally exiting the cell. The envelope glycoproteins exhibit a number of biologic properties; enumerating the function of which, is beyond the level of this course. Inner to it is the *tegument*, which is a space between the envelope and *capsid* and is comprised of various viral-encoded proteins, whose functions are yet to be elucidated. Moving inwards we have the nucleocapsid with icosahedron symmetry and consisting of 162 capsomeres (Fig. 12.5.4). The innermost layer is named the internal core and consists of the viral genome and proteins. Here the viral DNA is wound around the protein core.The nucleic acid replicates in the nucleus and characteristic Cowdry type A intranuclear inclusion bodies are present in all the infected cells.

Enumerate the structural differences between HHV-1 and 2 (including the clinical profle).

A.3 (e)

Table 12.5.1: Differences between HHV-1 and HHV-2

	HHV-1	**HHV-2**
Pock size on CAM	Small	Large
Temperature sensitivity (40°C)	-	+
Replication in chick embryo culture	Poor (plaques not produced)	Good (plaques produced)
Neurovirulence in mice	Less (less neurotropic)	More (more neurotropic)
Serological response	Specific antibodies to gG1 (glycoprotein G of HHV-1)	Specific antibodies to gG2 (glycoprotein G of HHV-2)
Restriction endonuclease analysis of viral DNA	Unique	Unique
Transmission	Primarily non-genital	Primarily genital
Urogenital infections	20% (approx)	80%
Non-genital infections	80% (approx)	20% (approx)
Neonatal infection	30%	70%

Serologic assays can distinguish reliably between antibody responses to HHV-1 and HHV-2; as by the assays mentioned above. Viral isolates can be most definitely be differentiated, by restriction endonuclease patterns of viral DNA.

What is the likely mechanism of this virus causing lifelong latent infections?

A.4 The exact mechanism for the genome of this virus to be repressed is not known. Probably low level or sporadic transcription of the early genes of this virus occurs, which may not be enough to initiate disease. Human herpes virus 1 infection of the neuron is unique, as no lysis of the cell occurs, despite replication.

The woman developed disorientation and mild neck rigidity, after four days of her initial consultation. A lumbar puncture was done, which revealed a leucocyte count of 120/microlitre with 82% mononuclear cells and 18% polymorphs.

What complication has she developed?

A.5 (a) The woman has likely developed a self limiting, aseptic meningitis, which can develop in approximately 33% of women having primary genital herpes. The human herpes virus 2 can be isolated from the CSF of this woman, if it is cultured.

Describe the pathogenesis of HHV-1 and 2 infections.

A.5 (b) Herpes viruses are fragile and survive for a limited period in the environment. As such *intimate contact* is required for their transmission. It is because of the prolonged intimate contact between mother and the baby during pregnancy and delivery, that herpes viruses are often associated with congenital and neonatal infections; for instance neonatal herpes and cytomegalovirus infections. Herpes viruses do not penetrate keratinized skin efficiently. These viruses induce disease primarily by direct destruction of tissue, by initiating immunopathologic response and/or by facilitating neoplastic transformation. Most herpes virus infections can be diagnosed clinically, but there exist several conditions, in which specific tests are necessary.

As mentioned previously, man is the only natural reservoir and intimate contact with infected secretions is the principal mode of spread. HHV-1 is transmitted primarily by contact with oral secretions, while HHV-2 is by contact with genital secretions. The primary infection occurs through damaged skin, oral/ urogenital mucosa or eyes. The neonate can get infection during passage through infected birth canal.

It is very important to distinguish between primary and recurrent herpetic infections. In *primary* infections, the HHV enters into the primary sites and replicates at the local site; for instance cells of epidermis and dermis in the skin sites. This results in the lysis of the local infected cells and initiation of a local inflammatory response. This leads to a series of events, which lead to the characteristic HHV lesions, which is a thin walled vesicle on an inflammatory base. Microscopically, the lesion is characterized by multinucleate giant cells with ballooning degeneration, oedema and characteristic Cowdry type A intranuclear inclusion bodies *(Tzanck cell)*. This picture is indistinguishable from a lesion caused by HHV-3 (Varicella zoster virus).

The *recurrent* infection is initiated by the intra-axonal transport of the virion from the nerve endings in the primary site to the nerve cell bodies in the ganglia. This is the site, where the viruses can enter a state of *latency*. The neuron appears to be a unique cell in that production of infectious virions (when produced) do not lyse the neuron.

The centrifugal migration of the infectious virions via peripheral (sensory) nerve from the ganglia to the skin/ mucosa explain, why large areas; which are distant from the original lesion may be involved in the recurrent infections. There are number of theories to explain the HHV latency and reactivation, but none are proven.

Antibodies to HHV-1 appear in early childhood and by adolescent in all. Antibodies to HHV-2 appear during adolescence with the initiation of the sexual activity. Cell mediated responses to HHV antigen are protective; as immunocompromised patient with CMI defects experience more severe and extensive herpetic lesions than those with defects in humoral immunity.

Describe the epidemiology of HHV-1 and 2 infections.

A.6 (a) HHV-1 and 2 infection occur *worldwide* and throughout *the year*. Transmission can occur both from overtly infected patients and from persons without clinical manifestation of infection, who are shedding HHV-1 and 2. Spread of HHV-1 infection from oral secretion to other skin areas is a hazard of certain professionals; as dentists and respiratory care unit personnel. Some studies have found frequency of HHV-2 antibodies amongst population to vary from approximately 3 percent in nuns to 70 percent in prostitutes. This is understandable, as shedding of HHV-2 is related to sexual activity. Studies using the PCR have shown that HHV reactivation on mucosal surface is more frequent than previously realized.

Compare and contrast the epidemiology of human herpes virus 1 (Herpes simplex virus type 1) and human herpes virus 2 (Herpes simplex virus type 2) infections.

A.6 (b) **Table 12.5.2:** Comparison of the epidemiology of HHV-1 and HHV-2

HHV-1	HHV-2
• Primarily an infection of the oropharyngeal mucosa	• Primarily an infection of the genital mucosa
• Transmitted primarily *by saliva*	• Transmitted primarily *by sexual contact*
• Latent infection occurs in the trigeminal ganglion	• Latent infection occurs in the lumbar and sacral ganglia
• Infections occur *primarily* on the face (although can cause genital infections)	• Infections occur *primarily* in the genital area (although can cause lesions on the face)
• Infections typically acquired in *childhood*	• Infections typically acquired, *after* individual becomes sexually active
• Both associated with central nervous system infections.	

If this clinical presentation had occurred to this woman, while she was in 3rd trimester of pregnancy, at what risk was her fetus susceptible to?

A.7 (a) The fetus was at risk of for developing neonatal herpes.

How can this complication be minimized to the fetus?

A.7 (b) Conducting the delivery of the baby by caesarian section (and not by normal vaginal delivery) can minimize the transmission of this disease.

What is the role of the condom usage in prevention of the HHV-2 transmission?

A.7 (c) Barrier form of contraception; as condoms can help to decrease the HHV-2 transmission.

Descibe laboratory diagnosis of HHV-1 and 2 infections.

A.8 Most herpetic virus infections can be diagnosed *clinically,* by the characteristic multiple vesicular lesions on an erythematous base. However, there are several situations, in which specific tests are necessary. For instance, in a case of suspected genital herpes, confirmatory test would exclude other similar diseases, allay anxiety, help behaviour modification and identify drug-resistant herpes viruses. Another instance, where laboratory diagnosis is crucial, is the management is a case of suspected herpetic encephalitis. Prognosis of an encephalitis case is usually poor, but if a herpetic encephalitis case is diagnosed early, antiviral administration results in excellent prognosis. In pregnant woman having suspected genital herpes, specific diagnosis is critical, as further course of management depends on diagnosis, as caesarian, section can prevent spread of genital herpes infection to infant.

An outline of the herpes virus infections is depicted at pg. 431, Chapter 10.

The *clinical specimens* to be taken would depend on the type of clinical disease presented. A genital herpes case may require the vesicle fluid to be aspirated. A smear could be made from the base of the vesicle, by scraping and staining with toluidine blue. It would reveal *Tzanck cells*, whose pathologic picture has already been discussed. The suggestive findings can be confirmed by antigen detection, E/M, molecular biology or viral culture studies. Spin amplified culture/ shell vial techniques have recently emerged.

A suspected case of herpes encephalitis could have its CSF, serum and brain biopsy (if possible) samples processed. HHV DNA PCR of CSF is being increasingly used and is more sensitive than viral culture. Direct immunofluorescence test of brain tissue is a reliable test.

Diagnosis of *neonatal infection* can be made sometimes, by demonstrating IgM HHV antibodies in the neonate. Measurement of IgM antibodies in children and adult may be helpful in diagnosing primary HHV infection but not of much value in recurrent infections. The serological methods are also useful for determination of disease susceptibility and potential for viral reactivation.

Which antiviral drugs can be administered to this woman (with HHV-2 infection)?

A.9 (a) Acyclovir can be administered. Currently the new antiviral drugs available are idoxuridine, famciclovir and valcyclovir.

What is the efficacy of these drugs?

A.9 (b) These drugs are quite efficacious. If these drugs are administered early in a case of meningitis due to human herpes viruses 1 and 2, the morbidity and mortality due to these agents is significantly reduced.

Has drug resistance been reported to these drugs?

A.9 (c) Yes. Human herpes virus 1 and 2 have been shown to have resistance to Acyclovir. Cross resistance to other drugs; as Famciclovir and Valacyclovir has also been reported.

Aspect related to case theme/examination assessment

Describe Herpesvirus simiae (Herpes B virus).

A.10 It is the simian (monkey) *counterpart* of HHV (HSV). It is named after Dr WB. who in 1932 was bitten on his left hand by a rhesus monkey, during studies on poliomyelitis and subsequently died due to ascending myelitis. Till now more than 40 such human infections have occurred and most of these have been fatal. Most of these occurred in the periods, when monkeys were in intense use, in the mid-1950s for polio vaccine development and in the 1980s for HIV studies. Human cases acquire infection, when *handling* infected monkeys and getting scratched or bitten and during the course of working directly with monkey tissue cell lines. The human infection may manifest *initially, as* skin lesions but the individual finally succumbs due to myelitis, encephalitis or concomitant multiorgan involvement. To prevent this infection, all monkeys should be considered infected and should always be handled with extensive arm and face protection.

Integrated Clinical Based Study of HHV-3 (Chicken Pox)/Skin Lesion

A 6 year old school going boy, Ashu presented with vesiculopustular lesions on his entire body. On examination, he was found to be febrile with clear lungs and no enlargement of liver or spleen. His chest radiograph was clear. His blood examination revealed a TLC of 20,800/cu. mm

Linkages: Pg. 368, 397, 432

What is the likely diagnosis in this case?

A.1 (a) The case is likely to have varicella (chicken pox) infection.

What is the differential diagnosis?

A.1 (b) The infectious diseases that could have presented this picture would include; varicella infection, impetigo (group A streptococcal infection), disseminated enteroviral infection and disseminated herpes simplex infection. The non-infectious diseases that could present a similar picture could be drug allergy, contact dermatitis and insect bites. The samples taken usually are vesicle fluid and scraping from base of lesion (also for zoster diagnosis).

How can the diagnosis of chicken pox be confirmed?

A.2 (a) A rapid technique would be to by make a Tzanck preparation with scraping from the base of the lesion; followed by staining the smear with Giemsa stain to demonstrate multinuclear giant cells (Tzanck cells) with intranuclear inclusion bodies. This is a simple technique, but has a low sensitivity of approximately 60%.

Direct fluorescent staining techniques on the smears from scrapings, increases the test sensitivity. Molecular biology tests; as PCR are also available to demonstrate the viral genome. The virus can also be cultured on cell line; as human fibroblasts, in which CPE can be demonstrated after 5-6 days of inoculation; as focal, refractile ballooning. Electron microscopy can reveal the virions and by this technique, they can be differentiated from the poxviruses. Serologic testing is used mainly to assess immunity status in unvaccinated health care workers, who may be exposed to patients with confirmed VZV infections. IgM specific antibodies can be detected by ELISA. A Fluorescent antibody to membrane (FAMA) test is also available, which detects antibody to membrane antigen.

Describe morphological properties of HHV-3.

A.2 (b) The morphological properties of HHV-3 are similar to the other viruses of herpesviridae family. It has a single serotype. Only enveloped virions of it are infectious, which may account for the lability of the virus.

Small pox is now eradicated from the world but the physician should be alert to an outbreak of this disease, due to frequent bioterrorism threats. How is small pox clinically differentiated from chicken pox?

A.3 The clinical differences between the two diseases are depicted in the table 12.6.1.

Table 12.6.1: Comparison of pathogenicity of smallpox and chickenpox

Smallpox	Chickenpox
Incubation: • About 12 days (range: 7-17 days)	• About 15 days (range: 7-21 days)
Prodromal symptoms: Severe	Usually mild
Distribution of rash: • Palms and soles frequently affected • Axilla usually not affected • Rash predominant on extensor surfaces and bony prominences.	• Seldom affected • Axilla affected • Rash mostly on flexor surfaces.

Contd.

Contd.

Characteristics of the rash:	
• Deep-seated	• Superficial
• Vesicles multilocular and umbilicated	• Unilocular
• Only one stage of rash may be seen at one unit time	• Rash pleomorphic, i.e., different stages of the rash evident at one given time, because rash appears in successive crops
• No inflammation is seen around the vesicles.	• Inflammation is seen around the vesicles.
Evolution of rash:	
• Evolution of rash is slow,passing through definite stages of macule, papule, vesicle and pustule. (Fig. 12.6.1)	• Evolution of rash is very rapid
• Scabs begin to form 10-14 days after the rash appears	• Scabs begin to form 4-7 days after the rash appears
Fever:	
• Fever subsides with the appearance of rash	• Temperature rises with each fresh crop of rash.

Human herpes virus 3 (Varicella zoster) virus will become latent in this boy, after the current infection episode is over, Can the virus get reactivated; when he grows up as an adult? What disease it causes then?

A.4 (a) Yes. Herpes zoster.

Describe the clinical presentation of this reactivation (Herpes zoster) infection.

A.4 (b) The herpes zoster (shingle) results from reactivation of the HHV-3 virus, which remains dominant in the dorsal root ganglia. The virus gets transported along the peripheral nerve to the skin, where it causes the lesions. The lesions involve unilateral dermatomes; usually T3 – L3. The lesions are classically vesicular. All age groups can have this disease but mainly the elderly get this disease.

How was it established that Chicken pox and zoster were caused by the same etiological agent?

A.4 (c) HHV-3 or varicella zoster causes two distinct clinical diseases, namely varicella (or more commonly called chicken pox) and herpes zoster (shingles). Since early twentieth century, similarities in epidemiologic and immunopathologic findings in chicken pox and shingles, suggested that varicella and herpes zoster were caused by the same etiological agent. It was isolation of the varicella zoster virus in 1958 and further molecular level work of the viral isolates, from the diverse lesions, that concluded the above hypothesis.

Can contact with chicken pox lead to herpes zoster?

A.4 (d) Varicella (chicken pox) is the primary infection with the virus in a susceptible individual (non-immune) while Herpes zoster is result the reactivation (recurrence) of the virus in the same individual, when its immunity has fallen. Thus contact with a zoster case may lead to chicken pox but contact with chicken pox won't lead to herpes zoster.

Describe the pathogenesis, epidemiology and clinical picture of herpes zoster.

A.4 (e) The mechanism that results in reactivation of HHV-3, leading to herpes zoster is unknown. Probably a fall in the immunity of the individual, which could be triggered due to different reasons, could activate the HHV-3 virus, which infected the dorsal root ganglia during chicken pox infection. The virus starts proliferating and starts descending down from nerves (centrifugally) to the skin, to cause the typical lesion. Histopathologically, lesions of both zoster and varicella are similar, being characterized by ballooning, degeneration, giant cell formation and intranuclear inclusion formation. The mechanisms by which the virus remains latent in the dorsal root ganglion and how it gets activated is a mystery.

Epidemiology

It involves the elderly with the highest incidence in individuals of the sixth decade and beyond. However, it can occur at any age including the newborn!*. Even an attack of herpes zoster fails to eliminate the HHV-3 virus from the dorsal root ganglion, this explain the 4% second attack of herpes zoster in these patients.

*The fetus could have had the chickenpox during pregnancy and reactivation in the first few months; as herpes zoster.

Clinical presentation

The incubation period of herpes zoster is difficult to determine. If the infection of the dorsal root ganglion is taken as the reference point, the virus after activation may take days to years to cause the classical disease.

The disease is characterized by unilateral vesicular eruption with a dermatomal distribution, often associated with severe pain (Fig. 12.6.2). The dermatomes usually involved are from T3 to L3. Like chicken pox, herpes zoster in immunocompromised

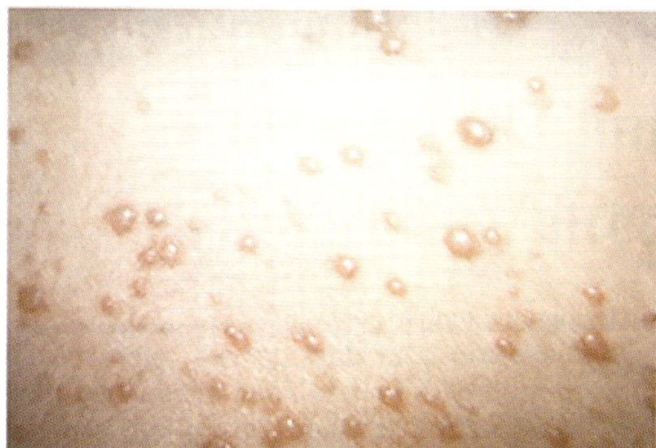

Fig.12.6.1: Varicella –Zoster Virus: Pustulovesicular rash due to VZV(HHV-3)
Courtesy: Joe Miller/CDC

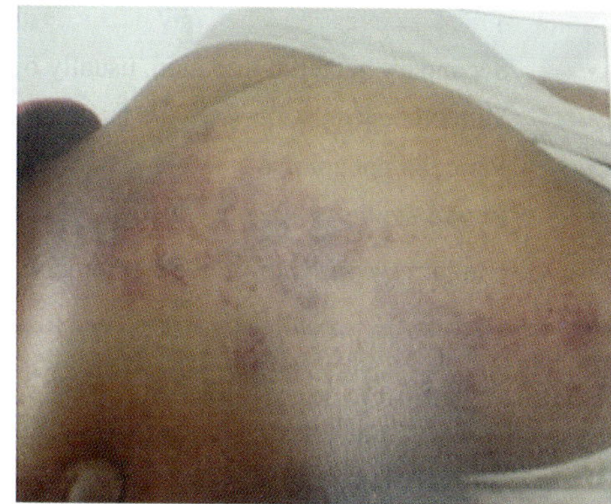

Fig.12.6.2: Herpes zoster-multi dermatomal Herpes zoster

HIV patients is more severe than normal population. The lesions may include hepatitis, pneumonitis, meningoencephalitis and other severe complications. Keratitis may be followed by severe iridocyclitis, or secondary glaucoma. So ophthalmologic consultation is requested in suspected in herpes zoster opthalmicus.

The complications of herpes zoster in normal individuals include:

- Herpes zoster opthalmicus [when 1st or 2nd branch of trigeminal nerve (fifth) involved]
- Ramsay Hunt syndrome (when geniculate ganglion involved presents; as pain and vesicles in external auditory meatus, loss of taste in anterior 2/3 tongue plus ipsilateral facial palsy)
- Transverse myelitis, Guillain Barré syndrome
- Lower motor neuron paralysis (occur as consequence of involvement of anterior horn cells of spinal cord; as involved in polio)

Describe the epidemiology of chickenpox?

A.5 (a) This disease is worldwide in distribution, being more common in temperate regions, where epidemic occurs in late winter and spring time. The disease is spread by the respiratory route. The disease is highly contagious with an attack rate of at least 90% amongst susceptible (seronegative). The incubation period is between 10-21 days. It is estimated that more than 90% of children in temperate regions get infected, by the time they become 10 years old.

Describe the pathogenesis of chicken pox.

A.5 (b) The disease is transmitted by the respiratory route (not by the cutaneous route). The transmission mode resembles that of small pox and is unlike the HHV 1 and 2 viruses. The entry of the virus into the respiratory tract is followed by the localized replication of the virus at undefined sites (likely in nasopharynx/upper respiratory tract, as PCR studies of this site have shown). This leads to the seeding of the reticuloendothelial system; resulting in viremia, which transports the virus to the skin, causing typical lesions. Simultaneously the dorsal root ganglia gets infected with the virus remaining in a latent state. Immunocompromised individuals may have visceral dissemination and severe disease.

Varicella virus is ubiquitous and it causes an extremely contagious disease. It occurs seasonally and in epidemic form. One attack leads to life long immunity. However; second attack may present; as subclinical and mild clinical form in immunocompromised individuals. Man is the only known reservoir of this virus. Chickenpox is a common infection of the childhood, although also seen in adults and involves both sexes. Intimate contact is the key determinant in the transmission of the disease. Secondary attack rates in susceptible siblings within a household range between 70 and 90 percent. Patients are infectious for a period of approximately 2 days before the vesicle formation and usually 4-5 days thereafter, until all lesions are crusted.

Describe the clinical profile of chicken pox.

A.5 (c) It is a benign illness, characterized by a generalized exanthematous rash. The clinical picture in contrast to the small pox; has been mentioned in table 12.6.1. The incubation period ranges between 10 to 21 days but is usually between 14-17 days. The longer incubation period in comparison to the primary HHV 1 and 2 lesions is understandable, as in the latter the infection is initiated by direct inoculation of the virus onto the affected site.

The rash which appears is usually a benign illness, progresses through macule, papule, vesicle, pustule and rash. It usually heals without complications. The successive crops appear over a short period of 2-4 days, which may explain the observation of seeing different stages of the rash on a patient. However, varicella is dangerous disease in immunocompromised neonates and children, as disease may become disseminated.

through the blood to infect the B lymphocytes, where the proliferation of EBV infected B cells along with reactive T cells, results in enlargement of lymphoid tissue. This produces immunopathological changes including diverse antibodies, which results in the syndrome of infectious mononucleosis. B lymphocyte remains the site, where EBV remains in latent state, probably for life.

What is the difference in symptomatology, when the EBV is contracted in childhood in contrast to being contracted in adolescence period?

A.5 Infections of HHV-4 (FBV) contracted in childhood are usually asymptomatic, whereas the infections acquired in adolescent period usually result in infectious mononucleosis.

Describe the clinical picture of EBV infection.

A.6 EBV produces a broad spectrum of illness ranging from asymptomatic state to classical heterophile positive infectious mononucleosis (glandular fever, kissing disease) syndrome with or without complications.

Most EBV infections in infants and children are asymptomatic or present; as mild pharyngitis with or without tonsillitis. In contrast the adults, have classic syndrome in greater majority of cases up to 75%. Complications in this syndrome are rare. Death occurs very rarely and could result due to splenic rupture, neurologic complications (as transverse myelitis or Guillain-Barré syndrome) or upper airway obstruction (hypertrophy of tonsils/adenoids with oedema of epiglottis/pharynx). Some studies have associated EBV with chronic fatigue syndrome.

The malignant diseases associated with this infection include Burkitt's lymphoma, anaplastic nasopharyngeal carcinoma and Hodgkin's disease. The other associated diseases include chronic fatigue syndrome, lymphoproliferative disorders and oral hairy leukoplakia (Fig. 12.7.1). (Disease association implies not a direct causation between the etiological agent and the disease but an increased association between the two)

The association of the virus with Burkitt's lymphoma is strong, which is seen in children of 5-8 years age in Africa; affecting their jaw, orbital cavities and gastrointestinal tract.

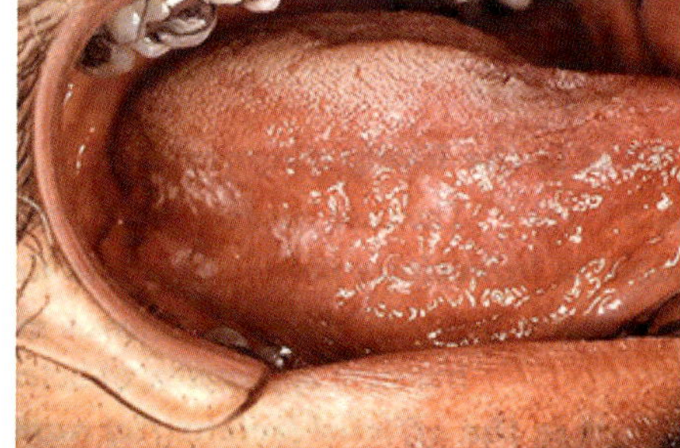

12.7.1: Leukoplakia: Patient with signs of early oral leukoplakia on the lateral border of the tongue

Courtesy: Sol Silver man/CDC

Describe the epidemiology of EBV infections?

A.7 This virus is present in salivary secretion and is believed to be acquired during kissing (kissing disease). A high incidence of this disease occurs in adolescent period. The disease is also transmitted less commonly through blood transfusion. The disease is unlikely to spread by fomites or aerosols; as the virus is labile and has not been isolated from environmental sources.

EBV infections occur worldwide, with no sex predilection. These infections are common in childhood and by adulthood, more than 90% of individuals are seen to be infected; as seen by seroepidemiologic studies. A peak in the incidence of I.M. is seen in adolescent period, which is explainable because of the increased sexual activity during the period. In developing countries, infections may occur at any early age, which may be explained by the lower standards of hygiene. Detailed information on the impact of this disease on the population is not available because this disease is not a reportable disease and in many cases get labeled as non-specific illness.

What is the role of cell culture in the diagnosis of infections mononucleosis (I.M.)?

A.8 (a) This virus can be isolated in cell culture. However; this technique is not utilized in the laboratory diagnosis for three reasons, namely the virus being ubiquitous (as this virus persists in the oropharynx and B cells for life) and the technique is laborious, as it involves a B cell line to cultivate the viruses. Thirdly it is difficult to detect the changes in the infected cells, which are transformed by EBV.

Which class and type of antibodies would be desirable to be demonstrated to make a diagnosis of acute infectious mononucleosis?

A.8 (b) Demonstration of IgM antibodies to viral capsid antigen (IgM-anti VCA) would be desirable to make a serological diagnosis for an acute episode of this infection.

Describe the laboratory diagnosis of Infectious mononucleosis (including the Paul Bunnel test).

A.8 (c) The laboratory diagnosis of infectious mononucleosis is essentially serologic as is evident from outline at pg. 432, Chapter 10. The initial blood picture is one of the leucopenia and later of leucocytosis. Atypical lymphocytes are the hematologic hallmark in the infection. Its range varies tremendously and may vary between 30-90% of the total lymphocyte count.

The only molecular biology technique that is available for this infection, is nucleic acid hybridization. It can demonstrate the virus particles in lymphoid tissue and blood.

The tests most often used in the diagnosis are serologic. One of the earliest test to be performed was the **Paul Bunnel test (classic heterophile test).** A commercial test called the '*monospot test*' with the same principle is also available, which has greater sensitivity than the classic test.

Principle (Paul Bunnel test)

This test is based on the presence of heterophile antibodies in the patients of IM. These antibodies were originally described by Paul and Bunnel, hence the name of this test. These antibodies appear in the serum against the EBV, but can also agglutinate (act against) the sheep RBCs. Such antibodies are however not specific, as these can also be seen in sera of normal uninfected individuals and in individuals who are exposed to serum; as in serum therapy. Infectious mononucleosis antibody can be differentiated from above categories, by agglutinin absorption tests. Infectious mononucleosis antibody has the characteristic of being absorbed by Ox RBCs but not by guinea pig kidney.

Procedure

The serum to be tested is inactivated, by heating the serum in a water bath at 56°C for 30 minutes. Doubling dilution of this serum is prepared in test tubes and equal volume of 1% sheep RBCs is added to all dilutions. The test tubes are incubated at 37°C for 4 hours. The tubes are observed for agglutination and a titer of 100 and above is suggestive of infectious mononucleosis.

To confirm the identity of the antibody, agglutinin absorption study is done as described above.

Interpretation

- 40% of I.M. cases have the heterophile antibodies in 1st week of infection.
- 80-90% of I.M. cases have the heterophile antibodies in the 3rd week of infection.
- Correlation of test with EBV specific serologic tests has a high correlation.

Limitation of test:

- Heterophile antibodies are not usually present in children
- Low positivity of the test in 1st week of infection

Epstein-Barr specific antibodies

Antibodies against number of EBV targets are detectable in patients; especially by ELISA. Two types of antibodies are of significance. One is the IgM anti-VCA (viral capsid antigen) antibodies, which are usually present at time of clinical presentation and persist for about 4-8 weeks. These antibodies have a good sensitivity and specificity. In contrast to this, the EBNA (Epstein-Barr nuclear antigen) antibodies indicate past infection, as these appear 3-4 weeks after clinical onset and persist lifelong.

D/D

- Heterophile negative I.M. (as by CMV)
- Viral hepatitis
- Acute toxoplasmosis, Streptococcal sore throat
- Primary HIV-1 infection

Does one attack of infectious mononucleosis, offer immunity to further attacks?

A.9 HHV-4 induced infectious mononucleosis can be contracted only once in a life time. It is not clear whether the protection is due to humoral and/or cellular immunity.

Are specific antiviral drugs available for this group of herpes virus infection; as are available for many other herpes viral infections?

A.10 (a) No, specific antiviral drugs are not available against this viral infection.

What advice would you give to this young cricketer?

A.10 (b) Since the case is professionally involved in a sporting activity, he should reduce the physical activity to minimize the complication of splenic rupture.

Outline the preventive aspects of this disease.

A.11 Isolation of patients with I.M. is unnecessary, as the transmission requires intimate contact

- Blood donation from I.M. patients may be delayed for some months, as virocytemia is demonstrable for several months after recovery.
- No vaccines available. Those under consideration must be carefully evaluated for potential oncogenicity, due to the nature of EBV.

Integrated Clinical Based Study of HHV-5 (CMV)/Pneumonitis

A 40 year old female, Bindu had an kidney transplant 5 months back. At the time of transplant, she was seronegative for HHV-5 (CMV), HIV, Hepatitis B and hepatitis C. Her kidney donor was CMV seropositive and negative for HBV, HCV and HIV serology. One week back, she got hospitalized on account of fever, fatigue and breathlessness. Her chest radiograph revealed diffuse infiltrates. A bronchoscopy was performed and bronchoalveolar lavage specimens were sent for bacterial, fungal, viral, mycobacterial cultures and transbronchial biopsy was sent for histopathologic and cytologic examination. The gram staining of the biopy specimen did not reveal any significant finding. All cultures did not yield any significant finding. The hematoxylin and eosin stain of the lung tissue revealed cytomegalic cells with characteristic 'owl eye' appearance.

Linkages: Pg. 368, 397, 432

What is the likely clinical diagnosis in this case?

A.1 (a) The case is likely to have HHV-5 (CMV) pneumonitis.

Comment on the derivation of the term 'Cytomegalovirus'.

A.1 (b) The term 'cytomegalovirus' was coined by Weller and colleagues to replace cytomegalic inclusion disease virus. The name 'cytomegalovirus' indicates the enlarged cytoplasm, the cells infected with the HHV-5 acquire (Fig. 12.5.3 at pg. 409). However, the inclusion bodies are present not only in the cytoplasm but also in the nucleus of the infected cell. HHV-5 cause a large number of disease syndromes in children and adults. Fitting in the theme of affairs! CMV has the largest genome amongst the herpes viruses, with viral particle about 150-200 nm (diameter).

Human CMV was first isolated by Smith, Rowe, Weller and colleagues in 1956. Virus replication is associated with production of enlarged cells (two to four times the surrounding cell), which have large intranuclear and smaller cytoplasmic inclusion. Clear halo around the intranuclear inclusion produce the 'owl's eye' appearance.

What is the likely mode of acquiring the infection in this case?

A.2 (a) This case is likely to have acquired this infection from the transplanted kidney. The CMV infected kidney could be the source of the infection.

Could this infection have been prevented (in the case under discussion)?

A.2 (b) This infection would have been prevented, had the selected donor been CMV seronegative.

Why it could not be prevented?

A.2 (c) It is not possible to always have organ donations from seronegative individuals; as the percentage of CMV positivity in the general population is high and there is shortage of organ donors.

What is the commonest clinical presentation of CMV disease in immunocompetent host?

A.3 (a) CMV mononucleosis.

What is the mode of acquiring CMV infection?

A.3 (b) This infection is acquired from exposure of secretions; as saliva, semen, urine and cervical from cases, who are HHV-5 (CMV) infected.

Describe the clinical profile of CMV infection (with special reference to various age categories).

A.3 (c) HHV-5 causes a wide spectrum of syndromes in infants, children and adults ranging from asymptomatic subclinical infection, fulminant congenital cytomegalic inclusion disease in infants, infectious mononucleosis syndrome in immunocompetent individuals to disseminated disease in immunocompromised patients. However, majority of the infected population; whether neonate, infant, children or adults remain asymptomatic. The reason for this phenomenon is not clear, though immunosuppression has been suggested to explain the causation of disease. But, this aspect does not explain everything; as many immunocompetent individuals present with the mononucleosis syndrome and many perinatal and congenital infections present asymptomatically initially, though some of them may present in later life with disabilities.

The various CMV syndromes, seen in the different age groups is depicted in table 12.8.1.

Table 12.8.1: Profile of CMV infections

	Mode of transmission	**Presentation**
Group		
Fetus	Transplacental/congenital	Congenital cytomegalic inclusion disease (CID)
Neonate	• During delivery • Breast milk feeding	Perinatal CMV infection (manifesting variedly; as hearing loss etc)
Children/adults	• Exposure to secretions as saliva, urine, semen, cervical secretions • Post-perfusion syndrome (repeated blood transfusion) • Post-transplantation (as kidney, bone marrow transplant) • Immunosuppression (following HIV or drugs)	CMV mononucleosis -do- Hepatitis, Interstitial pneumonitis, Meningioencephalitis Retinitis, colitis and others • CMV mononucleosis

As mentioned previously, CMV is a common cause of congenital defects in newborn. The congenital CMV infection may be asymptomatic at birth or present; as classic fulminant congenital cytomegalic inclusion disease (CID). The latter is characterized by jaundice, hepatosplenomegaly, petechial rash and multiple organ involvement (as microcephaly, retinitis and others).

The CMV mononucleosis presents variedly and its incubation period may vary from 20 to 60 days. Clinically, it is difficult to distinguish it from EBV induced mononucleosis. As the name mononucleosis indicates, there is relative and absolute mononucleosis.

Like most other infections, CMV causes severe manifestations in the immunocompromised patients. The patient may present clinically involving one or multiple organ system.

Describe the pathogenesis of CMV infections.

A.3 (d) Infection with CMV is a common event in the population, but the associated disease is a relatively rare event. An individual once infected with the virus carries the CMV for life. So CMV shares with the other herpes viruses, the capacity to remain latent in tissues, after recovery of the host from the disease. The precise sites of the latency of the virus in the body are not known, but the sites are likely to be monocytes, B lymphocytes, epithelial stromal cells of the bone marrow and body organs; as kidney. One should distinguish clearly between primary and secondary CMV infections. The *primary* infection occurs in the seronegative individual, while the *secondary* infection represent the activation of the virus in a seropositive (immune) individual. So a constant threat of CMV disease looms in an infected individual, anytime it becomes immunosuppressed. Most infected individuals remain asymptomatic but shed the virus in the secretions; as saliva and milk, as the virus can replicate in the ductal epithelial cells.

The virus can spread transplacentally in the pregnancy and cause congenital cytomegalic inclusion disease *(CID)*. The virus is a major cause of *congenital abnormalities* in the newborn. It can also transmit perinatally to neonate during the passage of the infant through the birth canal and later by breast feeding (through milk). In young children, the infection can spread by contact with saliva and urine and also by kissing (saliva being the mode). The virus can also be transmitted by sexual intercourse, as the virus is present in the cervix, semen and saliva. Blood transfusion and organ transplantation are other modes of its transmission. In the former, the risk of infection has been suggested to be proportional to the number of units transfused. As expected, immunocompromised individuals including AIDS patients have severe CMV disease. Cell mediated immunity is required for the resolution of the disease.

What is the subfamily to which this CMV belongs?

A.4 Beta herpesvirinae.

What are the challenges in incriminating HHV-5 (CMV), as an etiological agent in a suspected clinical case infected with this agent?

A.5 (a) Unlike HHV-1, HHV-2 and HHV-3, diagnosis of HHV-5 (CMV) infection cannot be made reliably clinically, so the microbiology plays an important role in the diagnosis. However, one must realize that incriminating CMV as an etiological agent even in the presence of clinical symptoms and the isolation of the virus from the sample may be misleading, as the virus is ubiquitous and often excreted subclinically.

Does the demonstration of cytomegalic cells or virus in samples; as urine/saliva from a suspected case of CMV infection be enough to incriminate it to be a cause of acute infection in the case?

A.5 (b) No, as the virus can be excreted from these sites for months to years after illness.

Which category of human population has nearly 100% CMV seropositivity?

A.6 (a) Female prostitutes and sexually active homosexual men.

Is clinical disease rate high in normal human population with high CMV seropositivity?

A.6 (b) No, clinical disease in immunocompetent individuals is rare, despite the population having a high CMV seropositivity.

Mention about epldemiology of CMV infections.

A.6 (c) The virus has a worldwide distribution, as indicated by the seroprevalence antibody studies. The prevalence is higher in developing countries, which have communal living and poor personal hygiene. The infection does not spread by casual contact, but requires prolonged and intimate exposure for transmission. Many body secretions contain the virus, which may lead to transmission of this virus. In developing countries, more than 50% of the population have been seen to be seropositive and 0.5-2% seropositivity is seen in the newborn.

Discuss the role of shell vial assay, in the diagnosis of CMV infection.

A.7 (a) *Shell vial assay* is a more sensitive and rapid technique in contrast to traditional viral culture technique with reference to HHV-5 (CMV) diagnosis. It employs fibroblasts cultivated; as monolayers on glass coverslips. Various clinical samples; as urine, tissues are inoculated onto it and centrifuged. Early CMV antigen expression can be detected on these cells, after 1 to 2 days of incubation, using fluorescent monoclonal antibodies.

Describe the laboratory diagnosis of CMV infections.

A.7 (b) Unlike HHV-1, HHV-2 and HHV-3, diagnosis of HHV-5 (CMV) infection cannot be made reliably clinically, so the microbiology laboratory plays an important role. However, one must realize that incriminating CMV as an etiological agent; even in the presence of clinical symptoms and the isolation of the virus from a sample may be misleading, as the virus is ubiquitous and often excreted subclinically. An outline of the diagnosis is depicted at pg. 432.

One of the earliest laboratory tests to diagnose this infection was the demonstration of cytomegalic cells; which are large, inclusion bearing cells (details pg. 409, fig. 12.5.2) in the urine sediment. This test is significant when positive and is based on the principle of virus being passed in the urine. Though the test is simple, however the test can be falsely negative.

An important test currently used is the demonstration of *CMV antigen* in peripheral blood leucocytes or *CMV DNA* in blood or other tissue/fluids of the patient. PCR assays are often employed to detect the latter. The limitation of this technique is that it cannot differentiate between latently infected cases and those having active infection.

Various samples; as urine, saliva and semen can be used to *isolate* the virus, using cell lines; as human fibroblast. However, the CPE may take 3-4 weeks to develop especially in samples, which have low viral titers, It manifests; as swollen refractile cells with granules in cytoplasm. Immunofluorescence technique or monoclonal antibodies can be used to confirm the identity of the virus, causing changes in the cell line. Shell vial assay is a better alternative technique than traditional viral cell culture technique.

Specific IgM antibodies can be detected in the infected individuals by ELISA techniques. This test is available; as a component of the panel available in the market as 'TORCH' Test. The titre of specific antibodies may remain positive for long and also presence of rheumatoid factor can give a false positive test.

Diagnosis of *congenital CMV* infection in the newborn requires expertise. Demonstration of viruria or specific IgM antibodies in the cord serum can be helpful.

Enumerate the antiviral drugs that can be used for treating this case (with CMV infection).

A.8 (a) Ganciclovir, Valganciclovir, Foscaranet and Cidfovir.

Has drug resistance been reported for any of these agents?

A.8 (b) Yes

Outline the preventive aspects for CMV infections.

A.9
- Caesarian section may be employed to decrease perinatal CMV infections.
- Antiviral; as Acyclovir can be used prophylactically in high risk cases, as renal transplantation recipients especially when the recipient is CMV seronegative and the donor is CMV seropositive.
- Use of blood and organs (as bone marrow) for transplantation from seronegative donors.
- CMV immunoglobulins can be used selectively, as its use in renal transplant recipients.
- Vaccines under trial.

Aspect related to case theme/examination assessment

Describe Human Herpesvirus 6.

A.10
- **Infects:** CD4+ T lymphocytes, macrophages
- **Transmission:** Mainly by saliva
- **Pathogenicity:**
  - Mostly asymptomatic
  - In children, causes sixth disease (exanthema subitum/roseola infantum)
  - In elderly group, associated with 'mononucleosis like' syndrome
- **Laboratory diagnosis:**
  - *Sample*-Peripheral blood mononuclear cells, serum
  - *Techniques*-Isolation of virus by co-cultivation with lymphocytes
    - Viral antigen demonstration by monoclonal antibodies using immunofluorescence
    - Antigen and antibody demonstration in patient serum by ELISA

Integrated Clinical Based Study of Hepatitis B Virus/Jaundice

A thirty year woman Shanti, presented with weakness and anorexia of 3 weeks duration. She had no history of any intravenous drug abuse or receiving any blood transfusions. Her eye examination revealed icteric (yellowish) sclera. Her hepatitis test profile revealed IgM HAV antibody, negative; HBV surface antigen, positive; IgM HBV core antibody, positive; and HBV surface antibody, negative.

Linkages: Pg. 368, 397, 432, 514

What is your presumptive diagnosis?

A.1 Acute hepatitis B infection.

How did she likely acquire this infection?

A.2 (a) She has no history of any blood transfusions or intravenous drug abuse. The infection episode is a recent one. In view of these circumstances, she has probably acquired the infection during sexual activity.

How was the HBV infection commonly acquired in the world war II period?

A.2 (b) In the beginning of this century, post transfusion HBV transmission was significant. In fact during the world war II, many US troops sent to yellow fever endemic area contracted this infection, as these were immunized with a live attenuated yellow fever vaccine that was 'stabilized' mistakenly with infective serum (having HBV).

Why did the incidence of HBV disease decrease in the subsequent period (to World War II it)?

A.2 (c) Mandatory HBsAg screening of the blood to be transfused started.

Can one rely totally on HBsAg demonstration for detecting HBV infected cases? If not, which additional test needs to be done?

A.2 (d) No. Some cases could be in the incubation period (all testing parameters negative), i.e., 'window period' in which HBsAg becomes undetectable, before the appearance of anti HBs antibodies. The individuals in this period could be detected, if anti HBc antibodies were assayed.

What was the role of the Blumberg in the discovery of the HBV?

A.3 (a) In 1995, Blumberg a geneticist and his colleagues found an antigen in the serum of an Australian aborigine. It reacted in a agar diffusion test with serum of a haemophiliac, who had received multiple blood transfusions, to form a precipitin line. Thus this antigen was called 'Australia antigen'. It was thought to be a host antigen and not in any way related to any infectious agent. After several years of investigation, this antigen was found to be associated with acute (serum) hepatitis and subsequently given the name of hepatitis B surface antigen. Its correct relation to hepatitis virus was realized with the discovery of hepatitis B by Dane and colleagues.

Who discovered the complete virion Hepatitis B and what technique was used for this purpose?

A.3 (b) Dane and colleagues in 1970 discovered virion of hepatitis B, by utilizing electronic microscopic techniques.

To which family does HBV belongs?

A.3 (c) Hepatitis B virus belongs to the family Hepadnaviridae. The fact that it is the only DNA virus in the group of hepatitis viruses (A to F) can be memorized by the presence of 'DNA' in hepadnaviridae.

Describe the structure of HBV and its role in pathogenesis.

A.3 (d) The general properties of this virus are those of the family, in which it belongs (Table 11.1.4, pg. 368). As it is a double stranded virus, the question of positive or negative polarity does not arise.

More detailed structural study of this virus than others is warranted, because the structure is complex and has implications in its laboratory diagnosis and vaccine production.

A line diagram of the complete virion and its incomplete particles is given in Fig. 12.9.1a. If serum from a HBV hepatitis patient is studied under electron microscopy, three types of virus particles can be seen. The least abundant of them; is the complete virion (see Figure 12.9.1b and 12.9.2) also called the Dane particles and the most abundant are the spherical particles

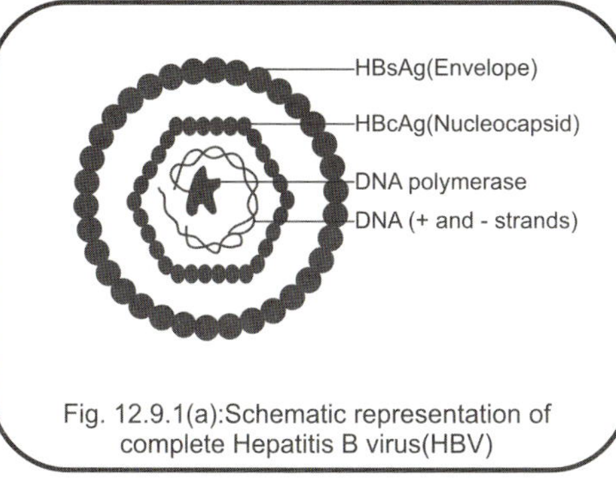

Fig. 12.9.1(a):Schematic representation of complete Hepatitis B virus(HBV)

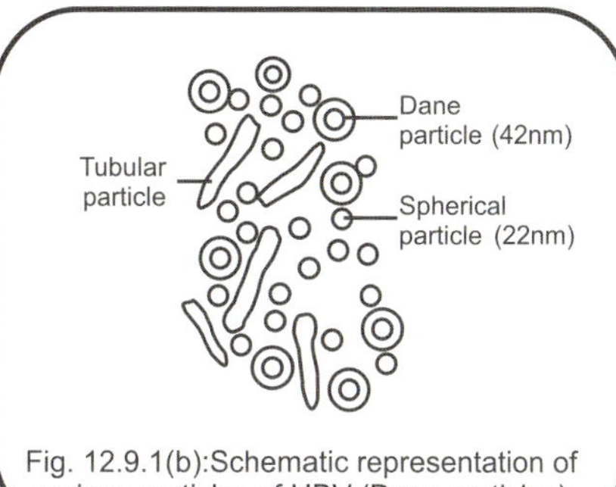

Fig. 12.9.1(b):Schematic representation of various particles of HBV (Dane particles)

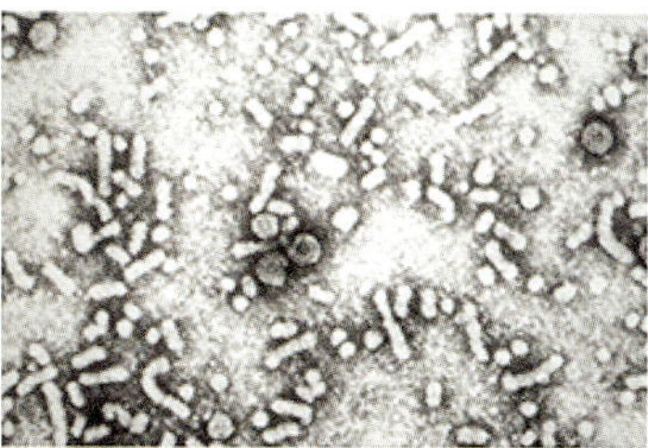

Fig.12.9.2: Hepatitis –B Virus: Electron micrograph depicting hepatitis virus virions(Dane particles)
Courtesy: Centers for Disease Control,Atlanta,USA

called Hepatitis B surface antigen (HBsAg). This may be responsible for the often reliance on HBsAg for diagnosis and also its earlier detection in hepatitis cases than the complete virion. The HBV DNA is unique in sense that it is partially double stranded, i.e., one strand is longer than the other. The short strand is the 'plus' strand and can vary in its length in comparison to the other 'minus' strand, which is complete. Another uniqueness of the genome is the overlapping of the four genes. The virus achieves genomic economy by this strategy of encoding proteins from 4 overlapping genes, i.e., if overlapping of genome had not occurred, a significantly larger genome would have been required. These are four proteins encoded by the four overlapping genes, as depicted in the table 12.9.1.

Table 12.9.1: Major genes coding for HBV antigens

Gene	Protein/antigen
S	HBsAg (Hepatitis B surface antigen)
C	HBcAg (Hepatitis B core antigen)
P	DNA polymerase
X	X protein (non structural, regulatory role)

There is another complexity of the genome, that there are two mRNA initiation sites in the capsid protein gene. Transcription and translation of one results in HBcAg and when differently processed, results in a variant known as HBeAg. The latter marker serves as a marker for active viral replication. HBcAg is not normally detectable in the serum, as antibodies formed against it, prevents its detection in the serum. It also remains mostly in the hepatocyte and its presence can be detected by immunofluorescence or immunohistochemical stains.

Is 'pure' HBsAg infectious? If not; why it is used in the diagnosis of HBV infection?

A.3 (e) No. An important concept of HBsAg, is that in pure form it is non-infectious!! They are used in diagnosis because they are abundant in amount, easier to detect than Dane particles and mostly associated with complete virion (which are difficult to demonstrate).

Enumerate the common antigenic type of HBV prevalent in India?

A.3 (f) Type 'ayw'.

Can HBV be cultured using traditional cell culture technique?

A.4 (a) HBV cannot be traditionally cultivated in the laboratory using cell lines.

If not, how is the antigen in bulk generated for the manufacture of current vaccine?

A.4 (b) Key genes of this virus have been cloned in yeast and bacteria. Hence large quantities of proteins (necessary) get produced by this technology.

Outline the steps involved in the production of the HBV vaccine.

A.4 (c) The recombinant HBV yeast vaccine is a classic successful example of how the recombinant DNA technology is serving millions of individuals at a global level. The non cultivability of the virus is not affecting the antigen production. It would be worthwhile to recall the steps required in the production of this vaccine.

(i) Viral DNA for HBsAg is identified and isolated.

(ii) This isolated viral DNA sequence is fused to yeast expression control sequence (because yeast would be later used for production) and built into a plasmid of *E.coli*.

(iii) The plasmid is introduced into yeast (*Saccharomyces cerevesiae*), enabling the transforming yeast cell to produce HBsAg.

(iv) The quantities of HBsAg that are recovered, purified and marketed by companies as 'Smithkline Beecham'.

What is the natural history of untreated HBV infection in an adult; as this?

A.5 (a)

- Mostly (in 90%) effective immune defense mechanisms, would lead to resolution of the infection.
- Occasionally (9%), the limited immune defense mechanisms, would lead to a chronic carrier state which would lead to severe chronic hepatitis (cirrhosis or hepatocellular carcinoma) or minimal chronic hepatitis (extra hepatic disease as 'serum sickness'Δ, glomerulonephritis, or polyarteritis nodosa).
- Rarely (1%) ineffective defective immune mechanisms could, lead to acute fulminant hepatitis, which may lead to death.

Δ Is a type III hypersenstivity disorder due to large amount of antigen in blood of chronic hepatitis cases.

Describe Hepatitis B carriers.

A.5 (b) As the name indicate, these are individuals, who carry hepatitis B virus in their body (without having disease).

Classification

(i) *Temporary/chronic: Temporary* carriers; as the name indicates, are individuals who carry the virus for short periods, i.e., few weeks to few months (less than 6 months), after getting infected. *Chronic* carriers are the individuals, as the name indicates; carry the virus for long periods, i.e., more than 6 months after getting infected.

(ii) *Simple/Super: Simple* carriers have low infectivity, as possess low levels of HBsAg and no HBeAg in blood. Hence, transmit the infection at a lower rate. The transmission from these individuals occurs only, if large amount of blood/serum from these cases is transferred. This category of carriers is commoner than the super carriers.

Super carriers have high infectivity and possess high level of HBsAg and possess HBeAg including DNA polymerase. Such individuals are designated as super carriers, as very minute amount of blood/serum from these individuals can transmit the infection.

Magnitude of the problem

Globally approximately 350 million individuals are carriers of hepatitis B. In developing countries the carrier rate is higher than the developed countries, where the rate is less than 1%. In India, the prevalence rate is 3.7% and it has approximately 40 million carriers.

Consequence

Chronic hepatitis carriers may remain healthy for their life time (approximately 30%) but others have significant possibility of developing hepatitis cirrhosis and hepatocellular carcinoma.

Laboratory diagnosis

see. table 12.9.2, pg. 429.

Describe the pathogenesis of HBV infection.

A.5 (c) HBV can be transmitted primarily by three routes. The most predominant is by *parenteral* mode, in which the virus enters by inoculation (often accidental) of even minute amount of infective blood, blood products, serum or other body fluids in various medical, surgical or dental procedures.

The other mode is by *perinatal* route, in which the infant gets infected during delivery with infected blood or secretions of mother.

As HBV is present in almost all fluids including semen and cervical secretions, *sexual* mode also plays a part in the transmission of HBV. It would include even casual kissing, in which infected saliva is exchanged.

Once the HBV reaches the liver via the blood stream, it multiplies principally in the hepatocytes. Copies of the HBV genome may integrate with the hepatocyte chromosome and may remain latent. HBcAg and viral DNA are present in the nucleus, the former can be detected by immunofluorescence. HBsAg and virions can be detected in the cytoplasm. The outcome of the acute hepatitis B depends essentially on the status of cell-mediated immunity and also on the age; at which infection is acquired. The importance of these can be gauged from the fact that

90% of infants borne to infected mother, would become chronic carriers of HBV because of immature immune defense mechanism (this figure may be contrasted with 9% conversion of acute hepatitis B infection to chronic carrier state in the other population). If there is deficient T cell response, symptoms may be mild, but it could lead to inability to resolve the infection, which could manifest as chronic carrier state and development of chronic hepatitis. To understand the sequence of humoral immune response in acute hepatitis, it is important to study the sequence of HBV antigens appearance and their relationship to various antibodies elicited. In figure 12.9.3a one can see that HBsAg is the first viral indicator to manifest in the late incubation period. Viral DNA and DNA polymerase appear transiently. The concentration of HBsAg and HBeAg increase in the acute viremic stage and these fall to baseline in the late acute viremia stage in a self limiting infectious case.

The first antiviral antibody to form is the IgM anti HBc in late incubation period. The fall in the HBeAg correlates with the rise of the anti-HBe antibodies. The anti HBs antibodies appear few weeks after disappearance of HBsAg and are the last to appear in the late convalescence and persist for many years.

Describe the epidemiology of HBV infection.

A.5 (d)

- **Agent:** Hepatitis B virus. The virus in of acid-sensitive category.
- **Reservoir of infection:** Man is the only reservoir of this infection with chronic carriers of HBsAg constituting the primary reservoir of infection. Globally, there are about 300 *million* carriers of HBV. India has about *45 million* such carriers.

  The carrier rates are higher in the tropics (5-15% or even greater) than in the most temperate countries (<0.1%) as U.S.A. and Europe. The carriers can be categorized into *super carrier* and *simple carrier*. Blood of the former category is *highly infectious*, because as little as 1 μg of it in the syringe can transmit the infection. These carriers show the presence of HBcAg, DNA polymerase and high titers of HBs Ag. In contrast the blood of simple carriers, is *less infectious* and the former two parameters are not detectable along with low titer of HBsAg.
- **Source of infection:**
  - Infected blood in the primary source, with infectious secretions; as saliva, vaginal secretions and semen also playing a part.
- **Modes of transmission:**

  (1) *Parenteral route:* In the beginning of this century, post transfusion HBV transmission was significant. In fact during the world war II, many of the US troops sent to yellow fever endemic area contracted this infection, as these were immunized with a live attenuated yellow fever vaccine that was 'stabilized' with infective serum. However the incidence of post transfusion hepatitis B has significantly dropped, since HBsAg screening of blood to be transfused became mandatory. However this risk can't be said to absent, as some cases who are donating blood could in the incubation period (routine testing parameters negative) designated as 'window period'. The transmission also occurs during usage of contaminated syringes/needles, dialysis and surgical/dental procedures. Certain social customs involving minute bleeding; as tattooing ear peering, nose peering and facial beautification, may also be involved in transmission of the infection.

  (2) *Perinatal transmission:* A HBeAg positive mother has a high probability of transmitting the infection to the neonate; most likely at the time of birth, as the neonate could swallow infected blood/fluids and get abrasions. (infection unlikely to be spread transplacentally).

  (3) *Sexual transmission:* As the virus is present in many secretions; especially saliva, sex with infected individuals can lead to transmission of the infection in promiscuous individuals and male homosexuals with varied sexual practices. These individuals have high incidence of this infection.

  (4) *Skin contact:* This route is seen in infected children in parts of the world other than Asia. This occurs when children have physical contact with infective skin conditions; as impetigo and scabies.
- **Host:** The infection is found worldwide, although the rates vary markedly.
  - *Age:* The infection is seen more in adults than children.

- *High risk groups:* The infection is an occupational risk in the medical and paramedical personal frequently exposed to blood; as surgeons, dentists, nurses' mortuary attendants, clinical laboratory technicans and scientists associated with serum work.

The incidence of this infection is also high in drug addicts taking illicit drugs intravenously, due to sharing of the needles. This infection could also be transmitted by recycled and improperly sterilized disposable syringes and needles. It is estimated that 10 percent of the 40 million people infected with HIV worldwide are coinfected with HBV. Presence of significant levels of anti-HBs antibodies in blood indicates immunity to this infection.

If this woman's hepatitis profile after 5 months; became anti-HBs positive from initially being negative, what impression you could make?

A.6 **(a)** The patient has become immune to natural infection.

Describe the sequence of humoral immune response in acute HBV infection

A.6 **(b)** See figure 12.9.3a

If this woman's hepatitis profile after 7 months was HBV surface antigen positive; IgM core antibody, negative; Anti-HBc, positive; What impression is conveyed?

A.7 **(a)** The patient has become chronically infected and is at increased risk of developing hepatic complications.

Illustrate the sequence of appearance of HBV antigens and antibodies in a chronic active hepatitis (CAH) case.

A.7 **(b)** In a chronic hepatitis case (Figure 12.9.3b), the HBsAg and HBeAg antigen levels rise and remain elevated, Only anti-HBc antibodies are formed. The absence of anti HBe and anti-HBs antibodies especially the latter, indicate the inability of the body to check the viral replication.

Tabulate the status of serologic and other markers in acute and chronic anti-HBS infection cases.

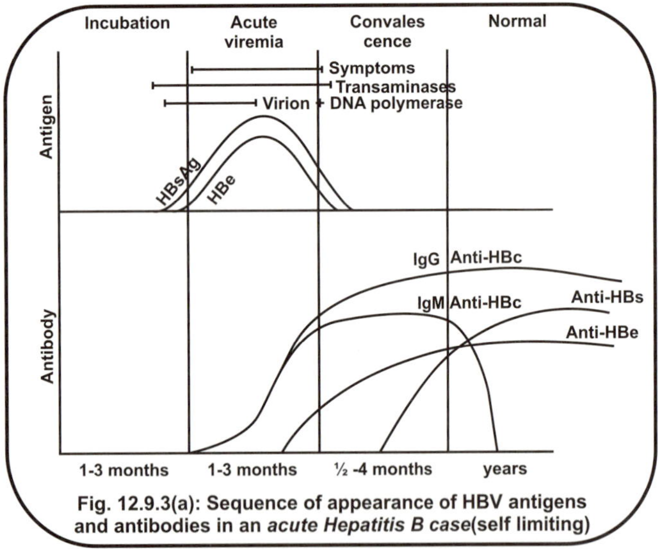

Fig. 12.9.3(a): Sequence of appearance of HBV antigens and antibodies in an *acute Hepatitis B case*(self limiting)

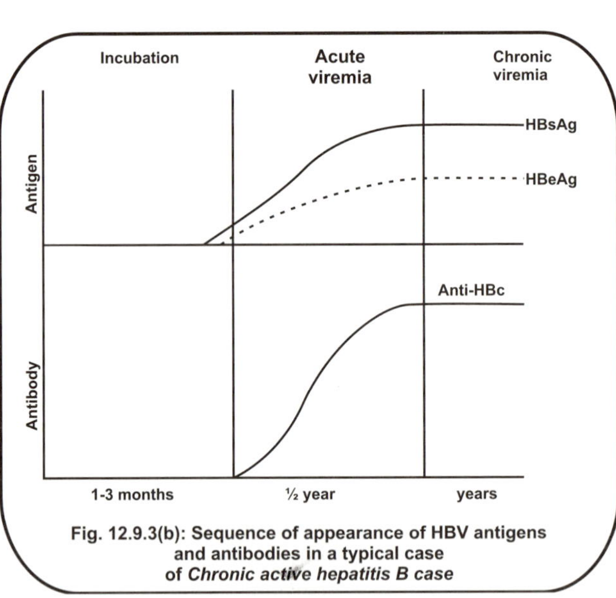

Fig. 12.9.3(b): Sequence of appearance of HBV antigens and antibodies in a typical case of *Chronic active hepatitis B case*

A.7 **(c)** The table 12.9.2 does not include all the variations, although an attempt has been made to convey some idea of the dynamic nature of infection, in which the various markers appear and/or disappear. The analysis of a single blood sample may provide an accurate diagnosis in many cases, however in some cases a second sample after some period may be required to make a diagnosis. For instance, falling HBsAg and HBeAg levels indicate early convalescence. Similarly to establish a chronic carrier state, HBsAg has to be present for at least six months. This parameter is often tested by latex agglutination test or ELISA techniques (window period aspect already discussed).

Table 12.9.2: Serologic markers in hepatitis B infection (Interpetation in various categories of HBV infection)

	HBsAg	HBeAg	Anti HBc		Anti HBe	Anti HBs
			IgG	IgM		
Acute infection						
Incubation	+	+	-	-	-	-
Acute phase	+	+	-	+	-	-
Early convalescence	+→-	+→-	+	+	-→+	-
Late convalescence	-	-	+	-	+	+
Past infection	-	-	+	-	+→-	+
Chronic infection						
Simple HBV carrier	+ (>6 months)	-	+	-	-	-
Super carrier	+	+	+	-	-	-
Chronic active hepatitis	+	+/-	++++	-	-	-
Other states						
Recent vaccination	-	-	-/+	-	-	++

NB: →, indicates a change occuring in a direction.

Enumerate the information the various HBV serological markers broadly convey?

A.8
- Remote infection – IgG anti HBc
- Recent infection-IgM anti HBc
- *Time of infection – IgM anti HBc (quantitative)
- Infection – HBsAg
- Infectivity – HBV-DNA
- Natural immunity – Anti HBe and anti HBs
- Immunity after vaccination – Anti HBs (quantitative)

What are the goals to be achieved in a therapy of a case with chronic hepatitis B infection? Compare the advantages and disadvantages of the two drugs namely; Lamivudine and alpha interferon used in the treatment?

A.9 The goal of the therapy is to minimize the progression of hepatic injury due to HBV infection. This could be seen as the case becoming a chronic carrier and/or resulting in histologic improvement of liver function, as evident by sequential liver biopsies.

Lamivudine can be easily given orally, has minimal side effects but is associated with HBV mutations, which limits the long term efficacy of the drug. On the other hand alpha interferon require parenteral administration, is not associated emergence of HBV mutations, but has high rate of adverse effects.

If this case; which was receiving Lamivudine had its HBV DNA levels initially decrease and then increase from 50,000 copies at 1 month to 300,000 copies at 4th month of therapy, what inference could be made about this case?

A.10 The case is going in for drug failure, as the case could have developed drug resistance HBV sub-populations likely through HBV polymerase mutation, making the drug ineffective. There is a also a possibility of poor drug compliance, i.e., the patient is taking the drug irregularly.

What advice should be given to this woman?

A.11 (a) The patient should be advised to have:

(i) regular hepatitis surface antigen estimation to monitor her hepatitis carrier status.

(ii) Not to donate blood

(iii) Personnel articles in contact with secretions, should not be shared

(iv) her dentist should be alerted about the HBsAg + status

(v) Her sexual partners should be advised to have hepatitis B vaccine

What are the indications for administration of the recombinant HBV vaccine?

A.11 (b) Indications

- **Pre-exposure** – Routinely all infant

- Medical staff (at risk of exposure)
  - o As dentists, surgeons, staff of haemodiaysis unit, blood bank personnel
- Clinical conditions
  - o Patients requiring frequent blood transfusion
  - o Haemophiliac patients on dialysis
  - o Inmates of mentally retarded and other conditions
  - o Immunologically impaired (usually double dose to that of adults administered)
- Behavioural conditions
  - o Male homosexuals with multiple sexual partners
  - o Drug addicts (as injecting drugs intravenously)

• **Post-exposure**
- Infant borne to HBsAg +ve mother
- 'Needle stick' injury
- Sexual partner

Describe passive immunization and combined immunization with reference to HBV.

A.11 (c) **Passive immunization** – Hyperimmune hepatitis B immunoglobulin (HBIG) may be basically used in two conditions (i) to perinatally exposed infants borne to HBsAg +ve mothers, immediately after birth (high infection rate in this age group) and (ii) to accidental needle stick injury cases; as surgeons, nurses and laboratory personnel. (iii) Sexual contacts of acute hepatitis B cases. This immunoglobulin is prepared from donor with high titers of antiHBs.

It is administered parenterally (intramuscular) in a dose of 300-500 IU, as early as possible after injury, but not later than 48 hours after the incident. It may not prevent the infection but prevents the disease and the development of its sequelae; as carrier state.

Combined vaccination–One example of an individual requiring this type of vaccine would be an accidental 'needle' stick injury case, who could receive the HBIG on one arm and then the vaccine dose at another site (three doses). Similarly the infant perinatally exposed from a HBsAg +ve mother individual, could receive the three doses of active vaccine, after the HBIG dose.

Enumerate the preventive and control strategies for HBV disease.

A.11 (d)

1. Blood banks must use highly sensitive kits to detect HBsAg and preferably also IgM anti HBc (as some hepatitis B positive cases could be in the window period) in blood of donors.
2. Proper sterilization of equipment and aseptic technique by surgeons, dentists, laboratory technicians, tattooists and personnel involved in ear/nose piercing.
3. Appropriate and timely use of HBIG in perinatally exposed infants, technicians involved in needle stick injuries and other exposure.
4. In hospitals and laboratories, where exposure with hepatitis B +ve clinical material is likely:
   (i) Gloves to be worn.
   (ii) Disposable rather than reusable equipment use.
   (iii) Protective clothing as gowns, masks and protective goggles may be worn, where splashing of potentially infective material is possible.
   (iv) Careful handwashing should be practised, after contact with any potential infected individual, if gloves are not used.
   (v) Mouth pipetting, eating, smoking and drinking be forbidden in laboratories, where infected material is being handled.
   (vi) Any spill of blood or other infective material be immediately disinfected with sodium hypochlorite solution etc. and be cleaned.
   (vii) Bed linen, towels and other material of HBsAg positive patients be disinfected, before usage for HBsAg negative patients.
5. HBsAg positive surgeons and dentists to be prudent in their work.
6. Behavioural changes in HBV carriers, e.g., pertaining to sexual practice.

An Outline of Laboratory Diagnosis of Key DNA Viruses

Virus/ Syndrome/ Approach	Specimens	Direct Demonstration of Viral Antigen/Genome/Particle In Clinical Specimen/Animal Inoculation/Egg Inoculation	Viral cell line	Growth/ Confirmation	Serological Tests	
					Type	Interpretation
Parvovirus B19	• RBCs • Bone-marrow • Serum • Liver (fetal)	• C.I.E.P • ELISA • RIA • Indirect immunofluorescence • Immunoenzyme staining with monoclonal antibodies • DNA - DNA Hybridization (nucleic acid) • P.C.R/ • Electron microscopy (from serum) • (Viremia usually lasts 7 -12 days)	Not cultivable in traditional cell lines	Can be cultured from cells in the presence of erythropoietin and IL-3	ELISA	No role in individual cases
Papilloma virus/ diagnosis is essentially clinical and histopathology confirms (internal polyps visualized by coloposcopy)	• Tissue : Fresh : Fixed • Exfoliated cells	• Immunofluorescence & Immunoperoxidase staining of fixed sections • DNA in sample by DNA-DNA hybridization & PCR • in situ DNA hybridization can identify & locate DNA in sample/ • Electronic microscopy can reveal particles, but rarely resorted to	Not cultivable	-	-	Serologic role is essentially epidemiologic
Polyoma Virus (JC/ BK)/ Diagnosis of PML is essentially histopathologic	• Brain biopsy/autopsy • Urine Cytological examination of exfoliated urinary epithelial cell, shows the presence of the enlarged deeply stained basophilic nuclei, with a single inclusion	• In brain biopsy by immunofluorescence • In urine, antigen can be detected by ELISA/ • DNA-DNA hybridization • in situ DNA hybridization • E/M can detect virion in brain tissue and urine	For BK, human fibroblast cell line required	Clinically not used	-	-
Adenoviruses/ Isolation of viruses from oropharynx & faeces should be interpreted with caution because of the asymptomatic intermittent shedding in these sites. If the significance is questionable, serologic testing of acute & convalescent sera may be necessary	Depending on lesion. • Conjunctival swab • Throat swab • Nasopharyngeal aspirate, transtracheal aspirates bronchial lavage, urine, faeces, genital secretion, biopsy	In different swab, viral antigen may be demonstrated using latex particles coated with antibody/ Viral DNA in faeces may be demonstrated by polyacrylamide gel electrophoresis/ Electron microscopy or Immuno electron microscopy can demonstrate virions in stool	• Hela • HEp2 (slow growing, growth takes few weeks)	CPE (as enlarged, round, grape-like clusters and intranuclear basophilic inclusion bodies)	CFT, HI, ELISA Demonstration of rise in titer of antibodies in paired sera is important	Useful sometimes in conjunction, not in isolation
Human herpesvirus 1 and 2 (HHV - 1 & HHV - 2) /Clinical picture characteristic	• Vesicle fluid • Skin swab • Conjuctival fluid • Corneal scraping • C.S.F • Brain biopsy	• In cell from base of lesion & in brain biopsy, antigen can be demonstrated by IF/HHV - DNA in C.S.F by P.C.R • D.N.A-D.N.A hybridization/by E/M(however cannot differentiate various herpes types)/ from base of lesion can demonstrate multinucleate giant cells & intranuclear inclusion bodies/ Newborn mice inoculated intracerebral or i/p develop encephalitis within a short period, staining of mouse brain exhibits Cowdry type A inclusion bodies (a multinucleate giant cells)/Using chorioallantoic membrane, it produces well defined small pocks within 3-4 days of inoculation (HHV -2 produces large & clear pocks)	• Human fibroblast • Vero cells • Rabbit kidney	Within few days rounding & balloning of cells, ground glass nuclei with characteristic intranuclear inclusion bodies & multinucleated giant cells Characteristic CPE _specific antisera to perform neutralization tests	• IgM, HHV 1 & 2 antibody test • IgG HHV - 1 & 2 antibodies (rising titre) by ELISA, Nt. test	High levels of HHV-1 antibody can interfere in detection of HHV-2 antibody

Contd.

Chapter 7

1. To which subfamily does HHV-4 (Epstein Barr) belong? A 3b., p. 417
2. What are the key characteristics of this sub-family? What is the basis of cytopathology seen in infection with HHV-4? A 3c, A4a., p. 417
3. Describe the epidemiology and pathogenesis of Infectious mononucleosis. A 4b., p. 417, A7., p. 418
4. Describe the laboratory diagnosis for Infectious mononucleosis. A 8c., p. 418-419
5. Describe Paul Bunnel test. A 8c., p. 419

Chapter 8

1. Comment on the derivation of the name 'Cytomegalovirus'. Alb., p. 420
2. Describe the clinical profile of infection with HHV-5 (CMV) with special reference to the various age categories. A 3c.,pgs. 397, 420, 421
3. What are the challenges in incriminating HHV-5 (CMV), as an etiological agent in a suspected clinical case. A 5a., p. 421
4. Describe the laboratory diagnosis of HHV-5 (CMV) infections. A 7b., p. 422
5. Describe Human Herpes virus 6. A 10., 423

Chapter 9

1. Classify Hepatitis viruses. To which family does the Hepatitis B virus (HBV) belong? Enumerate the differences between Hepatitis A and B. pg. 513-514, A3c., p. 424, (Table 14.4.5)., pg. 514
2. Describe the structure of HBV and mention its role in pathogenesis of disease. A 3d., p. 424-425
3. What is the natural history of untreated infection with HBV infection in an adult? A 5a., p. 426
4. Describe the epidemiology and pathogenesis of HBV infection. A 5c,d.,p. 426-428
5. Describe Hepatitis B carriers. A 5b., p. 426
6. Describe the sequence of humoral immune response in acute HBV infection. Mention the information the various HBV serological markers convey. A 7b., p. 428-429
7. Tabulate the status of serologic and other markers in acute and chronic HBV infection. A 7c., p. 428-429
8. Describe the laboratory diagnosis of infections caused by HBV. p. 432, A 5b., p. 426, A7c, A8., p. 428-429
9. What are the goals to be achieved in therapy of a case with Hepatitis B infection? Compare the advantages and disadvantages of the commonly used drugs. A 9., p. 729
10. Mention the steps involved in the production of the (recombinant) Hepatitis B vaccine. What are the indication of the usage of this vaccine. Describe passive and active immunization with reference to HBV. A 4c., p. 425-426, A 11b-d., p. 429-430

Section XIII: RNA Viruses

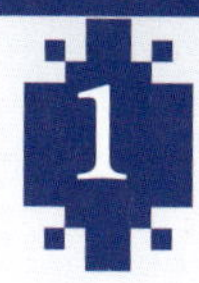

Overview of Clinical Profile (Pathogenicity) of RNA Viral Infections

Virus	*Disease*
Rotavirus	Acute diarrhoea (commonest viral agent for this disease, for children under 5 years) Details Chapter 2a, pg. 437-439.
Influenza virus (H1N1)	Influenza (details A2b,c, pg. 440)
'Swine' flu (H1N1)	Respiratory infection of pigs, can spread to human and result in outbreaks See Chapter 3, pg. 448-449
Influenza virus (H5N1, 'Avian' flu)	Respiratory infection of birds; as fowl, can spread to man, outbreak in India occurred in 2008 See Chapter 4, pg. 446-447
Parainfluenza viruses	Respiratory infections (See A11, pg. 451-452, Case 5)
Newcastle disease virus (Ranikhet virus)	Conjunctivitis (in individuals exposed to infected birds as poultry workers)
Respiratory syncytial virus	Respiratory syncytial virus infection See Chapter 5, pg. 451
Measles virus	Measles • See Chapter 6 A1, 2, p. 453
Mumps virus	Mumps Parotid gland enlargement in 95% cases (non suppurative parotitis) Complications; as meningitis, meningoencephalitis, panceatitis, orchitis and others
Human Metapneumovirus	Respiratory tract infection in children and adults
Rabies virus	Rabies • See Chapter 7, pg. 460, A5
Rabies related viruses as *Mokola virus, Duvenhage virus*	Human infection resembling rabies See Chapter 7, pg. 462 A.10
Filoviruses; as Marburg, Ebola	Haemorrhagic fever (feared for the high mortality rates)
Hepatitis A virus	Infectious Hepatitis • Details see Chapter 8, pg.463, A5
Enteroviruses	See A.1(e) Chapter 9, pg. 466
Poliovirus	Poliomyelitis • Details see Chapter 9, pg. 467., A.4,5
Coxsackieviruses	See A.7(b), See A.14 (ii), pg. 470
Echoviruses (Enteric cytopathogenic human orphan)	• Mostly cause asymptomatic infection • Some serotypes associated with aseptic meninigitis (common cause), pericarditis, myocarditis, infantile diarrhoea and encephalitis
Enterovirus type 70	Acute haemorrhagic conjunctivitis
Rhinoviruses	Common cold
Hepatitis E virus	Hepatitis • See Chapter 11, pg. 472-473
Caliciviruses; as *Norovirus* *Sapovirus* *Astrovirus*	 Gastroenteritis Gastroenteritis (children) Diarrhoea (in children)

Contd.

Contd.

Rubella virus	• Rubella • Congenital rubella syndrome. see Chapter 11, pg. 474., A1d) • Postnatal rubella, see A5; pg. 475
Dengue virus (4 serotypes)	Dengue ('break bone' fever) • Details see Chapter 12, pg.476., A5c,d
Japanese encephalitis virus	Encephalitis See Chapter 13, pg. 478., A3a)c) and chapter 4, section 14
Hepatitis C virus	Hepatitis Less severe disease than Hepatitis B and more than half of the cases develop chronic hepatitis. Cases can develop cirrhosis or hepatocelluar carcinoma. (details Chapter 14, pg. 482, A.5(b)
Coronaviruses	Common cold and associated with gastroenteritis
Eastern equine encephalitis virus	Encephalitis • see Chapter 4, pg. 512 (Section 14)
Western equine encephalitis virus	Encephalitis • see Chapter 4, pg. 512 (Section 14)
Chikungunya virus	Chickungunya (severe joint pain,fever, lyphadenopathy, conjunctivitis and rash), details see Chapter 13, A.7(iii), pg. 480
Human Immunodeficiency virus type 1 (HIV -1 virus)	Acquired immunodeficiency syndrome (AIDS) Details see Chapter 15, A.3(d), A.7, A.9(c), pg. 489, 490
Human Immunodeficiency virus type 2	Acquired immunodeficiency syndrome (often milder type)
Human T cell lymphotropic virus type 1 (HTLV-I)	Adult T cell leukemia and Spastic tropical paraparesis
Human T cell lymphotropic virus type II (HTLV-II)	Role not clear
Arenaviruses as: *Lymphocytic Choriomeningitis virus* *Lassa virus* *Junin virus* *Machupo virus*	 Occasionally influenza like illness and aseptic meningitis (Lymphocytic choriomeningitis) Lassa fever (haemorrhagic fever) Argentine haemorrhagic fever Bolivian hoaemorrhagic fever
Severe acute respiratory related coronavirus	Severe acute respiratory syndrome (SARS). Outbreak started in 2002 in South China to involve several countries; including India
Hepatitis D virus	Hepatitis • Details see Chapter 4, pg. 504-505, A1,4
*Prions**	Transmissible degenerative (spongiform) encephalopathies Details see Chapter 2, pg. 506-508, A2a.

* Is not a RNA virus, but proteinaceous particle.

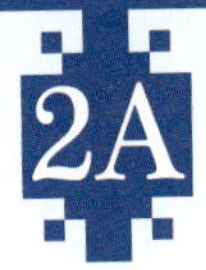

Integrated Clinical Based Study of Rotavirus/Diarrhoea

A 14 month male, Shinjan was admitted to the paediatric emergency with presentation of mild fever, severe diarrhoea and vomiting. The physical examination revealed severe dehydration. Microscopic stool examination revealed absence of leucocytes, ova, cyst or any parasites.

Linkages: Pg. 368, 435, 497

What is the bacterial and parasitic differential diagnosis in this case?

A.1 The acute diarrhea in this case could be bacterial, parasitic or viral in origin. Bacterial causes in this case could be Salmonella, Shigella, atypical *E coli*, *Yersinia enterocolitica.* Parasitic causes; as *E histolytica* are unlikely in the absence of pus cells in the stool. The parasitic causes in this case could be Giardia or Cryptosporidium species.

Subsequently stool culture for bacterial pathogens was performed, it did not reveal any bacterial pathogens.

What are the viruses that can be responsible for the presentation; in this case?

A.2 The viruses implicated in this case could be Rotavirus, Coronaviruses (enteric), Norwalk, Norwalk like viruses, adenoviruses (enteric), Calciviruses and Astroviruses.

Which is the commonest virus that can present a picture like the one in this case?

A.3 (a) Rotaviruses are the commonest viruses responsible for diarrhea in children less than 5 year of age.

What is the role of electron microscopy in demonstration of Rotavirus?

A.3 (b) Morphology of rotavirus is very distinctive in electron microscopy, characteristic 'wheel like' morphologic appearance is seen. However this approach is not practical and sensitive.

What approach is commonly used to demonstrate Rotavirus?

A.3 (c) The approach that is commonly used, is antigen detection in stool specimen. Simple methods; based on latex agglutination and reverse passive agglutination principle, are used to detect the specific antigen in the stool specimen.

What is the importance of rapid diagnosis test for Rotavirus infection?

A.3 (d) Rapid diagnostic tests for this etiological agent have implications in the diagnostic, therapeutic and control aspects. Once the rapid diagnosis of this disease is done, it obviates the need of other diagnostic tests. Use of antibacterial agents is avoided and the management focuses on rehydration. The children infected with this etiological agent can be cohorted, avoiding the use of isolation rooms; which can be used for other cases.

What is the role of demonstrating specific serum rotavirus antibodies in the diagnosis of a suspected case of rotavirus infection?

A.3 (e) Specific rotavirus serum antibodies can be demonstrated in the infected case, but these are not clinically useful.

To which family does Human rotavirus belong?

A.4 (a) Rotavirus belongs to family '*Reoviridae*'.

Comment on the origin of term 'reoviridae'.

A.4 (b) The name reovirus is an acronym and stands for 'respiratory enteric orphan virus'. These viruses inhabit the respiratory and enteric (gastrointestinal) tract and were considered orphans, as were not associated with any disease. However, this concept changed with the discovery of rotavirus in 1973 by Bishop in Melbourne (Australia), during electron microscopic examination of the duodenal biopsy of an infant. This agent was subsequently found to be important causes of infantile diarrhea worldwide.

Describe the morphology of Rotavirus.

A.4 (c) Rotavirus is non enveloped, double shelled icohsaehdral capsid resembling a 'wheel', with outer capsid attached by short spikes to the inner capsid. The viruses have double stranded segmented RNA genome, being constituted of 11 separate RNA molecules (segment). (Fig. 13.2.1 and 13.2.2)

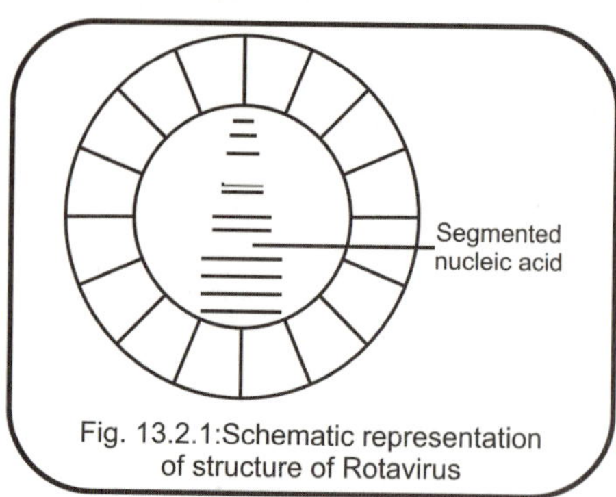

Fig. 13.2.1:Schematic representation of structure of Rotavirus

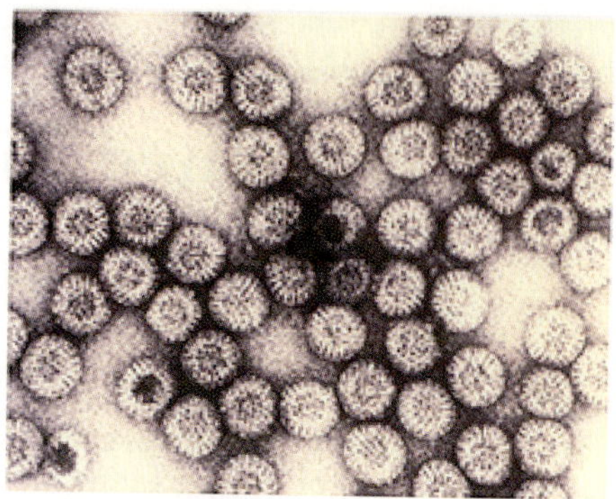
Fig.13.2.2: Rotavirus: Transmission electron micrograph revealing ultrastructural details of rotavirus icosaehdral protein capsid particles

Courtesy : Dr. Erskine I. Palmer/CDC

Do Rotaviruses of animal origin also exist?

A.4 (d) Rotaviruses of animal origin also occur. These present and produce acute gastroenteritis in a variety of animal species. Inter-species spread of this infection has not been demonstrated.

How many serotypes of Human rotavirus are known?

A.4 (e) Four

Describe the epidemiology of rotavirus diarrhoea?

A.5 (a) The rotavirus diarrheal disease is seen primarily in children *less than five* years of age, with most severe disease seen in children less than 2 years of age. Adults; especially who are caregivers to the infected child can get involved with this disease. The disease peaks in *winter months* in the temperate regions, which makes it to be referred as the 'winter vomiting disease'. It is a major cause of death in children less than 5 years in the developing countries; especially in the malnourished and the immunocompromised children.

The disease spreads primarily by the *faecal-oral* route. The nosocomial outbreaks are common in nurseries and day care centers. The spread can be controlled by paying attention to hygiene, which includes hand washing, disinfection and proper disposal of faecal contaminated articles; as diapers. The virus is resistant to chlorination.

Which is the serotype commonly involved in rotavirus infection?

A.5 (b) The rotaviruses are classified into seven serogroups. A-G, depending on the differences in the major group-specific capsid antigen VP6. Within group A, 14 serotypes; G1-G14 have been defined. Of these, G1-G4 are responsible for most of the severe cases globally.

Describe the pathogenesis of rotavirus diarrhea?

A.6 The pathogenesis of rotavirus diarrhea is *not completely* understood. This virus causes *blunting and atrophy* of the small intestinal villi. This results in the *reduction* of the absorptive surface of the intestine, which plays a part in the fluid accumulation in the intestine. The replacement of the absorptive cells by the immature cuboidal cells; also impairs enzymatic activity and molecule carrier activity, which results in loss of nutrients; as lactose and many ions; as sodium, potassium, chloride, bicarbonate and water.

If rotavirus infection had occured in this case, when it was a neonate; what would have been the clinical presentation?

A.7 Asymptomatic infection is the rule in neonates and this presentation is also common in adults.

How is rotavirus diarrhea treated?

A.8 No specific antiviral drugs are available. Fluids and electrolytes loss is to be replaced orally or parenterally (intravenously). If vomiting is not severe, oral administration should be preferred on account of ease of administration and low cost.

What control measures should be instituted in the ward, where this child with rotavirus diarrhea is admitted?

A.9 (a) This viral agent can remain viable on inanimate objects; as door handles for days and on hands for hours, so appropriate control measures need to be employed to prevent nosocomial outbreaks in day care centers and paediatric wards. Specific attention has to be given to strict hand hygiene and use of gloves by medical personnel.

What is electropherotyping? Describe its role in the control of this disease.

A.9 (b) *Electropherotypes* are patterns obtained, after polyacrylamide gel electrophoresis of viral RNA. In rotavirus, these reflect differences in the migration of the 11 RNA segments. This technique is valuable in the epidemiological study of rotavirus diarrohea.

Is there any need of Rotavirus vaccine?

A.10 (a) Yes. They would be required, as rotaviruses are highly infective and can spread fast in a family and in an institutional setting.

What should be the key characteristics that a successful rotavirus vaccine should have?

A.10 (b) A successful rotavirus vaccine should be able to be administered orally, induce protective gut immunity and should be especially effective in the first two years of childhood, when this infection is common.

Mention about the licensed rotavirus vaccine that had to be withdrawn, after reporting of a major side-effect?

A.10 (c) An attenuated recombinant rhesus rotavirus vaccine that was licensed for use in U.S.A. in 1998 had to be withdrawn on account of several reports of intussusception in the vaccinated children. Many of these cases required surgical intervention.

Mention about a current rotavirus vaccine in usage?

A.10 (d) An oral rotavirus vaccine is in usage for prophylaxis, in some of the developed countries. Three dosages at interval of few months are given in the early first year of age (see p. 634)

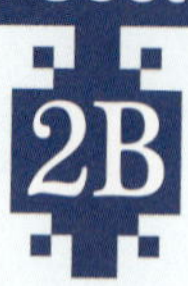

Integrated Clinical Based Study of Influenza Virus/Influenza

A 7 year old girl, Priti presented with high fever of 40°C that has rapidly risen in the last 12 hours, along with cough, rhinorrhea and severe myalgia in legs. Examination revealed bilateral conjuctivitis, but no rashes, lymphadenopathy or other signs. History revealed two days back a contact with a child in the school, who had breathing difficulty and ear discharge.

Linkages: Pg. 368, 435, 497

What is the differential diagnosis of this case?

A.1 The case is likely to have a respiratory infection, which could be caused by viruses; as Influenza A, Influenza B, Parainfluenza viruses, Respiratory syncytial virus or other respiratory viruses. The common bacteria that could be involved in such a case would include Group A streptococcus, *Mycoplasma pneumoniae* and other bacteria.

Is it easy to make a diagnosis of Influenza in the absence of an respiratory disease outbreak in the community?

A.2 **(a)** No, clinical diagnosis of Influenza is difficult to make in a community, unless an Influenza outbreak is present in the community.

What is the most likely diagnosis in the above case?

A.2 **(b)** The case is likely to have Influenza, considering the rapid rise of temperature and presence of severe systemic symptomatology. Influenza types A and B tend to cause severe illnesses, whereas Influenza type C causes mild infection. Influenza is essentially; an acute febrile respiratory infection. The incubation period is very brief; varying from just one day to three days. The disease is characterized by rapid and abrupt onset of fever, malaise, sore throat and cough. The onset can be so abrupt that the patient may be able to recall the time, the symptoms arose. The illness severity may reach a peak in 6-12 hours. The disease resolves usually in one week, if there are no complications.

Which is the populations at risk for developing complications of Influenza? Describe.

A.2 **(c)** The populations especially at risk for complications are the elderly, immunocompromised, those with cardiac and respiratory problems. These individuals have limited cardiovascular and pulmonary reserve, so respiratory infection can compromise, further the functioning of these vital organs, leading to death. Superinfection of lung with bacteria, primary viral pneumonia or mixed bacterial and viral infections of lungs, can be the other causes of death in this infected population. The other complications include myositis, Guillain Barré syndrome, encephalopathy, encephalitis and Reye's syndrome (characterized by fatty infiltration of liver and cerebral edema).

What rapid diagnostic test can be done to confirm diagnosis of Influenza?

A.2 **(d)** A rapid diagnostic test can be performed on nasopharyngeal specimen, utilizing specific fluorescent labelled antisera (Immunofluorescence test).

Outline the laboratory diagnosis of Influenza.

A.2 **(e)** See. pg. 497

How do you think the child likely acquired the Influenza infection?

A.3 **(a)** The I.P. of Influenza varies between 1-3 days. This case has likely contracted the disease from an infected child in the school.

Describe the pathogenesis of Influenza.

A.3 **(b)** The spread of infection from person to person is by inhalation of small aerosol droplets (smaller than 10 μm, highly efficient, generated by cough and sneezing). Hand to hand contact, other personal contact and even fomites may be involved in transmission of infection. It enters the body by upper respiratory tract, where the virus attaches to and infect the mucosal ciliated epithelial cells (primary sites of infection). The viral neuraminidase facilitates infection by dissolving the mucus film lining the respiratory mucosal cells and exposing the cell surface receptors of the latter cells. The virus replicates (multiplies) within 4-6 hours in the infected cells and gets released from it and infects adjacent cells, to slowly involve other parts of respiratory tract. The cellular damage remains confined to respiratory tract. Viremia rarely occurs and virus has been rarely been isolated from extrapulmonary sites. The systemic symptoms, are predominantly; caused by various cytokines released in response to infection. The secondary bacterial pneumonias that often occur in these patients are due to susceptibility to bacterial superinfection, resulting from loss of natural epithelial barriers. The recovery depends primarily upon interferon and cell-mediated immune response.

What are the key virulent factors of Influenza virus?

A.4 (a) There are two well characterized virulence factors on the surface of the virus; namely haemagglutinin and neuraminidase. *Haemagglutinin* is responsible for attachment of virus to sialic acid on glycoprotein receptors. Once the virus is endocytosed in the cell, haemagglutinin plays a key role in the formation of channels, through which the viral RNA enters host cell cytoplasm and initiates viral replication.

Neuraminidase is believed to help the viral penetration into the mucous layer overlying the infected respiratory cells. It also plays a part in the release and spread of the virus from infected cells to other cells.

Compare and contrast the features of Orthomyxoviruses and Paramyxoviruses.

A.4 (b)

Table 13.2.1: Features of Orthomyxoviruses and Paramyxoviruses

	Orthomyxoviruses	**Paramyxoviruses**
Members	Influenza virus	Parainfluenza virus Mumps virus Measles virus Respiratory syncytial virus
Diseases	Influenza	Parainfluenza, Mumps, Measles and Respiratory syncytial virus infection
Shape	Spherical/filamentous	Pleomorphic
Size	80-120 nm	100-300 nm
Genome	8 segment of RNA	Single piece of RNA
Nucleocapsid diameter	9 nm	18 nm
Antigenic variability	Significant	Minimal
Genetic recombination	Present	Absent

Highlight key historical features of Influenza infection.

A.4 (c) The study of Influenza virus seriously started, after the first pandemic of Influenza in 1918 at the end of 1st world war. The outbreak killed nearly 20 million people; more than the casualties of the war itself. The numerous techniques developed during its work, contributed significantly to the development of virology; as an exclusive important laboratory science.

The isolation of Influenza A in 1933 in Ferrets (an uncommon lab animal, used as model for Influenza) by Smith, Andrewes and Laidlaw was an important landmark. Burnett pioneered the use of embryonated egg for culture of viruses. This technique remained the standard system for study of viral multiplication and genetic interactions till early 1950s, when cell culture techniques became standard. The techniques of viral haemagglutination was accidentally discovered by Hirst, who tore a blood vessel (of the chick embryos), while harvesting Influenza-infected chick allantoic fluid.

Describe the types and subtypes of Influenza virus.

A.4 (d) Influenza virus has three genera, namely Influenza virus types A, B and C. The Influenza A is further subdivided into subtypes, based on H and N antigens. These subtypes are designated, according to the H & N antigens on their envelope, for instance H3N2 and H1N1. Of the hemagglutinins, three (H1, H2 and H3) and of neuraminidase, two (N1 and N2) appear to be of greatest importance in human infection.

Within each subtype, subtle differences in antigens (drifts) are designated by another nomenclature. The system includes the major Influenza virus type (as A/B), place of initial isolation, strain number, year of detection, followed by the antigenic subtypes, e.g., two strains of H3N2 of Influenza A virus that differ antigenically only slightly are called A/Beijing/1/78 (H3N2) and A/Hong Kong/1/79 (H3N2).

Diagrammatically depict the structure of Influenza virus.

A.5 (a)

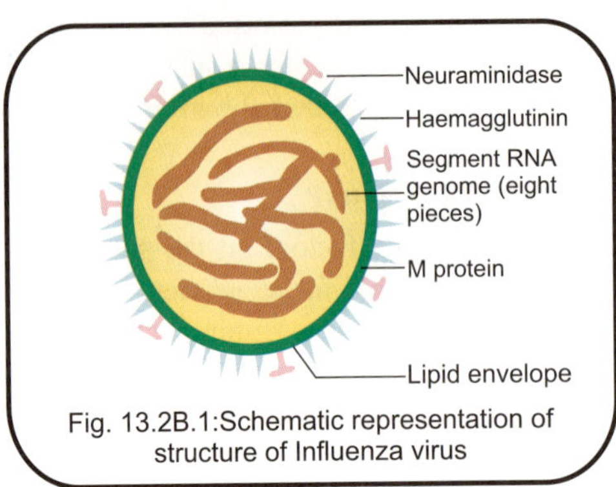

Fig. 13.2B.1:Schematic representation of structure of Influenza virus

Describe the structure of Influenza virus and enumerate the differences between haemagglutinin and neuraminidase.

A.5 (b) A schematic electron microscopic model of the virus is depicted in figure 13.2B.1. The shape of it is predominantly spherical or filamentous. The outermost layer is of the lipid bilayer of the envelope (from host cell, while budding), from which two types of spikes of peplomers project. The details of these peplomers; namely haemagglutinin and neuraminidase are covered in table 13.2.2. Inner to it; is the matrix (M) protein layer, which is believed to provide stability to the virion. Inside to the envelope are eight segmented pieces of RNA (seven in influenza virus type C). Each of this segments essentially, consists of negative sense single stranded RNA genome associated with nucleoprotein.

The Influenza virus share common internal proteins, as the nucleoproteins and membrane proteins but differ in their haemagglutinin (HA) and neuraminidase (NA) surface proteins. The characteristics of the HA and NA proteins is depicted in table 13.2.2.

Table 13.2.2: Characteristics of haemagglutinin and neuraminidase

HA	NA
• Present as triangular shaped projection	• Mushroom shaped projections
• 14 nm length	• 9 mm length
• More on virion (about 500 per virion)	• Number is less (about 100)
• Undergoes variation, which is of greater epidemiological importance	• Also undergoes variation
• 15 distinct subtypes (H1-H15)	• 9 subtypes (N1-N9)
• Causes stable haemagglutination at 4°C (of blood of many mammals and birds)	• Causes elution (reversal of haemagglutination, most rapid at 37°C, less active at lower temperature)
• Required for binding of virus to respiratory epithelial cells and RBC	Acts by destroying specific receptors on RBC, • Eluted viruses cannot agglutinate same RBC, i.e., process is irreversible, • Same virus can agglutinate fresh RBCs, • RBCs acted upon once by the virus, can again be re-agglutinated; by other viruses
• In *antigenic shift*, major changes in HA a.a. sequence. In *antigenic drift*, minor changes in HA a.a. sequence	• Major and Minor changes observed
• Antibodies are protective	• Antibodies are not that protective
• Antibodies act by preventing absorption of virus to cells	• It is postulated that these antibodies prevent release of virions from infected cells, thus limiting disease

Tabulate the differences between antigenic drift and shift.

A.6 (a)

Table 13.2.3: Differences between antigenic drift and shift

	Antigenic shift	**Antigenic drift**
	• Most antigenic determinants are altered	• Only certain antigenic determinant altered
	• Major alteration in H or N or both	• minor alteration in H or N or both
	• New subtype arises	• Remain same
Example	• In 1918, H1N1 arose from H3N8	• A/Beijing/1/78 (H3N2) arose from A/Hong Kong/ 1/79 (H3 N2)
In antigenic structure	• Sudden, drastic change	• Gradual, Sequential change
	• At Irregular interval	• At frequent intervals
**Due to*	• genetic *recombination	• Mutation in HA & N antigen
Role of immunity of population	• Antibodies to previous influenza strains, have no role in their detection/'neutralization'	• Antibodies have influence in their 'neutralization'
Causes	• major (sudden) epidemics and pandemics	• Periodic epidemics
Occur	• approximately every 8-10 years	• Occur at shorter duration (every 2-3 years)
Reinfection with same strain	• can occur after passage of long interval, when protective immunity wanes	• Can occur at short interval

*A cell infected with different Influenza A subtypes may yield progeny with antigens, derived from either of the two subtypes (including animal and bird strains)

It is very important to study this aspect, as this virus causes frequent outbreaks, epidemics and pandemics, with new antigenic strains; to which the population has no immunity. Hence; the enforcing authorities have always to be on the alert. Influenza A virus is most often associated with epidemics and pandemics. This is because Influenza A undergoes; frequent and almost annual antigenic variations. Influenza B virus is less often associated with epidemics and influenza C virus is not associated with epidemics.

Describe the epidemiology of influenza.

A.6 (b)

- **Source of infection:** Respiratory secretions of case or a subclinical case. The patient remains contagious 24 hours before the onset of clinical symptoms till about 48 hours after onset of symptoms.
- **Mode of transmission:** It is spread primarily, from one person to another; by droplet nuclei created by sneezing, coughing or talking.
- **Host:**
  - The infection occurs worldwide, although the rates vary markedly
  - *Age:* All ages are affected, although the mortality rate is higher in high risk groups; as elderly over 65 years of age and children under 18 months.
  - *Movement of man:* The modern modes of transport; as air result in fast spread of the infection.
  - *Immunity:* Resistance to infection is related to antibody against haemagglutinins. Man is susceptible to the new antigenic strains that emerge frequently.
- **Environment:**
  - *Season:* The epidemics usually occur in the winter months
  - *Overcrowding:* The attack rates are higher in close population groups; as schools colleges, other institutions etc.

NB: aspects of antigenic drift/shift and emergence of antigenic subtypes discussed in A.6a and 6c respectively.

Describe the emergence of antigenic subtypes of Influenza A in the last century.

A.6 (c) The epidemics that the mankind have experienced, since the last century are illustrated in table 13.2.4. It suggests an orderly recycling of the virus subtypes, as seen in one cycle that started in 1889-90, to be followed by a similar cycle starting in 1957-58.

Table 13.2.4: Emergence of antigenic subtypes of influenza A virus and their association with pandemics/epidemics

Year	Subtype	Antigenic variation	Severity of outbreak
1889-90	H2N2*	Antigenic shift	Pandemic
1900-03	H3N2*	Antigenic shift	Epidemic
1918-19	H1N1	Antigenic shift	Pandemic (severe)
1957-58	H2N2	Antigenic shift	Pandemic (severe)
1968-69	H3N2	Antigenic shift	Pandemic (moderate)
1977-78	H1N1	Antigenic shift	Pandemic (mild)
2009-10	H1N1**	Antigenic shift	Pandemic (severe)

*Based on retrospective serologic study of individuals alive during those years

**First major influenza outbreak of the 21st century (named 'swine' flu)

– Considerable evidence exists that 1918 strain arose from swine, 1957 and 1968 strains arose from birds (avian strain).

Usually severe pandemics occur, when major changes occur in both the major surface antigens of the virus, i.e., HA and NA. This was seen in the years 1918-19 and 1957-58. Such an event probably did not occur in 1977-78 probably because much of the world's population of the H1N1 era of 1918-1957 was alive and possessed protective immunity.

The designation of H2N2 of the strain that arose in 1957-58 was given to distinguish it from the previously prevalent strains of H1N1, to which it had no antigenic similarity. The strain that arose in 1968-69 had only a change in the HA antigen in comparison to strain previously endemic. In 1977, the changes occurred in both the major antigen, but it resembled a previously recognized strain, hence the name H1N1.

Explain the emergence of antigenic drift and shift in a community using a hypothetical Influenza virus structure.

A.6 (d) In the period after a major shift, the virus undergoes antigenic drifts at steady rates. The human body, responds to a new viral isolate, by producing antibodies and getting immune to the new isolate. Let's study a hypothetical occurrence of Influenza epidemic with respect to immunity status in the population. Let's say the AHyNy virus causes pandemic. The immunity of the population to it, increases in the next few years. This makes conditions favourable for a strain of AHyNy with minor variations (antigenic drift) to emerge in the environment. This may or may not cause an outbreak. If it does, the population becomes immune to it, in the next few years. This process of new strains with minor antigenic variation arising and causing outbreak/ epidemics in the population (with subsequent immunity) continues for 10-20 years. At this stage, the immunity level to all minor variants of virus is high. This creates favourable conditions for a new subtype (major variant) of influenza virus A Hz Nz to arise, which may not have circulated for many decades amongst the humans. This arises; as accumulated changes in antigenic sites are no longer neutralized by existing antibody. This cause another pandemic. This process may take a decade or longer.

Could antiviral drugs be used in this case of Influenza?

A.7 (a) As the case has presented early and has systemic presentation, antiviral drugs may play a part in decreasing the severity of the disease.

Enumerate the drugs available against Influenza and mention their mechanism of action.

A.7 (b) Specific antiviral drugs; as amantadine and rimantadine are available, for use early in disease (within in 48 hours of onset). These agents prevent viral penetration of target cells (or uncoating, target of action is M2 protein). They can reduce the duration of systemic and respiratory symptoms of influenza by ~ 50%. However; minor CNS side effects; such as insomnia and dizziness have been reported in some cases. Resistance in Influenza A to the above two drugs have been reported.

- Zanamivir and Oseltamivir, which are neuraminidase inhibitors are available for Influenza A and B
- Antibacterial drugs should be reserved for secondary bacterial pneumonias, if they develop.

Why should aspirin not be used, as antipyretic agent in children with viral infections?

A.7 (c) It may cause Reye's syndrome in children with viral infections. So, antipyretics; as acetaminophen should be used in them.

Could this infection of Influenza have been prevented?

A.8 (a) Yes, the infection could have been prevented, if the case had received Influenza vaccine. But usually, the children are not administered these vaccines, as these may not be cost effective, their administration would add to the number of vaccine injections to be adminstered, besides other reasons.

What should be the composition of Influenza vaccines commonly available?

A.8 (b) The vaccine has to be administered annually and the strains to be included should be subtypes HIN1 and H3N2 of

Influenza A and Influenza B, respectively. The antigenic composition of the vaccine should be determined by the types of viruses in circulation in the previous season.

Details: Pg. 634-635, Section 17

What role such vaccine can have in the promoting the economy of the country?

A.8 (c) Administration of Influenza vaccines can decrease the morbidity and mortality, due to this viral agent. This could save millions of rupees that would have been lost, as a result of loss of working human hours and investment to fight the sporadic and outbreak Influenza infections.

Enumerate key preventive strategies for Influenza.

A.9 (a) (i) Adequate respiratory hygiene

(ii) Chemoprophylaxis in high risk population (with amantadine etc)

(iii) Antiviral vaccine adminstration

(iv) Global surveillance of Influenza virus in human and other reservoirs

(v) Yearly manufacture of vaccine with the existing prevalent strain

(vi) Prediction of the antigenic drift and shift in the Influenza virus

(vii) Adequate hygiene

What is the basis of the hypothesis that has led to the recommendation of keeping pigs, birds and humans separately, as far as possible to prevent development of Influenza pandemic?

A.9 (b) The major antigenic shifts result in pandemics because the population has no immunity to the 'new' viruses. The antigenic shifts result in the introduction of a 'new' segment of RNA, resulting in new surface glycoprotein antigens. Genetic reassortment could explain these changes and this phenomenon has been seen in the Influenza A viruses in eggs and tissue cultures. But where does this process (reassortment) occur in nature? It is well recognized that human influenza A does not easily spread to birds and vice versa. So; it is likely that another species may act as intermediate host. This species is likely to be swine, which acts as host for both avian and human viruses. One unique feature of the 1957, 1968 and 1977 pandemics is that they all began in mainland China and then spread to both east and west. One hypothesis to explain this phenomenon, is that Influenza viruses in China can be isolated almost through out the year in the setting of swine, birds and humans living under the same roof, providing sufficient opportunity for the admixing of the avian and human Influenza viruses in swine. This hypothesis has led to the recommendation of keeping pigs, birds and humans separately, as far as possible.

Integrated Clinical Based Study of Influenza Virus/'Avian Flu'

In January 2008 in West Bengal (India), an outbreak occurred in poultry (hen and ducks), which resulted in over 1 lakh fowl deaths. To control the outbreak, over 10 lakh hens and ducks were culled (killed), by over 900 teams, that were sent by the Government of India in the same month. The livelihood of thousands of families got affected, who depended on 'backyard' poultry. Prices of chicken came crashing down to that below of vegetables and people stopped having their favorite chicken dish (including eggs) in restaurants and at home.

Linkages: Pg. 368, 435, 497

What was the virus that was implicated in the above outbreak?

A.1 (a) It was an avian subtype of influenza virus.

How is it designated?

A.1 (b) It is designated as H5N1, which is a subtype of influenza A virus. 'H' stands for haemagglutin and 'N' stands for neuraminidase. The numbers represent the subtypes for the two surface proteins.

Where was the diagnosis of the 'avian' influenza outbreak confirmed?

A.1 (c) The specimens from the infected birds were sent to high security animal disease laboratories (HSADL) in Bhopal and National Institutes of Virology in Pune, where laboratory confirmation of this disease occurred.

Why do only few labs perform such confirmatory tests?

A.1 (d) The laboratory should have a high biosecurity level (BSL); as exists in the above two labs, so that the laboratory personnel don't get infected with exotic viral agents and the local environment also doesn't get contaminated with it. The (HSADL) lab at Bhopal has BSL 4 facility.

What is a common differential diagnosis of this disease?

A.1 (e) Ranikhet disease

Why was there so much concern about the 'avian' influenza outbreak?

A.2 It was due to the following reasons:

(i) Economic loss to people

(ii) Ecological imbalance with loss of so many birds

(iii) Spread of the disease to neighbouring states and countries and possible emergence of a pandemic (if reassortment of genes between epidemic human strain and lethal avian strain occured)

(iv) Spread to human from infected birds

(v) Possibility of high case fatality rate in man, as man may not have protective (antibodies) immunity against this virus.

(vi) Possible spread of infection from human to human, if the virus undergoes reassortment of genes and/or has mutation.

(vii) No human vaccine is in common usage.

What was the reason for culling of these birds?

A.3 (a) The infected birds represented the animal reservoir for this virus.* Culling of the birds would reduce the risk of spread of the virus to other birds and humans. This would also prevent the emergence of a new virus by reassortment and/or mutation.

*culling means a deliberate killing of animal

What technique was employed to cull the infected birds?

A.3 (b) The neck of the bird was pulled and then twisted to silently kill the birds. The process resulted in a deliberate dislocation of the cervical vertebral column of the animal; resulting in the destruction of its spinal cord.

What was the advantages of this technique?

A.3 (c) The advantage of this technique was that no blood spill occurred; which minimized the risk of viral contamination.

What were the culling teams equipped with?

A.4 Each member of the culling team was equipped with a personnel protective equipment kit, which consisted of N95 mask (filters particles larger than 1micrometer with efficiency of 95%), gloves and oseltamivir (tamiflu) tablets.

How were the culled birds disposed?

A.5 (a) The culled birds were put in a pit, which was at least nine feet deep. It was then covered with lime and sodium hypochlorite, which was then covered with a thick layer of earth.

What was the importance of following this technique?

A.5 (b) The importance of this technique was that the virions of the killed birds are destroyed and their spread was minimized.

How were the local people motivated to hand over their live birds; which were the source of livelihood, to the government personnel for culling?

A.6 (a) In camps set up near the villages, the local people were encashed of the compensation slips, they were given in exchange for the hen. For a hen producing egg, the compensation slip was Indian Rupees 40.

What advise was given to poultry workers on sick farms?

A.6 (b) They were advised to wear gown, face-mask and goggles for protection. The poultry workers could wear shoe covers, so that shoes did not carry the virus.

How can such 'outbreak' scenario be prevented in the future?

A.7 The susceptible birds can be vaccinated against this virus. This wouldn't result in the elimination of this virus from the birds but would prevent new birds from this disease, by the induced protective antibodies. There has to be an effective surveillance that should result in improved communication network; between the villages, the veterinary hospitals and laboratories, so that an outbreak can be nipped at the early stage, before it becomes a big problem. This approach has been followed in China, Hongkong and other places.

What is the I.P. of 'avian' influenza?

A.8 1-5 days

How do you define a probable human case of 'avian' influenza (H5N1) infection?

A.9 A possible case of influenza has limited laboratory evidence of influenza A/H5 infection (positive laboratory confirmation of influenza A infection but insufficient evidence of H5N1) or no evidence of another cause of disease.

What advice do you give to international traveler visiting a place having an 'avian' influenza outbreak?

A.10 The traveller should avoid poultry farm and contact with animals in live food market; including surfaces that are contaminated with faeces of poultry or other animals.

Respirovirus and serotypes 2,4a and 4b belong to genus Rubula virus. It is an enveloped, single stranded RNA virus with minus sense and helical symmetry.

- **Pathogenesis:** The transmission occurs by droplets and contact with respiratory secretions. The incubation period is a few days. The virus multiplies and is responsible for various respiratory syndromes.
- **Pathogenicity:** One of the important syndromes caused by it in infants and young children, is laryngotracheobronchitis (croup). The patient can present with fever, cough and respiratory obstruction, so may require emergency tracheostomy. Pneumonia is also occasionally caused by these viruses. Adults and older children also get affected, in whom the presentation is milder.
- **Laboratory diagnosis:**
  - *Specimens:* Exfoliated cells from respiratory samples; as BAL and lung tissue
  - *Direct demonstration of virus:* By immunofluorescence staining, using monoclonal antibodies
  - *Isolation of virus:* Primary monkey kidney cell line is used for isolation. However there is little (or no) cytopathogenetc effect on the cells. The viral growth is detected by haemadsorption, using guinea pig erythrocytes or shell vial technique
  - *Serology:* ELISA or haemagglutination inhibition test can be used to demonstrate specific IgM antibodies or four fold rise of IgG antibodies
- **Vaccines:** Trials are in progress. No specific antiviral drugs are available.

Describe:

(i) Nipah virus, (ii) Hendra virus, (iii) Human metapneumovirus

A.12 (i) Nipah virus

- *Features:* Similar to Paramyxoviruses. It was first identified in 1999 in a pig farm in Malaysia.

It caused a neurological and respiratory outbreak in pigs, which also spread to man and caused more than 200 deaths. To control this outbreak, one million pigs were culled (killed). Subsequently outbreaks in Bangladesh and neighbouring parts of India has been reported. An outbreak in Kerala (India) occurred in May, 2018.

- *Reservoir:* Fruit bats (flying fox)
- *Transmission:* Close contact with infected pigs
- *Pathogenicity:* To be considered, as a rare cause of encephalitis. The disease can be mistaken; as Japanese encephalitis.
- *Importance:* The virus is of public health concern, as associated with high mortality. For the same reason, it has been categorized as a biosafety level 4 pathogen.

(ii) Hendra virus

- *Features:* They are similar to Paramyxovirus. It was first discovered in Hendra, a suburb of Brisbane, Australia. It caused a respiratory disease outbreak in horses, which later also led to death of the horse trainer.
- *Reservoir:* Fruit bats (Flying fox).
- *Transmission:* Exposure to infected secretions of horses.
- *Pathogenicity:* Outbreaks in horses recorded.
- *Importance:* Public health concern.

(iii) Human Metapneumovirus

- *Features:* It is a single stranded RNA virus, like Paramyxovirus.
- *Distribution:* It appears to be distributed worldwide.
- *Pathogenicity:* It is a respiratory pathogen, first reported in 2001. It causes respiratory tract infection in children and adults, a disease similar to one caused by Respiratory syncytial virus.
- *Laboratory diagnosis:* Sample-Respiratory secretion
  Techniques-RT –PCR used for diagnosis
  -Cultivation of virus is difficult
  -Direct IF test available (to demonstrate viral specific antigens in nasopharyngeal secretions)
- *Treatment:* No specific drugs or vaccine is available

Integrated Clinical Based Study of Measles Virus/Skin Rash

A seven year old girl, Sarita presented to the paediatric OPD with fever, cough, coryza and macular rashes on the head. Her chest radiograph didn't reveal any abnormal finding. Her throat swab sent for bacterial culture did not yield any pathogens. Her blood was drawn for viral serologic examination. Acute and convalescent phase (obtained 3 weeks later) sera samples were collected.

Linkages: Pg. 368, 435, 498

What is the differential diagnosis of this case?

A.1 (a) The *viruses* that can produce macular/maculopapular lesions; as seen in this case could be due to Measles, Rubella virus, Human herpes virus type 6, Human herpes virus type 4 (E.B.virus), Human herpes virus type 5 (CMV), enteroviruses and parvovrus B19. The *bacterial* diseases that could produce similar picture would include infective endocarditis, secondary syphilis, scarlet fever, meningococcal infection, *Mycoplasma pneumoniae* infection and rocky mountain spotted fever. Toxoplasmosis and drug eruption can also mimic this picture.

Can a vaccination history of the case, help in making a clinical diagnosis?

A.1 (b) Yes; for instance, if the child has had measles vaccination, the girl is unlikely to have this infection.

What key complications can occur in a measles case?

A.1 (c) Commonly the case could have secondary bacterial respiratory infection, that could manifest; as pneumonia or otitis media. This could result due to loss of ciliary function and development of oedema in respiratory epithelium. The case could also have diarrhoea, as a result, of secondary bacterial infection. The most dangerous complication is *encephalomyelitis*, which occurs in about one in every 1000 cases, has a mortality of 15% and permanent neurological sequelae in many survivors. A very late rare (approximately one in every million cases) severe complication, that may develop is *subacute sclerosing panencephalitis* (SSPE). This may be caused by a defective measles virus or a variant of measles virus. It may progress slowly over months to years and present; as seizures, motor function disorders, coma and death. The case could also have a suppression of cell mediated immunity, which may manifest as activation of latent tuberculosis.

The paediatrician looks for an buccal lesion, the presence of which can help to make a specific clinical diagnosis.

What is the lesion that is expected? Describe it.

A.2 The paediatrician is looking for *Kopliks spots*, which is pathognomic of measles. They are described; as bluish spots on red base on buccal mucosa opposite first or second upper molar. They appear a day or two before the appearance of the rash and disappear, as the rash spreads from the head to the trunk and finally to the periphery.

The lesion is present in this case.

What rapid diagnostic tests can help to confirm the diagnosis of measles?

A.3 (a) (i) Giemsa staining of the nasal secretions would reveal, multinucleated giant cells (Warthin-Finkeldey cells) and inclusion bodies in nucleus and cytoplasm.

(ii) Measles antigen can be demonstrated, using fluorescent microscopy on respiration secretions; using specific fluorescent monoclonal antibodies tagged to fluorescein dye.

Describe the role of direct demonstration of virus and cultivation of virus in the laboratory diagnosis of measles.

A.3 (b) In respiratory secretion sample; as aspirate from nasopharynx,viral antigen can be demonstrated by fluorescent stain, using specific monoclonal antibodies.

The cell line that can be used for culture is monkey kidney or human kidney. CPE; as multinucleate giant cells can be seen in about 7-10 days. The isolate can be provisionally categorized; as measles, if haemadsorption occurs with chick RBCs and can be confirmed with fluorescent monoclonal antibodies.

Outline the serological techniques used in the diagnosis of measles.

A.3 (c) Serological techniques; as CFT, HI and IgM capture ELISA techniques are available.

Outline the laboratory diagnosis of SSPE.

A.3 (d)
- EEG (Typical changes) and MRI (brain).
- Direct demonstration test of viral antigen, based on fluorescent antibody test on neural tissue. (besides typical histologic finding)
- For isolation of measles virus, a co-cultivation technique is used. The isolation is difficult; as the virus is a defective one. Here a layer of affected brain cells are layered onto monkey kidney or other susceptible cells.
- High titers of complement fixing antibodies to measles in serum and CSF suggest, that these are produced in brain. (Also see pg. 498].

To which family and genus, does the measles virus belong to?

A.4 (a) Measles virus belongs to family Paramyxoviridae and genus Morbillivirus.

Mention the virion projections peplomers of the virion, that play key part in the pathogenesis of this infection.

A.4 (b) The haemagglutin (conical shaped) spikes mediates adsorption to cell surfaces and F protein (dumb-bell shaped) mediates cell fusion (Fig. 13.6.1). No neuraminidase spikes are present, so in laboratory work, the haemagglutination of RBCs, is not followed by elution.

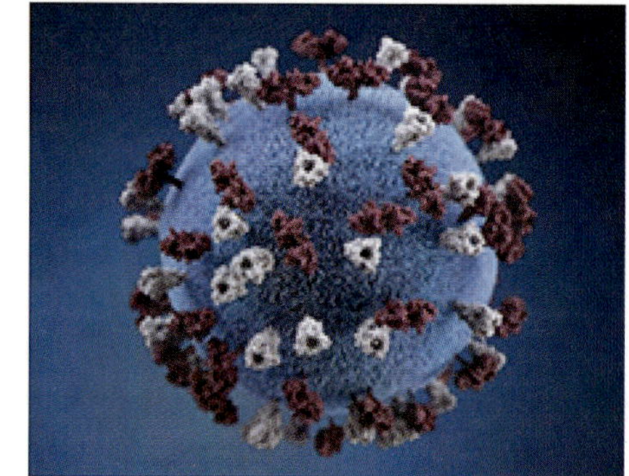

13.6.1: Measles Virus:A 3D graphical representation of a spherical-shaped measles virus, studded with H-proteins(haemagglutinin, tubercular studs, colored maroon) and F- proteins (fusion proteins, colored grey).These studs are embedded in envelope`s lipid bilayer

Courtesy: Allison M. Maiuri/CDC

Describe the pathogenesis of measles.

A.5 The infection spreads by respiratory secretions. The virus multiplies in the upper respiratory tract, local lymph nodes and enters blood stream *(primary viraemia)*. The virus then enters the reticuloendothelial system resulting in *secondary viremia*. The virus then reaches epithelial surface of skin, respiratory tract and conjunctiva. The rash is believed to be due to type IV hypersensitivity to viral antigens. The specific antibodies persist for decades making individual immune to reinfection.

How would you manage a case of measles (this case)?

A.6 (a) *Ribavirin* administered intravenously or an aerosol has been evaluated in immunocompromised individuals and severely affected adults. No, specific antiviral drugs exist for this disease and the case has to be managed symptomatically.

Does the supplementation of a diet with a particular vitamin have any role in reducing mortality, due to Measles infection?

A.6 (b) Yes, administration of vitamin A to children with measles can significantly decrease the severity of measles complications and reduce the mortality rate. In some countries, fortification of food items as bread, ghee/oil (margarine) and sugar has been done with vitamin A.

Mention about the epidemiology of measles.

A.7 (a) Man is the only natural host to the virus. The infected person is infectious, 3 days before the onset of symptoms till rash desquamates. The incubation period of the disease varies between 10-12 days.

What is the epidemiologic status of measles in the developed countries?

A.7 (b) In developed countries; as U.S.A., the incidence of measles is minimal. Many of the few cases that get reported in these places are seen in the immigrants to the population. This trend is attributable to more than 95% vaccine coverage amongst children entering school.

Can measles be eradicated?

A.7 (c) Yes, the disease is believed to be amenable to eradication. It would require one dose of the vaccine, which should cover at least 96% of the children aged less than 1 year. The accumulation of the immunization gap has to be prevented.

Discuss the logistics of the age, at which the measles vaccine should be administered.

A.7 (d) Antimeasles maternal antibodies can interfere with the seroconversion efficacy of the measles vaccine, if administered in infancy period. So, in developed countries, this vaccine is administered after 1 year. However, in developing countries, many cases of measles occur in infants, so a compromise is made and the vaccine is administered at 9 months. Such cases, may require another booster of the vaccine later on.

Describe the composition, indications, mechanism, side effects and contraindications of the measles vaccine.

A.7 (e) see pg. 635 Section 17

Can a child with measles infection be managed in a general paediatric ward?

A.8 No, as measles is a highly contagious disease and requires respiratory infection control measures, to prevent other children and staff from contracting this infection.

Aspect related to case theme/examination assessment

Describe Mumps.

A.9 Mumps

The mumps virus causes parotid gland enlargement (epidemic parotitis) and occasionally in severe cases; orchitis and aseptic meningitis. The term ‘mumps’ has been derived from the ‘mumbling’ speech of the patient.

- **Classification:** The virus belongs to family *Paramyxoviridae* and genus *Rubulavirus*. It is an enveloped, single stranded RNA virus with minus sense and helical symmery. It has a single serotype.
- **Epidemiology:** Man is the only reservoir. The infection spreads by direct contact with infected saliva or aerosol. It is less infectious than measles or chicken pox. Children between 5-10 year age group are more affected than adults, but when the latter get affected, the disease is more severe and complicated.
- **Immunology:** Immunity is life long after single attack either by infection or vaccine. A single serotype of this virus exists.
- **Pathogenesis:** The I.P. varies between 16-18 days. The virus after entry via the respiratory tract multiplies in the epithelial cells of the nasal and upper respiratory tract. Viraemia results and the virus spreads to salivary gland, testes, brain and other sites.
- **Pathogenicity:** Bilateral *parotid gland* enlargement is the commonest presentation occurring in 70-80% of cases. This results in a distorted face, having difficulty in eating and a mumbling speech. Epididymo-orchitis is the next common presentation of mumps. This is followed by complications such; as meningitis, meningoencephalitis, pancreatitis, polyarthritis and nephritis.

  In about one third cases, the case remains asymptomatic.
- **Laboratory diagnosis:** The case is usually classical and does not require laboratory help. The atypical case with meningoencephalitis presents a diagnostic challenge. The outline of the diagnosis is depicted p. 498.

  Specimen: Saliva, oral swab, swab from orifice of Stensen’s duct, throat swab, urine (one of the rare viruses to be isolated from it) and CSF.

  Direct viral antigen demonstration: In samples of saliva or throat swab by immunofluorescence staining.

  Viral isolation: Monkey kidney cell line or HEp2 lines are traditionally used. The CPE appears in the cell line in 7-10 days in the form of multinucleated giant cells, representing both intranuclear and intracytoplasmic inclusion bodies. Haemadsorption can also be demonstrated with chick/guinea pig RBCs.

  Serology: Traditionally CFT and haemagglutination tests were used to demonstrate specific antibodies but these are seldom used now. Different ELISA formats are used to detect specific IgM and IgG antibodies.

  Molecular biology test: Reverse trancriptase PCR is available to detect specific mRNA from clinical samples.
- **Treatment:** No specific antiviral drugs are available
- **Vaccine:** see pg. 636, Section 17

7 Integrated Clinical Based Study of Rabies Virus/Rabies

A 6 year old girl, Shabana staying in a village of the Kanha area of Madhya Pradesh (a state in central India) reported to the primary health center with myalgia, episodes of hyperactivity and aggression. The parents report that she was bitten by a cat three weeks back, the animal was not traceable. The physician suspects it to be a case of rabies.

ZERO BY 30 (Goal of zero human deaths from canine rabies by 2030—WHO

Linkages: Pg. 368, 435, 498

What is the differential diagnosis of this case?

A.1 (a) The differential diagnosis in this case is rabies, and other causes of encephalitis caused by herpesviruses, enteroviruses (as Coxsackie, Echo) and arboviruses (as Japanese encephalitis).

Describe the structure of the rabies virus.

A.1 (b) The basic characteristics of the virus are represented in Figs. 13.7.1 and 13.7.2. The bullet shaped virion has one end conical/spherical and the other end flat (measures 180/75 nm approximately). Outermost is the bilayered lipoprotein *envelope*, derived primarily from the host cell membrane (virus buds from cytoplasmic membrane). From this, project knob like *spikes* (9 nm long); composed of glycoprotein covers the entire surface of the virion except the planar end. The importance of these, is that these are utilized in the production of the subunit rabies vaccine. Inside to it is the helical nucleoprotein (nucleocapsid) core consisting of numerous (30-35) coils. The importance of this is that the Negri bodies are essentially composed of this nucleoprotein. So antinucleocapsid antibodies are useful in detecting rabies specific intracytoplasmic inclusions (Negri bodies) by immunofluorescence techniques.

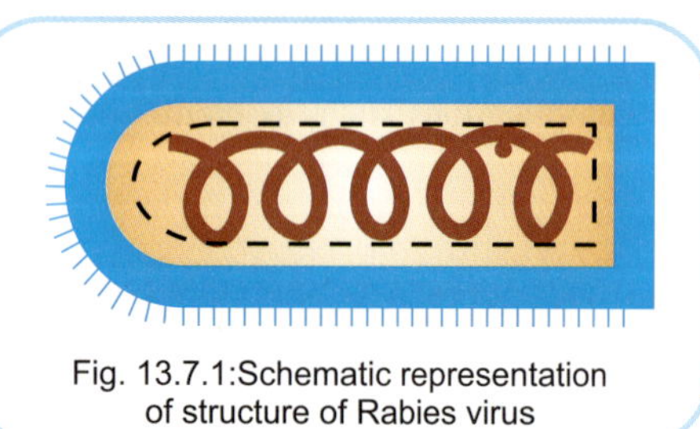

Fig. 13.7.1:Schematic representation of structure of Rabies virus

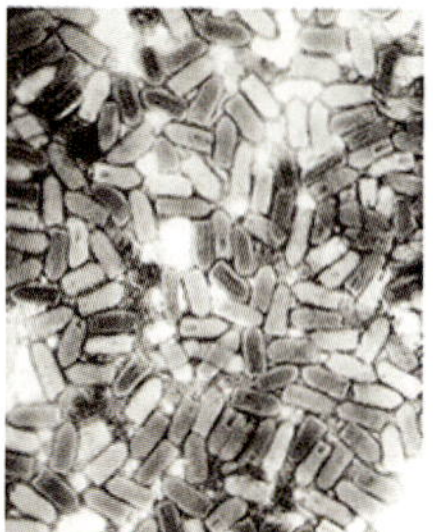

Fig.13.7.2: Rabies: Electron microscopic image

Courtesy: Fred A. Murphy/CDC

Differentiate between the two forms of the rabies virus.

A.1 (c) The rabies virus exists in two forms. One is the *street virus,* which has been isolated from natural human or animal infection cases. The other is the *fixed virus,* which has been obtained after several intracerebral passages in rabbit and becomes fixed as far as the incubation period is concerned. The differences between the two are depicted in table 13.7.1.

Table 13.7.1: Characteristics of Street and Fixed rabies viruses

Street virus	Fixed virus
• Can cause fatal encephalitis in laboratory animal by any route	• More neurotropic (Less infective by other routes)
• Fatal encephalitis produced after long and variable IP of 1-2 weeks	• I.P. is fixed, 6-7 days
• Cause neuroparalysis	• Loses neuroparalytic potential
• Not used for vaccine production	• Used for vaccine production
• Negri bodies can be demonstrated in animal infected and dying of 'street virus' infection.	• Negri bodies are not usually demonstrable in animal dying of 'fixed virus' infection

To which family does rabies virus belong? Describe briefly.

A.2 (d) Rabies virus along with the other rhabdoviruses, belongs to the family *Rhabdoviridae*. The latter family has viruses, which infect not only many vertebrates, but also insects and plants. Two genera exist in this family, namely:

1. *Vesiculovirus* – includes vesicular stomatitis viruses, Chandipura (arbovirus), Mokola and other viruses.
2. *Lyssavirus* (Lyssa, means rage or madness) – this genus contains rabies virus (rabidus, means mad), which causes rabies.

Describe the epidemiology of rabies.

A.2 (a) Rabies is primarily a *zoonotic* disease. Human rabies is reported from all continents except Australia and Antarctica. In India, Andaman and Nicobar island and Lakshadweep islands are free of rabies. Many countries including the United Kingdom, Japan, Sweden and some other countries have been reported to be free of human rabies. A rabies free area is defined; as an area in which no case of indigenously acquired rabies has occurred in man or any animal species for 2 years. This has been possible because of control on import on animal (including pets) and stray animals (as dog) and mandatory vaccination of pets.

However this data should be considered relative due to many reasons; including potential animal translocation events, capacity of rabies reservoir animals; as bats to travel long distances, lack of adequate diagnostic facilities in these places and reluctance of the national authorities to change respectable position of rabies free country status.

The *reservoir* of this virus are wild animals; as mustelids and viverrids (most warm blooded animals). The virus is ubiquitous in distribution except for some islands. These are three epidemiologic forms of rabies. One is the *sylvatic (jungle) rabies*, which accounts for maintenance of the reservoir of this virus. The virus survives in the reservoir population by remaining in a latent stage, with occasional activation, to be shed partly at any one time. From these reservoir species, the wild vectors, as foxes and jackals acquire the infection and infect in turn the domestic animals. This is responsible for the rabies in domestic dogs, cats and some high risk individuals, who come in contact with these wild animals. The high risk individuals include army people, hunters and veterinary personnel, who must take antirabies vaccine.

The other type is the *urban rabies* propagated chiefly by the bite of unimmunized (rabid) pet dogs and cats. The *third type* is the rabies, which is seen in certain Latin American countries; as Brazil and Mexico. Here the transmission to man has been reported in caves infested with bats via aerosol route.

Besides wild animals, vampire bats are a major reservoir of rabies in South America. They are responsible for death of thousands of cattle annually in that region because of their bite. These bats have been also responsible for causing occasional rabies in speleologists (who study scientifically the caves) of USA and S. America, who inhale their secretions; while working in the infested caves.

Modes of transmission:

(1) *Animal bites*: In India, most of the human rabies cases occur from dog bites. In USA, cat rabies is more prevalent. The possibility of contraction of rabies occasionally from other animals, as monkey and sheep should be borne in mind.

(2) *Licks*: Licks on abraded skin and mucosa, by dogs can transmit the disease.

(3) *Aerosol*: Such transmission has been reported in some countries; with caves infested with bats.

(4) *Transplantation*: Report of transmission by corneal transplants has been reported.

(5) Man to man: In man the disease is a 'dead end' but few case reports of such transmission are reported. All age groups are susceptible, however the disease in most common in children.

(6) Consumption of milk of infected animals (anecdotal reports).

Is rabies transmitted by cats?

A.2 (b) Yes, Warm blooded animals as cats, foxes etc. can transmit this infection, although in our country dogs are the commonest animals involved in transmission of human rabies.

In which country is rabies transmission by cats, commoner than by dogs?

A.2 (c) In U.S.A.

What bacteria can be transmitted to man by a cat bite?

A.2 (d) *Pasteurella multocida* and *Bartonella henselae*

Which countries are considered rabies free? How is a 'rabies' free area defined?

A.3 (a) Mammals of Antarctica are free of rabies. Some island countries; as Australia are considered to be *rabies-free. A few cases have however been reported from these countries.

*A 'rabies free' area is defined; as an area in which no case of indigenously acquired rabies has occurred in man or animal species for 2 years.

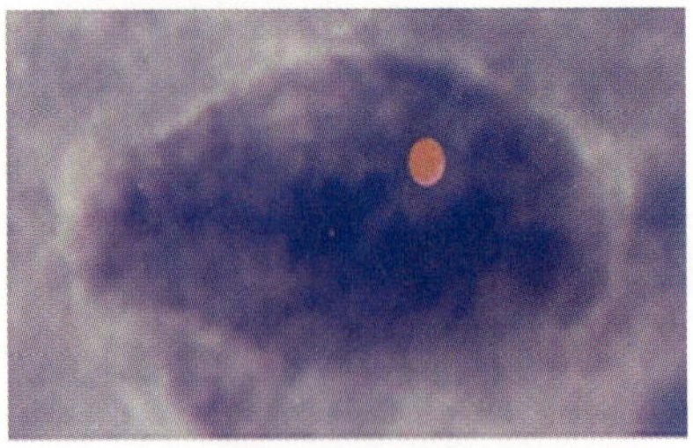

Fig.13.7.3: Negri body (Intracytoplasmic acidophilic inclusion body)

Which areas in India are considered rabies free?

A.3 (b) In India, Andaman and Nicobar islands and Lakshwadeep islands (U.T.) are considered to be rabies free.

Which part of the CNS in this case appears to be infected?

A.4 (a) The extreme behavioural changes in the case, indicate that the limbic system of the brain has got predominantly affected.

Tabulate the features of pathognomic lesion of rabies.

A.4 (b) The pathognomic lesion of rabies in the CNS is the Negri body (Fig. 13.7.3), whose features are listed in table 13.7.2.

Table 13.7.2: Features of *Negri body*

Characteristic	• Intracytoplasmic acidophilic inclusion body
Prevalence	• Present in 80% of rabies cases
Sites of brain, where most abundant	• Hippocampus and cerebellum
Size	• 3-27 µm
Shape	• Round/oval
Characteristic	• Pink structure with characteristic basophilic inner structures
Staining technique used	• Seller's (basic fuschin and methylene blue) – technique also result in fixation
Presence	• Mostly intracellular, however may be also extracellular
D/D	• Canine distemper (lacks inner structures)
Confirmation	• By IF technique using monoclonal antibodies (to nucleoprotein)
Diagnostic limitation	• May be absent in 20% cases having rabies

Note: Fixed virus usually does not produce Negri bodies in laboratory animal

Describe the pathogenesis of rabies in this case?

A.4 (c) The cat bite has likely driven the rabies virus-laden saliva into the striated muscles and/or the peripheral nervous system nerve cell endings, where the virion attaches and internalizes. The virus then spread up the nerves and spread centripetally to the anterior horn of spinal cord. From there, it reached the limbic system of the brain.

Describe the pathogenesis of rabies.

A.4 (d) Man essentially acquires the infection by bite of infected dog (in USA, cat rabies is more prevalent). Rabies can occasionally also be acquired by aerosol route, as has been seen in caves of S, America infested by bats. These are also reports of transmission by corneal transplant.

The *incubation period* of it varies from 7 days to >1 year (mean 1-2 months). Rarely cases with extended IP varying from 2-7 years have also been reported. The factors that could influence the length of IP; include the amount of virus introduced, quantum of host tissue involved (in the bite), host defense mechanisms and the actual distance that the virion has to travel to reach the central nervous system. The rates of infection and mortality are highest from the bites on the face and lowest from the bites on the legs.

The path taken by the highly neurotropic virus from the inoculation site to CNS is depicted in Figure 13.7.4 and 13.7.4a.

When the virion has multiplied and reached enough concentration to cross the n/m junction to enter the nervous system, it is not possible to halt the infection by immunization.

There is no haematogenous spread.

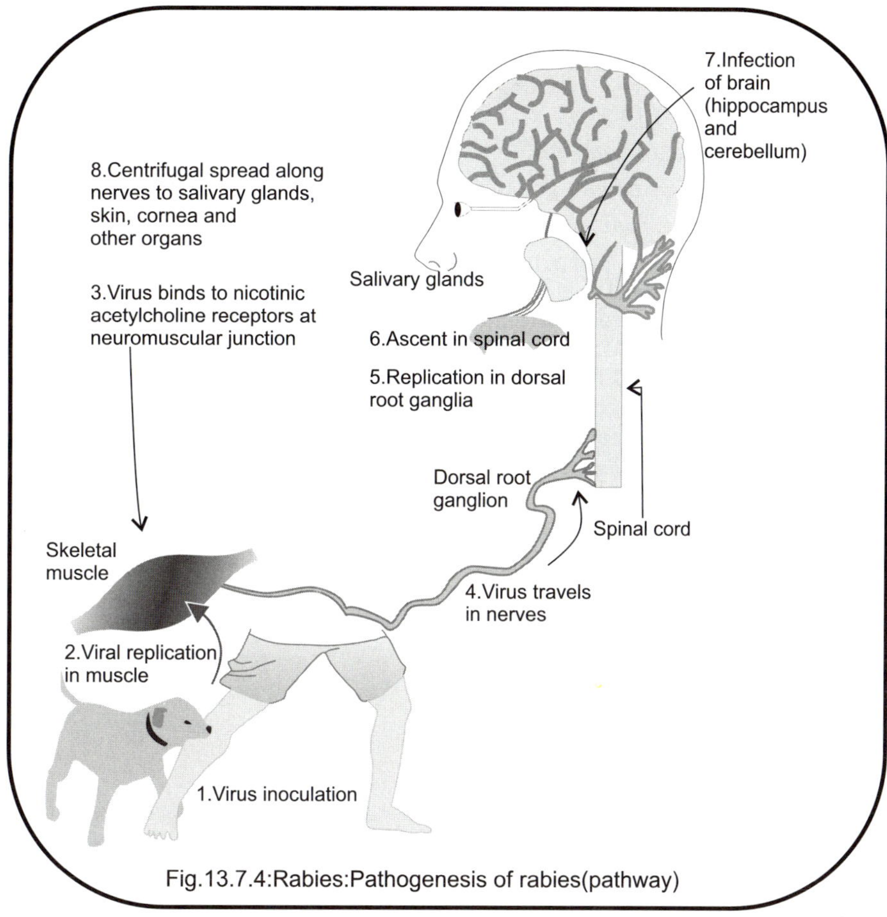

Fig.13.7.4:Rabies:Pathogenesis of rabies(pathway)

Virus introduced by bite of rabid dog in skin or deposited on mucous membrane.

↓

Viral replication in (striated) muscle (variability in IP is because virus can lie quiescently in muscle cell for varying periods)

↓

Virus enters peripheral nerves (travels 12-24 mm/day)

↓

Replication in dorsal ganglion

↓

Virus reaches (250-400 mm/day) anterior horn of spinal cord (after it, rapid ascent)

↓

Moves centripetally and reaches brain (including brain stem and cerebellum)
(Replication of it results in it hydrophobia, seizures and other CNS sign and symptom)

↓

Further virus descends and moves *centrifugally* to involve salivary glands, skin (as nape of neck) and other organs (results in perpetuation of the disease to other animal).

Fig. 13.7.4a: Ascending and descending path of rabies virus

Describe the basis of 10 day observation of suspected rabid dog.

A.4 (e) *In Dogs*: studying the sequence of events leading to acquiring clinical rabies is important, as it helps in accomplishing efficaciously the individual vaccination schedule of a rabies suspected case.

The event are summarized in table 13.7.3:

Table 13.7.3: Sequence of events in dog acquiring rabies

Day 1:	Dog bitten by a rabid animal
Day 6:	Rabies virus reaches dog's CNS (starting from peripheral nerves)
Day 9:	Virus reaches dog's salivary gland
Day 12:	Dog develops early signs of rabies and dies after 4-5 days.
	This data implies that animal takes about 3 days to develop signs of rabies after virus reaches it's salivary gland. So if a dog is observed for 10 days and doesn't develop any sign of rabies, it can be assumed that rabies virus wasn't present in the saliva of dog at the time of dog bite. Hence the basis of 10 days observation of a suspect rabid animal. *However* one must keep in mind, that occasional cases of human rabies have occurred in developing countries, where the dog remained apparently healthy for the 10 day observation (quarantine) period. There are *also reports* of asymptomatic long time rabies virus excretor in the dogs of India and Egypt.

Describe the clinical profile of rabies.

A.5 The disease presents; as an acute fulminant fatal encephalitis with rare survival. Classically the presentation is of the furious type. However, occasionally a paralytic (dumb) type of rabies may present; as an ascending paralysis resembling Gullian-Barré syndrome.

The clinical manifestations can be divided into four stages:

1. *Prodromal* (non-specific)
2. *Acute encephalitis*
3. *Brain stem dysfunction* and
4. *Death* (rarely recovery)

The symptoms of the prodromal stage probably reflect the virus entry into the CNS; usually at the dorsal root ganglion. Then picture is of *paresthesia and/or fasciculation around the site of inoculation of the virus, which is related to the virus multiplication at the ganglion. The other symptoms are fever, nausea, vomiting and headache.

*Abnormal sensation at bite site reflects localized nerve involvement.

Death is an eventuality in most rabies cases. The number of cases who have recovered are countable. The modern management; as intensive respiratory support can only prolong the life of the patient by few weeks. Death is usually due to respiratory paralysis (while the patient is conscious).

How can rabies infection be proved in the cat involved in this case?

A.6 (a) The cat in this case has to be isolated and sacrificed. An autopsy of the cat has to be performed in a biological safety cabinet, as it is a risky work. One part of the brain is put in 50% glycerol saline for isolation of virus. The other part is placed in Zenker's fixative (which has potassium dichromate and mercuric chloride) for Negri body demonstration.

What is the role of direct fluorescent antibody testing of the brain tissue in the diagnosis of rabies?

A.6 (b) Without performing this test, rabies cannot be ruled out from any animal tissue. In about 20% of rabies cases, however Negri body may not be demonstrated in the brain of the rabies cases.

Outline the laboratory diagnosis of rabies.

A.6 (c) See pg. 498, Chapter 16

What samples should be taken to confirm the diagnosis of rabies in the girl? Mention the tests that can be performed.

A.6 (d) The antemortem samples could; include corneal smear, conjuctival smear, saliva and full thickness skin biopsy from the nape of neck and/or face (including hair follicle).

The tests that can be run on these include direct fluorescent antibody test to detect rabies specific antigen and specific viral RNA/mRNA by reverse transcriptase PCR technique.

What is the basis of using saliva and conjunctival smear; as specimens in making an antemortem diagnosis of rabies?

A.6 (e) After the brain becomes infected by the virus, these sites are the first to get infected by the virus during its centrifugal spread, hence used in the antemortem diagnosis. The virus in these sites precedes or can accompany the development of early signs and symptoms.

What is the treatment approach for a case presenting with suspected bite with rabid animal?

A.7 (a)
- Wound immediately washed/flushed for 15 minutes (aim is to drive out any unbound virus).
- Wound can be disinfected with detergent, ethanol, tincture iodine or other virucidal substance.
- May infiltrate wound with specific antirabies serum in severe wound (antibodies may complex with virion and inactivate it).
- Tetanus toxoid.
- Antibiotic prophylaxis (if indicated).
- Wound to remain unsutured.
- No specific antiviral drugs available.
- Vaccine can be effective, if administered before the virus reaches the peripheral nerve, i.e., before the clinical onset. The administration of the vaccine, after the disease onset has no role, in fact the antibodies generated by it, may contribute to disease pathology.

What is the role of treatment in this case?

A.7 (b) The treatment in this case may only be helpful in alleviating the symptoms and would have no role in controling the viral infection or affecting the most likely fatal outcome in this case. In only six rabies cases till now, survival has been documented, after treatment was initiated.

What safety precautions should be taken, while handling a human rabies case?

A.7 (c) Safety precaution: person to person rabies transmission is rare but the aim is to prevent hospital staff exposure to rabies virus, which may be present in patient's saliva, tears, urine, and other body fluids. Standard precautions and respiration precautions; for respiratory suctioning are recommended. Health care workers (HCWs) with any cuts or other lesions should not be entrusted to look after rabies patient. The attendant should wear protective clothing; like apron, face-mask, rubber gloves and goggles, if warranted. Patient's secretions should be carefully swabbed and suitably disposed (as by incineration).

Why does this case appear to have poor prognosis?

A.7 (d) The virus has infected the central nervous system and the centrifugal spread of the virus in the body has most likely started. The infection has caused irreversible damage of the key neuronal anatomical areas.

What could have been done in this case that could have improved the chances of survival of this case?

A.8 (a) The girl should have been started on anti-rabies vaccine, immediately after the cat bite. As in this case, the cat is not available for observation, complete anti-rabies vaccine should be administered. The passive immunization should also have been started (see A8e)

Describe the first historical successful attempt of introduction of rabies vaccine.

A.8 (b) Before Pasteur developed the rabies vaccine, the management of the dog bites, included spine chilling cauterization of the wound by hot iron rod. This was probably, what moved Pasteur a chemist by training (not a physician) to use all his skills to develop the vaccine. Initially; the vaccine consisted of inactived brain and spinal cord of a rabies infected rabbit. Pasteur publicly demonstrated the efficacy of his vaccine, by saving the life of a peasant boy; named Joseph Meister in 1888 (bitten by rabid dog).

Classify categories of animal exposure and mention their significance.

A.8 (c) Classification of exposure

Category I	• Lick on intact skin • Touching/feeding of animals	No action, if reliable history is available
Category II	• Licks on broken skin • Minor scratch/abrasion	*Vaccination initiation + observe animals for 10 days
Category III	• Single/multiple transdermal bites • Contamination of mucous membrane with saliva	*Vaccination + RI_g as soon as possible, at distant site • Different 5 dose regimens available

* Gluteal region not to be used

Aim of classification

1. To decide plan of action and in past to decide dosage of nervous tissue vaccine. (WHO has now recommended discontinuation of nerve tissue vaccine)
2. To decide, if RIg is required

Classify the rabies vaccines in usage and mention about the intradermal regimen for rabies post-exposure-prophylaxis.

A.8 (d) see vaccine table at pg. 636, Chapter 10, Section 17

Conventionally the rabies vaccines are administered by intramuscular route. The intradermal regimen requires a reduced volume of vaccine to be utilized than any of the intramuscular regimens, resulting in reducing vaccine cost by 60-80%. This method may be considered in resource constraint situations.

Describe passive immunization in rabies.

A.8 (e) Passive immunization – Give Human rabies immunoglobulin (HRIG) – 20 IU/kg body weight

Or Equine rabies immunoglobulin (ERIG) (if human immunoglobulin not available)

Source of HRIG - obtained from rabies immunized human donors (is free of adverse effects; as anaphylaxis and serum sickness).

Indications

- All cases of category III exposure
- Can be considered in immunocompromised individuals of category II.

Sites

- As much as 50% of the calculated dose is to be infiltrated around wound site (if wound site is very small, amount to be infiltrated should be reduced).
- Other half approximately give intramuscularly (in thigh or arm), distant from that of the vaccination inoculation.

Omission of HRIG

(i) If case has received previously pre-exposure or post-exposure antirabies vaccine

(ii) If antirabies vaccination has been initiated and for about 2 weeks, HRIG has not been given. Late administration of HRIG is unnecessary, as by that time active antibody synthesis has started

What is the mechanism of action of rabies tissue culture vaccines?

A.8 (f) This vaccine generates an immune response; especially the antirabies antibodies, which impede the virus from reaching the central nervous system. The virus usually moves slowly in the nerve at a speed of approximately 3mm/hour. Rabies vaccine is a unique one, which helps to prevent the disease after exposure of the infectious agent has occurred.

What test is requested to assess the efficacy of pre-exposure rabies vaccine in a person?

A.8 (g) The post vaccine antirabies antibody titre should be estimated. If it is more than 0.5 I.U/ml in the serum, then one can assume that the vaccine administration has resulted in effective immune (protective) levels.

Enumerate strategies to control rabies.

A.9

- 'Leash laws' of pets (restriction of movement)
- Stray animal control ordinance
- Mandatory vaccination of pets
- Vaccine impregnated baits for wild animals
- Restriction on import of animals and quarantine
- Health education

Name some rabies related viruses.

A.10 They are antigenically different but give cross-reactivity with Rabies virus.

These do not appear to be protected by the rabies vaccine. The examples; include *Mokola virus* (report of two children infected with it), *Duvenhage virus* and others.

Integrated Clinical Based Study of Hepatitis A Virus/Jaundice

A 35 year old man, Sanjeev presented with passage of dark colored urine and clay colored stool. This was preceded by complaints of fatigue, fever and abdominal pain. The person gave an history of visit to Haridwar about three weeks back, where he often bathed in the Ganges river and consumed water that had not been filtered or chlorinrated. A hepatitis profile of tests were conducted on his serum, which revealed hepatitis B surface antigen, negative; hepatitis B surface antibody, positive; anti-HB core IgM antibody, negative; anti HAV IgM antibody, positive.

Linkages: Pg. 368, 435, 514

What is your clinical and microbiological diagnosis?

A.1 (a) The clinical diagnosis is one of jaundice. He is likely to have an acute hepatitis A infection (Infectious hepatitis); with past infection with hepatitis B.

Comment on the discovery and classification of Hepatitis A virus (HAV).

A.1 (b) Hepatitis A virus was discovered by Feinstone and colleagues in 1973 at the NIH, USA; from a patient's stool by immunoelectron microscopy. They found that these 27nm virions could be aggregated by convalescent, but not by preinfection serum of the patient. Subsequent biophysical and biochemical properties of it, led it to be classified as a member of Picornaviridae. Hence, it properties, resemble of the group (table 11.1.4, pg. 368 and Fig. 13.8.1). It was initially designated as 'enterovirus 72', but now due to its unique features is designated; as a new genus 'Hepatovirus'.

How many serotypes does HAV have? Mention the epidemiologic importance of this information.

A.1 (c) It has only one serotype throughout the world. This lack of serologic diversity has consequence in vaccine development and also explains the phenomenon of immune serum preparation to protect travellers from disease in various destinations. It also explains the lack of second HAV infection and lifelong immunity, after one attack of HAV infection.

What is the likely mode of his acquiring this infection?

A.2 (a) He is likely to have acquired this infection (I.P. 2-6weeks) through infected water, which would have gained entrance into him during bathing and/or drinking water.

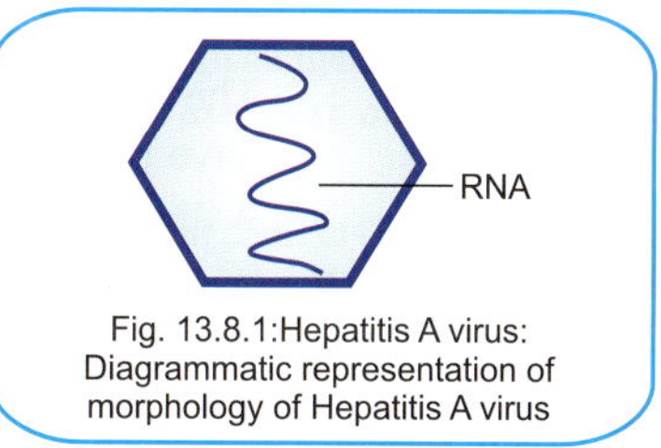

Fig. 13.8.1:Hepatitis A virus: Diagrammatic representation of morphology of Hepatitis A virus

Describe the pathogenesis of HAV infection.

A.2 (b) Its incubation period varies between 2-6 weeks, although determining this period is imprecise because the early symptoms are often vague and nonspecific. It spreads via the fecal-oral route. The virus is acid resistant and probably passes through the stomach unaffected and replicates somewhere lower in the intestinal epithelial cells. It spreads via blood to the liver, which is the major site of replication. The virus produced in the parenchymal cells and Kupffer's cell is excreted via the bile in large number (10^8 viral particles per ml) into the faeces; approximately 10 days before any signs and symptoms appear. From the faeces, it comes to the environment outside, where the virus can survive for weeks, in both fresh and salt water. Peak viral replication in hepatocytes is unlikely to explain the hepatocyte necrosis seen in the disease, as HAV is generally not cytopathic. The liver cell damage is likely to be explained by cell mediated immune response against the viral antigens. Exposure to HAV is almost 100% in developing countries before the age of 10 but the hepatitis in young children is usually subclinical and anicteric (without jaundice).

What is the cause of dark colored urine and of stool being clay colored in this case?

A.3 The dark color of the urine is due to bilirubinuria, besides; dehydration and clay colored stool is attributed to bile salts/ pigments normally present in stool.

9 Integrated Clinical Based Study of Poliovirus/Poliomyelitis

A 6 year old girl, Shanjana presented with acute onset of weakness/paralysis in her left leg in a remote place in western U.P., India in 2009. Examination of the case revealed fever and flaccidity (decreased tone of the muscle) of the limb but no sensory loss. The district authorities were very concerned.

Linkages: Pg. 368, 435, 500

What is your clinical and differential diagnosis of the above case? Discuss the possibility of case being one of poliomyelitis.

A.1 **(a)** The clinical diagnosis is one of acute flaccid paralysis. The differential diagnosis would include paralytic poliomyelitis, acute motor neuron disease (by enteroviruses other than polioviruses) and Guillain-Barré syndrome (symmetrical bilateral ascending paralysis with sensory loss).

Clinically; the case appears to be of paralytic poliomyelitis, as there is no sensory loss. The diagnosis of paralytic (spinal) poliomyelitis should be considered in any person, who has not received the polio vaccine, presents with fever, headache, back pain (including neck), asymmetric flaccid paralysis without sensory loss and pleocytosis (increased lymphocytes in CSF). The case could have been caused by the wild polio virus (PV) or could be one of vaccine derived paralytic poliomyelitis (especially in immunocompromised individual).

To which family does poliovirus belong?

A.1 **(b)** Picornaviridae (Pico, "small")

Classify picornaviruses, of medical importance.

A.1 **(c)** A.7b, pg. 368 Chapter 1, Section 11

Depict the structure of poliovirus.

A.1 **(d)** See figures 13.9.1 and 13.9.2

Classify the syndromes (diseases) associated with enteroviruses.

A.1 **(e)** **Table 13.9.1:** Syndromes associated with enteroviruses

Syndrome	Viruses
Neurologic	
Encephalitis	Many enteroviruses
Meningitis/Aseptic meningitis	Many enteroviruses
Paralysis	Polioviruses
Cardiac and Respiratory	
Myocarditis	Coxsackie B
	Coxsackie A (some)
	Echoviruses
Pleurodynia	Coxsackie B
Upper respiratory infection	Coxsackie A
Skin and mucosae	
Hand-foot and mouth disease	Coxsackie A
	Enterovirus 71
Herpangia	Coxsackie virus A
Ocular	
Acute haemorrhagic conjunctivitis	Coxsackie virus A, Enterovirus 71

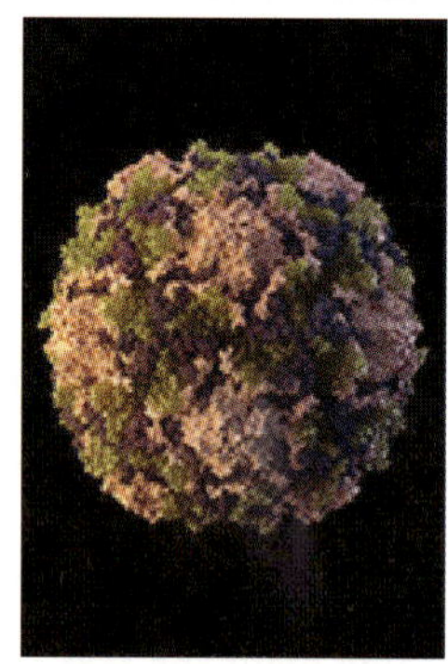

Fig.13.9.1: Poliovirus: A 3 dimensional representation of a single poliovirus virion. The capsid (protein shell) and RNA genome are illustrated clearly.

Courtesy: Meredith Boyter Newlore; James Archer/CDC

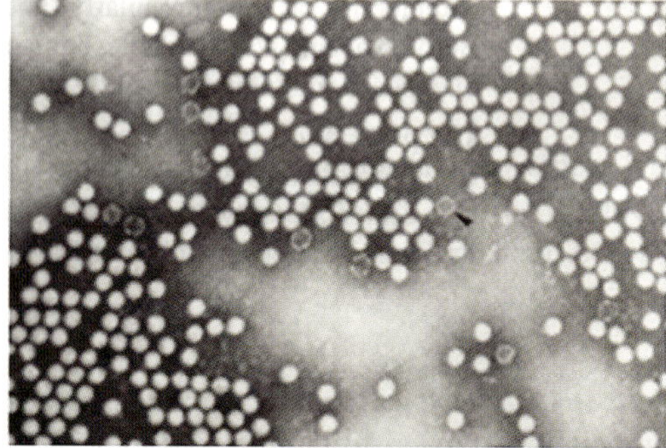

Fig.13.9.2: Poliovirus: Transmission electron micrograph of poliovirus

Courtesy: Dr.Joseph J. Esposito;F.A. Murphy/CDC

Why was the district health officer concerned?

A.2 (a) If the case was of paralytic poliomyelitis, it would have made India still be in the list of three polio-endemic countries. It would have indicated a lapse in Indian pulse polio programme. In 2014, India was declared as a polio free country, since no cases of wild polio were reported for three years.

Which were the polio endemic countries; as on 2014?

A.2 (b) Polio endemic area means, a place where wild poliovirus prospers and infects.

The three countries; as on 2014 were Nigeria, Afghanistan and Pakistan.

How can the diagnosis of poliomyelitis be made in this case?

A.3 From the case, faeces and stool swab can be taken and sent to the reference center for isolation of polioviruses. In the absence of a viral isolate, diagnosis of poliovirus can be established, serologically by demonstrating significant rise in the specific antibody titers in paired sera, using neutralization test. Serologic tests however cannot distinguish between wild type polio virus and vaccine virus infection. Outline at pg. 500, Chapter 16

How frequent is paralysis, as a presentation in poliomyelitis?

A.4 (a) It is a relatively infrequent complication of an otherwise trivial infection (seen in less than 1% of cases). Inapparent infection occurs in 90-95% of susceptible individuals following exposure.

Describe profile of minor illness and non paralytic poliomyelitis.

A.4 (b) About 5 percent of cases develop 'minor illness', which manifests as fever, malaise, sore throat and other associated symptoms.

Non paralytic poliomyelitis is seen in about 1-2 percent of cases, which manifests; as headache, neck stiffness and other symptoms indicative of aseptic meningitis.

Describe the pathogenesis of poliomyelitis.

A.5 (a) Man and some primates are susceptible to this infection. The spread, essentially occurs by ingestion; as depicted below

Ingestion (of virus)

↓

Multiplication in lymphatic tissue of oropharynx (tonsil) and peyer patch of gastrointestinal tract

↓

Reach regional lymph nodes (cervical and mesentric)

↓

Enter blood stream to cause primary viraemia

↓

Multiplication in R.E. system

↓

Secondary viremia

↓

Enter brain and spinal cord (by crossing blood brain barrier)

↓

Multiplication in neurons (essentially destruction of anterior horn cells of spinal cord)

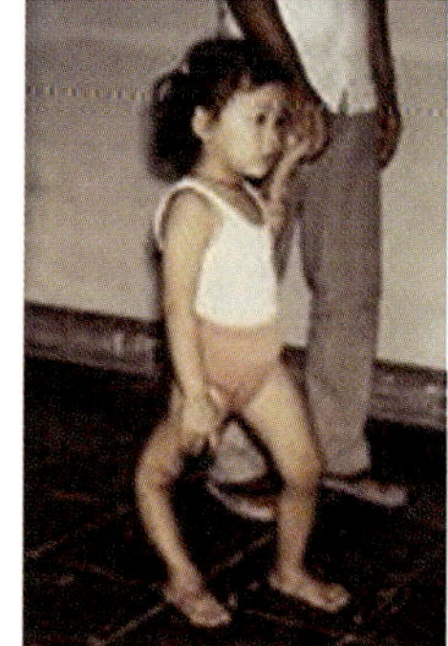

Fig.13.9.3: Child displaying a deformity in her limb due to polio

Courtesy: Centers for Disease Control, Atlanta, USA

Alternate route (rarely) is by entry of virus into motor neurons via peripheral neuromuscular junctions; as seen rarely after tonsillectomy cases in children.

Compare and contrast the presentation of spinal and bulbar paralytic poliomyelitis?

A.5 (b) *Spinal* paralytic poliomyelitis occurs essentially, due to lesions in the grey matter of the anterior horn of the spinal cord. The most characteristic feature is asymmetric distribution, affecting some muscles and sparing others. Clinically it manifests; as flaccid paralysis with usually no sensory loss. The most common pattern of involvement is single leg involvement followed by one arm. (Fig. 13.9.3)

The *bulbar* paralysis occurs, due to involvement of the motor nuclei of the pons and medulla. The cranial nerves most often involved are 9th, 10th and 12th. The manifestations; include dysphagia (difficulty in deglutiton), nasal speech and difficulty in breathing (dyspnoea). Rarely; the case can have combination of spinal and bulbar paralysis.

What is the most feared complication of paralytic poliomyelitis?

A.6 (a) It involves the respiratory tract and may manifest; as respiratory failure (occurs, when bulbar area is involved).

What is the cause of it?

A.6 (b) Respiratory failure may be caused by lesions of the respiratory centre, which may manifest; as irregular and shallow breathing. The other causes could be obstruction of airway, resulting from involvement of cranial nerve nuclei; especially of 9th, 10th cranial nerves or paralysis of respiratory muscles namely diaphragm and/or intercostal muscles.

How was respiratory paralysis managed in the past and how it is managed currently?

A.7 In the *past*, tank respirators (called 'iron lungs') were used to handle cases, having respiratory muscle paralysis. Despite the advantage of this approach not requiring tracheal intubation (which has complications), this technique is no more in use.

Currently techniques involving positive pressure ventilation are undertaken, which require tracheostomy. The latter procedure may involve many complications, but the technique permits an easy access to the patient.

Outline the laboratory diagnosis of poliomyelitis.

A.8 (a) See pg. 500, Chapter 16

Mention the molecular biology tests useful in laboratory diagnosis of polio.

A.8 (b) Nucleic acid sequencing and oligonucleotide fingerprinting, can be helpful in distinguishing a vaccine strain from a wild strain of polio/other enteroviruses.

PCR test can amplify viral RNA in clinical samples from CSF, urine, throat swab and can help in identification of enteroviruses other than polio viruses, from these samples.

What are the indications of using inactivated polio vaccine?

A.9 (a) This was used in some countries; as Sweden, Netherland, U.S.A. and other developed countries, where incidence of infection was low and risk of vaccine associated paralytic poliomyelitis outweighed advantages of oral polio vaccine. This vaccine was used in cases where oral polio vaccine is contraindicated; as immunocompromised individuals. This form of vaccine is preferred in persons over 18 years, as the risk of live virus associated paralysis is slightly higher in adults.

What are the indications of Salk (OPV) vaccine and mention its contraindications.

A.9 (b) The OPV (Sabin vaccine) is used in many countries in the immunization programme and in the epidemics.

The contraindications of its usage include

(i) Acute viral illness

(ii) Severe diarrohea and vomiting

(iii) Sensitivity to antibiotics used in vaccines; as streptomycin and neomycin

(iv) Severe reaction to previous dose

(v) Three weeks before or after the administration of normal immunoglobulins

(vi) Immunodeficency and malignancy cases

Compare and contrast the characteristics IPV and OPV (Sabin) vaccines

A.9 (c)

Table 13.9.2: Comparison of OPV and IPV vaccines

	OPV (Sabin)	**IPV (Salk)**
Route of administration	Oral	Parenteral
Type of vaccine	Live attenuated vaccine	Killed
Vaccination schedule	Initially three doses	Similar

Contd.

Contd.

Safety	Reversion to virulent form possible, resulting in disease; especially in immunodeficient	Reversion not possible
Economy	Economical	Expensive
Immunity	Systemic and local gut immunity	Only systemic immunity
Herd immunity induction	+	–
Immunity duration	Long	Requires boosters
Vaccine associated paralysis	+	–
Shelf life	Shorter	Longer
Sensitivity to heat	Extreme	Less
Control epidemic (ability)	+	–

What is vaccine associated paralytic poliomyelitis (VAPP)?

A.10 (a) As the name indicates, if the case has gets paralytic poliomyelitis, by the administered oral polio vaccine (instead of getting protected from the disease), it is designated VAPP. This can also occur is close contacts of vaccine recipients but does not cause community outbreaks.

What is the incidence of VAPP?

A.10 (b) The incidence is about 1 person acquiring per administration of 2.6 million OPV doses.

About 45% cases develop paralysis, after 7-21 days of the first dose.

What is the cause of VAPP?

A.10 (c) It is because of OPV vaccine strain gaining neurovirulence, as a result of nucleotide change in its genome, in the intestine of the vaccine recipient.

How do you differentiate a vaccine derived polio strain from a wild polio strain?

A.10 (d) It is essentially by RNA hybridization assay/Viral RNA sequencing.

Other tests that may be useful are:

(i) Virulence test in monkey: Administration of wild virulent strain intraspinally into monkey induces paralysis

(ii) Some markers; as wild strain grow well at 40°C, while vaccine strains do not.

What is the likelihood that in future no cases of polio would occur?

A.11 It is unlikely that no case of paralysis polio would be reported in the future, although their numbers would be negligible. This is because; as now the sewage water has high number of vaccine polio strains, at the cost of wild polio virus strain, so there is always a probability of the vaccine strains reverting to virulent state, infecting and causing polio. There is also a fear of importation of polio virus from countries, where polio has yet not been eradicated.

What was the requirement for India to be declared polio eradicated?

A.12 (a) India's prestigious 12000 crore pulse polio programme has made the polio eradication in India possible. The country needed to have no report of polio for three consecutive years to be declared polio eradicated.

What is Global polio eradication initiative?

A.12 (b) The global polio eradication initiative is an endgame strategic plan, which plans to deliver a polio free world by 2018.

Why is polio vaccination stil continuing?

A.12 (c) As the world is not free of polio and polio may re-emerge.

Many enteroviruses (other than polio and Coxsackie) exist, what approach is followed to diagnose them?

A.13 (i) Serologic diagnosis is limited due to large number of serotypes and lack of common antigen.

(ii) PCR approach is good, in which (broad) single pair of primers are used (sensitivity >92% and specificity 80%).

Aspects related to case theme/examination assessment

Describe:

(i) Echoviruses ***(ii) Coxsackie viruses***

(iii) Rhinoviruses ***(iv) Acute haemorrhagic conjunctivitis***

A.14 (i) Echoviruses

The term 'Echoviruses' represents enteric cytopathogenic human orphan viruses. As the name indicates, these viruses essentially infect only the humans.

- **Classification:** These are categorized into 28 serotypes, based on the neutralization tests.
- **Epidemiology:** Like other enteroviruses, they are spread primarily by the faecal-oral route.
- **Pathogenicity:** These were essentially designated as orphan viruses, because at the time of their discovery, no disease could be attributed to them. Currently these viruses are associated with encephalitis, aseptic meningitis, respiratory disease and myocarditis.
- **Laboratory diagnosis:**

  Specimens: CSF, Throat swab, Stool

  Techniques: They are broadly similar to as performed for the coxsackie viruses (excepting the infant mouse inoculation technique). Serologic diagnosis is challenging, due to numerous serotypes.

A.14 (ii) Coxsackie viruses

These viruses are named after the place of discovery, namely Coxsackie village, USA.

Classification: These are classified into two groups, namely group A and group B (table 13.9.3)

Table 13.9.3: Key characteristics of Coxsackie viruses

	Group A	Group B
Number of serotypes	21	6
Pathological changes after intracerebral inoculation into suckling mice	- Flaccid paralysis - Generalized myositis	- Spastic paralysis - Patchy focal myositis

- **Epidemiology:** Like other enteroviruses, the spread is primarily by faecal–oral route. Droplet spread is also known.
- **Pathogenicity:**
  - *Group A Coxsackie viruses*
    (i) Aseptic meningitis
    (ii) Herpangia (vesicular pharyngitis)
    (iii) Herpangia. Severe febrile pharyngitis, characterized by vesicles or nodules on the soft palate. (This entity should not be confused with pathogenicity of Herpes viruses)
  - *Group B Coxsackie viruses*
    (i) Aseptic meningitis
    (ii) Pleurodynia (Bornholm disease): It is essentially, myositis characterized by paroxysms of stabbing pain in chest and abdomen.
    (iii) Myocarditis and pericarditis: This is seen in all the age groups
    (iv) Juvenile diabetes: An association is seen with this entity
    (v) Neonatal infections: These can be acquired prenatally, natally or postnatally (from mother or nosocomially)
    (vi) Chronic (postviral) fatigue syndrome (epidemic neuromyasthenia, myalgic encephalomyelitis): An association has been seen with this entity.
- **Laboratory diagnosis**

  Samples: Blood, CSF, Faeces, conjunctival sample, vesicle fluid and others

  Techniques:

  (i) Infant mouse intracerebral inoculation (technique is diminishing)
  (ii) Cell culture of simian or human cell type. Characteristic CPE, as rounded refractile cells visible
  (iii) PCR-(broad-based primers)
  (iv) IgM serology
  (v) Neutralization tests-This is a technique used to type the isolates

A.14 (iii) Rhinoviruses

They are small RNA viruses that resemble picornaviruses, but differ in being more acid labile and heat stable. The virus has been named after 'rhine' (nose), the primary organ, which gets infected with this virus. Rhinoviruses grow optimally at 33°C, which is the temperature of the nose. The virus was isolated by Tyrell and colleagues in 1960.

- **Diseases:** They are incriminated in common cold, but the rhinoviruses are responsible for only about 50% of all the colds. More than 100 serotypes of this virus are known.
- **Pathogenesis:**

  The incubation period is 2-4 days. The disease spreads by respiratory secretion and via fomites from hands to nose and to the eyes. The viruses remain localized in the upper respiratory tract and cause inflammation, oedema and profuse exudation at the local site.
- **Immunity:** The person acquires specific immunity to the infecting serotype, which correlates to the local IgA antibodies. This immunity is however not beneficial, as the individual can get infected with rest of the (more than 100) serotypes and also get infected by the other viruses.
- **Clinical profile:** The case usually presents with sneezing, profuse watery discharge, nasal obstruction but no fever. The secondary attack rate is around 50%.
- **Laboratory diagnosis:** There is hardly ever a request to the laboratory diagnosis, as the disease is trivial and no specific antiviral drugs are available. However; the virus can be cultivated on human and monkey cell lines by incubating at 33°C. The viral antigen and RNA can also be demonstrated in the respiratory secretions by ELISA and PCR, respectively. Serology has only epidemiologic significance.
- **Treatment:** It is only supportive, as no specific antiviral drugs are available. This is really an enigma, as the medical science has progressed phenomenally, but has not yet been able to find a cure for common cold. However many pharmaceutical companies are pursuing the goal of finding a cure, as the prospects of earning is great.
- **Vaccine:** None is available

A.14 (iv) Acute haemorrhagic conjunctivitis

- **Historical:** In 1969, an outbreak of a new disease, namely acute haemorrhagic conjunctivitis was reported in West Africa. From this place, the disease spread to Asia including Japan, affecting more than 50 million people in a span of 2 years. At the time of the outbreak, the etiological agent could not be identified.
- **Epidemiology:** Many outbreak of this entity have subsequently been reported. The etiological agent of the outbreak of 1969 was later identified; as Enterovirus 70. The extremely short incubation period of less than 24 hours of this disease, may be one of the factors responsible for the occurrence of outbreaks with this viral agent. More than one million cases were involved in the 1971 outbreak of conjunctivitis in Mumbai, India.
- **Pathogenicity:** The disease is a self limiting one and as the name suggests associated with subconjunctival haemmorhage. Occasionally, transient involvement of the cornea (keratitis) occurs. Complete recovery of the case occurs within a week.
- **Complication:** In the outbreak, which involved India, radiculomyelitis was reported in a few cases.
- **Treatment:** No specific antiviral drugs are available. Only symptomatic management is possible.
- **Prevention:** As the disease is extremely communicable, implementation of hygiene is critical.

Section XIII: RNA Viruses

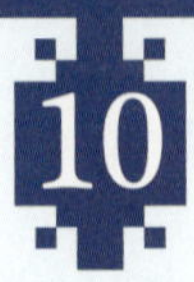

Integrated Clinical Based Study of Hepatitis E Virus/Outbreak

An outbreak of hepatitis occurred in Delhi in 1955-56, in which approximately 29,000 cases occured. The agent was then categorized; as enterically transmitted non-A, non-B hepatitis virus.

Linkages: Pg. 368, 435, 499, 514

What event led to the occurrence of this large outbreak?

A.1 (a) It resulted; as a result of the bursting of main sewerage line, which resulted in the contamination of the major drinking water source.

Why was the agent categorized, as epidemic of 'enterically transmitted non-A non –B hepatitis'?

A.1 (b) The cases who had this hepatitis had it an setting of an epidemic, related to ingestion and were negative for HAV and HBV.

Which virus was responsible for this outbreak?

A.2 (a) Hepatitis E virus was responsible for this outbreak.

Which group of workers were responsible for its discovery and what technique was used for its demonstration?

A.2 (b) *Balayan et al.* (1983) was responsible for the discovery. The technique that was used was immune electron microscopy of the infected stool, just like it had been used in HAV. However; there was an interesting aspect that the stool sample in which the HEV was demonstrated, was one of the investigators of the Balayan MS team, who had ingested the stool infiltrate, which was collected during an outbreak.

HEV was discovered in 1983, how can an outbreak of jaundice in 1955-56 be ascribed to this virus?

A.2 (c) The study of sera of the 1955-56 cases stored in deep freeze at the time of outbreak, revealed; when tested to be positive for HEV.

Describe the structure of HEV.

A.2 (d) This virus belongs to the family *Hepeviridae* (previously Caliciviridae) and genus Hepevirus. All the characteristics of the group were demonstrable in this virus, i.e., it is a single stranded, positive sense, non-enveloped virus with icosahedral symmetry. It is about 30 nm in diameter and spherical in shape. The genome is approximately 7.2 kilobases in length. It has not been cultivated in the conventional cell culture system.

What is the primary reservoir of HEV?

A.3 (a) The natural host is human, but water contaminated with sewage is the primary reservoir of this virus.

What is the likely reason for the low secondary attack rate of HEV infection in contacts of family members?

A.3 (b) It may be due to the increased lability of HEV virus in the environment.

Describe the clinical profile of HEV infection.

A.4 (a) The incubation period varies between 2-8 weeks. The presentation is one of acute self limited disease, that is often due to cholestasis. It does not lead to chronic hepatitis, malignancy or chronic carrier state. It is notorious for causing fulminant hepatitis and DIC in pregnant women, causing high mortality.

Compare and contrast the key clinico-epidemiological features of HAV and HEV infection.

A.4 (b) Infection with HEV has certain characteristics, though it resembles clinico-epidemiologically HAV:

- (i) It can cause large outbreaks; unlike HAV.
- (ii) Affects predominantly the adult population, unlike the HAV which affects the children and adults.
- (iii) Secondary attack rate is low, unlike in HAV infections.
- (iv) High mortality rate in pregnant women; unlike HAV infections.

(v) Sewage contaminated water is the primary reservoir in HEV infections.In HAV infection, spread occurs essentially from person to person by faeco-oral route.

Describe the pathogenesis of HEV infection.

A.4 **(c)** Infection spreads principally by the faeco-oral route. The natural host is human but water contaminated with sewage is the primary reservoir of this virus. The virus enters the body by ingestion, but it's route to liver from GIT is not known. The virus replicates in the cytoplasm of the liver. Most of the virus shed in the faeces is probably replicated in the liver. The virus is present in the bile and faeces during the late incubation period and one week after onset of illness. The pathogenesis of fulminant hepatitis and disseminated intravascular coagulation in pregnant women, especially during the third trimester is not known.

Describe the laboratory diagnosis of of HEV infection.

A.5 An outline of the diagnosis as depicted at pg. 499, Chapter 16. The diagnosis of acute hepatitis is essentially serologic, depending on demonstration of IgM-HEV antibodies or demonstrating a change of titers of IgG antibodies by ELISA.

The nucleic acid amplification assays may be rarely required in demonstrating the HEV-RNA in faeces and is detectable usually 2-7 weeks after onset. IEM demonstration of virions, does not have much role in a clinical diagnosis laboratory.

Are there any specific antiviral drugs or vaccine available for HEV?

A.6 No specific antiviral drugs or vaccine are available against this virus.

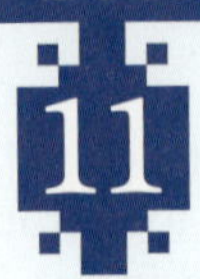

Integrated Clinical Based Study of Rubella Virus/Congenital Rubella

Examination of a two week old male neonate, Shrishti revealed cataract and hearing loss. The antenatal history of the mother was uneventful and TORCH investigation was not performed for her.

Linkages: Pg. 368, 436, 499

What is the likely clinical diagnosis in the above case?

A.1 (a) The case is likely to be one of *congenital rubella syndrome*.

To which genus, does the virus implicated in this case belong to?

A.1 (b) The rubella (German measles) virus belongs to *Togaviridae* (toga, greek for "mantle") family and to the '*Rubivirus*' genus. This virus unlike other viruses of Togaviridae, does not require a vector for transmission.

What is the likely pathogenetic mechanism involved in this case?

A.1 (c) Maternal rubella viremia during pregnancy, results in the infection of the placenta and the fetus. The cause of damage to cells and organs in this syndrome is not clear. The virus may just slow down the rate of cell division in the fetus. The slowing of the mitotic rate at critical stages in ontogeny, may affect the development of organs.

What is the classic triad of congenital rubella syndrome? Mention any other system commonly involved in it?

A.1 (d) The classic triad consists of cataract, deafness and cardiac abnormalities (commonly patent ductus arteriosus). Fig. 13.11.1, 13.11.2 The central nervous system commonly gets involved and can present as moderate to profound mental retardation.

What is the effect of the time of rubella fetal infection on the extent of teratogenicity?

A.1 (e) Maternal rubella viremia during the pregnancy may result in the infection of the placenta and fetus. Generally the earlier in the pregnancy the infection occurs, greater is the damage to the fetus. It is estimated that infection in the first trimester of pregnancy, results in fetal abnormalities in approximately 85 percent of cases in contrast to about 16% abnormalities; when infection acquired in the second trimester.

What is the microbiological approach to confirm the rubella diagnosis in the above case?

A.2 Congenital rubella can be diagnosed, by isolating the rubella virus or by detecting specific IgM antibodies in single serum sample or by demonstrating a significant rise of specific IgG antibodies in paired serum samples of infant. In biopsied tissue and/or other clinical samples; as CSF, rubella antigen can be demonstrated with monoclonal antibodies or rubella RNA can be demonstrated by 'in situ hydridization' or polymerase chain reaction. Intrauterine rubella infection is associated with persistence of virus in the newborn. At birth; virus can be easily isolated from throat swab, urine and other samples.

Could this disease have been prevented?

A.3 (a) Yes, this disease could have been prevented, if the mother of this neonate had received rubella vaccine. Details see pg. 639, Section 17

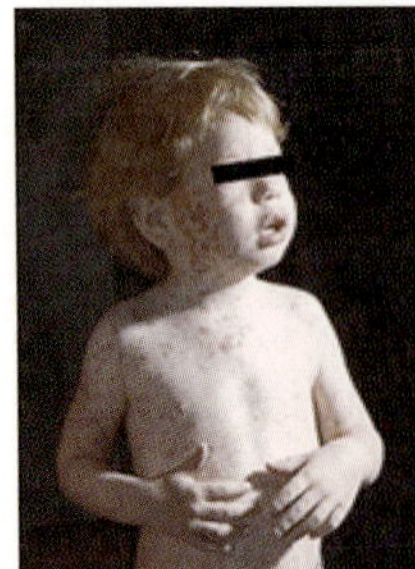

Fig.13.11.1:Child with Rubella rash
Courtesy: Centers for Disease Control, Atlanta, USA

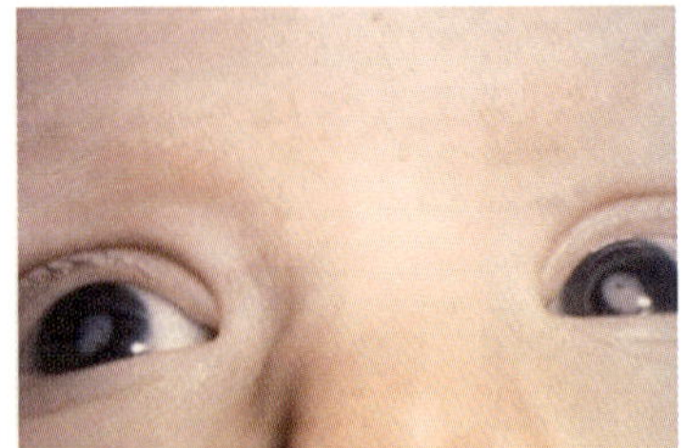

Fig.13.11.2: Congenital Rubella Syndrome: Photograph depicts cataract in the child's eye due to CRS
Courtesy: Centers for Disease Control, Atlanta, USA

What is the mechanism of action of the rubella vaccine?

A.3 (b) The vaccine is believed to be effective by producing specific antibodies against this virus. After many years of immunization, the antibody level wanes and then the cell mediated immunity is likely to play a part.

What is the aim of the rubella vaccination? Mention the impact this vaccination has had in the U.S.

A.3 (c) The aim of the rubella vaccination is to prevent the congenital rubella syndrome. The first priority is to protect the women of the child bearing age and then to interrupt the transmission by vaccinating the children. There have been no major epidemics in U.S., after the introduction of the vaccine there, although small outbreaks is certain settings have been reported.

Rubella was eliminated from the U.S. in 2001. Before the rubella vaccination programme which started in 1969, rubella was widespread in U.S.

What was the basis of the 'Rubella parties' that were organized in the past?

A.4 (a) These were formerly practiced in Australia, where pubescent girls were deliberately exposed to active rubella cases. The strategy was to stimulate the natural immunity of young adolescent girls. This strategy was in contrast to the other strategy, where immunity of all young children (boys and girls) was addressed.

What is the limitation of such an approach?

A.4 (b) As the population that is going to benefit is the teenagers, the benefit could only occur in the later years. These individuals could acquire the infection in the early period of their life and could present with postnatally acquired rubella.

What is postnatal rubella?

A.5 (a) This is rubella infection, which is acquired after birth and usually results in mild or subclinical illness. This is in contrast with the congenital rubella infection, which occurs in the foetus and often results in severe disease especially, if contracted in the first trimester.

Describe the epidemiology of postnatal rubella

A.5 (b) The rubella infection occurs worldwide with a peak incidence in the spring. The infection is spread by the respiratory route. Epidemics occur every 6-10 years; with one worldwide epidemic occurying in 1962-65, involving over 12 million cases in the USA, with over 20,000 children borne with congenital rubella syndrome.

What are the complications that are associated with postnatal rubella?

A.5 (c) The complications include arthritis exclusively in women, haemorrhage due to thrombocytopenia , vascular damage and encephalitis.

Describe laboratory diagnosis of postnatal rubella?

A.5 (d) The rash and the other features of rubella are not pathognomic, unless an epidemic is occurying at that time. So one has to rely on the laboratory for the diagnosis. Serological tests are often relied upon. ELISA tests are preferred. Haemagglutination test is also a standard test, however it requires that the serum be pretreated to remove non specific inhibitors; before testing. To confirm a recent rubella infection, rubella specific IgM antibodies have to be demonstrated.

The virus can also be cultivated from the nasopharyngeal swabs, or throat swabs, taken 6 days before and after onset of rash. Monkey or rabbit origin cell line can be used, in which inconspicuous cytoplasmic CPE occurs. *Shell vial technique gives result in 3-4 days post inoculation.

* see A.12a (iii), pg. 378 Section 11

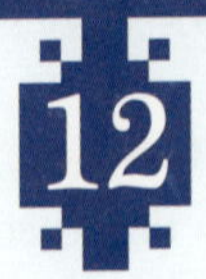

Integrated Clinical Based Study of Dengue Virus/Dengue Haemorrhagic Fever

A 40 year old executive, Anil staying in a farmhouse; equipped with swimming pool reported with three day history of high grade fever, severe myalgias and diffuse rash on the trunk. Blood examination revealed a TLC count of 3,000/mm³.

Linkages: Pg. 368, 436, 638

What is the clinical differential diagnosis of this case?

A.1 The differential diagnosis includes Dengue haemmorhagic fever, Chickungunya viral infection and other viral infections; as measles and Yellow fever. The bacterial infections could be meningococcal septicaemia or Leptospirosis.

A rapid diagnostic test for Dengue non-structural protein 1 (NSI) has been positive (in high titer) in this case. What is the likely diagnosis?

A.2 Acute Dengue infection.

To which family does Dengue belong?

A.3 (a) *Flaviviridae* (Flavi = yellow)

Name an important virus which belongs to Flaviviridae, but is not arthropod borne and spreads by blood transfusion.

A.3 (b) Hepatitis C virus.

Enumerate viral infections transmitted by Aedes mosquito.

A.3 (c) Chickungunya, Dengue (*Aedes aegypti*), Yellow fever and Rift valley fever.

What is unique about epidemiology of Dengue?

A.3 (d) It is an unique arboviral infection, in which no non vertebrate reservoir has been identified and man gets accidentally infected.

Why does one not rely on a test based on specific antibody demonstration in the early stage of dengue?

A.4 (a) In the early stage of infection, rise of specific IgM antibodies cannot be demonstrated, which occurs after 7-10 days of infection. In the early period of infection, one relies on *antigen detection* based test. The antibodies persist for 1-3 months, which can be detected by ELISA or immunochromatographic based tests.

What other category of tests can one reply upon in the early stage of dengue?

A.4 (b) During this stage, viral isolation can be attempted, though only possible in reference laboratories.Viral nucleic acid can be also be demonstrated by techniques; as RT-PCR.

What are the factors that have made dengue that was a mild illness in the nineteenth century, present only in the tropics, to have now increased manifold and put nearly half of the world's population at risk for this infection?

A.5 (a) Many changes have been responsible for this change. One is the rapid urbanization and the increased global travel. The increased urbanization has led to poverty at many places, with improper waste management and accumulation of water in vessels. All this has led to spread and adaptation of the *Aedes aegypti* to more places (which is a vector of this disease). The mosquito control/eradication programme has also suffered many setbacks.

Does Dengue virus have an animal reservoir?

A.5 (b) No

Describe the character of rash in dengue. Why is the fever in dengue called 'breakbone fever'?

A.5 (c) The I.P. is 5-8days. The rash is maculopapular in character and appears on 3rd or 4th day of infection. The fever lasts for for about 10 days. It is called 'break bone' fever because of severe pain in muscles and joints.

What are the two severe complications that can occur in dengue?

A.5 (d) Dengue haemorrhagic fever *(DHF)* and Dengue shock syndrome *(DSS)*.

How many times can one contract dengue infection in a life time?

A.6 (a) Four times, as this virus has four serotypes. Each infection provides immunity to the serotype, to which one was infected.

Does infection with one serotype, offer cross-protection to second infection by another serotype of dengue virus?

A.6 (b) It does *not*! It is expected that immunity achieved by an individual against one serotype of Dengue virus should offer protection against other serotypes, but there is evidence to the contrary. There is evidence that second dengue infection increases the chances of DHF, upon infection with a different serotype, than the one which infected originally. The mechanism of this phenomenon is not clear, but appears to result from antibody dependent enhancement of dengue virus infection. The earlier antibodies are probably not sufficient to neutralize new virus. Possibly the antibodies against the previous serotype bind more avidly against the new dengue serotype and are taken up via Fc receptors, by monocyte-macrophage of the host, in which it replicates best. The immune complex (including the virus) is taken more easily into the host cell than the virus without the antibody.

According to the WHO definition, what are the criteria, a case should have to categorized; as having DHF?

A.7 The following four criteria are to be met namely:

(i) Acute sudden onset of high fever for 2-7 days.

(ii) Hemmorhagic manifestations with; atleast a positive tourniquet test (>20 petechiae/square inch), presence of petechiae or others.

(iii) Platelet count <100,000/mm^3.

(iv) Hemoconcentration (rising packed cell volume) >20% or other evidences of plasma leakage; as ascites.

When did the last major outbreak of dengue occur in Delhi and what was the magnitude of this outbreak?

A.8 The last major outbreak in Delhi occurred in 1996, in which more than 10,000 cases occurred and 423 deaths occurred.

The case (in discussion) is being managed symptomatically and after 15 days the platelet count rises to 1.5 lakh/mm^3. Does this bear a favourable prognosis?

A.9 (a) A rise in platelet count in a case of DHF, indicates recovery from the infection.

If the platelet count in the case had continued to fall, what intervention would have been necessary?

A.9 (b) Platelet concentrate would have to be infused.

Can aspirin be used in a dengue case to manage fever and pain?

A.10 Aspirin is contraindicated in a case of Dengue, due to its anticoagulant properties.

Mention control measures of key importance, as no antivirals or vaccine against dengue is available.

A.10 (b)

(i) Using protective clothing and remaining in air conditioned environment.

(ii) Use of mosquito repellants; as N-N-diethyl-m-toluamide (DEET) during the time (of day), when Aedes mosquitos are most active.

(iii) Covering domestic water containers with foil to block transmission of Aedes.

(iv) As biological control; can use Mesocyclops, which is a natural predator of Aedes.

(v) mosquito eradication/control programme.

13 Integrated Clinical Based Study of Japanese Encephalitis Virus/Japanese Encephalitis

An outbreak of Japanese encephalitis occured in northern India; affecting mainly the states of U.P. and Bihar in 2005. Approximately 5000 cases were reported and 1300 deaths occurred.

Linkages: Pg. 368, 436, 638

Is diagnosis of arboviral infection, as Japanese encephalitis (JE) easy?

A.1 (a) No, unless there is an outbreak. The reasons include lack of clinical suspicion of these infections, difficulty in culturing arboviruses and lack of serological (antibody and antigen) based diagnostic kits.

What is the differential diagnosis of Japanese encephalitis?

A.1 (b) The differential diagnosis of Japanese encephalitis includes encephalitis due to other viruses, Human monocytic ehrlichiosis, human granulocytic anaplasmosis, acute HIV infection, Tularemia and Lyme disease.

Why is this disease named as 'Japanese encephalitis'?

A.2 (a) This disease was first recognized in the Japan in late nineteenth century (since 1871). The virus was designated as Japanese 'B' encephalitis to distinguish it from Japanese 'A' encephalitis virus, which was prevalent at that time.

Describe the spread of the disease in India?

A.2 (b) This disease was first reported in India during an encephalitis outbreak in Vellore (Tamil Nadu), in 1955. Since then it has spread to involve sporadically all states and union territories. Outbreaks have been reported from Tamil Nadu, Karnataka, Assam, UP (Gorakhpur) and West Bengal.

What could be the reasons for spread of this disease in India?

A.2 (c) Improvement in the irrigation system in the country has been instrumental in the increased rice cultivation. This has resulted in the proliferation of *Culex tritaeniorhyncus,* a principal vector that breeds in water.

What could be a possible factor for limited JE infection in India?

A.2 (d) It could be the high cattle to pig ratio.

Depict the life cycle of J.E. virus in the environment.

A.2 (e)

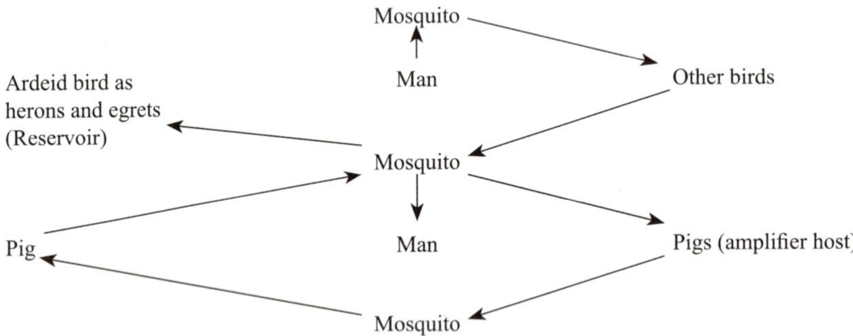

Is J.E. infection mostly symptomatic?

A.3 (a) No, the infection is mostly asymptomatic.

If not, then what is the cause of scare in reporting this disease?

A.3 (b) In some outbreaks due to this infection, the mortality ratio have been 37% and in few it even touched 50%. So, the disease assumes major public health importance.

What is the clinical profile of J.E. infection in symptomatic cases?

A.3 (c) The initial symptoms often include fever, headache, diarrhoea, vomiting and myalgias. After few days, movement disorders, convulsions and altered sensorium are reported.

Why are pigs considered amplifier hosts, as far as J.E. infection is concerned?

A.4 (a) Amplifier host indicate that they maintain cycle (of the microbe) not only within themselves, but also augment availability of the microbe to vector.

The pigs not only get infected with this virus, which can present; as encephalitis and abortions in them but this infection cycle also augments the availability of this virus to vectors.

What are the consequences of the above factor in the control of J.E. infection?

A.4 (b) (i) The pigs need to be moved away from human inhabitation, as often these are reared close to human dwellings.

(ii) Pigs need to be vaccinated against J.E.

(iii) In case of an outbreak, sacrificing (slaughtering) pigs could be done, as means to controlling the outbreaks; as has been done in avian influenza outbreaks, where birds were slaughtered.

As other animals also acts as hosts in J.E., this would imply that the complex ecology of this virus would make eradication of this disease unlikely in contrast to viral infections; as smallpox and polio.

Which vaccines are available in India against J.E.?

A.5 (a)

- A mouse brain killed vaccine is available, which is produced by growing Nakayama strain in mouse brain and then inactivating it with formalin. Two doses of this vaccine are administered subcutaneously at interval of 2 weeks followed by booster at 6-12 months.
- The inactivated mouse brain vaccine is being replaced by a cell culture-based vaccines. One of it is a live attenuated vaccine based on the SA 14-14-2 strain of J.E. virus.

Describe a J.E. vaccine being manufactured in India?

A.5 (b) In 2013, a vero cell-derived purified inactivated JE vaccine was launched. This indigenous vaccine is being manufactured in a public-private partnership mode between the Indians Council of Medical Research and Bharat Bioech. It has increased immunogenicity, superior safety and can be administered even during an epidemic.

What are the indications for J.E. vaccination?

A.5 (c) In endemic areas, mass vaccination can be practised, as has been done in rich countries; as Japan, Taiwan and Korea, where such measures have resulted in diminishing this disease. Opinions vary, if travelers to endemic areas should be vaccinated (visitors to endemic areas, spending atleast one month can consider vaccination).

What are the serious adverse effects reported with J.E. vaccine?

A.5 (d) Uncommonly systemic allergic reaction and rarely neurological effect.

Aspects related to case theme/examination assessment

Enumerate viruses of family Bunyaviridae of medical importance and describe their properties.

A.6 Bunyaviridae

It is one of the largest family of viruses infecting mammals. Most of the members are arthropod-borne and many persist in their arthropod vectors via transovarial transmission.

General properties: These are depicted in table 13.13.1

Table 13.13.1: Viruses of Family Bunyaviridae associated with disease in man:

Genus	Virus/Disease	Geographical distribution	Arthropod vector	Reservoir	Human Disease
Phelbovirus	Rift valley fever	Africa	Mosquito	Sheep, cattle, goats	Fever, retinitis, Haemorrhagic fever
Phelbovirus	Sandfly fever*	Mediterranean, S. America	Sandfly	Forest rodents	Fever, Conjunctivitis
Nairovirus	Crimean-Congo haemorrhagic fever	Asia, Eastern Europe, Africa	Tick	Sheep, cattle, goats	Haemorrhagic fever
Hantavirus	Hantaan and others; as Puumala, Belgrade, and Seoul	Africa, Europe	None	Rodents	Haemorrhagic fever, nephropathy
Bunyavirus	- California encephalitis virus - Chittor	USA, India	Mosquito	-	Encephalitis

The nucleic acid is segmented and genetic reassortment is demonstrable in cells coinfected with related bunyaviruses. The replication of the virus occurs in cytoplasm.

- **Classification:** The family Bunyaviridae is divided into four genera (see table 13.13.1). Man is infected by the bite of arthropods except Hantaviruses, for which the reservoir is the rodents and man gets infected, when it gets in contact with them.

- **Laboratory diagnosis:** Most Bunyaviruses can be cultivated easily in vertebrate cells (as BHK-21) or invertebrate cells (as mosquito cell line). They can also be isolated by intracerebral inoculation of suckling mice. Blood or autopsy tissue of the case can be used as sample. Serologic diagnosis is often used, as specific IgM assays using complement fixation or EIA technique.

*This virus is associated; as the name suggests, transmission by sandfly and the syndrome is designated; as sandfly fever. The disease is prevalent in countries around the Mediterranean sea, Central Asia and India.

Describe:

(i) Nairovirus/Crimean-Congo haemorrhagic fever (ii) Hantaan virus (iii) Chickengunya virus

A.7 (i) Nairovirus:

This is predominantly associated with the Crimean-Congo Haemorrhagic fever.

- *Distribution:* This disease is primarily seen in the Central Asia and eastern Europe. Outbreaks in India in 2011 from Gujarat in medical personnel have been reported.
- *Epidemiology:* This disease is transmitted by the tick of the genus Hyalomma. The vertebrate are key amplifier hosts.
- *Pathogenicity:* The disease starts; as fever, headache and severe back pain. As the name of the disease suggests, haemorrhage from the skin and the internal organs is reported. Case fatality rate uptil 50% have been recorded.
- *Control:* • Tick control measures, • Strict isolation of the patient with strict barrier measures

A.7 (ii) Hantaan virus:

This virus is associated with a hemorrhagic fever with renal syndrome. This was noted for the first time in the Korean was of 1950s, when thousands of UN troops developed fever and renal failure, with case fatality rate of 5-10%.

- *Epidemiology:* the mystery of the disease was solved in 1978, when Hantaan virus was isolated in Korea from the field rodent, named *Apodemus agrarius*. The virus belonged to the bunyavirus group. This virus is not transmitted by arthropod vector transmitted to man but by inhalation of aerosolized rodent urine or direct contact with rodent excreta. In 1993 in USA, a pulmonary syndrome has been documented to be associated with another Hantavirus.
- *Pathogenicity:* The renal syndrome often presents; as lumbar abdominal pain, haemorrhagic fever with severe renal tubular involvement. The person may go into a hypotensive shock due to excessive haemorrhage.
- *Laboratory diagnosis:* The diagnosis is essentially serologic with demonstration of specific IgM antibodies by ELISA.
- *Control:* (i) Rodent control, (ii) An inactivated suckling mice brain vaccine for human use is available.

A.7 (iii) Chickungunya virus:

The virus causes fever associated with arthralgia, myalgia and rash. The name 'chickungunya' implies bent up/folded posture, which the patient acquires, due to severe joint pain occurring during the disease. The virus belongs to the family Togaviridae and genus Alphavirus.

- *Epidemiology:* (i) Geographical distribution: Africa, South Asia, Philippines
  (ii) Vertebrate reservoir-Monkeys, Man
  (iii) Vector-*Aedes aegypti* (recently some changes in the vector have been reported)

  Several outbreaks have been reported with this virus. A mutation in the virus has been claimed to be responsible for the changing epidemiology associated with this virus. This disease is being currently categorized as a re-emerging disease. The disease is endemic in India with the first outbreak being reported in Kolkata in 1963. The disease behaves as an urban epidemic like dengue. In 2016, an outbreak in Delhi occurred.
- *Pathogenicity:* Fever, arthralgia, myalgia and rash. The fever is typically biphasic, also described as 'saddle back'. The characteristic of the disease is the crippling joint pain, occasionally persisting for many months.
- *Laboratory diagnosis:* The diagnosis is essentially serologic. For diagnosis in early period (0-7 days), good results are obtained by RT-PCR. Specific IgM antibody appears after 4 days of infection and lasts for few months. ELISA kits in India are provided by N.I.V., Pune to the government institutes.
- *Treatment:* No antiviral drugs are available. Symptomatic treatment is instituted.
- *Vaccine:* None is available

Integrated Clinical Based Study of Hepatitis C Virus/Jaundice

A 30 year woman, Sri Devi presented with nausea, vomiting and pain in right upper quadrant. Her abdominal examination revealed enlarged liver. She gave history of receiving frequent blood transfusions on account of low haemoglobin levels, due to undiagnosed bone marrow disease. Her hepatitis serologic tests profile revealed hepatitis C antibody test positive, by enzyme immunoassay technique.

Linkages: Pg. 368, 436, 514

Which infectious agent is the woman infected with? Mention the likely mode of her acquiring the infection.

A.1 She is infected with Hepatitis C virus. She is likely to have acquired this infection through the infected blood units, she has received.

Is it possible for the woman to have acquired the infection by infected blood, assuming that all the blood units transfused were tested negative/non reactive for HCV antibody?

A.2 The commonly performed test on blood units in a blood bank, is an antibody detection test, based on enzyme immunoassay technique. These tests have sensitivity of approximately 97%. It is possible for one of the many blood units that this woman received to be HCV infected and being undetected by the kit that was used (i.e., a false negative test having occurred).

Mention the year HCV was discovered and the approach used to detect it.

A.3 (a) HCV was recognized in 1989, as a result of molecular cloning of the genome of this virus. So, this virus has not been detected by an electron microscopic demonstration or by a culture technique.

The work occurred at the Michael Houghton's laboratory at Chiron coroporation along with Daniel Bradley's lab at CDC, Atlanta (USA)

Mention the classification and structure of HCV.

A.3 (b) This virus belongs to the family *Flaviviridae*, hence its properties are of this group (see p. 368). This virus is spherical with an approximate diameter of 50 nm and with the genome 9.7 kilo bases (approx) in length; encoding several proteins. The envelope has numerous glycoproteins.

This virus till now has not been cultivated, i.e., there exists no cell culture system that permits its replication but it has been cloned in *E.coli*.

Mention the role of HCV heterogeneity in its epidemiology, treatment and vaccine development.

A.3 (c) The HCV displays tremendous *heterogeneity*, which results in the existence of at least six genotypes and more than 80 subtypes. It exhibits another unique variation called *quasispecies variation*, which implies that multiple HCV variants (mutants) can be recovered from the plasma and liver of an infected individual at one given time. This heterogeneity occurs because of the high level of virion turnover along with the presence of reverse transcriptase enzyme, which lacks normal mechanisms of genetic proof reading, which leads to mutations. The tremendous genetic heterogeneity could be responsible for varying epidemiology, clinical severity and response to the therapy in this disease (as genotype 1 requires longer treatment with interferon α). Vaccine development is a challenge, due to the numerous genotypes and subtypes.

Is it important to do this confirmation?

A.4 (a) It is important to confirm the diagnosis, as with immunoassays (for antibody detection), false positive results are possible, as it is a screening test. The aim of screening test is to pickup maximum number of infected individuals. This test however cannot distinguish between acute, chronic or resolved (past) infections.

What tests can be performed to confirm HCV infection?

A.4 (b) A recombinant protein immunoblot assay can be performed, which is a more specific test for demonstration of specific antibodies than other immunoassays. $^{\Delta}$The HCV RNA can also be demonstrated by RT PCR technique or some other molecular amplification technique. This technique has the advantage of not only being more specific but also detecting the infection, before the case develops an antibody response.

Δ The presence of antibodies to HCV only indicate an exposure to HCV. The CDC recommends that all positive antibody tests to be followed by a HCV RNA test, that details viral RNA in the blood to determine whether or not the person has an active infection.

What other assessments are recommended in a HCV infected case?

A.4 (c) The liver can be assessed by an ultrasound scanning and liver biopsy to assess the development of cirrhosis, portal hypertension and/or hepatocellular carcinoma, if any.

Describe the laboratory diagnosis of HCV infection?

A.4 (d) One thing to consider in the diagnosis, is that HCV RNA can be detected in blood within two weeks of exposure. So; this parameter is detectable before antibody can be detected, which takes about 10 weeks to become detectable. So in initial stage of disease, reliance cannot be laid on the economical serological tests. Reliance should be laid on ALT (SGPT) to monitor the progression of a case, as its level fluctuates episodically.

The samples that aid in the diagnosis are serum and liver biopsy. The histologic examination of the liver helps to exclude other liver disease; as alcoholic hepatotoxicity or hemochromatosis. The biopsy is also the best index to stage the hepatitis besides being used to demonstrate the HCV antigen by immunofluorescence and 'in situ' hybridization.

Nucleic acid amplification technique; as RT-PCR commonly demonstrate the HCV-RNA in blood. A recent new technique, branched DNA (DNA) assay, which is a direct hybridization assay using a branch–chained DNA probe and enzymatic amplification of the hybridization signal, though a less sensitive technique. The advantages of the nucleic acid amplification test is

(i) They are the first test to become +ve in HCV infection.

(ii) Can detect viral load

(iii) Can determine genotype of HCV

(iv) Can monitor clearance of virus, after initiation of treatment

(v) No need of any confirmatory test, as required after antibody screening method.

The serological tests are based on demonstrating antibodies to HCV antigens. As mentioned previously, these tests are not demonstrable in the first ten weeks following exposure. However the fourth generation dot blot assays based on core viral antigens, (NS3, NS4 and NS5) can detect HCV antibody within 6-8 weeks of exposure. All the results that come positive by the EIA technology must be confirmed by the recombinant immunoblot assay (RIBA). This is a blot assay based on recombinant antigens; as the name indicates and is more specific test, so helps to exclude the false positive reports.

What are the routes of HCV transmission, besides blood transfusion?

A.5 (a) HCV can be transmitted by:

(i) Sharing of needles,syringes etc during illicit intravenous drug abuse

(ii) During sexual practices

(iii) Mucus membrane exposure to infected blood

(iv) Needle stick injury

(v) Blood transfusion

Describe the pathogenesis of HCV infection.

A.5 (b) Man (infected) is the natural reservoir of this virus. The infection is spread by percutaneous exposure to blood and plasma derivatives, e.g., needle stick injury, intravenous drug usage or tattooing. Sexual and perinatal transmission play a small role.

The incubation period of acute hepatitis C is about 7 weeks, so is intermediate between that of hepatitis A and that of hepatitis B. Majority of the acute cases are symptomatic (about 75%).

The long term complications; as cirrhosis and hepatocellular carcinoma usually occur more than 20 years after the onset of infection, though rapid cases of progression have been reported. The immunological and other factors associated with this progression are not clear. HCV RNA has been found in tears, semen, urine and some other fluids. So these may play a role in infection.

If this woman has history of intravenous drug abuse, to which other infectious agents, would she be at increased risk of contracting?

A.6 (a) Intravenous drug abuse makes this woman at risk for other blood borne diseases; as HBV, HDV and HIV. The woman is also prone to bacterial and fungal endocarditis and its complications. The woman may also be prone to other STDs, if she is involved in promiscuous sexual practices, often seen in individuals involved with drug abuse.

Describe the epidemiology of HCV infection.

A.6 (b) The infection occurs globally with about 170 million people estimated to be infected. The age group of 30-49 years old adults have a high frequency of infection. The carrier rates range from 10-20%.

Few Indian studies report the prevalence to be 15%. In India, the commonest prevalent genotypes are 2 and 3.

Egypt has a high prevalence of about 20% HCV infection. This is related to the unsafe injection practices and use of contaminated equipment. HCV accounts for about 40% of chronic liver disease. It is the most frequent cause requiring liver transplantation.

What is the role of genotyping of HCV in its the treatment?

A.7 (a) Currently six genotypes, one through six are known for HCV. Many subtypes are also known.

Infection with different genotype has varying disease profiles. For instance; infection with genotype one, requires extended therapy and despite it, has lower cure rate. Significant variations in viral nucleic acid sequences is seen, as a result of high mutation rates, which result in variation of viral envelope proteins, which may be important in the virus escaping from the immune system and in causation of chronic infections.

What drugs are used in the treatment of HCV infection?

A.7 (b) Till now recombinant interferon alpha was approved by FDA along with ribavirin.

Recently Sofosbuvir introduced in the west is giving good results

What approaches can be utilized to prevent HCV infection?

A.8 (i) Programmes to prevent needle-stick injuries in health care workers

(ii) Minimize mucus membrane exposure to blood

(iii) Screen HCV infection in high risk populations; as those attending STD clinic and indulging in intravenous drug abuse.

(iv) Mandatory HCV testing, before blood transfusion

Aspects related to case theme/examination assessment

Describe Kyasanur Forest disease.

A.9 Kyasanur Forest disease

It is locally known as 'Monkey fever'. Besides India, this disease has not been reported from any other country. The virus has been named after the place of its first isolation, i.e., Kyasanur forest in Karnataka, India. The isolation was done in N.I.V., Pune.

- *Etiological agent:* KFD virus, is antigenically related to the Russian-spring-summer encephalitis (RSSE) complex. The virus belongs to family *Flaviviridae* and genus *Flavivirus*.
- *Vector:* Hard tick (*Haemaphysalis spinigera*). The tick once infected, remains so for life.
- *Reservoir:* Forest birds and small animals are believed to be the reservoir for this virus.
- *Epidemiology:* The first outbreak of this haemorrhagic disease occurred in 1957, primarily as a fatal outbreak in the monkeys. Another major outbreak occurred in the 1982, also in Karnataka, resulted in deaths of more than 100 persons.
- *Clinical presentation:* The onset is usually with high fever and can present as bleeding from several sites.
- *Laboratory diagnosis:*
  - Essentially serologic
  - Viral isolation and real time PCR techniques are available.
- *Treatment:* No specific antivirals are available
- *Vaccine:* Killed vaccine developed at Haffkine Institute, Mumbai available (some protection)

Section XIII: RNA Viruses

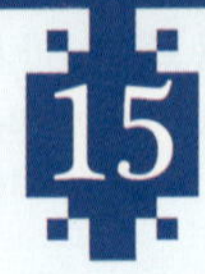

Integrated Clinical Based Study of Human Immunodeficiency Virus/AIDS

A 25 year old male, Shantanu was well about 7days back; when he complained of fever, cough and diffuse body aches. Throat examination revealed acute pharyngitis. He gave history of having anal intercourse with a parenteral drug abuser about 6 weeks back. Hepatitis A, B and C virus and HIV serologic tests were negative (non reactive). His chest X-ray did not reveal any abnormality. His TLC count was 2,500/cu. mm. and DLC revealed 60% polymorphonuclear leucocytes, 32% lymphocytes and 7% *atypical* lymphocytes.

Linkages: Pg. 368, 436, 639

What syndrome is the case is likely to have?

A.1 The case is having an infectious mononucleosis like syndrome.

The physician suspects the case to be HIV infected, despite HIV antibody test being non reactive. What test can be ordered to confirm his suspicion?

A.2 The physician can order for a HIV antigen detection test; as p24 level in his blood sample or a viral nucleic acid based test. HIV culture is performed only in reference research laboratories.

What is the I.P. of AIDS?

A.3 (a) The incubation period of AIDS varies from many months to many years (exceeding decades at times) .

What is the natural history of AIDS.

A.3 (b) Before one studies the pathogenesis, it would be worthwhile to study the natural history of HIV infection, so that the overview remains in the mind.

Exposure	Infection	Disease
Is physical contact to an infectious agent in manner, that may enable the infection to occur	Entry and subsequent replication of an infectious agent in a biological host	Clinical signs and symptoms, which are directly/indirectly due to the disease causing agent
e.g. sexual intercourse with an infected individual		
Not all exposure result in *infection*	Most infected individuals after a varying latent period, enter the *disease* stage.	
Many individuals are anxious at this stage to know, if they have acquired the infection. Many may present in a panic state Advise of lab test	*Window period* is time taken from infection till appearance of detectable antibodies. They are usually detectable within 6-12 weeks of infection (antibodies develop a week after the presentation of the 'glandular' fever).	

Describe (in detail) the pathogenesis of AIDS, emphasizing the four stages of HIV infection.

A.3 (c) The case typically passes through stages of *acute infection, clinical latency, ARC* (Aids related complex) and *AIDS*. The whole cycle can be completed in few months or can take decades. In the first year of infection, the infected case enters a 'steady state' level of HIV RNA, which primarily determines the rate at which CD4+ T lymphocytes decline. The simultaneous measurement of plasma HIV RNA levels and CD4 cell counts can predict disease progression (Fig. 13.15.1).

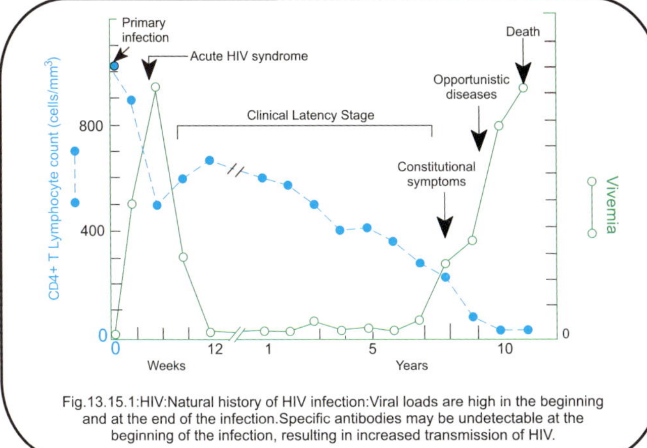

Fig.13.15.1:HIV:Natural history of HIV infection:Viral loads are high in the beginning and at the end of the infection.Specific antibodies may be undetectable at the beginning of the infection, resulting in increased transmission of HIV.

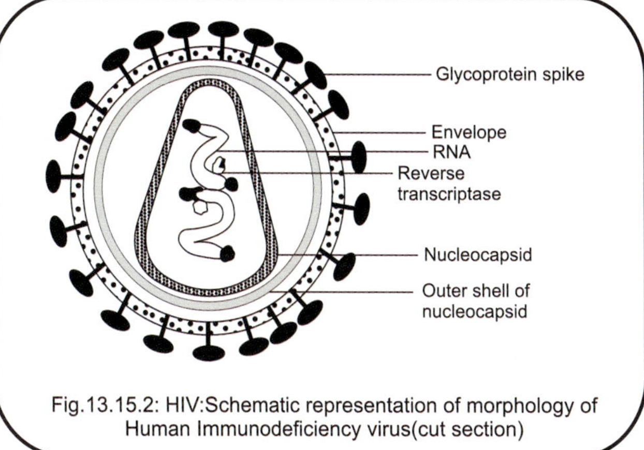

Fig.13.15.2: HIV:Schematic representation of morphology of Human Immunodeficiency virus(cut section)

The process of HIV replication and activation of provirus is depicted in the following flow diagram.

HIV gp 120 (of virion) (Fig. 13.15.2) binds to CD4 molecule on target cells (as lymphocytes, dendritic cells)

↓

Fusion of virion with target cell membrane (facilitated by co-receptors of HIV, gp 41)

↓

HIV virion enters target cells (nucleocapsid)

↓

HIV RNA and enzymes released (following removal of core proteins)

↓

ssRNA converted to RNA-DNA hybrid (using viral reverse transcriptase enzyme)

↓

ssDNA (original RNA degraded partially by ribonuclease H)

↓

dsDNA (using DNA dependent RNA polymerase)

↓

dsDNA translocates (reaches) the cell nucleus and integrated to the target cell chromosomal DNA by the viral integrase enzyme

↓

Becomes provirus (it may remain latent for long periods)

Activation of provirus

↓

Transcription of proviral DNA

↓

Production of several mRNAs

↓

Viral mRNAs transported to cytoplasm of target cell

↓

Synthesis of viral precursor proteins (by target cell ribosome)

↓

Viral proteins after cleavage of precursor protein by viral proteases

↓

HIV ssRNA and other components of HIV virion assemble in host cell

↓

The target cell buds out forming the viral envelope

↓

Virus particles complete maturation and bud out from cell surface

The human being can be exposed to HIV virus in various ways. However, it is important to know that not all exposures lead to HIV infection. The highest transmission rate of about 90% would be in blood transfusion of infected HIV positive blood to less than 1% transmission in infected needle stick injuries. In infected blood, virus in the serum and the numerous blood cells is the source of infection. Newborns can acquire the infection through the virus present in the secretions of the genital tract. The infant can acquire the virus through the infected breast milk. In sexual practices, the source of the virus is the infected semen, cervical and vaginal secretions.

The initial infection in cases of 'local' HIV entry (as opposed to infection by blood transfusion) is characterized by infection of mucosal lymphocytes, macrophages or dendritic cells of the rectum, vagina or urethra, during intercourse or of the upper alimentary canal from swallowing infected breast milk or saliva (rarely). From these localized sites, the virus spreads in the body through blood or draining lymph nodes. The lymphoid tissue of the body become infected by initial localizing of the virus in the dendritic cells and later the infection of the CD4 lymphocytes.

The HIV infection can be categorized into 4 stages:

1. **Acute HIV disease:** In the primary HIV infection, viral infection in the CD4 lymphocytes intensifies, leading to a burst of viremia (see peak in Fig. 13.15.1) and rapid spread of virus to other body tissues (including brain). As many as 5×10^3 infectious virions per ml in plasma, can be found during this stage.

   This leads to a initiation of strong HIV specific immune responses, which bring the viremia levels to almost baseline. This stage is also called *acute disease syndrome* (acute phase viraemia), which presents; as acute mononucleosis like syndrome (like flu) in about 50% of individuals with primary infection. Almost all patients develop some degree of viraemia during this stage, though some may remain asymptomatic or cannot recall symptoms. One must be aware of the *window period* in this stage, which is the interval period between HIV infection and appearance of specific antibodies in the serum. This period can last a couple of weeks. The importance of this is; that an infected person in this stage can transmit the infection, as by his blood donation but is negative by specific antibody detection test for HIV. The person finally undergoes seroconversion during this stage.

2. **Asymptomatic stage [Clinical latency]:** In this stage of clinical latency (minimal clinical symptoms), virus levels in the body remain at very low levels, however it is not eliminated from the body. In the body, persistent viral replication occurs at very low rates.The majority (about 90%) of the HIV proviruses are transcriptionally inactive, which indicates that only ten percent of the infected cells with HIV DNA (provirus) also contain viral mRNA and/or viral proteins. The untreated patient in this stage stays for a median period of 10 years, before patient becomes clinically sick. The CD4 level in the case, however continues to fall. The overall cellular immune status ranges from normal to moderate deficency. The mechanisms by which the virus is able to evade the immune response are not known, but the ability of HIV to mutate plays a part in the evasion.

Student cartoon three

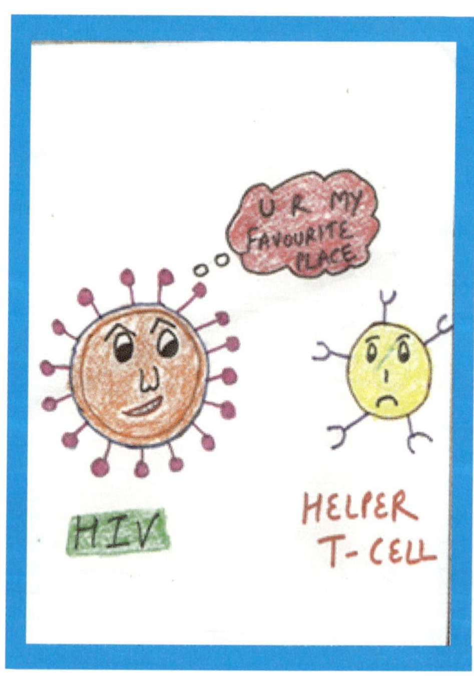

3. **Aids related complex (including ♦PGL):** The continuously decreasing CD4 levels and a sudden increase in plasma viral levels lead to state in the individual called the AIDS related complex.The patient here manifests; non-specific signs and symptoms; as night sweets diarrhoea, weight loss, PGL (persistent generalized lymphadenopathy) and some opportunistic infection; as herpes zoster and candidiasis, which indicate impaired immunity.

4. **AIDS:** It takes a period varying from few months to some years for a case to present; as a fully blown case of AIDS. The falling CD4 levels (especially below 200 cells/cu.mm) and increasing viremia▲ levels

♦ PGL is defined; as enlarged lymph nodes of greater than 1 cm in size, in two or more non-contiguous sites, persisting for atleast 3 months. This entity must be differentiated from other causes of lymphadenopathy; as lymphomas.

▲ HIV load is typically undetectable below levels of 40-75 copies per ml. The goal of the HIV therapy is to lower load below detectable level.

contribute to this state. The patient manifests here AIDS defining illnesses; as pneumocystis pneumonia, Crysptosporidiosis (see table 13.15.3, p. 390) and malignancies; as Kaposi's sarcoma. The cellular immune deficit in this state is severe and irreversible.

Mention the stages of WHO clinical staging of HIV/AIDS for adults and adolescent with confirmed HIV infection.

A.3 (d) There are four clinical stages from clinical stage 1 to clinical stage 4 (details consult a clinical textbook)

Classify retroviruses of human importance.

A.4 (a) Retroviruses of human importance

Subfamily	Genus	Virus	Disease
Oncovirinae	Delta retrovirus	HTLV-1	• Adult T cell leukemia, • Spastic tropical paraparesis
		HTLV-2	Role not clear (can transform CD4+ cells 'in vitro' like HTLV-1)
Lentivirinae	Lentivirus	HIV-1	AIDS
		HIV-2 (resembles Simian immunodeficiency virus, SIV which causes SAIDS, disease observed in Asian macaques, kept in captivity)	AIDS (Less severe form)
Spumavirinae	Spumavirus	Human foamy virus (named so, as causes 'foamy pathology' in infected cells)	Not associated with any disease

NB: SAIDS is Simian AIDS

Mention the diseases caused by caused by HTLV 1 and 2.

A.4 (b) Human T-lymphotropic virus 1 (HTLV 1) was the first retrovirus found to be infecting man and causing* adult T-cell leukemia. It is a rare malignancy found only in Japan, Africa and Caribbean. It also causes spastic tropical paraparesis, a neurologic disease with spastic features. HTLV-2 can also transform CD4+ T cells 'in vitro' like HTLV-1, but its pathogenetic role is not clear.

*spread by blood,sexual intercourse

Describe the emergence of AIDS.

A.5 As recently as the late 1970s, the belief that was getting formed was, that infectious diseases were not a threat to the developed world and the public health challenges stemmed mainly from malignancies, cardiovascular diseases and degenerative diseases. However, certain events in early 1980s, redefined how the world currently looks at the infectious diseases. It would not be too much of an exaggeration to talk of period previous to 1980s as the pre-HIV era.

In 1981, a new disease (clinically) was described in the male homosexual population of certain US cities (as New York, San Francisco and Los Angeles), who had unexplained high occurrence of *Pneumocystis carinii* (now jirovecii)pneumonia and Kaposi sarcoma. These cases appeared to be infectious and were immunosuppressed, hence the syndrome was described as acquired immunodeficiency syndrome. Initially, there was a backlash against the gay (homosexual) community, as it was realized that even blood donated by them was infectious. However, shortly the disease was also recognized in intravenous drug users (male and female), and in recipients of blood transfusions from certain population. Despite lot of diagnostic work on these cases, the etiological agent of this syndrome could not be isolated and identified for about two years. Credit for first isolating the incriminating virus from these cases went to Luc Montagnier and his team (Pasteur Institute of France), who isolated it from a male homosexual, who was suffering from lymphadenopathy in 1983. They called it the lymphadenopathy associated virus (LAV) for obvious reasons. Subsequently,* Robert C Gallo and his team of US (next year) also isolated a virus named Human T cell lymphotropic virus III (HTLV III) in a malignant cell line, with samples from several cases of AIDS. Although AIDS was first recognized as a clinical entity in 1981,the earliest record of HIV-1 infection, now comes from a serum sample obtained in 1959 from a Bantu resident (male) of Kinshasa in Republic of Congo. This early period till 1985, when routine HIV antibody testing was not established in the U.S. and some industrialized countries, led to HIV transmission to many blood recipient cases; especially haemophiliacs. This occurred, as this mode of transmission was not known initially.

Since this virus was named differently in different studies, International committee on virus nomenclature, gave a generic name 'Human immunodeficiency virus' to this virus. Subsequently after tremendous analysis of epidemiologic data including blood transfusion data, laboratory animal work and experimental work, by 1984, it was proven that the etiological agent of AIDS was a virus (HIV).

Subsequently, in 1985, the development of ELISA kits, showed this infection to be also prevalent in the developing countries. The same year, serological findings revealed the presence of another related virus in the prostitutes of the West Africa and this human retrovirus was designated HTLV-IV (now designated HIV-2). This was phylogenetically more close to Simian Immunodeficency virus (SIV), which caused SAIDS, but clinically causes less severe manifestations than HIV-1.

*Finally however his team was not given the credit for this discovery and in 2008 only Luc Montagnier was awarded the Nobel Prize for this discovery

Describe in detail the structure of HIV virus highlighting the functional aspects.

A.6 (a) The HIV virus belongs to the family Retroviridiae (Table 11.1.4, so the general properties of the group hold true for this virus). Basically the structure can be divided into three regions, from outermost to innermost; as envelope, core (nucleocapsid) and nucleic acid (Figures 13.15.2 and 13.15.3). The virus is spherical in shape with a diameter of 90-120 nm and has icosahedral symmetry. The outermost layer is the envelope, lipoprotein in nature, from which 72 spiked knobs project from 72 transmembrane protein (fusion protein), named gp 120 and gp 41 respectively. The gp 120 is derived from an initial, bigger, precursor, structure of virus, namely gp 160; by lysis. The alphabets designation refers to its glycoprotein nature and the number to its originally determined molecular weight in kilo Daltons (kDa). The role of the gp 120 is in the initial binding of the HIV to the host cell receptors; consisting of CD4 molecules. The role of gp 41 is as a fusion protein

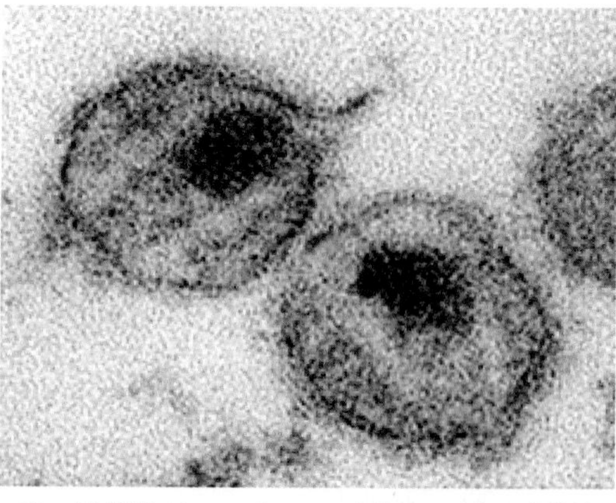

Fig. 13.15.3: Human Immunodeficency Virus (HIV): Transmission electron micrograph depicts ultrastructural details of this virus

Courtesy: A. Harrison:and Dr. P. Feorino/CDC

The icosahedral core consists of an outer matrix, protein layer of P17 and an inner major capsid protein layer of p24 protein.

The innermost structure in the virion consists of two identical positive strands of RNA. The innermost structure also consists of copies of reverse transcriptase and some enzymes; as integrase.

The length of the HIV genome is 9.2 kb. It contains 9 genes, out of these, three are major (or structural), namely *env*, *gag* and *pol,* which yield the envelope/core proteins, nucleocapsid core proteins and enzymes required for replication, respectively (Table 13.15.1). The remaining six genes code for regulatory proteins and have a major role in controlling viral expression (Table 13.15.1).

RT reverses the normal transcription process and makes a DNA copy of the viral RNA genomc. This copy which is called provirus is integrated into the cell genome and is replicated along with the cell DNA.

Table 13.15.1: Genomic organization and function of important genes (simplified) of HIV

Gene	Antigens/protein coded	Functions
Gag	53-kDa precursor	
	p17	Forms outer core protein layer
	p24	Forms inner core protein layer
Pol	100-kDa precursor	
	p64	Has reverse transcriptase and RNase activity
	Other with protease and integrase activity	Endonuclease for integrating viral DNA into host chromosome
Env	gp 120 (gp 160-kDa is precursor)	Protrudes from viral envelope and binds CD4
	gp 41	Transmembrane protein required for fusion
Tat	Discussion beyond UG level	Transactivator of transcription
Rev		Regulator of protein expression
Nef		Negative regulatory factor
Vpu		Viral protein, promotes maturation & release of virus
Vif		Viral infectivity protein
Vpr		Viral protein, stimulates promoter region

Mention about the molecular heterogeneity of HIV virus.

A.6 (b) Molecular heterogeneity of HIV

Two distinct types of HIV have been recognized; namely HIV-1 and HIV-2. The latter can also result in severe immunosuppression and serious opportunistic infections, though often causes less severe disease. HIV-2 was first reported in W. Africa in 1986, it has also been reported from Mumbai in India and its prevalence in US is extremely low. It has 40% approximately sequence homology with HIV-1, which results in frequent cross-reactions between the two. Its transmission is similar to HIV-1. HIV-2 EIA test is available for its detection. Dual infection with both HIV-1 and HIV-2 have been reported. In India, blood banks test for evidence of both HIV-1 and HIV-2 antibodies, before certifying the sample as non-reactive for AIDS. The first case of HIV-2 infection in India was reported from Mumbai in 1990. Now there are reports of its isolation from several states.

Tremendous molecular heterogeneity has been seen in HIV-1. HIV-1 has been divided into 3 groups, namely HIV-1M (major group), HIV-1 O (outlier) and HIV-1N (new virus). The group M is responsible for most of the infections in the world. This group comprises of nine *subtypes* or *clades* designated from A to K (without E and I). These are regional preponderances of these types.

Mention the 1993 CDC (Centre for Disease Control, Atlanta, USA) AIDS surveillance case definition and classification system.

A.7 **CDC definition** (where appropriate diagnostic facilities are available)

It is defined as a illness characterized by

- One or more of the opportunistic infections (listed) that are at least moderately indicative of underlying cellular immunodeficiency causes and observed for all other causes of reduced resistance reported to be associated with atleast one of those opportunistic infection.
- Absence of all known underlying cause of cellular immunodeficiency other than HIV.
- Positive antibody to HIV 1/2 or positive viral culture or other positive laboratory parameter.

Currently the CDC (in 1993) has revised its case definition to place HIV-infected individuals according to clinical and CD4 cell level groupings as follows:

Table 13.15.2: 1993 CDC Classification system for HIV-Infected adults and adolescent

CD4 cell categories	**Clinical categories**		
	A	B	C
	Asymptomatic, acute HIV or PGL	**Symptomatic conditions**	**AIDS–indicator conditions e.g., esophageal candidiasis**
>499/µl	A1	B1	C1
200-499//µl	A2	B2	C2
<200//µl	A3	B3	C3

PGL- progressive generalized lymphadenopathy

*A list exists with the CDC for categories, B and C

Source: CDC guidelines for AIDS diagnosis, 1993 revision

In which country is homosexual rather than heterosexual sex, the primary mode of HIV transmission?

A.8 **(a)** U.S.A.

What populations is at increased risk for acquiring HIV infection.

A.8 **(b)** The HIV spreads primarily sexually, by contact with infected blood and vertically from mother to fetus. In the sexual mode, the transmission can occur by vaginal, anal intercourse and oral-genital contact. So the populations at increased risk of HIV infection include promiscuous men and women, homosexuals, intravenous drug users, children born to HIV positive mothers and individuals, who have received frequent blood transfusions.

Describe the epidemiology of AIDS.

A.8 **(c)** **Etiological agent:** HIV- I and HIV- II

- Clades categories:

Reservoir of infection: Cases and carriers of HIV infection, once a person is HIV infected, the virus remains in the body life-long.

Source of infection: Significant amounts of the virus are found in blood, semen and CSF. It has been isolated from all body fluids (excepting sweat); as plasma (including PBMC), semen, vaginal fluid, cervical fluid, milk, tears and bronchial fluids. However it is only the former three, that are mainly involved in transmission of HIV. It may be mentioned that in the developing countries, the HIV positive mothers are recommended to give the breast milk to their babies, for reasons mentioned subsequently.

Adminstration of clotting factor preparations, pooled immunoglobulin, albumin and hepatitis B vaccine does not result in transmission of HIV-1, as the production step; as heat treatment of clotting factors destroys the virus.

Modes of transmission:

HIV can be transmitted primarily by three modes namely *sexual* transmission, *blood* contact and *perinatally* (maternal-fetal and mother- child)

Globally, heterosexual sex is the primary (70-75%) mode of HIV transmission; excepting in the United States where homosexual sex is the primary (approximately 49%) mode of transmission. Any type of sex; namely oral,vaginal or anal can spread AIDS The vast majority of the HIV transmission is by penetrative vaginal or anal sexual intercourse. The transmission can occur from an infected man to woman, from an infective woman to man or from an infected man to man.

The relative risk per exposure varies from 0.1-1%. The risk of acquiring HIV infection in enhanced, by presence of genital diseases; as syphilis and gonorrhoea. In general, an infected male transmits the infection more efficiently than an infected female. One of the reasons for this, may be the longer period the infected semen remains in contact with the female genital mucosa. The highest risk of transmission in sexual contact would be in receptive anal intercourse (of male to male). In this case, the rectal mucosa remains exposed to the infected deposited semen.

In parenteral transmission, transfusion of the blood and blood products is an important mode in the transmission of HIV. Infected unsterile syringes and needles often used by i/v drug users; as in Manipur (India), also result in transmission of infection. The medical and paramedical personnel are exposed to the risk of needle stick injuries (relative risk per exposure is about 1%). Transplantation of tissue and organs is unlikely to result in transmission, due to testing of donors for HIV.

An HIV infected woman can transmit the infection to the fetus transplacentally or to the newborn during passage through the birth canal. The transmission on to the neonates and infant can also occur through feeding the infected breast milk. The rates of transmission by this mode vary from 20-25 percent. In developing countries as ours, the breast milk may be the only source of nutrition for the infants, such feeding may be permitted, unlike in the developed countries.

Host:

AIDS is a global pandemic with virtually every country in the world reporting it. Globally, about 40 million people are infected with HIV/AIDS (Dec 2005). The area with the highest infection is the Sub-Saharan Africa (25.6 million). The epidemic in India and China has lagged behind that of Africa.

Age: Most cases have occurred among sexually active person aged 20-49 years. Children make up a small fraction of the total quantum.

In North America, Europe and Australia, approximately 51% of cases are homosexuals. The high risk individuals are male homosexuals and bisexuals, promiscuous individuals; including prostitutes, intravenous drug abusers and individuals, who are long standing recipients of blood and bloods products.

In India, the first AIDS patient was reported in 1986 (from Mumbai). The incidence of HIV infection is highest in Manipur (178 per thousand), to be followed by Maharashtra. The high rate in the Manipur is because of high i/v drug abusers number and proximity of the state to the 'golden triangle'. In India, according to NACO in 2006, there were 5.2 million HIV cases.

What is the importance of suspecting HIV in the early stage of infection?

A.9 (a) An expert physician should be able to pick up HIV cases in their early infection stage. The diagnosis of primary HIV diagnosis is often missed. The acute mononucleosis like syndrome (flu like) is seen typically in about 50% of cases with primary infection. The cases in this early stage can be managed with minimal morbidity, as the viral load is less and the immune system has not undergone functional derangement.

How do you explain the HIV serology (antibody) being negative (non reactive) in this case?

A.9 (b) After viral infection, the antibody takes few weeks to rise. Hence in the initial period of infection ('window period'), the viral infection can be demonstrated by tests, that are based on HIV antigen and/or nucleic acid demonstration.

Enumerate the opportunistic infections associated with AIDS.

A.9 (c) See Table 13.15.3

Table 13.15.3: Opportunist infections associated with AIDS

CATEGORY	INFECTION/SYNDROME
Bacterial	• Salmonellosis (especially recurrent), • Mycobacteriosis, • Recurrent and multiple bacterial infections
Fungal	• Visceral candidiasis, • Cryptococcosis (disseminated), • Coccidioidomycosis (extrapulmonary), • Histoplasmosis (extrapulmonary), • *Pneumocystis jivovecii* pneumonia
Viral	• HHV-1 to HHV-6 and HHV-8 infection
Protozoal	• Amoebiasis, • Giardiasis, • Isosporiasis (causing diarrhoea), • Chronic cryptosporidiosis, • Toxoplasmosis (of brain)
Helminthic	• Strongyloidiasis (disseminated)
Malignancies	• Kaposi`s sarcoma, • B cell lymphoma, • Hodgkin's lymphoma
Others	• HIV dementia (subacute encephalitis), • Wasting syndrome (due to HIV), • Progressive multifocal leukoencephalopathy

Describe the laboratory diagnosis of AIDS.

A.9 **(d)** The laboratory diagnosis of AIDS can be studied in the following four categories namely:

I. Lab diagnosis of suspected cases (including blood sample, organ donors)

II. Lab diagnosis of cases in 'window period'

III. Lab diagnosis of HIV infection in new born (congenital/perinatal)

IV. Laboratory monitoring of HIV positive case

I. Laboratory diagnosis of suspected cases

Non specific markers

- Lymphopaenia
- Reduced CD4/CD8 ratio
- Thrombocytopenia (occasionally reported)
- Hypergammaglobulinemia

The profile of tests available in laboratory diagnosis is depicted table 13.5.4 and 13.5.5

I. Detection of anti HIV antibodies, constitute the mainstay of diagnosis of HIV. Reliance is often placed on the screening assays as EIA/rapid/simple test.

If specimen is reactive, repeatedly with two of the above tests, using different antigen and different testing/detecting system, it is retested with a third test (above category) using different antigen and different testing system. The screening assay may be followed by supplemental tests. They detect antibodies with high specificity and are Western blot/Immmunofluorescence tests, which are difficult to use in the Indian setting, as the tests are expensive, time consuming and need expertise.

Table 13.15.4: Classification of tests used to diagnose HIV infection based on microbiological principle of test

Antibody detection
• Classical ELISA test (3-4 hours)
• Simple tests – EIA (1/2 – 1 hr) based
• Rapid test (takes few minutes)
o Dot blot assays
o Latex agglutination (particle)
o HIV spot and comb tests
• Western blot
Antigen detection
• P24 antigen assay (immune complex dissociation assay)
• Antigen sandwich ELISA
• Antigen capture ELISA
HIV culture
• HIV I and II isolated (require HT cell line (T-cell), IL-2, reverse transcriptase)
Nucleic acid detection$^{\Delta}$
DNA–PCR amplification of HIV proviral DNA from peripheral blood mononuclear cells
RNA (quantified)– HIV RNA PCR (cDNA from HIV RNA amplified)
• HIV RNA amplification by branched DNA assay (signal amplfied, instead of target)
• Nucleic acid sequence based amplification (NASBA)
CD4 count
(i) Flow cytometer (often used), (ii) EIA assay (available), (iii) Microsphere assay
Δ Role of nucleic acid detection tests (as PCR)
• Early, acute HIV infection diagnosis
• If Western blot test is indeterminate
• Determine HIV status in window period
• Diagnosis of HIV in newborn
• To monitor antiretroviral therapy (by monitoring viral load)
• Subtyping of HIV virus (by Real time PCR)

NB: In host cells, HIV remains integrated as DNA

Table 13.15.5: *Classification of antigens used in various generations of ELISA*

First generation: Antigen used are derived from disruption of viruses (as by detergent) grown in human lymphocytes.
Second generation: Uses artificially obtained recombinant antigens, expressed from microbes (including yeasts).
Third generation: Uses synthetic oligopeptides
Fourth generation: Simultaneous detection of p24 antigen and HIV antibody.

Sequence of testing:

If EIA indeterminate → Perform Western Blot → (if indeterminate) Perform Nucleic acid test or culture

Can repeat sample after 3-6 months, if clinically indicated

II. Lab diagnosis of HIV infection in window period

Window period is the period following entry of HIV into the body and the appearance of detectable levels of antibodies with an available test. The p24 antigen capture assay developed in 1996, decreased the interval between infection and detection (window period from 21 days for antibody testing to 16 days with p24 antigen tests and subsequently to 12 days with nucleic acid testing)

The tests available for this category include PCR, viral culture and p24 antigen assay (positive in about 40% cases).

Nb-During acute infection, p24 antigenemia, precedes seroconversion usually by 2-3 weeks.

III. Lab diagnosis of HIV infection in newborn

Diagnosis of HIV infection in a child before 18 months is difficult, if born to a seropositive mother. This is because transplacental transmission of HIV antibodies from mother to foetus can occur as early as 8 weeks of gestation or may be even earlier. The transplancentally acquired maternal antibodies can persist in the child upto 18 months of age. So, in a child less than 18 months of age, diagnosis should not be made by routine serum antibody tests. In this age category, diagnosis can be made with the help of detecting specific IgA and/or IgM antibodies, as these do not cross placenta. Tests based on detecting p24 antigen in serum and PCR technique are also useful.

IV. Laboratory monitoring of HIV positive case

The various tests that may be required to diagnose the various infections that a HIV case may be having would depend on the clinical profile of case, as it may be stool examination for parasites in a case with gastrointestinal pathology. However, two tests are to be performed at regular intervals in all cases, to determine and monitor prognosis; namely CD4 T Cell count and HIV RNA levels in serum or plasma. Two tests commonly performed to quantify RNA in serum are quantitative RT-PCR assay (Real time PCR) and branched DNA assay. With an efficacious anti-retroviral therapy, these levels should fall. Patients with CD4 T cell count of <200/µl and <50/µl are indications of pneumocystis and MAC (*Mycobacterium avium* complex) prophylaxis.

Beta-2 microglobulin and neopterin can be used as markers of disease progression, as their levels are low in clinical latency stage (asymptomatic) and rise with progression of HIV disease.

Recently, resistance to antiretroviral drugs has been reported. To detect this resistance, various assays are available.

The status of the various tests in relation to the different stages of AIDS is illustrated in table 13.15.6.

Table 13.15.6: Tests status in different stages of AIDS

Test	Primary infection (window period)	Acute HIV syndrome	Clinical latency stage (asymptomatic period)	AIDS/ARS
Antibody demonstration; as by ELISA	-	+	+	+
p24 antigen detection	+*	+	-	+
Virus culture	+	+	+-#	++
PCR test (viral RNA/DNA) Δ	+^	++	+	+++

*(positive in about 40%)

^Has highest sensitivity (92-100%)

#1 in 50,000 PBMC in asymptomatic patients and 1 in 4,000 PBMC in symptomatic cases carry infectious HIV.

Δ NAATs detects the HIV earliest in the blood. This test is expensive and not used in routine screening unless person had a recent high-risk exposure.

Discuss the strategies of HIV testing in India.

A.9 **(e)** Table 13.15.7: Strategies of HIV testing in India

	Indication	Technique	Interpretation
Strategy I	• Use in blood banks (for transfusion safety) • Organ donation (as tissues, sperms)	- Sample (blood/serum) subjected to single E/R tests for HIV	If sample reactive (positive), sample is discarded (destroyed)
Strategy II-A	• HIV surveillance	• Sample tested by another E/R test, if sample reported reactive (positive) by first test	- Sample reported (positive), only if second test reports reactive (positive) - If first report is reactive (positive) and second report is negative, sample is reported non-reactive (negative)
II-B	HIV diagnosis in symptomatic case	• Sample tested as per strategy II A. If sample is positive (reactive) by first assay, non reactive (negative) by second assay, then a third 'tie breaker' test is put.	- If third assay is negative, then sample is reported as negative (non reactive), but if it is positive, then sample is reported as indeterminate (and case is retested, after an interval of 2-4 weeks)
Strategy III	• HIV diagnosis in asymptomatic individuals	- Sample tested by three E/R/ tests (Fig. 13.15.4) - Strategy similar to IIB, but to report positive, if first two tests are positive, third one still needs to be put, which should also be positive	- Sample has to be reported positive by all three tests to be designated as positive - Sample reported as negative by first test is not tested further and reported as such - Sample reported as positive by first test but negative by either second or third is finally reported as indeterminate (equivocal). Such samples have to be retested after 2-4 weeks (see Fig. 13.15.4)

NB: E-ELISA, R-Rapid, S-Supplemental

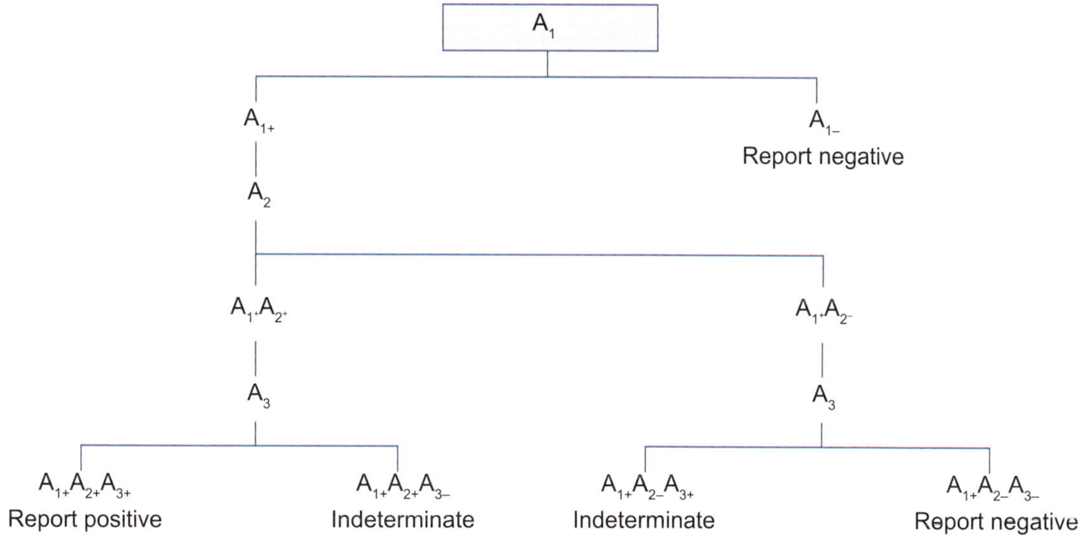

• All reports are given after post-test counselling

Fig. 13.15.4: Strategy III: To detect HIV infection in asymptomatic individuals

NB: Assays A1, A2, A3 represent 3 different assays based on different principles or different antigenic compositions

Nb: Antibody based report is given as reactive/non reactive rather than positive/negative, as the report has to be interpreted in relation to various clinical parameters.

The basic principle utilized in the HIV testing strategies, is that a test used in blood transfusion should have the highest sensitivity, as one cannot afford to miss a positive (reactive) blood sample in such testing. If such strategy is not enforced, it could result in transfusion of a HIV infected blood. So, it does not matter much, if such a test gives few false positive reports, such blood bags would just be discarded.

However, when one is concerned in making a diagnosis of an individual case, one cannot afford to give a false positive report, as this would result in tremendous trauma and other consequences to the individual. So tests performed on individuals should have high specificity (such tests would have very low false positive results). The best strategy in such scenario, is to first use test of highest sensitivity and then use tests of higher specificity in second and third strategies.

How should this case be managed with specific reference to his behaviour and administration of antiviral drugs?

A.10 (a) The case should be counseled and explained that if he has sexual contact with others, they could get HIV infected. The case should receive combined antiretroviral therapy.

Has drugs resistance been reported to antiretroviral drugs?

A.10 (b) Yes.

Describe the concept of ART and classify antiretroviral drugs.

A.10 (c) Several anti-retroviral agents are available currently, that form the mainstay of the anti-retroviral therapy (ART)- table 13.15.8. Current treatment for AIDS uses a combination of drugs, these regimens are designated HAART (Highly active anti-retroviral drugs).

The anti-retroviral drugs available currently block the life cycle of HIV replication at several steps. The recently licensed *enfuvirtide* is a fusion inhibitor and prevents the virus from entering the target cell. The second target in the HIV life cycle, for which effective anti-retroviral drugs are available, is the reverse transcription of viral RNA onto cDNA (see Figure 11.1.3 and Table 13.15.8). These drugs inhibit the production of cDNA (viral DNA) by competitive inhibition and chain termination. The third and last category of anti-retroviral drugs that are available act by blocking the cleavage of precursor proteins into units, required for construction of a new mature virion and are called *protease inhibitors* (table 13.15.8).

An important indication of the anti-retroviral drugs, besides use in the HIV infected individuals and decrease the viral load, is the use in mother to prevent HIV infection of infant. This could prevent the virus transmission during childbirth or viral transfer in milk, during breast feeding.

NB: ideally the drugs should be HIV specific, interfere minimally with normal cell processes and should have high therapeutic index (ratio of the toxic dose to effective dose)

Table 13.15.8: Some anti-HIV drugs in clinical use

Fusion inhibitors

Enfuvirtide – administered by subcutaneous injection.

Reverse transcriptase inhibitors (nucleoside inhibitors)

- Zidovudine (azidothymidine) – administered orally
- Lamivudine – administered orally
- Stavudine – administered orally

Reverse transcriptase inhibitors (non-nucleoside inhibitors)

- Neviparine – administered orally
- Efavirenz – administered orally

Protease inhibitors

- Indinavir – administered orally
- Nelfinavir – administered orally
- Ritonavir – administered orally

The use of immune modulators such as recombinant IL-2 in conjunction with HAART is being examined to reconstitute the immune system and restore normal functioning.

Describe post-exposure prophylaxis (with reference to suspected HIV exposure).

A.11 Post-exposure prophylaxis

It is a strategy of prevent HIV infection, following suspected high risk HIV exposure, which could be in the form of a sexual activity, needle stick injury or other exposure. It implies intake of antiretroviral drugs to prevent HIV from replicating and spreading within the body. The drugs should be started at the earliest within 2 hours of exposure but not later than 72 hours. The baseline HIV test of the exposed individual should be done at the time of exposure. If it is negative; then the test is repeated at 6 weeks, 3 months and 6 months post exposure.

Health care workers and physicians (including dentists and surgeons) are normally at a very low risk of acquiring HIV infection during management of the infected patient. The occupational exposure that may place a medical personnel at risk of HIV infection; includes percutaneous injury, contact of mucous membrane or contact of skin with blood, tissue or other body fluids. The risk of acquiring infection, depends on many factors; including the amount of infected fluid (usually blood) involved in the exposure, the quantum (amount) of virus in patients fluid at the time of exposure and if post exposure prophylaxis was taken within the recommended period (72 hours). The average risk of HIV transmission, following needle stick injury is about 0.3% in contrast to HBV transmission following needle stick injury, which is about 6-30%.

Following occupational exposure, the post-exposure prophylaxis (PEP) should be instituted depending on the exposure code (EC1 to EC3) and HIV status code (HIV SC) of the source (table 13.15.9). To reduce the risk of HIV transmission, care of the wound including washing and use of antiseptics, may be undertaken.

Table 13.15.9: Determination of PEP recommendation

EC	HIV SC	PEP regimen
1 (mild)	1 (High CD4 T cell count and low viral load	PEP not warranted
1	2 (Low CD4 T cell count and high viral load)	*Basic regimen
2 (moderate)	1	*Basic regimen
2	2	**Expanded regimen
3 (severe)	1 or 2	**Expanded regimen

EC-Exposure code, HIV SC-HIV status code, PEP- postexposure prophylaxis

*Zidovudine 300mg BD + Lamivudine 150mg BD – 4 weeks

**Basic regimen + Indinavir 800 mg TDS – 4 weeks

Mention about the current status of the AIDS vaccine.

A.12 No effective vaccine is available presently, but that does not reflect truly the efforts and money that have gone in to develop a HIV vaccine. The role this approach may play in the future, to halt the HIV pandemic could be phenomenal.

Till now several agents have undergone phase I trials, some have undergone phase II trials and one sub unit agent has undergone phase III trial. In India, the National AIDS research institute (NARI) of the ICMR, at Pune has been selected, as one of sites for the AIDS vaccine development and evaluation.

The reasons, why despite tremendous effort globally, no vaccine is available are many. Firstly this virus, integrates with genome of different tissues of the human body and can remain latent for years. Secondly, it infects primarily the very cells, that play a paramount role in the immunity, i.e., CD4 cells. Thirdly, no natural immunity is seen after HIV infection, which a vaccine may aim to achieve.

Fourthly the infection exposure may occur daily in some individuals at high risk, making the immune response ineffective.

Describe the various strategies for AIDS prevention.

A.13 *Education, counselling* and *behaviour modification* are the cornerstone in the programme.

Prevention of sexual transmission

- "Safer sex" (abstinence, monogamy, avoid sexual promiscuous behaviour)
- Use of condoms (10% failure rate)
- Treatment of all STDs
- Counselling in marriage, if one partner is HIV positive
- Testing of HIV status, before marriage
- Avoid unnatural practices; as anal intercourse
- Fellatio (oral sex) has some risk of contracting infection
- Kissing is relatively safe
- Behaviour modification of individuals practicing high risk behaviour; as having multiple partners, performing anal intercourse etc.

Prevention of transmission through blood and other tissues

- Standard/"Universal precautions" to be practised by all medical personnel, while handling blood and blood containing fluids from all patients. Any patient may harbour the HIV virus and other pathogens, so consider body fluids from all patients to be hazardous.
- All blood and blood products to be screened for HIV antibody assay (preferably by p24 antigen assay also)
- Sexually promiscuous (prostitutes) and i/v drug users should restrict from donating blood
- Screening of bone marrow, semen etc for HIV before use
- Consideration of new technology, as use of two pairs of gloves, "needleless" intravenous delivery system.

Prevention of infection among IDUs (injection drug users)

- Stop usage of the illegal drugs
- No sharing of syringes or needles
- If syringes/needles in short supply, boil for 20 minutes or use virucidal solution; as undiluted house bleach (sodium hypochlorite)

Prevention of perinatal infection

- HIV testing, before marriage
- ART of HIV infected individuals (antiretroviral therapy, mother during pregnancy)
- ART of infant born to HIV positive mother within 48 hours of birth
- Avoidance of breast feeding of HIV positive mother to her child in developed countries
- ART of infected women

Prevention of transmission in health care sitting

- Standard precautions (Universal precautions) to be followed by all medical personnel (hand washing and protective barriers)
- Care in use of needles and other sharp instruments
- Use of impervious needle disposal
- Use of PEP in indicated individuals (see A.11)
- Routine serologic surveillance of HCWs
- Employees sustaining adverse exposures should have HIV testing at 0 day (for baseline), 6 weeks, 12 weeks and 6 months, after exposure (CDC recommendation).

An Outline of Laboratory Diagnosis of Key RNA Viruses

Virus/ Syndrome/Approach	Specimens	Direct Demonstration Of Viral Antigen/ Genome/Particle In Clinical Specimen/ Animal Inoculation/Chicken Egg Inoculation	Viral cell line	Growth/ Confirmation	Serological Tests	
					Type	Interpretation
Rotavirus	Faeces Serum	Detected by latex agglutination test, RPHA, ELISA/Polyacrylamide gel electrophoresis analysis of viral RNA permits, discrimination between strain (4 serotypes)/ During acute stage about 10^{11} virus particles per ml are present in faeces, can be detected by E/M I.E.M	Primary monkey kidney lines as MA	CPE is not characteristic	Serum antibody can be measured by EIA, RIA, HI or CF	Not refined to the extent to be used in routine diagnosis
Influenza viruses A, B, C	• Nasal / throat washing • Swab of nasopharynx/throat • Sputum • Lung (at autopsy) is collected using suitable buffered salt solution. Specimen should be processed immediately. If short delay is expected, store at 4°C. If longer delay is expected store at 70°C. The specimen is treated with antibiotics to destroy bacteria	*Direct fluorescent test* can demonstrate antigen in epithelial cells within 2 hours. In nasal wash specimen,both IFA and EIA are rapid techniques • Chick embryo can be inoculated by intramniotic or intraallantoic routes (this technique was standard about 3 decades back, nowadays chick embryo essentially used for vaccine production, though in some cases, it may have better sensitivity) • After 2-3 days of incubation viral haemagglutination can be demonstrated in the fluid • Further typing and subtyping of influenza isolates	• Primary monkey kidney • Human embryo kidney cells • MDCK (Madin- Darby canine kidney continuous cell line) Note: culture should have trypsin to split neuraminidase	• Growth of virus at 33°C to 35°C in cultured cells is recognized by haemoadsorption of guinea pig red blood cells, after few days (3-7) • Isolate is then identified by haemagglutination inhibition • Some strains of influenza A can agglutinate only guinea pig RBC's, while influenza B can agglutinate both guinea pig & fowl RBC's. Influenza C can agglutinate only fowl RBC at 4°C. • Fresh isolates of influenza fail to produce CPE in monkey kidney cell culture.	• Complement fixation, haemagglutination inhibition and Neutralization test can be used • Novel subtypes arising by antigenic shift may have novel neuraminidase as well as new haemagglutinin, so the isolate should be tested to detect major & minor changes, arising by antigenic 'shift' or drift, using reference antisera against purified HA and NA.	• Four fold or higher rise of antibody titre between acute and convalescent phase sera has to be demonstrated (use in epidemiological studies) • The problem of 'original sin' complicates the identification of strain-specific antibodies (where the key antibodies elicited by the current strain of virus are against the first strain of influenza virus, one experienced years earlier and represent anamnestic response)
Parainfluenza viruses 1-4	• Mouth washing • Throat swab (esp. posterior pharynx) • Exfoliated cells, aspirated from respiratory tract • Respiratory mucus (must be adequately solubilized for elaborating antigen for ELISA)	• Immunofluorescent staining of exfoliated cells from respiratory tract • Detection of antigen in mucus by ELISA or RIA	Primary monkey kidney or human kidney	• Inoculated cells incubated at 33-36°C (Roller apparatus gives better result) • Little CPE, except by Parainfluenza type 2, which induce syncytium formation • Viral growth is detected by haemadsorption of guinea pig RBC's (4 and 25°C) • Differentiation from other haemadsorbing respiratory viruses is done by fluorescent antibody staining or by haemagglutination inhibition, using virus from cell culture supernatant	ELISA, CFT test	Demonstrate rise in titre

Contd.

Contd.

Measles (Rubeola virus)/ Most cases are diagnosed clinically, laboratory diagnosis may be necessary in cases of atypical measles	• Respiratory secretion • Serum	In aspirate can demonstrate viral antigen, by using fluorescent staining, monoclonal antibody Giemsa staining of sample will show Cowdry type A inclusion body and giant cells (Warthin-Finkeldey cells)	Monkey/human kidney cell line	• Multinucleate giant cells produced in 7-10 days (both intranuclear and intracytoplasmic inclusion bodies) • Can confirm with fluorescent monoclonal antibody or haemadsorption with chick RBC	CFT, HI, NT, IgM capture ELISA	Rising titre or measles-specific IgM antibody is significant
SSPE	• Serum • CSF • Brain biopsy	*Fluorescent antibody test* on neural tissue	Monkey kidney or other susceptible cell (isolation from a brain of patient is difficult)	Co-cultivation technique used - layer affected brain cells onto the monkey kidney cell line	CFT in serum; especially CSF	High titre of antibodies especially in CSF, suggest that these antibodies are produced in brain and have not crossed blood-brain barrier
Mumps/ Atypical cases and presentation; as meningo-encephalitis require laboratory help	• Saliva (or swab from orifice of Stensen's duct) • Throat secretion • Urine • CSF	*Immunofluorescence test* can demonstrate viral antigen	Monkey kidney or HEp2 line	becomes +ve in 3-5 days, identified by cell line haemadsorption	• Traditionally CFT (using soluble(s) and viral (v) antigens –IgM ELISA • HI (Used to monitor immune status in vaccination studies	
Respiratory syncytial virus/ Typically patient is 1-3 month infant with respiratory symptoms, who may progress quickly to cyanosis	Nasal secretion, Pharyngeal secretion (nasopharyngeal aspirate). Virus is extremely fragile, so sample should be added without delay and freezing (some even recommend bed side inoculation)	*Immunofluorescence* test with conjugated monoclonal antibodies can give result in less than 1 hour (Direct & Indirect)	Hela, HEp2, monkey cell cultures	• Growth occurs in 5-15 days with development of giant cells and syncytia. • Monoclonal antibodies can detect CPE earlier • Absence of haemadsorption distinguishes RSV from all other paramyxoviruses • Immunofluorescence test can also identify definitively	• CFT • Neutralization test	Test not very useful, as babies have poor immune response
Rabies/ *In Animals* - Commonly required to know, if the animal known to have inflicted the bite is rabid *In Man* - Antemortem Postmortem	• Animal sacrificed and hippocampus, brain stem or cerebellum region can be processed If can examine within 2 days, can refrigerate (If longer delay, can transport on dry ice or in 50% glycerol saline) • Corneal smear • Corneal biopsy • Saliva • Skin biopsy from (a) nape of neck (b) bite site • CSF _Serum(to assess response to vaccination) • Salivary glands • Hippocampus • Brain stem • Cerebellum	E/M can demonstrate viral particle/ • In skin biopsy, corneal smear or saliva can demonstrate genomic RNA or viral mRNA by PCR or dot-blot hybridization assay (with 32P labelled nucleic acid probes) • Giemsa's stain or Sellers technique can demonstrate inclusion body (Negri body may be absent in 20% of patients)/ Mouse pathogenicity test- intracerebral inoculation of sample into suckling mice, observe for 28 days	• Vero monkey kidney • BHK (Baby hamster kidney) • Mouse neuro-blastoma	No CPE occurs After 18-24 hrs of inoculation, presence can be demonstrated by fluorescent antibody test	In serum and CSF, specific antibodies can be demonstrated by ELISA	• These occur usually late in disease, not relevant. • Vaccination can cause confusion (vaccinated individuals have low titres of < 1:64 of neutralizing antibodies)
Marburg & Ebola/ Filoviruses are classified as Biosafety Level 4 pathogens, so utmost care in isolation. Prompt notification of public health authorities is mandatory for suspected cases, before any diagnostic attempts are made	• Serum • Blood • Autopsy specimens e.g. from liver Samples must be refrigerated & packed according to IATA regulation to world's few containment facilities	Virions can be demonstrated in blood, liver, lungs by E/M & staining fluorescent antibody (following precautionary irradiation)	Vero cell cultures Virus culture must be attempted only in maximum security laboratories	-	Antibody by immunofluorescence & RIA	Antibody are demonstrable 7-10 days, after infection (is an exotic antigen)

Contd.

Contd.

Lymphocytic choriomeningitis virus/ Diagnosis is suggested by history of rodent contact No person to person transmission of infection has been documented	• Serum • Blood • C.S.F.	Intracerebral inoculation of Blood/CSF to weaning (1 month old mice or young guinea pig)	-	-	Rising titre of serum antibodies by indirect IF, C.F.T, Nt tests	
Calciviruses	• Faeces • Serum	Viral antigen detected by ELISA/ by Immunoelectron microscopy viral particle can be demonstrated		-	IgG and IgM specific antibodies by ELISA	
Hepatitis E/ Serologic & viral antigen demonstration approach is resorted to (previously exclusion approach)	• Faeces • Serum	Viral antigen in stool/ RT. PCR can demonstrate viral genome/ Viral concentration in stool is usually low & is present only during first week, after onset of jaundice *Immune electron microscopy* can demonstrate aggregated Calicivirus like particles using Monoclonal antibodies	Virus not cultivable	-	IgG - anti HEV IgM - anti HEV IgG and IgM antibodies by ELISA and western blot assay	
Rubella (German measles)/ Indications for diagnosis 1. A woman considering vaccination wants to know her immune status 2. An unimmunized woman in 1st trimester of pregnancy develops rash, want to know, if she has contracted disease & should have an abortion 3. A baby is born with signs suggestive of rubella syndrome(in latter two conditions culture can have role)	• Throat swab • Serum • Cord blood • Amniotic fluid in pregnant woman by amniocentesis *Infants with CRS* • Throat swab • Urine in new born • C.S.F • Leucocytes	-	• Vero • Rabbit kidney (RK-13, SIRC)	CPE is inconspicuous Infection detected by interference technique in which inoculated monkey kidney cells are challenged by Coxsackie A Culture not used routinely, as is expensive, tedious & may require as long as 2 weeks for demonstrable effect	Traditionally haemagglutination inhibition(H.I.)was the test & gold standard IgG &IgM specific antibodies by ELISA	Presence indicate immunity(as single serotype) For confirming primary rubella, 4 fold rise to be demonstrated between acute & convalescent sera Becomes +ve 1 week after appearance of rash & can remain positive for few months
HIV I & II (AIDS)/diagnosis essentially serologic initial screening tests ELISA/ rapid ICT based (Immunochromatographic based tests common) *Confirmation* of result done by repeating the serological test of different type Bacterial, Viral, Parasitic, Fungal infection & malignancies may need to be identified Other non-specific indicators are: • Lymphopenia: • Lowering of CD4 : CD8 ratio (even reversal): • Hypergammaglobulinemia: • Deficient C.M.I	• Serum • Blood • Other specimens according to opportunistic infections	1. *p24 levels* (can be detected in serum by ELISA in 30% patients during 'window' period i.e. have role before specific antibodies are detectable. Levels can also help in monitoring ART. *P.C.R* role in: (a) Early infection(before antibodies appear) (b) Retesting viral load, so monitoring treatment (by RT-PCR) (c) In diagnosing babies borne to infected mothers (d) In diagnosing double infection (e) Detecting sequence variabilities of HIV genome (by gene sequencing)	Culture a research tool Lymphocyte culture co-cultivation done: Patient's peripheral lymphocytes inoculated in presence of mitogens; as PHA & interleukin-2 (T cell growth factor), can be isolated from all the stages & numerous specimens; as bone-marrow, lymph node etc.	Growth identified by: (i) RT activity (ii) E/M to detect viral particle (iii) P24 in supernatant (iv) Indirect immunofluoresence, using specific monoclonal antibodies to detect HIV proteins	HIV1 & 2 detected with separate tests (combined kits also available) Negative when patient in 'window periods' *Screening tests:* ELISA : Rapid test: (i) Latex agglutination test (ii) Dot blot (ICT based test): *Confirmatory tests* repeat test of different type: Western blot (antibodies to specific viral proteins detected) Appropriate HIV testing strategy to be applied Details: p. 491-494	-Highly senstive & specific Require expensive equipment & about 4 hrs. - Time required is less than 30 mins. Easy interpretation More expensive -Antibodies to: core protein: reverse transcriptase: surface antigen, detected(sometimes test is ambiguous, then designated as indeterminate & then repeated after 6 months)

Contd.

Contd.

Poliomyelitis	• Faeces • Throat swab • C.S.F.(Difficult to isolate from it) • Serum Laboratory diagnosis is important, unless epidemiologic support exists It is important to differentiate wild virulent strain from attenuated vaccine strain	Nucleic acid hybridization to differentiate from vaccine strain(as nucleic acid sequences of both strains are known) Direct electron microscopy/Immune electron microscopy can demonstrate viral particle/ Intraspinal inoculation of monkey was done to differentiate wild strain from vaccine strains (develop typical sign & symptoms)	Any human/simian cell line	C.P.E develops within a few days, early changes include cell retraction, increased refractility, cytoplasmic granularity & nuclear pyknosis Neutralization tests with standard sera of 3 types	• Neutralizing antibody • C.F.T	Paired sera are required for interpretation
Coxsackie group A-23 serotype group B - 6 serotype	• Faeces(isolation from it should be interpreted cautiously, as asymptomatic shedding can persist) • Throat swab • C.S.F.	Intracranial inoculation into suckling mice Pathological changes in suckling mice *Group A*: - flaccid paralysis; - Generalized myositis; - Death within a week *Group B*: - spastic paralysis; - focal myositis; - localized lesions within liver, pancreas & other organs	Human diploid embyonic lung fibroblast, human rhabdomyosarcoma cell line	• C.P.E resemble those of polioviruses but develop slowly • Identification involve, several pools of reference sera	Not much role	

Section XIII: RNA Viruses

17 Assessment/Examination Questions

Chapter 2a

1. Classify viruses which cause gastroenteritis. To which family does Human Rotavirus belong? How has the name of the family been derived? Pg. 513, A4a, b., p. 437
2. Describe the morphology of the Rotavirus. Describe the epidemiology of rotavirus diarrohea. A 4c., p. 437, A 5a., p. 438
3. Describe the pathogenesis of rotavirus diarrohea. A 6., p. 438
4. What approach is commonly made to demonstrate this etiological agent? Describe the laboratory diagnosis of rotavirus diarrohea. A 3b-e., p. 437, p. 497

Chapter 2b

1. Mention key historical features in relation to Influenza. Compare and contrast the features of the Orthomyxoviruses and Paramyxoviruses. A 4c., p. 441, A 4b., p. 441
2. Illustrate the structure of the Influenza virus (in a figure). Briefly describe the structure of Influenza virus and tabulate the differences between haemagglutinin and neuraminidase. A 5b., p. 443
3. Describe the types and subtypes of Influenza virus. A 4d., p. 441-442
4. What are the key virulent factors of Influenza virus? Describe the pathogenesis of Influenza. A 4a., p. 441, A 3b., p. 440-441
5. Describe the epidemiology of Influenza. Describe the emergence of antigenic subtypes of Influenza A in the last century. A 6b, c., p. 443-444
6. Explain the emergence of antigenic drift and shift in a community using a hypothetical viralstructure. Tabulate the differences between antigenic drift and shift. A 6d., p. 444, A 6a., p. 443
7. Describe the laboratory diagnosis of Influenza. Pg. 497, P. 440
8. Describe vaccines used for prevention of Influenza. A 8a-c., p. 444-445, pg. 634-635
9. Enumerate key preventive strategies with reference to Influenza. What is the basis of the hypothesis that has led to the recommendation of keeping pigs, birds and human separately as for as possible? A 9a,b., p. 445

Chapter 3

1. Describe 'avian' (Bird flu) Influenza. P.446-447
2. During the recent outbreak of 'avian influenza', why was there so much scare? P. 446, A 2., p. 446
3. Why were the birds 'culled' (killed) during the outbreak? A 3a., p. 446
4. How can such 'outbreak' scenario be prevented in the future? A 7., p. 447

Chapter 4

1. Describe 'Swine flu'. P. 448, 449
2. What is 'swine flu' in pigs? Does 'swine Influenza virus', normally cause human infection? A 1, A2., p. 448
3. What was the likely origin of the 'swine influenza strain' that was involved in the outbreak in 2009? A 3., p. 448
4. Why was there a scare during the 'swine flu' outbreak progression? A4., p. 448
5. How was a confirmed case of 'swine flu' infection defined? A 5., p. 448
6. Is it safe to eat pork that is likely to be infected with this virus? A 10., p. 449

Chapter 5

1. Classify Paramyxoviruses. Describe morphology of Paramyxoviruses. A 3c., p. 450, A3b., p. 450 and p. 368
2. Write briefly on Parainfluenza viruses. A 3c., p. 450
3. To which family does RSV belong to? What are the viral envelope characteristics of this virus? A 3a., p. 450, A 3b
4. Describe pathophysiology of wheezing in RSV disease. A 2., p. 450
5. Describe Respiratory Syncytial virus including its laboratory diagnosis. P. 450-451
6. Describe briefly the following viruses namely Metapneumovirus, Nipah and Hendra viruses. A 12., p. 452

Chapter 6

1. To which family and genus, does the measles virus belong to? Describe the morphology of this virus including the virion projection peplomers and mention their part in the pathogenesis of the infection. A 4a., p. 454, A 4b., p. 45
2. Describe Measles virus including its laboratory diagnosis. Chapter 6., p. 453-455
3. Describe MMR vaccine. P. 636
4. Describe briefly SSPE. P. 498

Chapter 7

1. To which family does rabies virus belong? Describe briefly. P. 368 and A2d., p. 457
2. Describe the structure of rabies virus incorporating a diagram. Differentiate between the two forms of rabies virus (street and fixed virus). A 1b, c., p. 456, 457
3. Describe Negri body incorporating a diagram and tabulating the features. A 4b., p. 458
4. Describe in detail the pathogenesis of rabies. A4d., p. 458
5. Describe the basis of 10 day observation of suspected rabid dog. A 4e., p. 459-460
6. What is the basis of using saliva and conjuctival smear; as specimens in making an antemortem diagnosis of rabies. Describe the laboratory diagnosis of rabies. A 6e., p. 461, p. 498 (outline), A 6 a-e., p. 460-461
7. Classify categories of animal exposure and its importance. Classify the rabies vaccines in usage and describe them. A 8c,d ., p. 461-462
8. Describe passive immunization in rabies. A 8c., p. 462

Chapter 8

1. Comment on the discovery and classification of Hepatitis A virus (HAV). A 1b., p. 463
2. Enumerate the viruses involving the liver. Tabulate the differences amongst the various Hepatitis viruses. P. 513-514
3. How many serotypes does HAV have? What is the epidemiologic importance of this information? A 1c., p. 463
4. Describe the epidemiology of HAV and explain why do outbreaks due to this agent spread slowly and require months to peak and spread? A 4b., p. 464
5. Describe laboratory diagnosis of HAV infection. Mention briefly about HAV vaccine. A 6., p. 464-465

Chapter 9

1. Classify picornaviruses of medical importance. A 1c., p. 466
2. To which family does poliovirus belong? Briefly describe structure of poliovirus. A 1b., p. 466, A 1e., p. 466
3. How frequent is paralysis as a presentation of poliomyelitis? A 4a., p. 467
4. Describe pathogenesis of poliomyelitis. A 5a., p. 467
5. What is the most scared complication of paralytic poliomyelitis? What is the cause of it? How was paralytic poliomyelitis managed in the past and how it is managed currently? A 6a,b, 7., p. 468
6. Describe the laboratory diagnosis of poliomyelitis.
7. Describe the vaccines used against poliomyelitis. Compare and contrast the IPV and OPV vaccines. P. 637-638 and A 9c., p. 468-469
8. Write briefly on VAPP. A 10a., p. 469
9. Enumerate the enteroviruses of public health importance and mention the diseases caused by them. A 1e., p. 466
10. Describe briefly the following namely Echoviruses, Coxsackieviruses, Rhinoviruses and acute haemorrhagic conjunctivitis. A 14i-iv, p. 469-471
11. What approach is followed to diagnose the many enteroviruses (other than polio and coxsackie)? A 13., p. 469

Chapter 10

1. Which virus was responsible for the outbreak in Delhi in 1955-56 in which approximately 29,000 cases occurred? Describe the unique aspects about the HEV discovery including the technique used. A 2b., p. 472
2. What is the likely reason for the low secondary attack rate of the HEV infection in contacts of family members? Compare and contrast the key clinic-epidemiological features of HEV infection with that caused by HAV. A 3b, A4b., p. 472-473
3. Describe HEV including its laboratory diagnosis. p. 472-473

Chapter 11

1. Classify congenital and viral infections. To which family and genus, does rubella virus belong to? p. 514-515, A 1b., p. 474
2. Describe the pathogenicity and laboratory diagnosis of congenital rubella syndrome. A 1c., p. 474, A2., p. 474

3. Describe epidemiology and laboratory diagnosis of postnatal rubella. A 5b., p. 475, A 5d., p. 475
4. Describe rubella vaccine including the possible role of the 'Rubella parties' in the control of this disease. A 3a-c, A 4a,b., p. 474-475

Chapter 12

1. Classify (including definition) the arboviruses. Enumerate the diseases caused by them and mention the vector involved. Mention the common arboviral disease in India. p. 515-516
2. To which family does dengue virus belong? Enumerate viral infections transmitted by Aedes mosquito. A 3a., p. 476, A 9b., p. 599
3. What are the factors that have made dengue that was a mild infection in the nineteenth century; present only in the tropics, to have increased manifold and put nearly half of the world's population at risk for this infection? How many times one can contract dengue in a life time? A5a, A 6a., p. 476-477
4. Why does one not rely on a test based on specific antibody demonstration in the early stage of dengue? Describe the laboratory diagnosis of dengue. A 4a., p. 476, A 4b., p. 476, A 7., p. 477
5. Enumerate the arboviruses that cause haemorrhagic fever. Describe Dengue haemorrhagic fever (DHF). p. 515, A 5d, A7

Chapter 13

1. To which family does the Japanese encephalitis virus belong to? p. 368
2. Describe the role of pigs as amplifier host in the transmission of this disease. A 4a., p. 478-479
3. Most of the infections with this virus are aymptomatic, then why does report of this disease cause fear amongst the public? A 3a, b., p. 479
4. Describe Japanese B encephalitis vaccine. A 5a-d., p. 479, p. 638
5. Describe the following namely Bunyaviruses, and Hantavirus, Chickungunya virus. A 6, A7.

Chapter 14

1. Name an important virus which belongs to the Flaviviridae family, which is not arthropod borne but spreads by blood transfusion. p. 481
2. Briefly describe the morphology of the HCV. Mention the role of the HCV heterogeneity in its epidemiology, treatment and vaccine development. p. 368, A 3c., p. 481
3. Which technique can detect HCV infection, before the individual develops antibody to the virus? Describe the laboratory diagnosis of HCV infection. A 4b., p. 481-482, A 4d., p. 482
4. What is the role of genotyping of this virus in the treatment of this infection? Describe the drugs used in the treatment of HCV infection. A 7a., p. 483, A 7b., p. 483
5. Describe HCV including its epidemiology and pathogenesis. A 6b., p. 483, A 5b., p. 481
6. Describe Kyasanur Forest disease.

Chapter 15

1. Classify retroviruses of human importance. A 4a., p. 487
2. Describe in detail the structure of the HIV virus highlighting the functional aspects (including the genes encoding the HIV antigens). A 6., p. 488
3. What is the I.P. of AIDS? What is the natural history of AIDS? A 3a, A3b., p. 484
4. Describe the emergence of AIDS as an entity. A 5., p. 487
5. Describe in detail the epidemiology of AIDS; emphasizing the modes of transmission. A 8c., p. 489-490
6. Describe in detail the pathogenesis of AIDS. A 3c., p. 484-487
7. What is the importance in suspecting HIV in early stage of infection? Can HIV serology (antibody) be negative in a early case? A 9a., p. 490, A9b., p. 490
8. Enumerate the opportunistic infections associated with AIDS. A 9c., p. 490
9. Describe in detail the laboratory diagnosis of AIDS. p.499, A9d., p. 491-493
10. Describe strategies of HIV testing in India. A 9c., p. 493-494
11. Describe post exposure prophylaxis in a suspected HIV exposed case. All., p. 494-495
12. Describe in detail the strategies for AIDS prevention. A 13., p. 495-496

Section XIV: Miscellaneous Virology

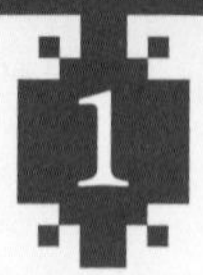

Integrated Clinical Case Based Study of HDV/Jaundice

Shanti (case of HBV infection) improved after receiving treatment for 6 months. Subsequently, she received three blood transfusions on account of low haemoglobin levels. She continued on the treatment but reported back to hospital after 18 months with worsened condition and liver biopsy revealing severe cirrhosis.

How could the fast progression of liver cirrhosis in this case be explained?

A.1 The case would have got infected with HDV during the blood transfusion, she was receiving.

Investigation of this case revealed presence of IgM – HDV antibodies in the serum.

What is the diagnosis of the case based on the current findings?

A.2 The case is having a HDV *superinfection*. This is a more common presentation than the *coinfection* category. Here a chronic hepatitis B case or a carrier gets infected with HDV. These cases can also present acutely, as above. Here more than 70% of the cases, finally result in chronic hepatitis. When HDV infection is transmitted from donor with one HBsAg subtype to an HBsAg +ve recipient of another subtype, HDV assumes HBsAg of recipient.

One (bad) characteristic of the chronic delta hepatitis is that it hastens the progression of cirrhosis, as what a HBV infection take about 15 years to develop cirrhosis; might be shortened to 2 years.

How can the diagnosis of HDV infection be confirmed?

A.3 Rising titres of specific HDV antibodies indicate acute infection, while sustained high titres indicates chronic infection.

The diagnosis can be confirmed by demonstrating the delta antigen and/or RNA in serum/liver.

How does co-infection of HBV case with HDV infection present?

A.4 This is a less common situation than super-infection, in which the patients gets simultaneous infection of HDV and HBV. Acute delta hepatitis tends to present as a severe illness with a high mortality of 2-20%. Most of the cases resolve and less than 5% of these cases can result in chronic delta hepatitis, in contrast to more than 70% of cases in super-infection category. The latter category occurs; when a chronic carrier of Hepatitis B gets infected with HDV.

Mention the discovery of HDV.

A.5 In 1977, Rizzetto and his colleagues in Italy described a new antigen in the nuclei of hepatocytes of HBsAg carriers by an immunofluorescence based technique. It was called delta antigen. Subsequently; this antigen was found in 36nm diameter, virus like particles, the capsid of which was indistinguishable from HBsAg. This was named hepatitis D virus. Some believe it to be a satellite hepatitis B virus. One of the unusual and absolute requirement of this virus, is the coinfection with hepatitis B virus, that it requires. So, it is a defective virus with insufficient genetic material to code for the various antigens, including delta, clearly HBV provides the genetic information to provide the various enzymes required for replication and expression.

Describe the structure of HDV.

A.6 Hepatitis D belongs to genus *Deltavirus*, it is a spherical virus of 36nm diameter with single stranded positive sense RNA strand.

It has an outermost coat of HBsAg encoded by the HBV genome. Inner to it is the HDag coat, encoded by the HDV with help from the HBV genome. Innermost is the RNA of the HDV. So it is a fascinating relationship of an DNA and a RNA virus in an infected hepatocyte.

How is HDV infection acquired?

A.7 The infection occurs primarily by the parenteral route and requires that the recipient person must be HBV infected. For other routes of transmission, there is little information. The incubation period varies between 2-12 weeks.

Mention about the epidemiology of HDV infection.

A.8 All areas with prevalence of HBV are not equally affected by HDV. High prevalence of HDV have been seen in Amazon basin of South America, Central Africa, Italy (Southern) and middle Eastern countries. The reasons for areas; as China and Southeast Asia not having a high prevalence of HDV is not known, though these areas have high HBV prevalence.

The infection is commonly seen in persons, who have multiple blood transfusions; as haemophiliacs or who are intravenous drug users.

How can HDV infection be controlled?

A.9 (i) Screening of blood for HBV can limit HDV transmission also

(ii) HBV immunization can prevent HDV infection; as HBV is necessary for HDV replication.

2 Integrated Clinical Case Based Study – Prions/ Outbreak of Bovine Spongiform Encephalopathy (BSE)

An outbreak of bovine spongiform encephalopathy ('mad cow disease') occurred in U.K. in 1987, which spread to involve more than 1.5 lakh cows by 1995. It resulted in sacrificing of even unaffected cattle. The beef industry was in shambles. Other countries stopped beef import and beef became a taboo.

What group of infectious agent was responsible for this outbreak?

A.1 Prions (Proteinaceous infectious particles).

How are prions defined?

A. 1 (b) These are unique infectious protein particles, not requiring nucleic acid for infectivity.

Classify the animal and human diseases implicated to prions?

A.2 (a)

Disease of Animals			
Disease	**Host**	**I.P.**	**Pathology**
Scrapie	Sheeps, Goat Mice	Months to years	Spongiform encephalopathy
Bovine spongiform encephalopathy	Cattle	Months to years	Spongiform encephalopathy
Mink encephalopathy (resembles scrapie)	Minks	Months to years	Spongiform encephalopathy
Disease of Man			
Disease	**Host**	**I.P.**	**Pathology**
Creutzfeldt-Jakob disease	Human, Chimpanzees	Months to years	Spongiform encephalopathy
Kuru	Human, Chimpanzees	Months to years	Spongiform encephalopathy
Gerstmann-Straussler Scheinker syndrome	Human, Chimpanzees	Months to years	Spongiform encephalopathy
Fatal familial insomnia	Human, Chimpanzees	Months to years	Spongiform encephalopathy

To what category are these diseases categorized?

A.2 (b) These are categorized; as Transmissible degenerative (spongiform) encephalopathies. These are also categorized as slow virus diseases.

Enumerate other chronic persistent viral infections (by conventional viruses).

A.2 (c) In animals – Visna (seen in the sheep, the etiological agent is a retrovirus)
– Maedi (seen in the sheep, etiological agent is a retrovirus)
In man – Subacute sclerosing pan-encephalitis (SSPE, by Measles virus)
– Progressive multifocal leucoencephalopathy (by Papova virus)

What is the pathology of prion mediated lesions?

A.2 (d) Varying degrees of neuronal loss,spongiform neuronal changes and astrocyte proliferation is seen.

How do these diseases spread?

A.2 (e) It is very important to determine, how prions mediated diseases spread, for one can then control the spread of disease. However, the process is not clear. It is believed that prions may cause some copies of normal protein to fold abnormally. Prion protein (PrP) has been identified on human chromosome 20 and has been cloned (MW 27-30 kD). The normal prion protein is designated as PrP^{c} (superscript 'c' designates cellular). Under some conditions, abnormal form of protein may be produced by conformational change, designated as PrP^{sc} (superscript 'sc' designates abnormal scrapie form). Prion are believed to be altered product of normal gene and specific prion mRNA is found both in normal and infected tissue. So these findings may negate the theory that prions are infectious agents. The prion mediated diseases postulate a unique concept in biology, where protein without nucleic acid is associated with disease transmission and replication. It is an exception to the central dogma of molecular biology. An abnormal isoform of the prion protein is believed to be the component of the prion protein to be associated with disease and transmissibility. The *abnormal* isoform differs from the the normal cellular form by the high beta sheet content, being insoluble in detergents, propensity to aggregate and relative resistance to proteolysis. One hypothesis to explain the reproduction of the prion proteins is, that the PrPsc forms heterodimer with PrPc serving as a template, which alters the folding of the latter to PrPsc. Because of their resistance to digestion, these forms accumulate (aggregate); as in scrapie into birefringent rods and fibrils in membranes, giving rise to pathology.

What are the biological and physical properties of prions?

A.2 (f)
- Are filterable with estimated diameter of <5 nm
- no virion like structure visible by electron microscope.
- unusual resistance to UV radiation, boiling (so for sterilization by autoclave, increased temperature and/or time required; as 134°C for 1.5 hour or chemicals; as 10% formalin for one hour)
- Transmissibilty to experimental animals.

What are the characteristic of prion mediated diseases?

A.2 (g) **General:** Inherited (10-15%), Infectious and sporadic disorders

Anatomical localization: Confined to nervous system

Pathology: Prion proteins accumulate within the nervous system; as amyloid plaques.

- Lesion characterized by progressive vaculoation in neurons (so; designated spongiform), extensive astroglial hypertrophy, proliferation and spongy change in grey matter.

Immunology
- Absence (minimal) of inflammatory/immune response
- No alteration in pathogenesis by immunosuppressants.

Clinical features
- Long incubation period (months to years)
- Chronic progressive pathology
- Usually fatal

Transmission to experimental animals: Intracerebral route of inoculation brings the most rapid onset of disease.

Resistance of these infective agents: To formaldehyde,Ionizing radiation and Dry heat.

How to sterilize articles suspected to have prions: (i) 134 -138°C for 1.5 hours (ii) Sodium hypochlorite (25% sodium hypochloride) for 1 hour.

What was the cause of the bovine spongiform encephalopathy 'BSE' outbreak?

A.3 It was through protein supplements, to cattle containing bonemeat, from sheep carcasses containing scrapie agent, which was inadequately treated to destroy its infectivity. The use of this feed is now prohibited since 1988.

Why were the unaffected cattle sacrificed in the 'BSE' outbreak?

A.4 The unaffected cattle might have been subclinically affected by this disease and would represent an unknown reservoir of this infection.

Can 'BSE' spread to man?

A.5 It isn't very clear, if the transmission occurs; as the incubation period may extend many years. However; a histopathological study of a 'new variant' of CJD cases, indicates that transfer from animal to human does occur. This entity has been designated as variant Creutzfeldt-Jakob disease, which can affect the younger population also.

Who got the nobel prize for work on prions?

A.6 Stanley Pruisner in 1997.

Aspects related to case theme/examination assessment

Describe Creutzfeldt–Jakob disease and Kuru?

A.7 **Classical Creutzfeldt–Jakob disease (CJD)**-It is characterized by dementia, as a result of spongiform degeneration of brain.

It has been characterized into three types, namely sporadic, inherited and acquired. The *sporadic* CJD is characterized by rapidly progressive disease with death within a few months. The *inherited* CJD has a autosomal dominant mode of inheritance. Two forms in it are Germann-Straussler-Schinker's syndrome and fatal familial insomnia. The acquired category comprises of two types, namely variant CJD (discussed in Q5 of this clinical case, p. 507) and *iatrogenic* CJD. The latter occurs after corneal transplant, contaminated injection of pituitary growth hormone and human dural grafts used in head injury.

Kuru-It is a human disease caused by prions and is characterized by cerebellar ataxia and tremors. It has an incubation of period of many years and ends fatally in 3-6 months. It is seen predominantly in women and children of eastern highlands of New Guinea, who indulge in the practice of cannibalism (eating of dead bodies of relatives, after an ritual). This disease is disappearing with the prohibition of ritual cannibalism. This disease can be transmitted experimentally to chimpanzees by inoculation of infected brain of Kuru patients. C. Gajdusek was awarded a nobel prize for his work in this disease.

The diagnosis of prion diseases in man is a challenge. PrP^{sc} can be demonstrated only in a research laboratory in a tissue. Sophisticate immunoassay is available for their demonstration. Indirect histopathological studies including immunochemical studies can indicate the disease process. Brain MRI can also be suggestive.

Describe Subacute sclerosing panencephalitis (SSPE) and Progressive multifocal Leuko-encephalopathy (PML).

A.8 **SSPE:**

- *Disease:* Is a rare fatal and slowly progressive degenerative disease of the central nervous system.
- *Follows:* Measles infection many years after initial infection. Death may occur 1-3 years, after onset of symptoms. It occurs very rarely after measles vaccination and very rarely after rubella infection.
- *Pathology:* A slow demyelination of the CNS with gradual degeneration of the mental and motor functions.
- *Diagnosis:*
  - Electron microscopic evidence of virus in the brain cells.
  - Serological evidence in serum and CSF (high titers of measles antibodies).
  - CMI to measles virus lacking.
  - Defective virus resembling measles virus can be cultivated from brain cells by a co-cultivation technique using Hela cells.

PML

- *Disease:* Is a rare subacute demyelinating disease of the elderly.
- *Follows:* Infection of the oligodendrocytes by Papova virus.
- *Pathology:* Disease occurs in elderly, whose immune system is impaired because of immunosuppressants or malignancy. The disease is characterized by progressive loss of motor functions, vision and speech. Death may occur after few months.
- *Diagnosis:*
  - Demonstration of virus by electron microscopy in brain tissue.
  - Demonstration of viral nucleic acid by PCR in CSF or brain tissue.

Oncogenic Viruses

Cancer deaths will be eliminated for all under 80 by 2050. — University College London and King's College, London

Cancer cells may be viewed; as the altered self cells, that are not in the control of normal growth regulating mechanisms. It is estimated that viruses are etiologically involved in about 10-15% of all human cancer cases. Let's study the current scenario.

Which were the transmissible cancers in the early 20th century, known to have a viral etiology.

A.1 (a) These were animal cancers; namely avian (fowl) leukosis and avian sarcoma.

Who were the scientific workers associated with this discovery?

A.1 (b) Credit goes to Ellerman and Bang and Peyton Roux for these demonstrations. The work on the avian (fowl sarcoma) fibrosarcoma occurred in 1919, when the workers excised this tumor from chicken ground it and injected the filtrate into another chicken to replicate the tumor.

Who was awarded the nobel prize for the work on viral oncogenesis?

A.2 Peyton Roux in 1966 for work in avian sarcoma.

Name the process by which cells acquire properties of cancer.

A.3 (a) Transformation

Compare the process of transformation of cells by DNA and RNA oncogenic viruses.

A.3 (b) In *DNA viruses*, the viral genome (provirus) or a portion of the viral genome (provirus) gets integrated with the host cell; except in cases of Papillomaviruses and Herpesviruses, where the provirus usually remains episomal. Usually, no infectious virus is produced by the host cell, as the integrated viral DNA is incomplete or 'defective' but new proteins may get encoded, which can disrupt regulation of cell processes and result in neoplastic transformation.

The commonest examples of *RNA viruses* implicated in cancer are retroviruses. The viral RNA is converted into double stranded DNA by reverse trascriptase (RNA directed DNA polymerase) enzyme, which gets integrated with host cell genome, as provirus. This may remain latent for long periods, but often transcribe a complete range of viral proteins and new virions, which may bud from the host cell plasma membrane. The process of transformation is usually slow and the tumor is often seen after long latent period.

Enumerate the characteristic of cells transformed by viruses.

A.3 (c)

Table 14.3.1: Characteristics of cell transformed by viruses

Genomic changes	• Viral genome usually integrated with chromosome (rarely exists; as plasmid) • Chromosomal alterations (may) express poorly/not present
Changes in antigen	• Apperance; sometimes of tumor-specific transplantation antigen (TSTA) and/or new intracellular antigens; as T antigen
Morphological changes	• Cells usually get rounded and pile up (as cell contact inhibition is lost)
Growth changes	• Increased growth rate • May divide indefinitely in cultures

Does the process of transformation of cells in culture is always accompanied by formation of tumors in animals? Give example.

A.3 (d) No, e.g., HHV-4 (Epstein Barr virus) causes immortalization of human B cell but that is only one of the many processes, that can result in the development of Burkitt's lymphoma.

e.g., Infection of the liver cell by hepatitis B virus results in increased proliferation of these cells, however this is only one of the processes that can lead to hepatocellular carcinoma.

Enumerate the mechanisms by which oncogenic viruses transform cells.

A.4 (a)
- Activating or supplying growth-stimulating genes
- Removing the mechanisms, that inhibit growth; as loss of p 53
- Preventing apoptosis

What is v-onc (viral oncogene), c-onc, protooncogene and tumor suppressor gene? Briefly explain their importance.

A.4 (b)
- *v-onc* (viral oncogene): These are genes of viruses, which induce the transformation of a normal cell into a tumor cell. Currently more than about 60 such v-onc genes are known (Table 14.3.2).
- *c-onc* (cellular oncogene): It is the normal cellular gene corresponding to more than the 60 v-onc genes (Table 14.3.2)
- *Proto-oncogene:* It implies the normal cellular genes corresponding to the v-onc genes, having a origin in the retroviruses.
- *Tumor suppressor gene* (anti-oncogene): As the name indicates; are genes that by their protein products, are involved in negative regulation of growth. They were discovered in 1989 and if these are inactivated by mutation, excessive growth, resulting in tumor may occur eg retinoblastoma gene (whose loss leads to the development of retinoblastoma). These genes are recessive, so both copies of the genes have to be inactivated for excessive cellular activity to occur. It must be realized that the process of conversion of a normal cell into a tumor cell is a multistep process.

Table 14.3.2: Relationship between viral and cellular oncogenes

VIRAL ONCOGENE	Origin	Tumor in natural host	CELLULAR ONCOGENE	Chromosomal location in man
v-src	Chicken	sarcoma	c-src	20
v-ras	Rat	sarcoma	c-ras	11
v-myc	Chicken	myelomatosis	c-myc	08

NB: src-sarcoma of chicken, myc-myelomatosis of chicken and v-myc is myelomatosis of chicken

Enumerate viruses associated with animal cancers.

A.5 By *DNA viruses*
- Benign histiocytomas (in monkeys, by Yaba virus)
- Sarcomas in new born hamsters (associated with adenovirus)
- Marek's disease (associated with herpes virus, is neurolymphomatosis of chicken)
- Lucke's tumor of frog (associated with herpes virus, is adrenal adenocarcinoma)
- Sarcoma in rodents (associated with SV 40)
- Lymphoma (or reticulum cell carcinoma) of animals, e.g., monkey's kidney (associated with Herpes virus *samiri*)

By *RNA viruses* (retroviruses)
- Avian sarcoma leukosis complex
- Murine leukosis viruses
- Leukosis –sarcoma virus

Enumerate DNA and RNA viruses implicated in human cancer.

A.6 **Table 14.3.3:** DNA and RNA viruses implicated in human cancer.

DNA viruses

	Virus	**Malignancy**
Family		
Papovaviridae	Papilloma	Warts (genital; as penile and cervical) which may become malignant
	Polyoma	Carcinomas and sarcomas
	BK and JC	Polyoma
Poxviridae	Molluscum contagiosum	Nodular epidermal Hyperplasia
	Shopa fibroma	Fibroma
	Yabavirus	Nodular fibromatous hyperplasia
	HHV-4	Nasopharyngeal carcinoma, Burkitt's lymphoma, B cell lymphoma
	HHV- 8	Kaposi sarcoma
Hepadnaviridae	Hepatitis B	Carcinoma of liver

RNA viruses

Flaviviridae	Hepatitis C	Carcinoma liver
Retroviridae	Human T cell lymphotropic viruses 1 & 2	T cell leukemia/lymphoma
	Human immunodeficiency virus	Associated with non-Hodgkin lymphoma

NB: Certain adenoviruses can cause sarcomas in hamsters but do not cause cancer in man

Mention a human genital cancer for which a vaccine has become recently available. Briefly describe its composition and mechanism of action.

A.7 – Cervical cancer (in women). Vaccine details see pg. 633, Section 17.

Table 14.4.5: Characteristics of Hepatitis Viruses

Virus	HAV	HBV	HCV	HDV	HEV
Discoverer	Feinstone et.al	Blumberg (HBsAg), Dane et.al. (virion)	Bradley Lab (at CDC)	Rizzeto and colleagues	Balayan and colleagues
Year	1973	1965, 1970	1989	1977	1983
Family/Genus	Picornaviridae/ Hepatovirus	Hepadnavirdae/ Orthohepadnaviridae	Flaviviridae/ Hepacivirus	Unclassified/ Deltavirus	Hepeviridae/ Hepevirus
Virion (diameter)	27 nm	42 nm	60 nm	35 nm	30 nm
Envelope	-	+(HBsAg)	+	+(HBsAg)	-
Genome Size	7.5 kb	3.2 kb	9.4 kb	1.7 kb	7.6 kb
Transmission (primary mode)	Fecal-oral	Parenteral, Sexual, perinatal	Parenteral	Parenteral	Fecal-oral
Prevalence	High	High	Moderate	Low	Regional
I.P. (weeks)	2-6 (weeks)	2-6 (months)	6-8 (weeks)	2-12 (weeks)	6-8 (weeks)
Antigen in Blood	HAV	HBsAg, HBeAg	HCV	HDAg	HEV
Antibody in blood	Anti-HAV	Anti-HBs, Anti-HBc, Anti-HBe	Anti-HCV	Anti-HDV	Anti-HEV
Chronic Disease	None	Often	Often	Often	None
Oncogenic potential	No	Yes	Yes	No	No
Extrahepatic Lesion	+	+	+	-	-
Mortality	<1%	1-10%	Variable with genotype	1-10%	1–2% (high in pregnancy)
Vaccine	+	+	+	+ (for HBV)	-

VIRAL INFECTIONS OF THE GENITOURINARY SYSTEM

These diseases are depicted in table 14.4.6. Genital herpes and warts are important sexually transmittted diseases, whose incidence has increased with change of the sexual practices. The viruses infecting the urinary tract are depicted in table 14.4.6, fortunately these rarely infect this system.

Table 14.4.6: Viral Diseases of the Genitourinary System

Disease	Virus
GENITAL	
Genital herpes	HHV -2>HHV-1
Genital warts	HPVs 6 & 11
Genital carcinomas	HPVs 6, 11, 16, 18 & 31
Cervicitis	Adenovirus 37
Mollusum contagiosum	Molluscum contagiosum virus
URINARY	
Urethritis	HHV-2, Adenovirus 37
Acute hemmorhagic cystitis	Adenovirus 11, 21
Glomerulonephritis (immune complex mediated)	Hepatitis B virus
Nephropathy	HHV-5 (CMV), Hantan virus

CONGENITAL AND PERINATAL VIRAL INFECTIONS

These infections are depicted in Table 14.4.7 Congenital (*Prenatal*) infectious are those that are acquired by the fetus transplacentally before birth. The *perinatal* (natal or intrapartum) infection are those, that are acquired during passage of the baby through an infected genital tract or infection from faeces. The *postnatal* infections are as the name indicates, those that are acquired after delivery.

Table 14.4.7: Congenital and Perinatal Viral Infections

	Virus	Disease
Prenatal	HHV-3 (Varicella)	Congenital varicella syndrome
	HHV-5 (CMV)	Cytomegalic inclusion disease
	Rubella	Congenital rubella syndrome (CRS)
Intrapartum	HHV-2(HSV-2)	Neonatal Herpes
	Coxsackie B	Myocarditis (newborn)
	HHV-3 (Varicella)	Disseminated varicella zoster
	HHV-5 (CMV)	Pneumonia
Perinatal	Hepatitis B/C	Hepatitis B/C, carrier state
	HIV-1 & 2	AIDS
	HTLV-1	Leukemia

ARBOVIRUSES

Arboviral illnesses are viral illnesses transmitted to vertebrates (including man) by bite of arthropod vectors. Arboviral classification is based on epidemiologic grounds and is being maintained, as is useful biologically (in the field). This group contains viruses belonging to different viral families, so this classification is not taxonomically acceptable.

Table 14.4.8: Arboviruses and their association with clinical syndromes

Virus	Genus/Family	Geographical distribution	Vector	Reservoir
Fever with or without rash and arthralgia				
Chikungunya	Alpha virus/Togaviridae	Africa, Asia (including India)	*Aedes aegypti*	Not Known ?(Monkey)
Sindbis	Alphavirus/Togaviridae	Africa, Asia	Mosquito	Birds, Mammals
Dengue	Flavivirus/Flaviviridae	South east Asia (especially Thailand and India)	*Aedes aegypti*	Not Known ?(Monkey)
West nile	Flavivirus/Flaviviridae	Asia, Africa and USA	Mosquito	Birds
Sandfly fever	Bunyavirus/Bunyaviridae	Mediterranean, Asia and Tropical America	Sand fly	Not known
Colorado tick fever	Orbivirus/Reoviridae	USA	Tick	Rodents
Encephalitis				
Eastern equine encephalitis	Alphavirus/Togaviridae	Americas	Mosquito	Birds
Western equine encephalitis	Alphavirus/Togaviridae	Americas	Mosquito	Reptiles
West nile	Flavivirus/Flaviviridae	Asia, Africa and USA	Mosquito	Birds
Japanese encephalitis	Flavivirus/Flaviviridae	East and South East Asia	Culicine Mosquito	Wild birds, Pigs
Russian Spring-Summer Encephalitis	Flavivirus/Flaviviridae	East Europe, Russia (formerly)	Tick	Mammals (including Rodents), Birds and Ticks
Haemorrhagic Fever				
Crimean Congo Hemorrhagic fever	Nairovirus/Bunyaviridae	Africa, Middle East, Asia (including India)	Tick	Small mammals
Chikungunya	Alphavirus/Flaviviridae	Africa, Asia (include India)	*Aedes aegypti*	Not known (?monkey)
Dengue	Flavivirus/Flaviviridae	South-east Asia (especially Thailand and India)	*Aedes aegypti*	Not known (?monkey)
Kyasanur Forest Disease	Flavivirus/Flaviviridae	Karnataka (India)	*Ixodes ricinus*	Forest birds and animals
Yellow fever	Flavivirus/Flaviviridae	Africa, South America	Culicine mosquitos	Monkey, man

VIRAL HAEMORRHAGIC FEVER

This category of diseases are a heterogenous group but share a characteristic of widespread hemorrhages from the body's epithelial surfaces including GIT and skin. The diseases are depicted in table 14.4.9.

Table 14.4.9: Viral Haemorrhagic Fevers

Virus/Family	Disease	Distribution
Dengue/Flaviviridae	Dengue, DHF, DSS	South east Asia (especially Thailand and India)
Kyasanur Forest/Flaviviridae	Kyasanur forest disease	Karnataka (India)
Yellow fever/Flaviviridae	Yellow fever	Africa, South America
Crimean–Congo Haemorrhagic fever/Bunyaviridae	Crimean haemorrhagic fever	Africa, Middle east, Asia (including India)
Lassa/Arenaviridae	Lassa fever	Africa
Marburg/Filoviridae	Hemorrhagic fever	Africa
Ebola/Filoviridae	Hemorrhagic fever	Africa
Hantan or Haantan/Bunyaviridae	Rodent-borne nephropathy	Asia, Europe
Rift Valley Fever/Bunyaviridae	Rift valley fever	Africa, Middle East
Junin/Arenaviridae	Argentine haemmorhagic fever	Argentina
Machupo/Arenaviridae	Bolivian hemmorhagic fever	Bolivia

Note: Arboviruses common in India include Chickungunya, Dengue, J.E., K.F.D., Sindbis, Chandipura, Chittoor, Gunjam and Vellore.

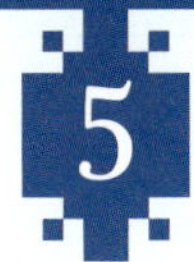

Antiviral Drugs

High Throughput Screening (HTS) is a drug-discovery process widely used in pharmaceutical industry. It allows the assaying of a large number of potential modulators against disease targets to identify 'hits'. Let's hope this technology and other techniques bring us close to the control the viral diseases.

Mention about the initial development of antiviral drugs.

A.1 In the beginning, most of the available successful antiviral drugs were nucleoside analogs and were effective against herpes group of infections. The first antiviral drug to be licensed for the treatment of systemic herpes group of infections was *Adenine arabinoside*, being synthesized in 1960. However like any cytotoxic anticancer drug, it had the limitation of causing severe side effects on parentral administration. A major success in antiviral chemotherapy occurred in 1974, when Acycloguanosine (Acylovir) was discovered. Its full potential as an antiherpes drug was, however only realized in mid 1980s. It can be administered both locally and systemically. It has the advantage over adenine arabinoside in requiring a herpes virus coded enzyme to activate it, thus reducing its toxicity on non-infected host cells, as only virally infected cells would have the enzyme.

Discuss the reasons for decreased availability of antiviral drugs.

A.2 The availability of antiviral drugs has been scarce for many reasons. *One*, many viral infection are trivial in nature, short lasting and heal without causing any major morbidity. So the acute need of antiviral drugs is sometimes not felt. *Secondly*, viruses are absolutely dependent on the host metabolic pathway for their survival (including replication), so most antiviral drugs would have some toxicity on the host cell, a feature that is not welcome. For the same reason, antiviral drugs must be able to enter* human cells for their activity. *Thirdly,* presence of viral mutants to antiviral drugs is discouraging. Viral mutant resistant to every manufactured antiviral drug have been detected. This problem gets accentuated, when extended drug therapy (months to years) is required for chronic infections; as HBV, HCV, herpes infections and HIV. *Fourthly,* antiviral drugs must be extremely efficacious and should be almost 100% efficient in blocking viral growth. For minimal replication in the presence of an antiviral drug, provides the environment for resistant mutants to prosper. Such a situation can occur in inadequate administration of antiviral drugs. The simultaneous use of two or more antiviral drugs can combat the drug resistance problem, e.g., ART combinations in AIDS and IFN-α + ribavivin in HCV treatment. The combination may also reduce the drug toxicity. *Lastly* the cost of bringing an new antiviral drug to market can be in the range of $ 100 million to $ 500 million (Rs. 500 crore-2500 crore).

*Except those that would be acting at the level of viral attachment, penetration, uncoating and those that act at release of virus.

Tabulate the currently available antiviral drugs, their usage and their mechanism of action.

A.3

Table 14.5.1: Currently available antiviral drugs and their mechanism of action

Name of drug	Category	Usage	Mechanisms
Amantidine/Rimantidine	Matrix protein M2 inhibitor	In Influenza A infection	Inhibits viral entry and penetration
Ribavirin	Synthetic analog of nucleoside guanosine	In ^RSV, HBV, HCV, Lassa virus and others	Inhibits nucleic acid synthesis, block capping of mRNA
–	Antisense RNA (expression by vector)	Papillomaviruses	Inhibit mRNA synthesis
Acyclovir	Purine analog	Herpes simplex, Varicella zoster	Inhibits viral DNA polymerase
Vidarabine	Purine analog	Herpes simplex, Varicella zoster	Inhibits viral DNA polymerase

Contd.

Contd.

Valacyclovir	Purine analog	Herpes	Inhibits viral DNA polymerase
Ganciclovir	Purine analog	Cytomegalovirus	Inhibits viral DNA polymerase
Idoxuridine	Pyrimidine analog	Herpes	Inhibits viral DNA polymerase
Zidovudine (azidothymidine)	Nucleoside reverse transcriptase inhibitor-NRTI (Structural analog of thymidine)	HIV	Reverse transcriptase inhibitor
Zalcitabine/ Dideoxycytidine	NRTI	HIV	Reverse transcriptase inhibitor
Didanosine/ Dideoxyinosine	NRTI	HIV	Reverse transcriptase inhibitor
Stavudine	NRTI	HIV	R.T. inhibitor
Lamivudine	NRTI	HIV, HBV	Nucleoside reverse transcriptase inhibitor
Nevirapine	Non-nucleoside reverse transcriptase inhibitor (NNRTI)	HIV	Nucleoside reverse transcriptase inhibitor
Saquinavir *Ritonavir* *Indinavir* *Nelfinavir*	Protease inhibitors	HIV	Δ Proteases essential for production of mature infectious viral particles and/or their release
Zanamivir (Relenza), Oseltamivir (Tamiflu)	Neuraminidase inhibitor	Influenza A and B infection	ΘNeuraminidase enzyme is involved in maturity of new virion and budding of virus from host cell
IFNα 2a	Interferon	HBV, HCV	Multiple effects including inhibition of viral protein synthesis
IFNα- 2b		HCV, HBV, HPV (condylomata acuminata)	
Interferon alpha 2b		Condylomata acuminata	
Palvizumab	Chimeric monoclonal antibody (human and murine)	RSV	Neutralizes RSV and inhibits its fusion with host cell membrane
Pleconaril		Picornaviruses	Block uncoating of picornaviruses
Raltegravir	Integrase inhibitor	HIV	Block integration of cDNA of HIV into host chromosome
Maraviroc	CCR5 co-reception antagonist	HIV	C-C chemokine receptor 5 binding by drug leads to blocking of HIV binding to macrophages
Enfuvirtide	Fusion inhibitor	HIV	Block penetralion and uncoating of HIV

^ Given as aerosol form, mechanism not clear

Θ So, inhibition of neuraminidase activity would prevent the release of the virus and block viral spread

Δ Many HIV proteins which are synthesized by viral mRNA, need to be cleaved by viral protease, before mature HIV is produced.

NB: Protease inhibitors are given in combination with RT inhibitors to prevent (minimize) the development of drug resistance.

6 Assessment/Examination Questions

Chapter 1

1. Describe Hepatitis D virus. P. 504-505

Chapter 2

1. Classify the animal and human diseases implicated to prions. A 2a., p. 506
2. Enumerate chronic persistent viral infections caused by agents other than prions. A 2c., p. 506
3. What are the biological and physical properties of these unconventional agents? A 2f., p. 507
4. What are the characteristic of prion mediated diseases? A 2g., p. 507
5. During the 'mad cow disease' outbreak of 1990s, why were the unaffected cattle sacrificed? A 4., p. 507
6. Describe the following diseases namely: Creutzfeldt–Jacob disease, Kuru, SSPE and PML. A 7, A8., p. 508

Chapter 3

1. Who was awarded the nobel prize for work in viral oncogenesis? A 2., p. 509
2. Enumerate the viruses associated with animal cancer. A 5., p. 510
3. Enumerate the viruses associated with human cancer. A 6., p. 510-511
4. Describe oncogenes. A 4b., p. 510
5. Discuss the mechanisms involved in viral oncogenesis. A 3a-d and A 4a,b., p. 509-510

Chapter 4

1. Outline the viruses associated with central nervous system diseases. Table 14.4.1., p. 512
2. Outline the viruses associated with eye diseases. Table 14.4.2., p. 512
3. Outline the viruses associated with genitourinary system diseases. Table 14.4.6., p. 514

Chapter 5

1. Discuss the reasons for the scarcity in the availability of the antiviral drugs for viral infections. A 2., p. 517
2. Enumerate the currently available antiviral drugs and their mechanism of action. A 3., p. 517-518
3. Describe anti-retroviral agents. A3., p. 517-518., and Table 13.15.8., p. 494
4. What are interferons? Describe their role as antiviral agents. A 3., p. 518

Section XV: Mycology

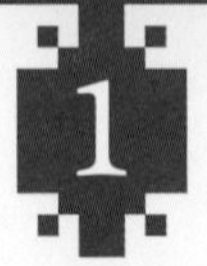

General Aspects Including Classification and Laboratory Diagnosis

Medical mycology ('mykos' means mushroom) deals with the study of fungi that are of relevance to human beings; especially as agents of disease. Fungi have now globally emerged as important causes of human infectious diseases. However the impression shouldn't go that they are only harmful to man. They have been useful to man; as a model for study of genetics (*Neurospora crassa*), source of food (edible mushroom), industrial use in the production of alcohol/wine (Saccharomyces), production of antibiotics (penicillin from *P. notatum*), drug (ergot from Claviceps) and vaccines (*Saccharomyces cerevisiae*-in recombinant hepatitis B vaccine). Let's study this category of infectious agents.

How are fungi differentiated from bacteria (prokaryotes)?

A.1(a) These are eukaryotes and can be differentiated from bacteria (prokaryotes) by (i) being both multicellular or unicellular (ii) possessing rigid cell wall containing chitin, mannan (as in candida) and other polysaccharides (unlike peptidoglycan in bacteria) (iii) cell membrane containing ergosterol (in bacteria; sterols are present only in mycoplasma (iv) the cell cytoplasm contains true nucleus, mitochondria and endoplasmic reticulum (v) divide by both sexual and asexual processes (vi) spores (sexual and asexual) are formed for reproduction, not as a means to escape unfavourable conditions. Most fungal spores are of asexual category and the two types are conidia and sporangiospores. Conidia (microconidia and macroconidia) are formed externally by mitosis on a specialized hyphal structure called conidiophore, whereas sporangiospores are formed internally within specialized structures called sporangia.

How are fungi differentiated from other eukaryotes?

A.1(b) Fungi possess a rigid cell wall composed of chitin and glucan and a cell membrane, in which instead of cholestrol, ergosterol is present.

Why are fungi often overlooked as etiological agents for human disease?

A.2 Fungi; as etiological agents are often overlooked in the medical science because routine microbiological cultures and investigations are usually bacterial based. The identification of most fungi requires skilled human observation rather than automated machines. The traditional culture techniques are also time consuming and require many weeks for isolation of the fungi. For this reason, the diagnosis of fungal diseases is often by exclusion and the failure of the antibacterial antibiotics to give a favourable outcome. The patient could get maximum benefit, if the medical mycologist, pathologist and the clinician work in close harmonious collaboration, in management of cases with fungal diseases.

What are the reasons for the emergence of fungal infections?

A.3 The reasons for the emergence of fungal infections are many. One, the bacterial infections have been controlled in the developed countries. Secondly, the factors that have led to an increase in the life span of man; as usage of antimicrobial agents, steroids, immunosuppressive agents and anti-cancer drugs, all predispose to fungal infections. Thirdly, the current life style disorders; as diabetes mellitus also predispose the individual to fungal diseases.

Describe the epidemiology of fungal infections.

A.4 Most fungi that are pathogenic to man are saprophytic in nature. Most fungal infections arise from contact with environmental reservoir. These diseases are fortunately not communicable from one person to another. The exceptions being Candida species, which may form part of person's microbial flora and some superficial mycoses, which can be transmitted by close personal contact; as sharing of personal usage items; as combs and nail cutters.

Many human fungal infections are mild and self limiting, due to strong innate immunity to fungi. Neutrophils serve to phagocytize and kill fungi. T-cell mediated immunity is a key factor in protection from fungal disease. The natural habitat of most fungi is soil or water, containing decaying organic matter. The fungi obtain soluble nutrients by secreting degradative enzymes; as cellulases and proteases into their surrounding environment. Some fungi; as Candida species can be parasitic in nature but they are mostly endogenous in origin, i.e., originate from persons own microbial flora. The optimal temperature for growth of most fungi (yeasts and molds) is 25-30°C. The notable exceptions being *Cryptococcus neoformans* and *Tricophyton verrucosum,* which grow optimally at 37°C.

Describe the morphological classification of fungi.

A.5 Fungi can be classified in several ways. One of the simplest classifications is the morphological classification based on the morphology of the fungal cell and colony. It divides the fungi into four categories (as depicted in flow-diagram 1)

Flow Diagram 1: *Morphological classification of fungi* (based on morphology of cells)

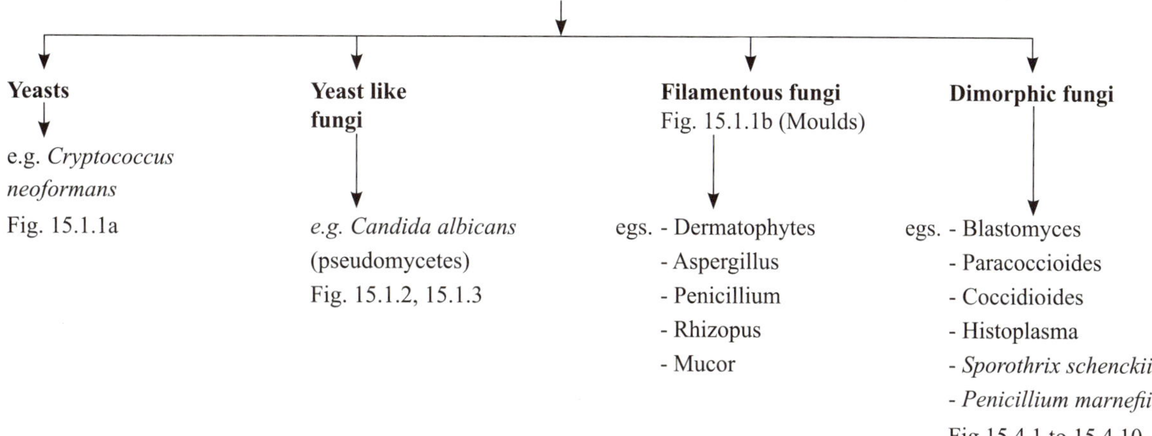

At one extreme are the simple structures known as the **yeasts**, which are unicellular organisms, that are spherical or ellipsoidal in shape (Fig 15.1.1a) and reproduce asexually by budding or by fission to produce daughter cells. The daughter cells (or progeny) may elongate to produce structures designated as *pseudohyphae* (Fig. 15.1.2.). At the other extreme are the structures known as the **moulds** or **filamentous fungi**. These are multicellular structures consisting of tubular structures called *hyphae*. These grow and branch to form structure called *mycelium* (Fig. 15.1.1b).

The **second** category of fungi based on morphology is called **yeast-like-fungi**. This category arises, as some fungi apparently have characters of yeasts and moulds, e.g., some yeasts; as *C. albicans* develop filamentous component. The latter structure arises as this fungus divides by budding, but the buds fail to separate and these elongate to appear as hypha like structure is called *pseudohypha*. It is important to differentiate these two structures. (Table 15.1.1)

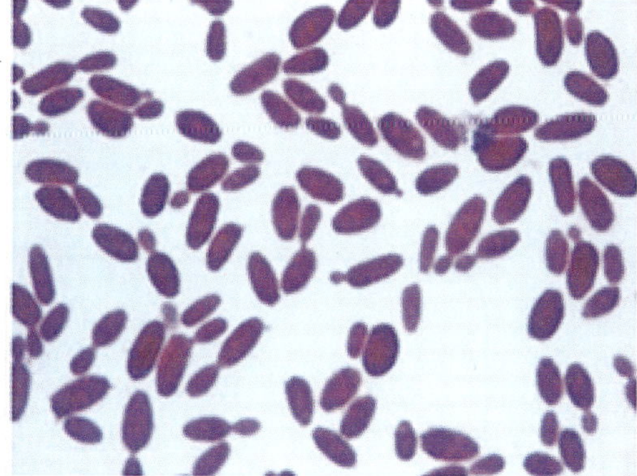

Fig.15.1.1 (a): Gram stained smear demonstrating budding yeast cells

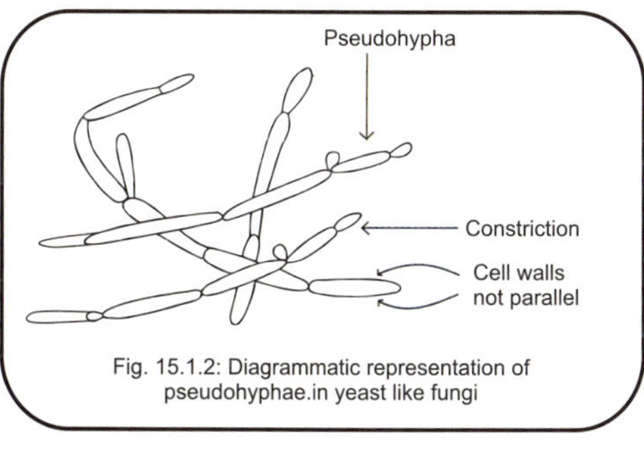

Fig. 15.1.2: Diagrammatic representation of pseudohyphae.in yeast like fungi

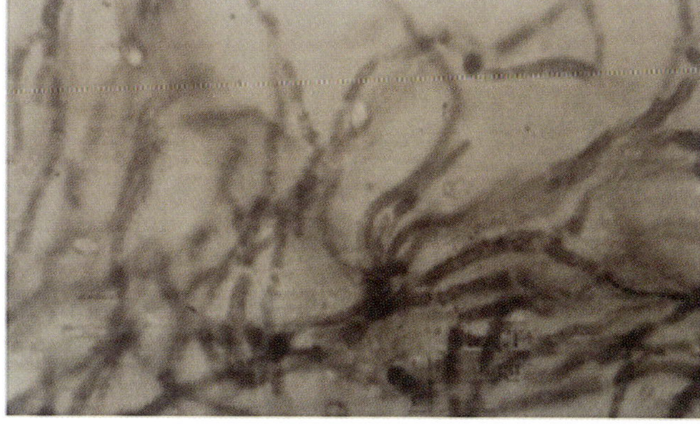

Fig.15.1.1 (b): Mycelium(intertwining of branched hyphae)-KOH preparation of skin scraping

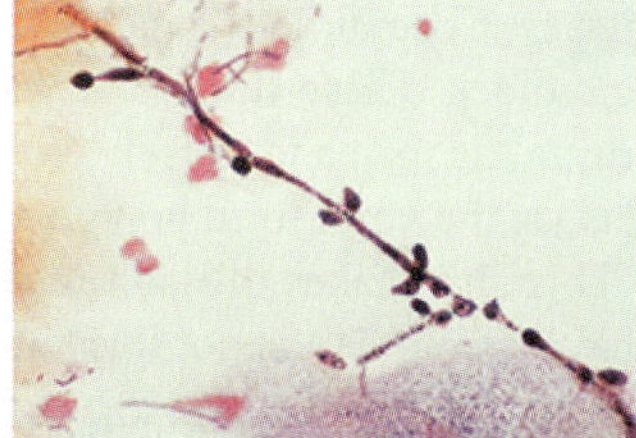

Fig.15.1.3: *Candida albicans*: Vaginal smear demonstrating pseudohyphae of this fungus

Courtesy: Dr. Stuart Brown/CDC

Table 15.1.1: Differences between hypha and pseudohypha

	Hypha	**Pseudohypha** (Fig. 15.1.2, 15.1.3)
Formed by	apical cell elongation	budding
Tip cell is	longer than preceding cell	not longer than preceding cell
Cell walls	are parallel to each other	not parallel
Septa between cells	are straight and parallel	Constriction seen between junction of two cells

Another example in this category of fungus is Trichosporon species, that are yeasts with filamentous extensions.

In the ***third*** category of fungi, i.e., *moulds (or filamentous fungi)*, the vegetative unit is long filament like structure with parallel walls and is called hypha (plural-hyphae). These may form colonies, often described as wooly. They reproduce by formation of different type of asexual (conidia and sporangiospores) and sexual spores (Figs. 15.1.4., 15.1.6, 15.1.7).

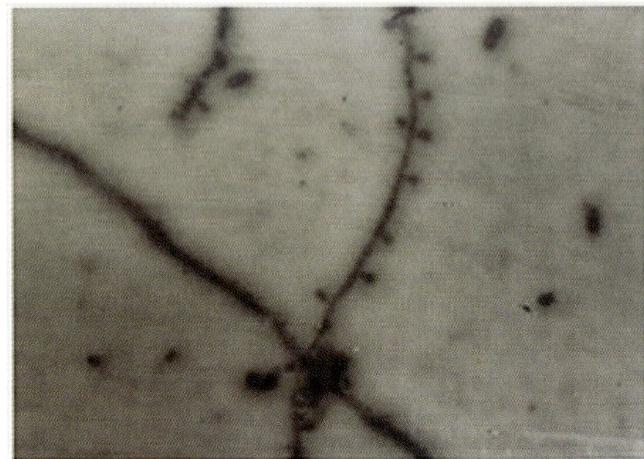

Fig. 15.1.4: Conidia borne on sides of hyphae (tear shaped microconidia of *T. rubrum*)

In favourable circumstances,the spore absorbs water and germinates by producing tube-like structures called germ tubes (Fig. 15.1.4 (a) and (b)). These elongate and become hypha (plural-hyphae). The hypha during its growth can get divided by formation of transverse walls or septa. Such hyphae are called *septate hyphae*. Those without these septa are called *non-septate hyphae*. The hyphae branch, rebranch and intertwine to form a structure called *mycelium*. The categorization of fungi on the basis of septate (having septa) and aseptate hypha is depicted below:

→*Septate (having septa)* (*15.1.5a*)
- *Hyaline* (non dematiaceous) - Aspergillus spp., Pencillium spp., Fusarium spp., Dermatophytes spp., Paecillomyces spp.
- *Dematiaceous* (pigmented) - Alternaria spp., Cladosporium spp., Fonsecaea spp., Phialophora spp., Wangiella spp, Bipolaris spp.

→*Aseptate (sparsely septate)* (Fig. 15.1.5b)-belong to Zygomycetes egs–Rhizopus spp., Mucor spp. and Rhizomucor spp.

The **fourth** category of the fungi based on morphology is **dimorphic fungi**. These express the extreme switching over, i.e., they exhibit mould form under one type of environmental conditions and yeast form in other conditions, e.g., systemic pathogens; as Blastomyces, Histoplasma, Coccidioides and Paracoccidioides. These fungi behave as moulds in the outside environment and on agar media at 25-30°C but form yeast form in the man and outside environment temperature of 37°C. The dimorphism provides a survival advantage to the fungus, as the yeast form being usually larger in size than conidia, is better able to resist the phagocytic attack than conidia. This also makes difficult the transmission of these fungi from one person to another; as the infective form of mould (having conidia) is not formed in the man except *C. immitis*.

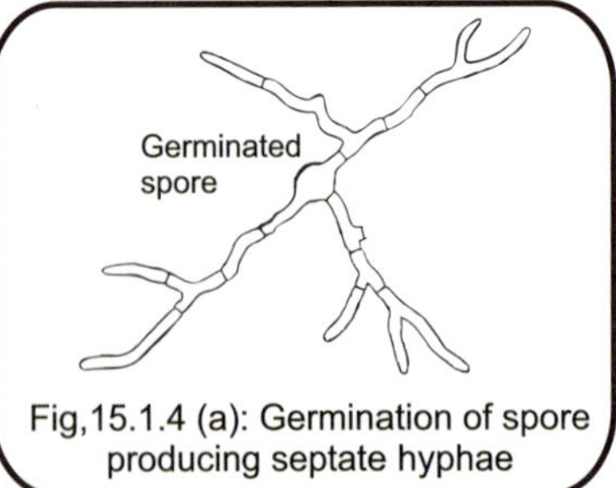

Fig,15.1.4 (a): Germination of spore producing septate hyphae

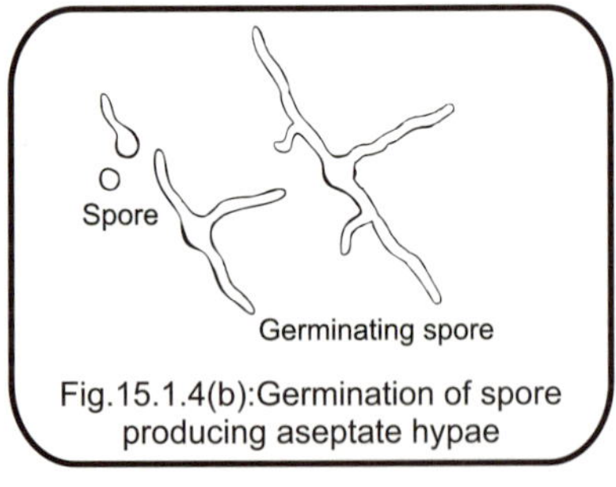

Fig.15.1.4(b):Germination of spore producing aseptate hypae

This aspect has a diagnostic implication also, as sometimes parallel cultures are to be put at 25°C and 37°C, to identify both phases in clinical samples; containing suspected dimorphic fungi. Sometimes conversion of mould stage to yeast phase is required for diagnostic confirmation of an isolate. This would require subculture onto an enriched medium; as brain heart infusion agar and incubation at 37°C.

Describe the taxonomical classification of fungi.

A.6 In the taxonomical classification, the fungi are categorized into four medically important classes (division), based on the nature of sexual spores and septation of hyphae (Flow diagram 2).

Flow Diagram 2: Medically important classes (divisions) of fungi

Classes

Zygomycetes	**Ascomycetes**	**Basidiomycetes**	**Deuteromycetes** (fungi imperfecti)
- Lower fungi, have non-septate hyphae	- Septate hyphae	-Septate hyphae	- Septate hyphae
- Sexual spores are known as *zygospores* - Asexual spores are called sporangiospores	- Sexual spores (*ascospores*) are present within a ascus (sac)	-Sexual spores (*basidiospores*) are borne on a basidium	- Lack sexual stage. Most medically important fungi belong to this class
egs Rhizopus, Absidia, Mucor	e.g., Saccharomyces *cerevisiae*	e.g., *Cryptococcus neoformans*	e.g., *Coccidioides immitis, Paracoccidioides brasilensis, Candida albicans*

A new class Pneumocystidiomycetes has been recently introduced to include *Pneumocystis jivovecii*

Sexual spores are formed less frequently and formed only, when some specific environmental condition are met. For this reason, these spores do not get formed, when fungi are cultivated in basal (ordinary) media.

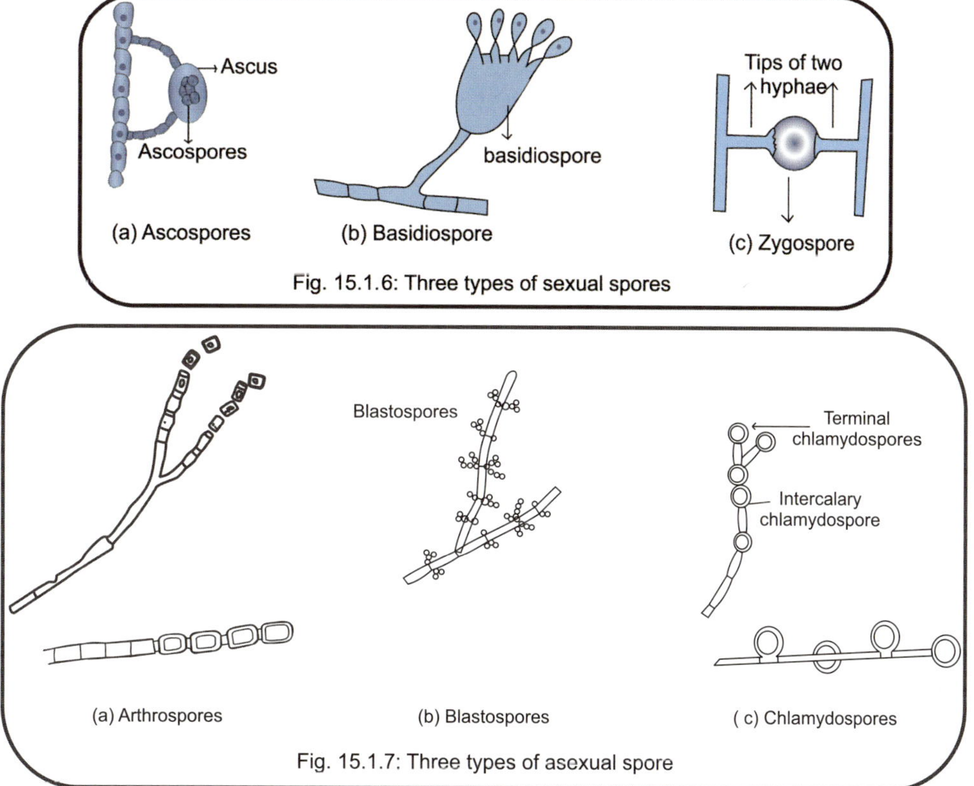

Fig. 15.1.6: Three types of sexual spores

Fig. 15.1.7: Three types of asexual spore

The process of sexual sporulation gets initiated, when haploid nucleus from each of the two compatible strains (of the same species) fuse to form zygote. The sexual spores are categorized into three types, namely (Fig. 15.1.6):

(i) **Ascospore** is sexual spore, formed inside; a sac called ascus, e.g., Aspergillus.

(ii) **Basidiospore** is sexual spore, formed at end of club shaped structure called basidium, e.g., Cryptococcus.

(iii) **Zygospore** is sexual spore, which has thick wall and is formed, as result of sexual conjugation, when tips of two adjacent hyphae approach each other and fuse to form a thick walled structure, e.g., zygomycetes.

The **asexual** spores are numerous and easily observed, however this classification is not based on them, although asexual spores can help in genus identification.

The asexual spore can be categorized into two groups, namely:

- Aerial spores
- Vegetative spores

Aerial spores: These can be of four types

(i) Conidia: borne on sides/tips of hyphae e.g. aspergillus conidia, Pg. 553.

(ii) Sporangiospores: formed within sporangium e.g. Rhizopus, Pg. 547.

(iii) Microconidia: Small and single; as Trichophyton, Dermatophytes.

(iv) Macroconidia: Large, multicellular and septate e.g. Microsporum.

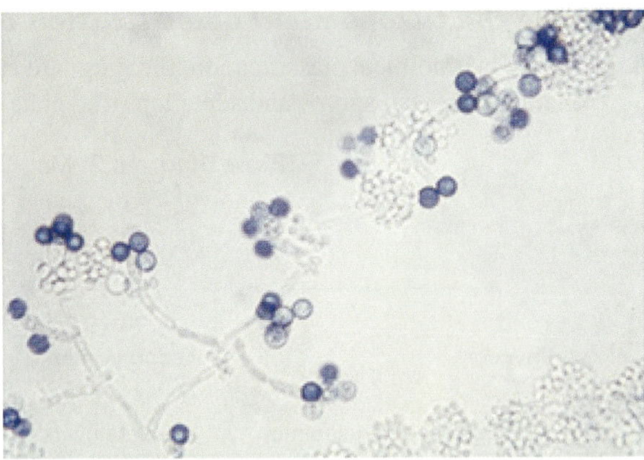

Fig.15.1.8: *Candida albicans:* Chlamydospore (thick walled reproductive structure) of this fungus

Courtesy: Dr. Gordon Roberstad/CDC

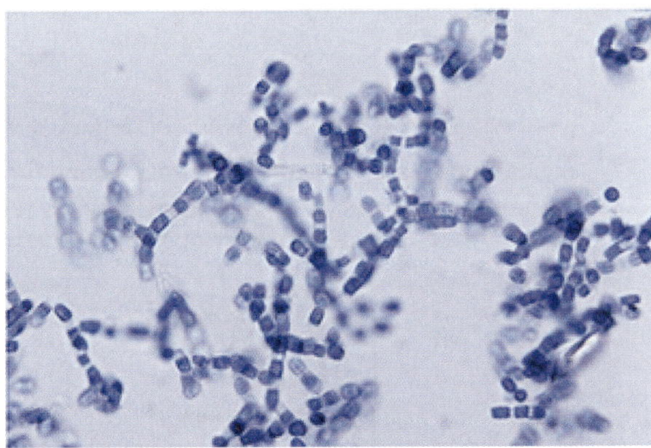

Fig.15.1.9: *Coccidioides immitis:* Photomicrograph reveals thin, septate and hyaline hyphae from which numerous thick walled and barrel shaped arthroconidia have sprouted

Courtesy: CDC, Atlanta

The **vegetative** asexual spores are broadly of three types, namely; **blastospore, chlamydospore** and **arthrospore** (Figs. 15.1.7-15.1.9). *Blastospore formation* is seen in Candida spp; where the buds break away from the parent cell (pseudomycelium), enlarge and reproduce in this fashion. *Chlamydospore* is formed, when the cell of hypha is converted into a thick-walled and dormant spore designated chlamydospore. These may be formed terminally or intercalary (when formed in the hypha). *Arthrospore* is seen in Coccidioides, when a part (rectangular) of the hypha is cut out of the parent cell to form arthrospore. Most of the medically important fungi lack sexual reproductive cycle and are allotted the class deuteromycetes. It is possible that the sexual cycle may have been lost during evolution, that may be reason for this class also to have a name as fungi 'imperfecti'. It is also possible that the sexual spores are so rarely produced that they go undetected.

Is it possible for a fungus to be known by the asexual form producing asexual spores (i.e., anamorph) to change its nomenclature, once its sexual phase producing sexual spores (i.e., telemorph) gets known? Yes! *Blastomyces dermatitidis, Histoplasma capsulatum, Cryptococcus neoformans* are the anamorphic names of the fungi, which are often used instead of their respective; telemorphic names, which were allotted later; as *Ajellomyces dermatidis, Ajellomyces capsulatus* and *Filobasidiella neoformans*, respectively. Another reason for anamorphic name to be used more often is that diagnostic laboratories don't use culture conditions, that would produce the telemorph.

Describe in general the laboratory diagnosis of fungal diseases.

A.7 Sample

Collection (when mycotic diseases suspected)

This aspect is being separately taken as mycological diagnosis is often missed and misdiagnosed. To make an accurate fungal diagnosis, it is important that a correct sample is taken appropriately.

Superficial mycoses

Skin: In case of suspected skin lesions, small scales can be scraped off from the margin of the lesion, by a round scalpel, after having decontaminated the skin by spirit. Cotton swabs from this site are *unacceptable* specimens.

Hair: The affected hair should be removed completely using epilation forceps. Clipped hair is unacceptable specimens.

Nail: Full thickness of the affected nail adjoining the apparently healthy nail needs to be taken. Superficial scraping or swabs are unacceptable specimens.

Mucous membrane (mouth, vagina etc). The suspected lesion should be scraped with a blunt scalpel. A dry swab from the site is an unacceptable specimen.

Subcutaneous mycoses

Pus/grain/biopsy: It should be collected aseptically into a vial. A swab from the site is an unacceptable specimen.

Systemic mycoses

- *Sputum:* Many pulmonary mycoses are missed and wrongly treated as pulmonary tuberculosis, so it is important that an appropriate sample is taken to isolate fungus.

  About 5 ml of sputum is taken preferably after early morning coughing spell, after vigorous washing of the mouth. It is collected in a sterile wide mouthed container.

  Twenty-four hour collection of sputum is unsuitable for mycological investigations, as they get overgrown by bacteria and saprophytic yeast like fungi. Throat swab is also an unacceptable specimen.
- *Cerebrospinal fluid/blood:* it should be remembered that insufficient quantity of sample, can result in a false negative result and increased sample inoculation; increases the chances of fungal recovery, however many times this is not practically feasible.
- *Urine:* About 25-50 ml of morning midstream urine is used as a specimen. A twenty-four collection is unacceptable, as it gets overgrown by bacteria and saprophytic fungi.

Transportation (of specimens, when fungal agents are suspected).

Generally specimens should be transported in container; which is sterile, humid and leak-proof. However; dermatological specimens should be transported in a dry container and should be stored between 15 to 30°C. Extreme heat and cold can affect fungal viability, hence room temperature transport and storage is recommended; excepting 30-37°C storage for CSF and 4°C extended storage for samples as urine, sputum, pleural fluid and peritoneal fluid, which are likely to be contaminated by bacteria.

Processing

The clinical samples that are required to be processed include all possible types of skin scrapings, tissue and other biopsy material, pus, sputum, blood and other sterile fluids.

Direct microscopy along with *culture* on a Sabouraud dextrose agar (SDA) surface would be the technique that could identify majority of the pathogenic fungi. The role of the wet mount examination in the identification of fungi from clinical samples cannot be over emphasized. One of the commonest techniques is to make the mount in ten percent potassium hydroxide. The alkali degrades the proteinaceous material of the tissue, leaving the fungal element unaffected and more prominent. The hyphae, yeasts and asexual spores may get demonstrated by this technique. However the sexual spores and fruiting bodies are uncommonly demonstrated, as the medically important fungi rarely undergo sexual sporulation. A technique that can facilitate the examination of fungi in clinical samples, is the KOH–*calcofluor staining,* that makes rapid fungi detection possible, due to bright fluorescence under UV light. However; the technique requires the availability of a fluorescent microscope. The stain binds to polysaccharides; as the chitin present in the fungal cell wall. *Gram staining* can stain some of the fungi, as yeasts; as gram positive structures, however many fungal structures remain faintly stained or unstained. India ink preparation can help in the demonstration of capsule of *C. neoformans* by the principle of negative staining.

Haematoxylin and eosin staining of tissue sections can reveal many pigmented fungi. However; Gomori's methenamine silver and *periodic acid-Schiff* (PAS) *staining* methods can stain almost all fungi (detect yeast cells and hyphae in tissue). In the former staining, the fungi appear black colored against green background, whereas in PAS staining the cell walls of fungi stain magenta colored. PAS staining is used to detect polysaccharide and mucosubstances; as glycoprotein and glycolipids in tissue. Such substances are found in connective tissue, mucus, glycocalyx and basal, laminae. In fungal infection, it stains cell walls of the live fungus as magenta/ deep pink, whereas the Gomori's methenamine silver stains both living and dead cells. Histologic examination of tissue helps to differentiate fungal infection from colonization (i.e. determine if, fungal invasion of tissue has occured or not).

Sabouraud dextrose agar is an enriched medium often used for the isolation of most fungi (may also page 53). Its lower pH of 5.5-5.6 and high sugar content; inhibits most bacteria. Addition of chloramphenicol (or other antibacterial) and cycloheximide (actidione) helps to inhibit growth of most bacteria and saprobic fungi, respectively. *Brain heart infusion* agar supplemented with antibiotics is also used for isolation of fungi. *CHROMagar* Candida is a selective, differential agar medium used for isolation and presumptive identification of some common Candida species. The 'chromogenic mix' in the medium stains, the different Candida species differentially. The addition of specific substrates/chromogen in the medium permits detection of specific enzymatic activities of specific yeast species. *Dermatophyte test medium* (DTM) is a selective medium used for isolation and identification of dermatophytes. The antibiotics in the medium; suppress the bacteria, saprobic yeasts and moulds and the alkaline by products, produced by dermatophytes change the phenol red indicator from yellow to red. The cultures are incubated at temperatures between 25°C-30°C. Paired cultures at 25 and 37°C may be used to demonstrate dimorphism. A technique used to study better the undisturbed morphology of the fungus is the *slide culture technique,* which involves inoculation of a small agar block with the fungal isolate.

The fungal growth once it occurs; is identified by the color, morphology of the colony, reverse pigmentation, assimilation studies, DNA probes and the exoantigen test. The microscopic morphology of the fungus is studied by making a lactophenol cotton blue (LPCB) mount. It involves teasing the fungus in the LPCB solution. The chief components of LPCB; include cotton blue to stain fungal elements and lactic acid to preserve morphology. *Assimilation studies* are a type of biochemical tests that are core to the identification of yeasts and aid in the identification of moulds. They are based on the ability of the isolate to use carbohydrate; as the sole source of carbon and of nitrate; as the source of nitrogen. Growth of the yeast is the end point of a positive test.

The *exoantigen test* is based on the isolation of soluble antigens, prepared from mycelial growth and identifying them with an immunodiffusion procedure. Some of the fungal isolates for which DNA probes, are now available include Blastomyces, Coccidiodes Cryptococcus and Histoplasma species.

Serological tests based on demonstration of antibodies in patient's serum or CSF, has role for only some fungi. This is because although serum antibodies are formed against numerous fungi, however the sensitivity and specificity of the tests is lacking to make them of clinical value. Complement fixation test is one of the classical tests available for the diagnosis of dimorphic fungal pathogens. Serological tests also have a role in the diagnosis of aspergillosis and cyptococcosis.

Antigen detection has a limited role in the diagnosis of fungi because of poor sensitivity of the technique. Latex agglutination test is available to demonstrate capsular polysaccharide of *C. neoformans* in CSF of patients. Candidal mannan and aspergillus galactomannan demonstration is useful in diagnosis of candidiasis and aspergillosis, respectively. MALD1-TOF MS detects specific peptides/proteins and may be useful in rapid diagnosis of fungi from clinical sample.

Antifungal susceptibility testing is now clinically required, as many antifungal agents are available and drug resistance to antifungal drugs is now common. However the standardization of technique has been hindered because of difficulty in standardizing inocula and growth conditions. Techniques for susceptibility testing of yeasts are available but for mould isolates are less well standardized.

Outline the clinical classification of mycoses.

A.8 The categories are **superficial and cutaneous mycoses** (details see pgs 527-531), **subcutaneous mycoses** (below skin) (details see pgs. 532-536), **systemic mycoses** (details see pgs 537 to 542), **opportunistic mycoses** (details see pgs 543 to 555) and the miscellaneous category (details see pgs. 556 to 557). Opportunistic mycoses include Candidosis, Cryptococcosis, Zygomycosis, Aspergillosis, Penicilliosis and infections due to *Penicillium marnefeii*. Fungi causing systemic mycoses include *Blastomyces dermatitidis, Histoplasma capsulatum, Coccidioides immitis* and *Paracoccidioides brasilensis*.

Tabulate the commonly used antifungals and mention there

A.9 **Table 15.1.2:** Most commonly used antifungal drugs

Agent	Mechanism	Indication
Grisans		
Griseofulvin	Binds to tubules, interfering with microtubule function, thus inhibiting mitosis	Dermatophytes
Polyenes		
Amphotericin B	Binds with ergosterol, a component of fungal cell membrane, disrupting its integrity	Most systemic fungi
Liposomal amphotericin B	Same as above	Same as above, Less toxic than above
Nystatin	do	systemic fungi
Imidazoles		
Clotrimazole	Inhibit ergosterol synthesis of fungi	Broad spectrum, topical use
Ketoconazole	Inhibil ergosterol synthesis of fungi	Broad spectrum, topical and systemic use
Triazoles		
Fluconazole	Selective inhibition of fungal cytochrome p450 enzyme (inhibiting conversion of lanosterol to ergosterol) i.e. ergosterol synthesis inhibitor	Candida spp., Cryptococcus spp.
Itraconazole	Same as above	Blastomyces spp., Histoplasma spp., Sporothrix spp., Candida spp. and others including Aspergillus spp.
Voriconazole	Same as above	Candida spp., Aspergillus spp., Fusarium spp. and others
***Echinocandins and other antifungals**		
Flucytosine	DNA and RNA synthesis inhibitor (antimetabolite)	Dermatophytes, systemic fungi and others Often used in combination with fluconazole and Amphotericin B
*Micafungin, caspofungin	is Echinocandin, which inhibits β-glucan synthesis in fungal cell wall	Systemic fungi
Terbinafine	Inhibit ergosterol synthesis of fungi.	local use (Dermatophytes)

2 Integrated Clinical Case Based Study on Superficial and Cutaneous Mycoses

An adolescent male, Kaniksh comes to a medical OPD with a roundish patch on the scalp, which is scaly and devoid of natural hair (Fig. 15.2.1).

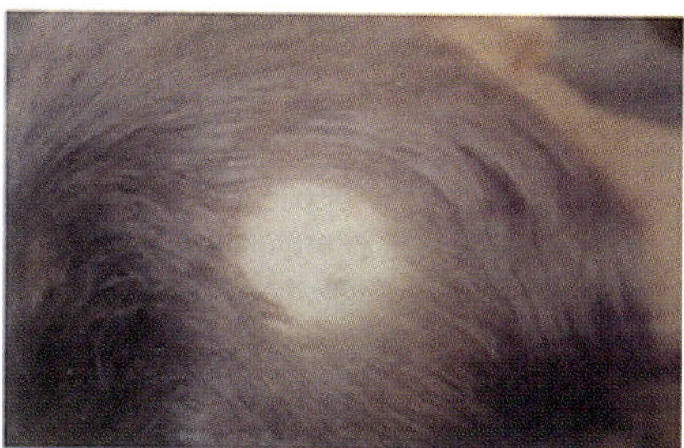

Fig. 15.2.1: An adolescent with a scaly, rounded patch, devoid of hair on the scalp (Tinea capitis)

What is your clinical diagnosis?

A.1 **(a)** Tinea capitis (ringworm) - details see A.7

What is the common term for this lesion?

A.1 **(b)** Ringworm

Mention the clinical category of mycoses, to which this case belongs

A.2 (c) Cutaneous mycoses

What clinical sample would you take to confirm your clinical diagnosis of the above case?

A.3 See A.7, p. 531

How do you manage this case?

A.4 **(a)** See A.7, p. 531

What is the prognosis of this case?

A.5 **(b)** Good. The affected area can again get regrowth of hair.

Enumerate and describe the superficial mycoses that can infect the skin and its appendages.

A.6 ***Superficial mycoses involve superficial layers of skin and hair,*** See table 15.2.1

Table 15.2.1: Superficial Mycoses

	Tinea versicolor* (Malassezia, Pityriasis versicolor)	**Tinea nigra,**	**White piedra**	**Black piedra**
Etiological agent	*Malassezia furfur* (*Pityrosporum orbiculare*)	*Hortaea werneckii*	*Trichosporon beigellii*	*Piedraia hortae*
Geographical distribution	Worldwide, but primarily in tropics	Essentially a tropical infection	S. America, Europe and Japan	Tropical infection
Epidemiology	- This fungus is a normal commensal of the skin - Occurs mainly in young adults	- Common saprophytic fungus	- Usually affects pubic and axillary hair - Temperate and semitropical climate	- usually affects scalp, hair
Pathogenesis	- Disease of dead layer of skin - No inflammatory response seen - Disease may be considered an opportunistic infection	- Thick keratinized sites as palms and soles involved	Infection of hair shaft, nodules are fungus elements cemented together on hair	Infection of hair shaft, nodules are fungus elements cemented together on hair
C.F. /Pathogenicity	Lesions on trunk and arms, varying from pink to yellow-brown (lesions may appear hypo or hyper-pigmented) (consultation sought for cosmetic reason)	Brown to black macular lesions usually on hands or feet	- White nodules attached to hair shaft	- Black nodules attached to hair shaft (Fig. 15.2.5)

Contd.

Knowing details of the microscopic characteristics of various dermatophytes is not expected at the undergraduate level.

Epidemiology:

These are distributed worldwide. The dermatophytes can be categorized into Anthropophilic (anthropo + G. phileo, to love), Zoophilic (prefering animals) species and geophilic (soil loving), table 15.2.4. The distribution of these could account for the ecologic and geographic differences in the occurrence of various dermatophytes.

Table 15.2.4: Distribution of dermatophytes according to habitat

Anthropophilic	Zoophilic	Geophilic
T. rubrum, T. violaceum, T. tonsurans, E. floccosum, M. audouinii *T. mentagrophytes*	*T. equinum* *M. canis* ('canis' derived from canine) *T. verrucosum* (in cattle)	*M. gypseum* *M. nanum*

Anthropophilic (prefer man to animals) species are essentially adapted to man and are transmitted from man to man, by desquamated skin and inanimate objects; as combs and nail cutters. The *zoophilic* species are adapted to animals as dogs, cats, cattle and are transmitted from animal to man directly and indirectly. *Geophilic* species are essentially found on soil from which they infect both man and animals.

Man to man transmission usually requires close contact with an infected subject (man or animal) or infected inanimate materials, as dermatophytes are of low infectivity and virulence. Transmission can occur in the context of a family set-up, beauty saloon, barber shop, a locker setup; or a swimming pool. These fungi thrive on warm and moist environment. It is essential that a medical attendant performs hand hygiene, after coming in contact with an infected patient.

Pathogenesis:

Dermatophytes grow only on the keratinized skin and its appendages. It doesn't penetrate the deeper layers of skin. The dermatophytoses begins, when minor traumatic *skin* lesions come in contact with the fungi. The fungal cell produces keratinolytic proteases, which help its entry into living cells. Invasion up to the level of stratum corneum can occur. The lateral spread of infection and the associated inflammation, produces the characteristic distinct advancing margins. The multiple skin lesions scan at times fuse to form unusual geometric patterns.

Nail bed infections initially cause, discoloration of the subungual tissue followed by hyperkeratosis and apparent discoloration of the nail plate, due to underlying infection (Fig. 15.2.13). Infection and subsequent disfigurement of the nail occurs later. This can lead to the subsequent compression of the adjacent soft tissue.

The infection of the *hair* usually begins; as an erythematous papule around the hair shaft, which subsequently results in scaling, discoloration and fracture of the shaft. Three types of hair infections are seen, namely *ectothrix* in which arthrospores are seen primarily on the surface of the hair shaft (Fig. 15.2.6), *endothrix* – in which arthrospores are seen primarily in the hair shaft and *Favus*; in which sparse hyphal growth and formation of air space occurs within the hair shaft.

Clinical picture: The presentation varies from inconspicuous colonization to chronic progressive eruptions, that may last many years with significant discomfort and disfiguration. Classically, the lesions are circular, which spread with an erythematous border with varying degrees of scaling and inflammation. The *Trichophyton* infects the skin hair and nail, while the *Epidermophyton* infects the skin and nail, whereas the *Microsporum* infects the skin and the hair. The various infections are designated according to the site of infection, e.g.,

Tinea capitis (scalp) (Fig. 15.2.10)

Tinea faciei (face excluding bearded area)

Tinea barbae (beard and moustache area)

Tinea corporis (nonhairy skin of body) (Fig. 15.2.11)

Tinea cruris (groin and perineum)

Tinea manuum (hands, onychomycosis) (Fig. 15.2.12)

Tinea unguium (nails) (Fig. 15.2.13)

Tinea pedis (feet, athlete's foot)

Tinea gladiatorum (gladiator = wrestler)

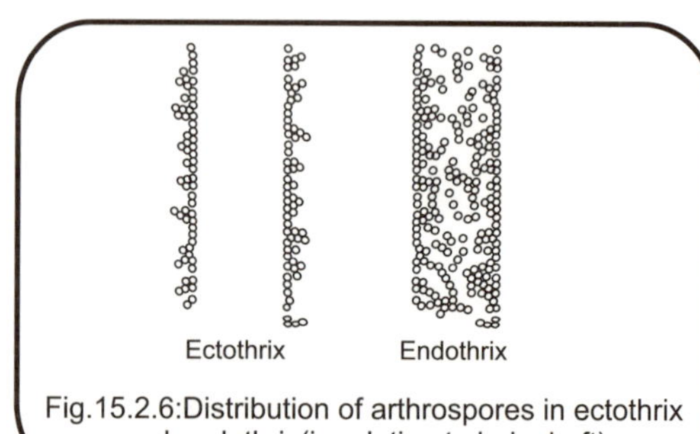

Fig.15.2.6:Distribution of arthrospores in ectothrix and endothrix(in relation to hair shaft)

Infection with *Tricophyton tonsurans*; transmitted by person-to-person contact, as the main source of transmission in wrestlers.

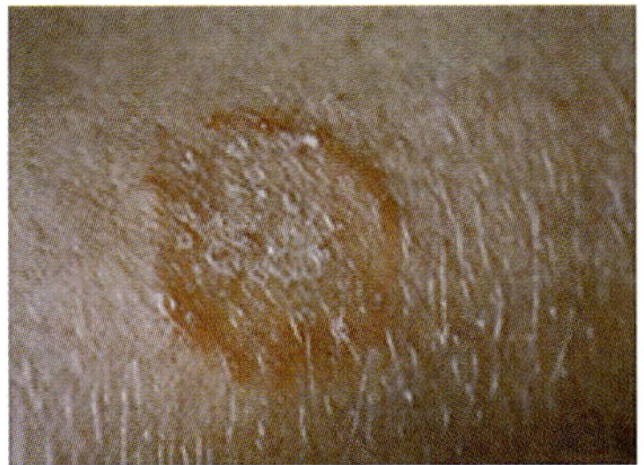

Fig.15.2.11: Ringworm: Tinea corporis(ringworm on the arm) due to *Tricophyton mentagrophytes*

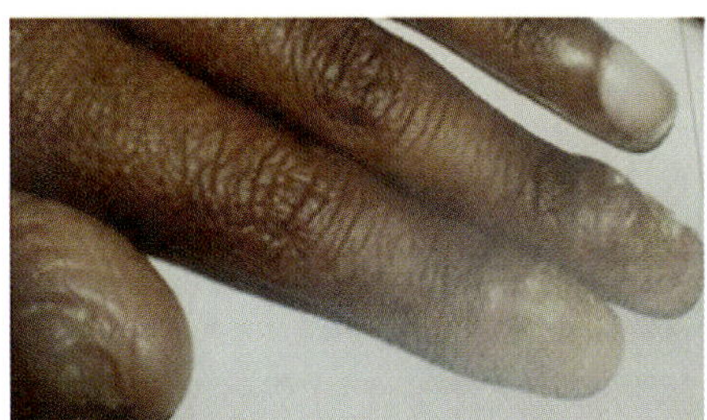

Fig.15.2.12: Tinea mannum

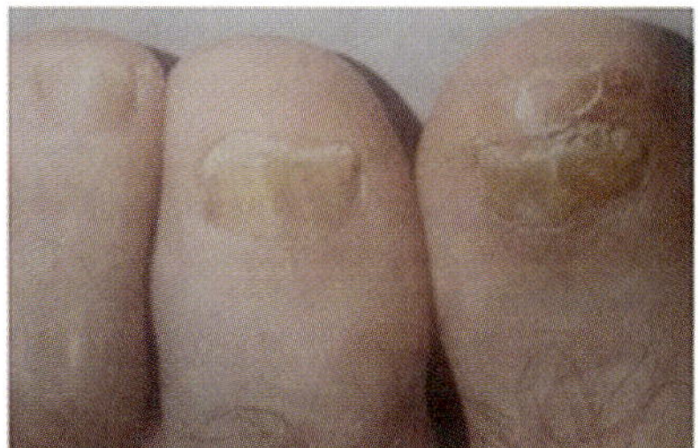

Fig.15.2.13: Tinea unguium

Dermatophytid (Derma = skin) or Id reaction: These are sterile lesions, distant from the primary dermatophyte lesion. The aetiology of this isn't clear but is likely due to hypersensitivity reaction to fungal antigen. These may be confused with an allergic drug reaction.

Laboratory diagnosis:

The chief goal of the diagnostic techniques is to distinguish dermatophytoses from other skin and appendage diseases caused by other fungi, bacteria and other non-infectious inflammatory skin disorders as; dermatophytids, contact dermatitis and psoriasis. An important task in the diagnosis is the proper collection of the samples, as inappropriate sample collection can result in false negative diagnosis.

- *Specimens:* (i) skin scraping from the edge of the lesion (ii) infected hair (iii) infected nail.
- *Collection:* (details chapter 1 Section 15, Page 525)
  - (i) Skin scraping: The infected area disinfected with spirit and the edge of the lesion, is scraped; using a blunt sterile scalpel. The scrapings are collected in a black paper.
  - (ii) Infected hair: It can be plucked using forceps or is cut with sterile scissors.
  - (iii) Infected nail: The infected nail part, which may be discolored or brittle, is collected using a scalpel or a nail cutter.
- *Transport:* The samples are collected into folded squares of black paper. It helps to preserve the specimen in a dry state for many weeks.
- *Wood's lamp examination:* The U.V. lamp examination of the infected hair helps in provisional diagnosis, as certain dermatophytic fungi; as *M. gypseum* and *M. canis* fluoresce under this light, while others do not.
- *Direct microscopy:* KOH examination is an important technique in the diagnosis and can demonstrate the branched hyalıne septate hyphae with arthroconidia (microconidia and macroconidia aren't seen here). The ectothrix and endothrix infection can also be differentiated. However; it is important that clearing (dissolving) of the sample must occur, which in skin and hair may occur in about 30 minutes but for nails may require hours (even 1-2 days).
- *Culture:* Culture of the sample mayn't be necessary, if the KOH preparation is positive, as the presumptive treatment can start and may not vary significantly with the identity of the isolated dermatophyte. However; if the clinical suspicion is high in case, where the KOH examination is negative and the sample has been appropriately collected, then the culture is warranted. S.D.A. with and without antibiotics is inoculated with the sample and incubated at 25-30°C for 3 weeks. The slants can be examined daily for growth. Grossly, the presence of red pigment indicates the presence of *T.rubrum,* while the presence of violet pigment indicates the presence of *T. violaceum*.

  The LPCB preparation of the growth, when it occurs can help in speciating the dermatophytes, by the characteristics of the microconidia and macroconidia. (Table 15.2.3, p. 529)

  Hair perforation test helps in differentiating *T. mentagrophytes* (positive) from *T. rubrum* (negative) and *M. canis* (positive) from *M. equinum* (negative). Detailed morphological features for identifying the dermatophytes at the species level is not expected at the U.G. level.
- **Treatment:**

  General hygiene, as regular baths and keeping the skin dry can prevent the infection.

  In mild infections, the skin lesions may resolve without chemotherapy. However topical clotrimazole or miconazole or tolnafate may be useful.

  Severe infections require the usage of oral griseofulvin, terbinafine/itraconazole, besides topical antifungal. Therapy must be continued for weeks to months, as relapses are common.

NB: Dermatophyte test medium can help to differentiate dermatophytes from bacterial contaminants. Dermatophytes turn the medium red by raising pH by metabolites; whereas other bacteria and fungi do not.

Integrated Clinical Case Based Study on Subcutaneous Mycoses

A 30 year woman from Himachal Pradesh (India), involved in farming, presented to the primary health center with two ulcers on the left leg. The women reported often getting hurt, by thorns during her work.

What is the differential diagnosis of the case, if it is a fungal disease?

A.1 (i) Mycetoma (initial stage) described from pgs. 532 to 533, Fig. 15.3.1 and 15.3.2 (ii) Sporotrichosis described from pgs. 533 to 534. Subcutaneous mycoses involve the deeper layers of skin including connective tissue and muscle.

What gross finding in the pus would point towards a diagnosis of mycetoma?

A.2 Presence of granules

What is the characteristic finding of the yeast stage of Sporothrix schenckii?

A.3 Detecting hyphae, with conidia at ends; borne as 'flower like clusters'. (Fig. 15.3.3 and 4)

What is the drug of choice for treating this infection (Sporotrichosis)?

A.4 Itraconazole.

(reference from A.1 (i) MYCETOMA (Madura foot, Maduramycosis)

It is a chronic, localized swollen lesion, usually on the foot or hand, involving the skin, subcutaneous tissue, fascia and bone, characterized by tumefaction (induration), suppuration and draining sinuses containing granules (or microcolonies) of the etiologic agent.

Etiological agents: Table 15.3.1 (these are basically saprophytic soil fungi)

Geographical distribution: Worldwide, but more common in the tropics. In India, Eumycetoma is more prevalent in North India in comparison to South India; whereas for Actinomycetoma the picture is reverse.

Epidemiology: The disease name 'Madura foot' has been based on the original report of this disease from Madurai in 1842 by Gill. The fungi for this disease occur in the soil and man acquires it by direct inoculation. The disease is commonest in the tropics especially, where chronic dampness leads to macerated skin. The disease occurs most commonly on the feet and legs, as they are the commonest to get injured and get contaminated by the soil fungi. The disease is common in young (20-40 years) active males; who are farmers, grazers, field workers and carpenters. The lesions on head, neck and back get party explained by the individuals carrying wooden sticks (for fuel burning) and other articles on these parts.

Pathogenesis: The Actinomycetes or the filamentous fungi enter through injuries; caused by thorns, sharp stone or wooden splinters. This infectious agent initiates an acute inflammatory response initially and may result in microabscesses in subcutaneous tissue. This lesion progresses slowly and involves deeper structures and produces characteristic abscesses. The center of the lesion may contain the tangled filaments or these may clump to form microcolonies (granules). Subsequently these abscesses burst open and present; as chronic multiple sinuses, discharging seropurulent fluid with characteristic granules.

Table 15.3.1: Etiological agents of Mycetoma

Actinomycetoma (Bacterial)	Eumycetoma (Eumycetes, Fungal)
- *A. israeli*	- *Madurella mycetomatis* (Brown to black granules)
- *A. bovis*	- *Madurella grisea* (,,)
- *Actinomadura pelletierii* (red granules)	- Exophiala (*Phialophora) jeanselmei* (,,)
- *Nocardia asteroides (*whitish granules*)*	
- *Actinomadura madurae*	

Clinical profile: The clinical picture is typical with the lesions, most often on the feet (Fig. 15.3.1) or legs; as already mentioned. Hands and upper limbs are less commonly affected.

Laboratory diagnosis:

The diagnosis is usually easy, as the clinical picture is characteristic on the lower limb.

Specimens: Pus, exudates (from sinuses), grains and biopsy of affected site.

Collection of specimen: The surrounding of the lesion is cleaned. The pus or exudates is collected in sterile water. After a few minutes, the granules sediment and can be collected by a Pasteur pipette.

The granules can also be collected by placing a gauze-piece on the lesion or manually picking by a loop from the lesion, if possible.

Direct microscopy: The *granules*, if obtained are examined for their size, color and texture. The color of the eumycetoma (fungal) granule is white or black The *granules* (grains) can be crushed between two slides and then heat-fixed and stained (Fig. 15.3.2). Knowing the detailed microscopic characteristics of these is not expected in the UG curriculum.

A KOH mount can help to differentiate between actinomycotic and eumycotic granules. The granules of the actinomycotic (bacterial) mycetomas have thin filaments ($\leq$ 1 µm wide), whereas the granules of eumycetoma (fungal) have thicker (wide) filaments, which may be septate and have chlamydospores. Gram staining can help to identify gram positive filamentous bacteria. Acid fast stain using 1% sulfuric acid can help to identify Nocardia.

Culture: The clinical samples for identification of the pathogens should be inoculated on media with and without antibiotics. The generic and species identification is possible by the culture. Knowing the gross and microscopic characteristics of these fungal agents is not expected in the U.G. curriculum.

Other tests: Serological, Nucleic acid probes have limited role.

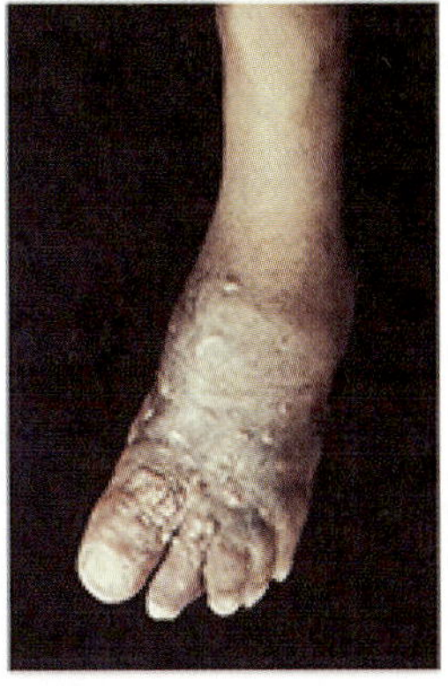

Fig.15.3.1: Mycetoma: Left foot (dorsal view) exhibiting pathologic changes indicative of a mycetoma

Courtesy: Dr. Victorial (Mexico); Dr. Lucille K. George/CDC Atlanta

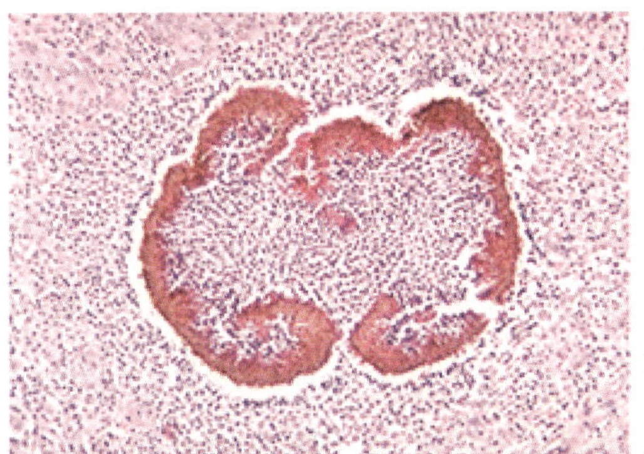

Fig.15.3.2: 'Black Grain Mycetoma': Micrograph depicts histopathologic changes due to *Exophiala salmonis*

Courtesy: Centers for disease control and prevention,Atlanta,USA

Treatment:

Actinomycotic mycetomas: Usually respond well to antibacterial antibiotics; as sulfonamides.

Eumycetoma (fungal mycetomas): These respond very poorly or not at all to antifungal drugs. Surgical management; as amputation is often required.

Botryomycosis: It is a mycetoma like condition caused by *S.aureus*.

NB: amputation is cut off by surgical operation (a part of the body)

(reference from A.1 (ii) SPOROTRICHOSIS (Rose Gardner's disease)

It is a chronic disease of skin and subcutaneous tissue characterized by nodules and ulcerations and caused by *S. schenckii*.

Etiological agent: *Sporothrix schenckii* (dimorphic fungi).

Geographical distribution: Worldwide including India (more prevalent in northern states)

Epidemiology: The fungus is a saprophyte found widely in soil, decaying organic material; as woods and on surfaces of various plants. The infection often occurs in young people because of the exposure to the sources. The fungus enters the body through skin by inoculation due to trauma. The individuals, who are at increased risk include gardeners, farmers, carpenters and rural workers; often traumatized by thorns. Majority (75%) case are males, but it is not known, if it is actually due to greater exposure of males to fungus in the environment. One outbreak of sporotrichosis involving 3000 miners was traced to the timber; used to support mine shafts.

Pathogenesis: The infection is initiated by the traumatic implantation of the spore usually in the hand or the forearm, e.g., by penetration of a thorn. The fungus spreads from the primary site through the lymphatics to the regional lymph nodes. Granulomatous inflammatory lesions occur at intervals. The organisms are scanty in the human lesions. Infection rarely spreads beyond the regional lymph nodes to involve the skeletal, pulmonary or the central nervous system. The dissemination of the fungus is likely to occur in the immunocompromised individuals.

Morphology: On SDA at 25°C, the colony grows in a mold form. It is blackish and shiny. Microscopically the hyphae are thin, septate with single celled conidia borne in clusters at tip of conidiophores (Fig. 15.3.3 and 15.3.4).

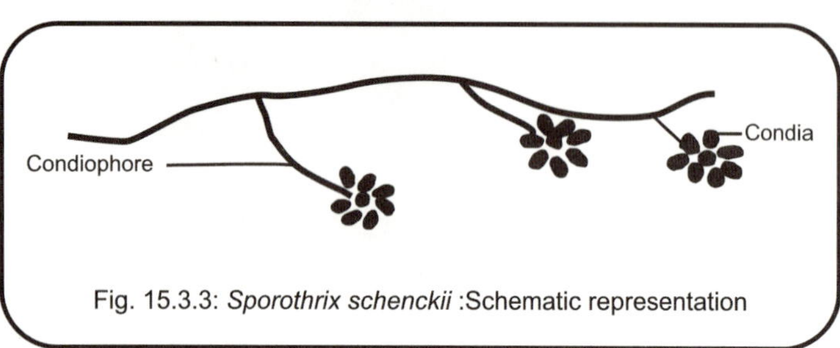

Fig. 15.3.3: *Sporothrix schenckii* :Schematic representation

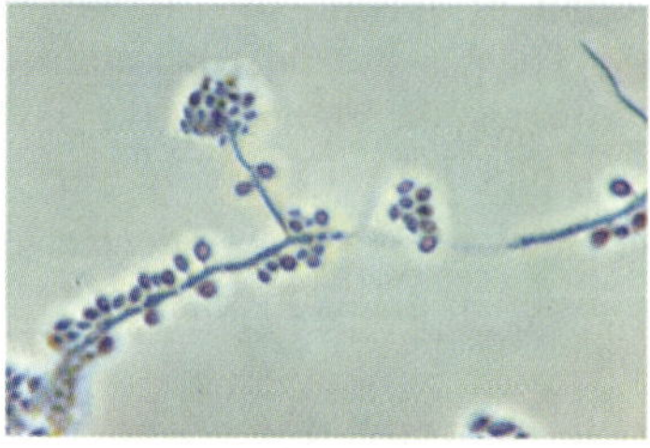

Fig. 15.3.4: *Sporothrix schenckii* :Mold form demonstrating thin septate hyphae with single celled conidia in flower –like sporulation

Courtesy:Dr Libero Ajello/CDC

The *mold form* can be converted to yeast form in BHI/blood agar at 37°C. The colonies are pasty, greyish and opaque. Microscopically the yeast cells are thin walled, often fusiform and show budding.

Clinical profile: The disease can occur in the following forms:

(a) *Lymphocutaneous sporotrichosis:* As the name indicates, there is a primary cutaneous nodule on the extremities; which may ulcerate. This is followed by the involvement of lymphatics, which results in indurated lymphatics and enlarged lymph nodes.

(b) *Fixed cutaneous sporotrichosis:* In this the primary nodule that occurs, doesn't spread.

(c) *Disseminated sporotrichosis:* In this, the other systems of the body get involved and are found in immunocompromised individuals.

Laboratory diagnosis: The organisms are usually scarce in the clinical specimens, so culture of the samples has a greater role in the diagnosis than direct microscopy.

Specimens:

1. Pus (aspirated from unruptured nodules) 2. Scraping from ulcer 3. Biopsies from edge of ulcer

Direct microscopy:

(i) KOH preparation: Uncommonly; spherical yeast cells (3-5 μm), sometimes fusiform or cigar shaped, observed.

(ii) Histopathological exam: In H & E and PAS staining, besides yeast cells, rarely the pathognomic 'asteroid body' may be demonstrable. It is composed of yeast cells surrounded by amorphous eosinophilic 'rays'.

Culture: The samples may be cultured on SDA with antibiotics at 25°C. The typical colonies come in 3-5 days. This form can be converted to the yeast form, by subculturing on BHI or blood agar at 37°C.

Specific Antigen and Antibody detection: Limited role.

Treatment: *Cutaneous* sporotrichosis-Potassium iodide given orally.

Systemic form: Itraconazole, ketoconazole.

Aspects related to case theme/examination assessment

Describe Chromomycosis.

A.5 (a) **CHROMOMYCOSIS** (chromo = color):

The term chromomycosis indicates infection by pigmented (dematiceous) fungi. It includes two entities namely Chromoblastomycosis and Phaeohyphomycosis.

Chromoblastomycosis:

It is a slowly progressive, chronic granulomatous infection of the skin and subcutaneous tissue.

Etiological agents: belong to three genera (are basically soil fungi) namely *Fonsecaea pedrosoi*, *F. compacta*, *Cladophialophora carionii* and *Phialophora verrucosa*.

Geographical distribution: tropical and subtropical countries.

Epidemiology: These fungi inhabit the soil and often infect the agricultural workers, who lack protective clothing and get infected by the fungi entering from the soil, The entity is common in barefoot workers.

Pathogenesis: The fungus is primarily acquired by traumatic inoculation into the extremities. The lesion is initially a papule at the site of trauma, which later slowly becomes warty or tumorlike (described as cauliflower like). Staining of the infected tissue (histological examination) reveals sclerotic bodies (Fig. 15.3.5). They are round or irregular, copper colored (dark brown) septate cells that appear to be dividing.

Morphology: These fungi grow on routine fungal media slowly taking weeks to demonstrate the characteristic conidia. Grossly the colonies are heaped up, darkly pigmented with the reverse side of the medium revealing black color. Knowing the characteristic microscopic features of the three genera in this group is beyond the U.G. curriculum.

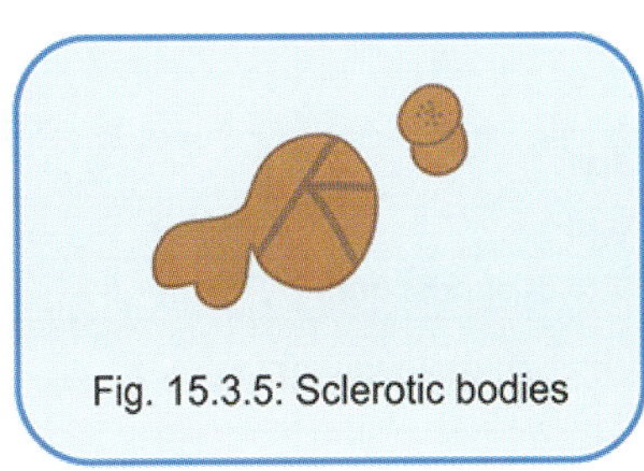
Fig. 15.3.5: Sclerotic bodies

Clinical profile: The characteristic lesion appears on the feet and legs but may involve other areas.

Laboratory diagnosis:

- *Specimen:* Scraping from crusty areas or biopsy from lesion.
- *Direct Microscopy:* KOH mount may reveal the characteristic sclerotic bodies (absent in phaeohyphomycosis). Stained infected tissue may also reveal the sclerotic bodies.
- *Culture:* The generic and the species identification of the fungi of this category require culture (their characteristic features are beyond the U.G. curriculum).
- *Serological and other tests:* Limited role.

Treatment: Surgery and antifungal drugs have a significant role to play.

Describe Phaeohyphomycosis

A.5 (b) Phaeohyphomycosis:

It is infection by the pigmented (dematiaceous) fungi that besides causing subcutaneous abscess; may also cause brain abscess, sinusitis, pulmonary and other systemic infections.

Etiological agents: Alternaria spp., Bipolaris spp., Curvularia spp., Exophiala spp. and Cladiophialophora spp.

The disease is often seen in immunocompromised individuals. The morphologic and microscopic characteristics of the etiological agents is beyond the U.G. curriculum.

Laboratory diagnosis: The KOH mount of the infected tissue may reveal pigmented hyphae. The staining of the infected tissue as by H & E stain reveals hyphae (however absence of sclerotic bodies). For generic and species identification, culture is required.

Describe Rhinosporidiosis.

A.6 Rhinosporidiosis

It is a chronic granulomatous disease of the subcutaneous tissue, characterized by polyp formation; usually in nose. Currently it is categorized as a parasite.

Etiological agent: *Rhinosporidium seeberi* (Seeber reported first case in 1900 from Argentina).

Geographical distribution: 90% of reported cases are from India and Srilanka. In India, it has been reported mostly from South India. The disease is also common in South America.

Epidemiology: Nothing definite is known about the source and mode of transmission of this disease. This organism has not been cultivated in inanimate media. The infection is common in children and young adults. It affects predominantly the males. The disease is more common in persons, who bathe in dirty stagnant pools of water, paddy cultivators and divers; who collect sand from riverbeds. The infection may be transmitted through water or dust. This organism may be associated with fishes.

Pathogenesis: The disease spreads through endospores, likely to be transmitted by water. The endospores when they reach an appropriate site, as mucous membranes, develop into sporangia. The course of disease is slow and chronic.

The fungus usually remains localized to the mucous membrane but rarely can spread haematogenously to the lungs and bones. It causes hyperplasia and chronic inflammatory reaction in the tissue.

Morphology: The classification of this organism is not clear. It has been cultivated in cell lines (epithelial cell), but not possible to cultivate it in inanimate media. Sporangia are seen in the epithelium and the stromal layers; about 200-300 µm in diameter (Figs. 15.3.6 and 15.3.7). It is important to differentiate it from spherules of *C. immitis,* as these two structures may be confused with each other (table 15.3.2). The sporangia are easily demonstrated in tissues stained with H & E or G.M.S (Gomori's methenamine silver) or P.A.S (periodic acid-Schiff). The sporangia are infiltrated with lymphocytes, plasma cells and macrophages. There are numerous endospores inside, which when the sporangium ruptures get released, can develop into new sporangia in appropriate sites.

Table 15.3.2: Comparison of morphology of ***R.seeberi*** and ***C.immitis***

	Sporangia of *R. seeberi*	**Spherules of *C. immitis***
Size	Larger (200-300 µm)	Smaller (15-80 µm)
Wall	Thicker	Thinner
Size of endospores	Larger (6-7 µm)	Smaller 2-5 µm

Clinical profile: The disease is characterized by friable polyp usually confined to nose, mouth or eye (conjunctiva). However the other sites; as genitalia, ears and other parts may get involved.

Laboratory diagnosis:

- *Sample:*
  1. Excised polyp
  2. Nasal aspirate (after injecting saline)
- *Direct microscopy:* The direct mount may reveal the sporangia. However the diagnosis is mostly made in tissues stained with H & E, which reveal the typical sporangia with endospores.
- *Culture:* On inanimate media not possible (however report of growth on animate media)
- *Serology:* Not useful.

Treatment:

1. Surgical – excision of the polyp
2. Treatment with dapsone has some role.

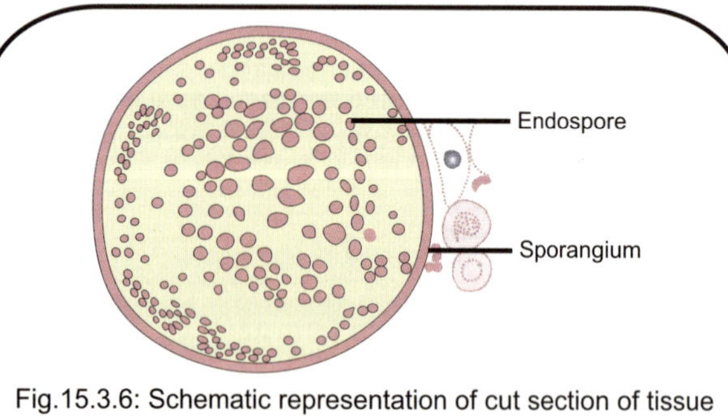

Fig.15.3.6: Schematic representation of cut section of tissue demonstrating sporangia of *Rhinosporidium seeberi*

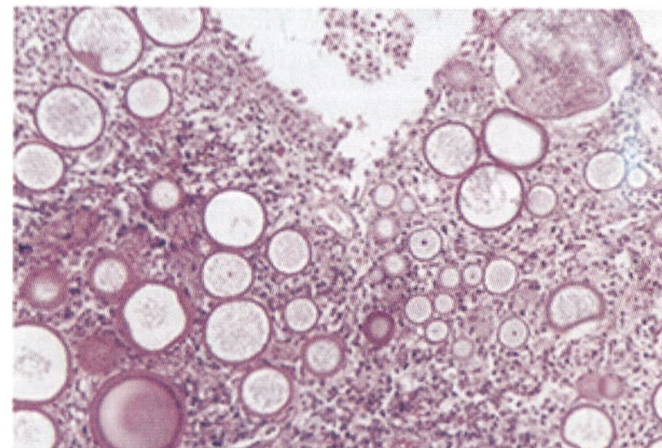

Fig. 15.3.7: *Rhinosporidium seeberi*: Micrograph depicts numerous sporangia of this fungus in a case of rhinosporidiosis of nose

Courtesy: Dr. Martin Hicklin/CDC

Integrated Clinical Case Based Study on Systemic Mycoses

A 26 years male from Gwalior, M.P. presented with fever, generalized weakness and dyspnoea. His chest X-ray revealed bilateral diffuse infiltrates. Ultrasound of abdomen revealed hepatosplenomegaly and lymphadenopathy. Conventional investigations; as sputum for culture revealed no clue.

What invasive specimen may be useful?

A.1 Bone marrow aspirate (BMA)

Fungal culture of BMA revealed septate hyphae with tuberculate macroconidia.

What is your diagnosis?

A.2 Disseminated histoplasmosis

Describe the morphology, epidemiology, pathogenesis, pathogenicity, laboratory diagnosis and treatment of infections caused by *Histoplasma capsulatum*

A.3 HISTOPLASMOSIS

Etiological Agent: *Histoplasma capsulatum* [Teleomorph stage (sexual stage) is known and named as *Ajellomyces capsulatus,* but the asexual name continues to be used in the medical literature] The designation *H. capsulatum* is a misnomer, as the organism has no capsule, the unstained areas around the organism in tissue sections is actually an artifact, formed during fixation and staining.

Geographical distribution:

Cases has been reported from India. It has worldwide distribution and more prevalent in central and eastern U.S.. This fungus is one of the common primary pulmonary and systemic pathogens.

Epidemiology:

Source: Soil fungus

Mode of infection: inhalation of spores (conidia)

H. capsulatum is a soil fungus, where it exists in a filamentous form. It prefers mostly surface soil; especially that is enriched by the droppings of certain birds, as pigeons and bats. This distribution of soil with such characteristics may explain the unique distribution of the disease. The fungus persists in the contaminated soil for years and becomes airborne, when the soil gets disturbed. Dust of places, where these birds live; as caves or old building, can also act as a source of the infection.

Pathogenesis:

The infection occurs by *inhalation of conida* (spores). The initial infection is pulmonary and involves conversion of the fungus to the yeast form. The primary lesion with lymphatic spread; resembles primary tuberculosis lesion.

The conversion of conidia to yeast stage occurs in the macrophages of the alveoli and the subsequent multiplication occurs within it. The hallmark the infection is the infection of the reticuloendothelial system. A disseminated form of histoplasmosis may occur in immunocompromised individuals; as those having AIDS.

Clinical presentation:

Most of the cases are *asymptomatic*. Some of the cases, who develop acute pulmonary infection, present with fever and cough and it is very difficult to distinguish these clinically and radiologically from tuberculosis. Lack of diagnostic workup of these cases, can result in administration of ATT to these cases, which can be disastrous. Dissemination is rare and involves reticuloendothelial system, which may present as hepatosplenomegaly, lymphadenopathy and anaemia. *Disseminated histoplasmosis* shares many features with disseminated tuberculosis cases.

Cutaneous and mucocutaneous forms of histoplasmosis are known, where granulomatous and ulcerative lesions occur on the skin and mucosal areas; as mouth and pharynx.

Morphology:

Mold form: Seen at 25°C-35°C, where colony grossly appears; as cottony growth, color varying from white to brown. Microscopically the hyphae are septate and bear characteristic macrocondia and microconidia. Macroconidia are 8-16 µm in diameter, spherical, thick-walled with tuberculation (Figs. 15.4.1, 15.4.2).

Yeast form: This forms on rich enriched media at 37°C. The colony is mucoid and creamish in color. Microscopically it reveals small, spherical/pyriform, 2-4 µm diameter yeast cells (Figs. 15.4.3, 15.4.4).

Laboratory diagnosis:

Specimens: Sputum, bone marrow aspirates, peripheral blood, tissue biopsy specimens and biopsy of oropharyngeal ulcers.

Direct microscopy:

Smears from sputum, blood, bone marrow and CSF can be fixed with methanol and stained with Giemsa stain. Yeast cells 2-4 µm would be seen typically within the cytoplasm of macrophages and monocytes.

Culture:

The Sabouraud's agar tube (with antibiotics) incubated at 25-30°C would reveal the *mold form* of fungus with characteristic microconidia and macroconidia. It would require an incubation period of at least 4 weeks, as the growth is slow.

This form can be *converted* to the yeast form by subculturing in an enriched medium and incubating at 37°C. The exoantigen test can also be performed for confirming identification of the mold stage. The nucleic acid probe may also be used for confirmation.

Serological tests:

CFT is available to demonstrate antibody against this fungus. Titers of $\geq$ 1:32 that persist or rise are indicative of active infection.

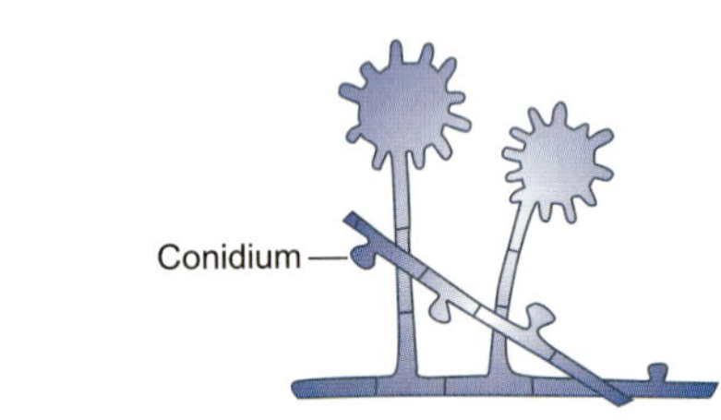

Fig. 15.4.1: Schematic representation of the mycelial form of *H. capsulatum*

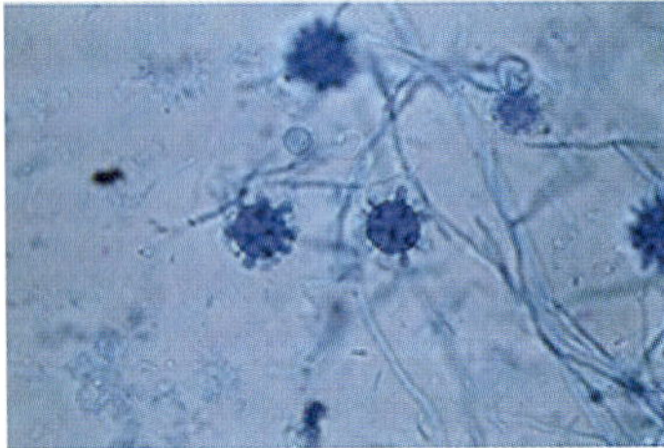

Fig.15.4.2: *Histoplasma capsulatum*: Photomicrograph demonstrating numerous tuberculate spheroidal macroconidia and diaphanous filamentous hyphae

Courtesy: Dr . Libero Ajello/CDC

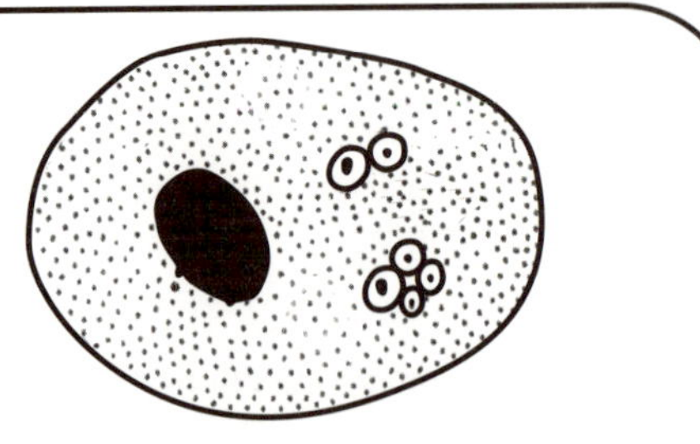

Fig. 15.4.3: Yeast cells (phase) in a macrophage

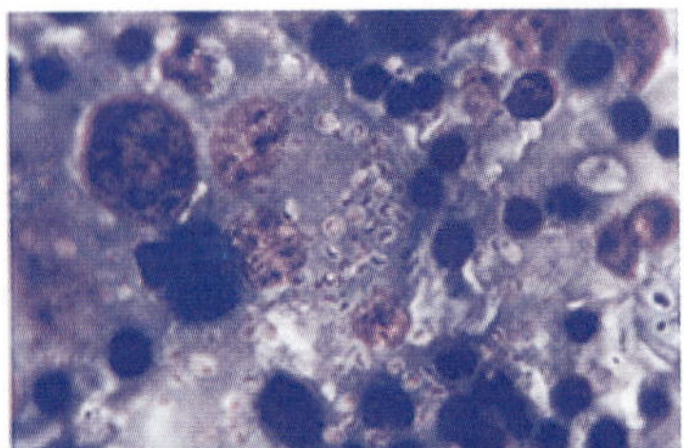

Fig. 15.4.4: Histoplasmosis: Photomicrograph depicting numerous yeast stage organisms of *H. capsulatum* in liver tissue specimen(Giemsa stained)

Courtesy :Dr, Lucille K. George

Histoplasmin skin test:

It is an intradermal skin test similar to the tuberculin test and is based on the principle of delayed hypersensitivity. The positive test indicates past or present infection. However a negative test doesn't rule out histoplasmosis. This test is of epidemiological value.

Treatment:

Most cases of pulmonary histoplasmosis are asymptomatic and require no treatment. In progressive disease cases, amphotericin B or Itraconazole can be used.

Aspects related to case theme/examination assessment

Enumerate other fungi causing systemic mycoses and describe them.

A.4 *Blastomyces dermatitidis* (Blastomycosis, pg. 539 to 540), *Coccidioides immitis* (Coccidioidomycosis, pg. 540 to 541), *Paracoccidioides* brasilensis (Paracoccidiodomycoses, pg. 541 to 542)

Blastomycosis (North American blastomycosis/Chicago's disease)

Etiological agent:

Blastomyces dermatitidis, the species name 'dermatitidis' indicates skin (dermis) to be the commonest (70%) secondary site to get involved, if rare dissemination occurs, after primary pulmonary involvement.

The sexual form, i.e., the teleomorph state of this fungus exists and is known as *Ajellomyces dermatitidis*.

Geographic distribution:

Cases have been reported from India

Widespread distribution include North, American continent (especially Ohio-Mississipi river vallcy), Africa and Asia.

Epidemiology:

Source: Soil

Male to female ratio: 10:1, Age distribution (most patients): 20-60 years

No occupational predisposition

Pathogenesis:

The spores (microconida), when become airborne enter lungs and inside it, get transformed to the yeast stage to cause pulmonary infection. The pulmonary lesion may heal spontaneously or becomes chronic. It rarely disseminates to other extrapulmonary sites, but when it does; skin, bones and genitourinary systems are the predominant organs (system) that get involved. The lesions are characterized by suppurative and granulomatous features.

Morphology:

Mold form: At 25-30°C, septate hyphae having terminal or lateral, spherical to pyriform microconidia (about 3-5 μm in diameter) (Fig. 15.4.5).

Yeast form: At 37°C, smooth cream colored colony. Yeast cell are spherical, thick walled, single bud attached to parent cell with broad base. Yeast cells are large (8-15 μm) in diameter in comparison to yeast cells of *Histoplasma capsulatum* (Fig. 15.4.6).

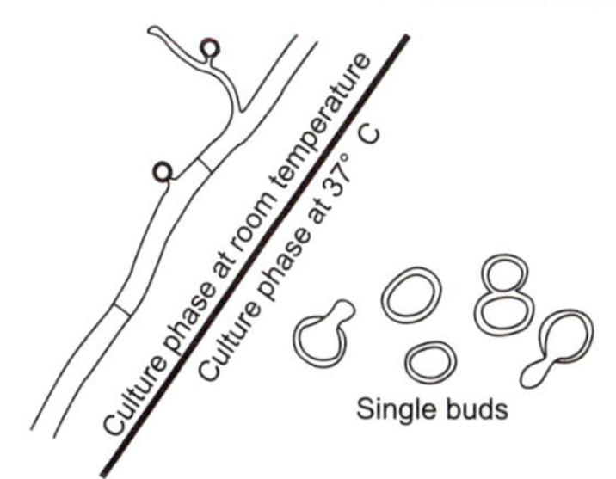

Fig. 15.4.5: Schematic representation of the mold and yeast phase of *B. dermatitidis*

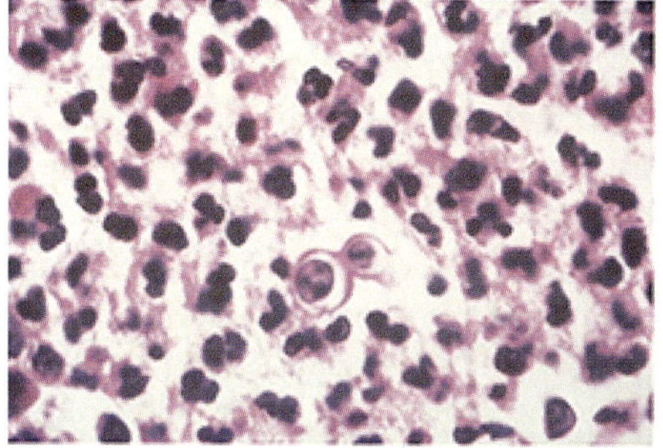

Fig.15.4.6: *Blastomyces dermatitidis*: Photomicrograph demonstrating budding cells of this fungus surrounded by neutrophils

Courtesy: Centers for disease control and prevention/Atlanta,USA

Clinical features/forms:

Asymptomatic (in more than 50% cases).

Pulmonary blastomycosis – most commonly present; as mild lower respiratory tract infection, sometimes as self-limited pneumonia.

Disseminated form (disseminated blastomycosis): Seen in immunocompromised individual; as having AIDS or transplant recipients receiving steroids or immunosuppressant drugs. Disseminates to many organs including bones.

Cutaneous form – Skin is a site often affected, if rarely dissemination, occurs after primary pulmonary infection. It affects the exposed parts of the body and the lesion presents as a papule, which subsequently breaks down to form an ulcerative lesion.

Laboratory diagnosis:

Specimens: Sputum, pus, skin scraping and biopsy of affected tissue.

Direct microscopy: In KOH mounts, thick walled yeast cells with broad based buds, 8-15 μm diameter could be demonstrated.

Such structures would also be demonstrated in tissue sections stained with H & E and PAS stains.

Culture:

Culture on SDA with antibiotics; as cycloheximide and gentamicin would demonstrate the mold form, with septate hyphae with round/oval microconidia.

For confirmation of the isolate, a subculture of the above has to be performed onto special enriched media at 37°C, which would reveal the characteristic yeast like colony with characteristics yeast form, i.e., conversion of mold form to yeast form. The exoantigen study can also confirm the identity of the isolate.

Serology:

Immunodiffusion test, CFT and ELISA tests are available to detect antibodies against 'A' antigen, which is considered specific for blastomyces.

Skin test:

Not considered significant, because of cross-reactivity.

Treatment:

Amphotericin B, Itraconazole and ketoconazole can be used for treatment.

COCCIDIOIDOMYCOSES (Valley/California Fever)

Etiological agent: *Coccidioides immitis*

Geographical distribution: Not autochthonous (local/indigerous/native) case yet reported from India

Restricted in southwestern regions of USA (as California, Texas), Mexico, Central and South America. Because of unique distribution of disease, also named as 'Valley fever' and 'California disease'.

Epidemiology:

- *Source:* Desert Soil (fungus exists as saprophyte)
- *Mode of infection:* Infection is initiated by inhalation of arthrospores from soil sites.

Infection doesn't exist outside the endemic areas. Persons in these areas are at high risk of infection. Individuals outside the endemic areas may contract the disease, during a short visit to the endemic areas.

Pathogenesis:

Inhaled arthrocondia are small in size to bypass the defense of the tracheobronchial tree to lodge in the alveoli. There the conversion to the spherule stage occurs. This represents the yeast phase of the dimorphic fungus, though exactly it isn't the yeast form. The spherule grows slowly to become the mature form with numerous endospores inside. On rupture of the spherule, the endospores get released.

These spread locally and can disseminate to the various extrapulmonary sites; as meninges and skeletal system. These are the infective forms and wherever they settle, they get transformed into spherules. This stage is not infective, so human to human transmission is not possible. Rarely, however hyphae may form in the tissues with arthrospores, then transmission to another case is possible.

Morphology of the fungus.

- *Hyphal (Mycelial) stage* [in vitro form]: For the demonstration of this stage, no special media are required. Here the hyphae are branched and septate, which can fragment into arthrospores (3-6 μm)

- *Yeast stage* [in vivo form]: For the demonstration of this form in laboratory, special enriched media; as BHI agar is required. As mentioned previously, this form is not exactly a yeast form, but a thick walled spherule (15-80 µm in size) with numerous endospores inside.

Clinical Feature:

- Asymptomatic (more than 50%)
- Pulmonary coccidioidomycosis (most common) – a self limited influenza like presentation
- Chronic meningitis
- Disseminated coccidioidomycosis (in less than 1% of infected persons; can involves bone, eyes etc.)

Lab diagnosis:

The laboratory requisition form must mention a suspected diagnosis of coccidioidomycosis, as the mold form often isolated in the laboratory, has arthrospores, which are extremely infectious.

Specimens: Sputum, CSF, Pus and biopsy specimens

Direct microscopy:

Charcteristic spherules may get demonstrated in the clinical specimen with KOH mount. Histopathological examination with H & E staining and PAS could demonstrate the typical spherule with or without endospores (Figs. 15.4.7, 15.4.8).

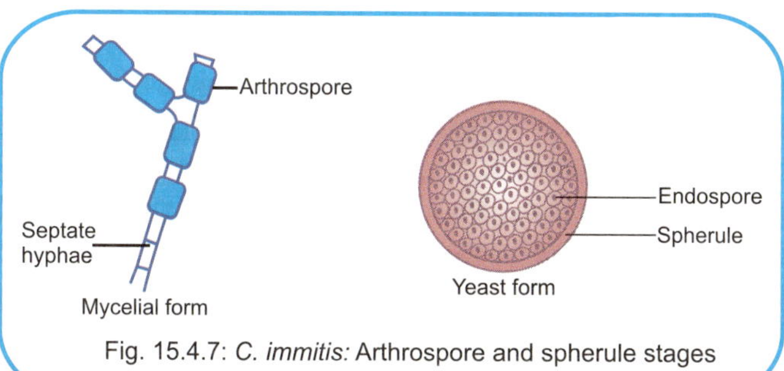

Fig. 15.4.7: *C. immitis:* Arthrospore and spherule stages

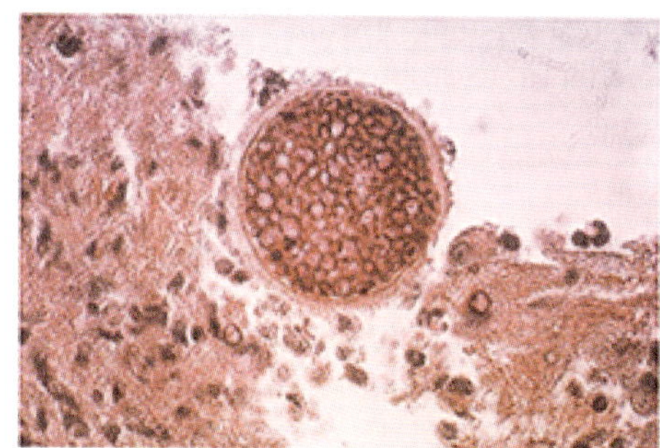

Fig.15.4.8: Coccidioides spp.: Photomicrograph demonstrating spherule of this fungus in a pas stained lymph node (480X)

Courtesy: Dr. Lucille K. Georg/CDC

Culture:

All culture work must be done with biohazard protection, as the mold form contains highly infective arthrospores.

Routine fungal media can be inoculated and incubated at 25-30°C. The specimens that contain the spherule would get converted to the filamentous form and could be demonstrated.

To confirm that the mold form is Coccidioides, the conversion to yeast form can be attempted by subculturing the fungus in enriched media and incubating at 37°C for few weeks or by animal inoculation.

The mold form can also be identified by *exoantigen test*.

Serological tests:

C. immitis is one of the few fungi, where serological tests are useful. Latex agglutination test and CFT are often performed for specific antibody demonstration.

Skin tests:

An intradermal test using 'Coccidioidin' an antigen from fungus is available and the test is based on delayed hypersensitivity reaction. It has a role in epidemiological studies and has limited role in individual diagnosis because of poor sensitivity and specificity.

Treatment:

Most cases of primary pulmonary Coccidioidomycosis usually resolve spontaneously. Treatment with intravenous amphotericin B followed by oral itraconazole or fluconazole is very much indicated in extrapulmonary and disseminated cases.

PARACOCCIDIODOMYCOSIS (South American Brazilian Blastomycoses)(Reference from P. 539-Q4

Etiological agent:

Paracoccidiodes brasilensis. The species name is derived from Brazil, where there is a high incidence of this disease.

Geographic distribution:

Not yet reported from India

Confined to Central and South America (common in Brazil).

Epidemiology:

- *Source:* Soil
- *Mode of infection:* Infection of spores (conidia)

Majority of patients with symptomatic disease are young males. Presence of oestrogen in females is likely to inhibit the formation of the yeast form. Person to person transmission is not known to occur.

Pathogenesis:

Infection occurs with the inhalation of the spores. The infection is chronic, granulomatous type and begins with primary pulmonary asymptomatic infection that can disseminate haematogenously to produce ulcerative granulomata in the mucosal surfaces of the nose, mouth, GIT tract, lymph nodes and other internal organs.

Morphology:

Mold form: It does not show any characteristic form, it is slow growing and hence culture requires prolonged incubation at 25°C for 3-4 weeks.

Yeast form: It is highly characteristic and gets produced by incubating at 37°C in enriched media. The yeast cell shows multipolar budding. This has been described as 'Mariner's wheel' appearance or 'Mickey mouse cap' appearance, this feature helps to differentiate this fungus from *B. dermatitidis* and other yeasts (Figs. 15.4.9, Fig. 15.4.10).

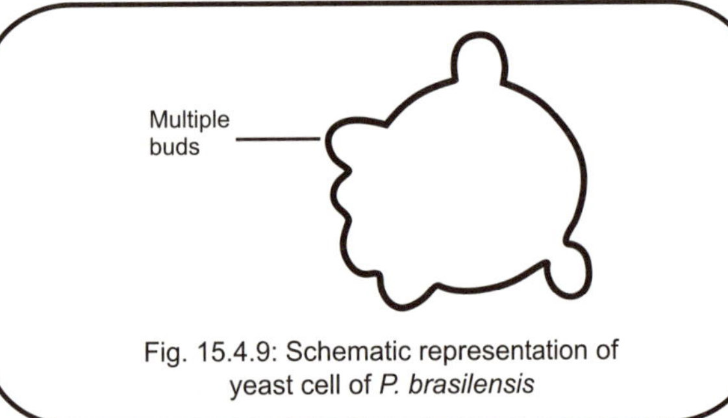

Fig. 15.4.9: Schematic representation of yeast cell of *P. brasilensis*

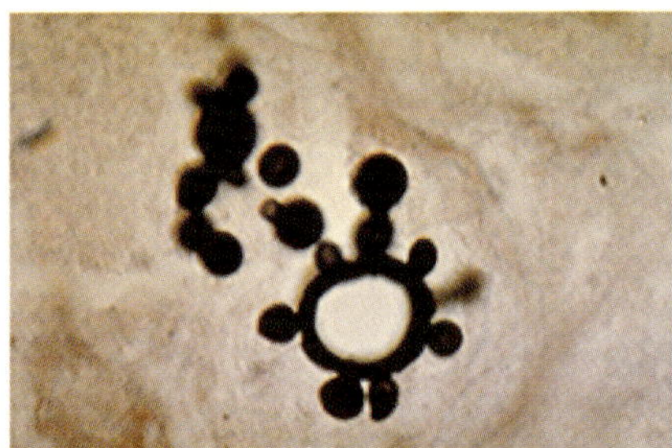

Fig.15.4.10: Paracoccidiodomycosis: Photomicrograph demonstrating budding cells of *P. brasilensis* (Methenamine silver staining)

Courtesy: Dr. Lucille K. Georg/CDC

Clinical features:

These resemble those of histoplasmosis except that the commonest secondary site of infection is mucocutaneous in nature including mouth and nose, where painful destructive lesions may be present.

Laboratory diagnosis:

Specimens: Sputum, pus and biopsies from lesions.

Direct microscopy: Typical multipolar yeast cells can be demonstrated in the KOH mount.

These typical finding may get demonstrated also in tissue sections with H & E staining.

Culture:

The culture tube incubated at 25-30°C with the clinical sample grows uncharacteristic hyphae. To make a diagnosis in culture, subculture of the growth at 37°C in enriched media is required, where characteristic yeast forms can be demonstrated (i.e., mycelial to yeast form conversion).

Serological test:

ELISA and CFT test are available. The former test has good sensitivity and specificity.

Treatment:

Itraconazole is the drug of choice. Fluconazole and Amphotericin B may also be used.

Integrated Clinical Case Based Studies On Opportunistic Mycoses

Currently the opportunistic* mycoses are common. Theoretically, any fungus can cause opportunistic fungal infection. Let's study this category of fungi focussing on three integrated clinical case based studies.

Integrated Clinical Case Base Study 1

A 16 year old girl Ashima having leukaemia, presented with fever of 5 days duration. She had no localizing symptoms and no other signs were elicited on her. She is on chemotherapy, which includes steroids.

How should this case be approached from a diagnostic angle?

A.1 As the case is likely to be immunocompromised, she is prone to common bacterial, fungal and viral infections. Such cases are likely to have minimal (muted) signs and symptoms, as the capability to mount inflammatory response is compromised. In such cases; broad spectrum antimicrobials may be administered after blood, stool and other relevant samples are taken.

This case was started on amoxicillin and gentamicin. Even after seven days of administration, no favorable response was seen in the case.

What is the likely cause of no response in this case?

A.2 (a) The case is likely to have a fungal infection.

Why was presumptive antifungal therapy not started in this case?

A.2 (b) Many of the antifungal drugs; as amphotericin B are toxic and these may not be a part of the initial empirical therapy regime.

A reassessment of the case revealed multiple whitish, adherent lesions on the right tonsil and posterior pharynx.

What clinical sample should be taken from this case? Mention the investigations that need to be performed.

A.3 Two swabs should be taken from the lesions and subjected to microscopic examination (after staining) and culture.

The gram stain of the smear revealed budding yeast cells with pseudohyphae (Fig. 15.1.3). The culture revealed growth of *C. albicans* (Fig. 15.5.1). This organism was also isolated from blood.

What is the natural habitat of C. albicans?

A.4 *Candida albicans* is a normal inhabitant of skin, gastrointestinal and genitourinary tract (details see epidemiology, in A.8)

Which systemic antifungal can be administered in this case?

A.5 Amphotericin B can be administered systemically with 5-fluorocytosine.

What are two common tests that can be performed to confirm the species of the Candida organism, as 'albicans'?

A.6 Germ tube test (Fig. 15.5.2) and Chlamydospore formation test on cornmeal agar.

Both these two tests are positive in *C. albicans*.

Can Candida infection be prevented by usage of certain agents?

A.7 No. Certain fungal infection, as Pneumocystosis can be prevented by prophylactic administration of Trimethoprim -sulfamethoxazole.

*. The fungi in this category are usually human commensals or are found is the environment. These fungi are of low virulence and cause disease in immunocompromised, debililated or persons with artificial devices/implants.

Miscellaneous Mycoses

Describe Otomycosis.

A.1 It is defined as the superficial fungal infection of the external auditory canal.

- **Etiological agents:** *A. fumigatus, A. niger, Penicillium sps, Candida albicans, C. tropicalis* and *C. krusei*.
- **Epidemiology:** It occurs commonly in warm, humid climate in individuals with poor hygienic conditions. Usage of topical agents and corticosteroids, predispose to this fungal infection.
- **Clinical profile:**

  The common symptoms are itching, irritation and pain. Complications may occur due to secondary bacterial infections with Proteus and Pseudomonas species and may result in perforation of eardrum.
- **Laboratory diagnosis:**

  Specimen: Ear swab from discharge or infected site.

  Direct microscopy: KOH preparation and gram stain of the sample, would reveal fungal elements; as pseudohyphae, hyphae and yeast cells.

  Culture: Two set of SDA media are inoculated and incubated at 25°C and 37°C; respectively to cultivate the incriminating fungi. LPCB preparation helps in the identification of the fungus.
- **Treatment:** Topical application of ointment or gel obtaining Nystatin or Imidazole is helpful, when used for few weeks.

Describe Keratomycosis (fungal keratitis)

A.2 It is defined as an invasive fungal infection of the cornea.

- **Etiological agents:** *A fumigatus, A niger*, Penicillium sps, Candida sps, Fusarium sps, Curvularia sps., Alternaria sps. and many other saprophytic fungi.
- **Epidemiology:** It usually follows corneal trauma. Use of contacts lens and increased use of topical steroids have led to an increased incidence of this entity (keratomycosis).
- **Pathogenesis:** The fungal spores colonize the injured tissue. Their germination leads to infection of the site, which may lead to hypopyon ulcer and endopthalmitis.
- **Clinical profile:** The person complains of foreign body sensation, blurred sensation and increased sensitivity to light (photophobia).
- **Laboratory diagnosis:**

  Specimen: Corneal scraping from the edge or base of the ulcer, may be taken using a local anaesthetic, by the ophthalmologist.

  Direct microscopy: KOH preparation and the gram stained preparation of the specimen may reveal fungal elements; as gram positive pseudohyphae, hyphae and yeast cells.

  Culture: Two sets of SDA media are inoculated and incubated at 25°C and 37°C, respectively to cultivate the incriminated fungi. LPCB preparation helps in the identification of the fungi.
- **Treatment:** Natamycin ointment or flucytosine drops are useful.

Describe mycotic poisoning.

A.3 When the fungus itself causes the disease, the entity is called *Mycetism* whereas; when specific products of the fungi cause the disease, it is called *mycotoxicosis*.

The commonest example of *mycetism* is the ingestion of the poisonous mushroom. The poisonous mushroom are difficult to differentiate from the edible variety. Fruiting bodies of mushrooms (Basidiomycetes) are highly adapted for the production and dissemination of spores. One of the most dangerous mushroom, is *Amanita phalloides* (common name "death cap"), since fatalities are most commonly associated with this species. The mycotoxin involved is Amatoxin and it acts primarily; at the gastrointestinal tract and parasympathetic system. Mortalities may exceed 50%, even when treatment is initiated early. Death results from heart failure. Besides *Amanita phalloides,* many other species of poisonous mushrooms exist. The mycotoxins produced by them include muscarine and gyromitrin.

Several mycotoxins known to be causing mycotoxicosis are known. The most potent and best characterized mycotoxin is *aflatoxin,* which is of eighty varieties and produced by *Aspergillus flavus*. This infection is frequently found in groundnut, corn (maize) and flour. It is important that grossly disfigured and infected food items be identified and not consumed. The two most potent aflatoxins are B-1 and G-1, which are converted by liver microsomal enzymes into active compounds, that bind to DNA and induce mutations. These toxins are tumorogenic and cause tumors in animals, however as yet no direct evidence of these for human disease exists.

The mycotoxins of importance are summarized in table 15.6.1.

Table 15.6.1: Mycotoxins

	Fungus incriminated	**Target organ**	**Source**
Mycotoxin			
Aflatoxin	*Aspergillus flavus*	Liver, brain, kidney	Nuts, corn, flour, oil seeds
Ochratoxin	*Aspergillus ochraceous*	Liver, kidney	Grains, rice
Trichothecenes	Fusarium spp and others	Skin, GIT, Eye	Maize
Fumonisins	Fusarium sps	In man, associated with oesophageal cancer	Maize
Muscarine	*Amanita muscaria*	Activation of parasympathetic system	Mushrooms
Ergot alkaloids	Claviceps spp.	Affect circulation and neurotransmission	Grains
Rubratoxin	*Penicillium rubrum*	Liver	-

7 Assessment/Examination Questions

Chapter 1

1. Can fungi also be useful to man? Explain. P. 520 (Vignette)
2. How are fungi different from bacteria (prokaryotes)? A 1a., p. 520
3. What are the reasons for the emergence of fungal infections? A 1b., p. 520
4. Why are fungi often overlooked, as agents for human disease? A 2., p. 520
5. Describe the epidemiology of fungal diseases. A 4., p. 520
6. Describe the morphological classification of fungi. A 5., p. 521
7. Describe Dimorphic fungi. A 5., p. 522
8. Outline the taxonomical classification of fungi. A 6., p. 523
9. Mention the principles of laboratory diagnosis of fungal infection. A 7., p. 524-526
10. Classify the commonly used antifungals. A 9., p. 526

Chapter 2

1. Tabulate the surface infections of superficial mycoses, that can infect the skin and its appendages and discuss their laboratory diagnosis (Tinea versicolor/Malassezia/Pityriasis. Tinea nigra, White Piedra and Black piedra). A 6., p. 527-528
2. Describe *Malassezia furfur* and *Trichosporon beigelli.* Table 15.2.1., p. 527-528
3. Describe the morphology, epidemiology, pathogenesis, laborarory diagnosis and treatment of cutaneous mycoses (Dermatophytes/Ringworm/Tinea). A 7., p. 528-531

Chapter 3

1. Describe subcutaneous mycoses. p. 532-536
2. Describe the following entities; namely (a) Mycetoma (b) Sporotrichosis (c) Chromomycosis (d) Rhinosporidiosis. Pgs. 532, 533, 534, 535

Chapter 4

1. Enumerate fungi causing systemic infection. A 4 and A2., p. 537
2. Decribe the following entities; namely (a) Blastomycosis (b) Histoplasmosis (c) Coccidioidomycosis (d) Paracoccidioidomycosis. Pg., 537-542

Chapter 5

1. Enumerate the fungi causing opportunistic fungal infections. Describe zygomycosis with special reference on diagnosing this entity at the earlest. Pg. 543 (introduction), case 2., pg. 546-548
2. Enumerate the common Candida species infecting man. Describe the epidemiology, pathogenicity and laboratory diagnosis of Candidiasis. A 8., pg. 544, introduction, Case one., pg. 544-546
3. Describe Aspergillosis and Penicilliosis. P. 552-554, A 6., P. 551-552
4. Describe *Penicillium marneffei* and *Pneumocystis jirovecii infections.* 551-552 and 554-555
5. Describe the epidemiology, pathogenesis and laboratory diagnosis of Cryptococcosis. A5., pg 549-550

Chapter 6

1. Describe the following entities; namely (a) Otomycosis (b) Keratomycosis and (c) Mycotic poisoning (Mycotoxins). A1-A3., p. 556-557

Section XVI: Clinical Microbiology

1 Specimen Collection and Transport

An optimal specimen collection is vital for a faster and accurate infectious disease diagnosis. A poor specimen can result in isolation of contaminants, failure to isolate the etiological (actual) microbe and/or incorrect diagnosis and treatment. So the role of proper sample collection cannot be overemphasized. Let's study this important laboratory technology, often overlooked by the technologists and clinicians.

Outline a classification strategy for the clinical samples, collected for microbiological processing.

A.1 (i) Direct sample: It implies sample is directly from the infected site

(ii) Indirect sample: the site of origin is usually sterile but likely to the contaminated during collection, e.g., expectorated sputum, urine collected through urethra.

(iii) Sample from the site of infection, which is in contact with normal flora, e.g., stool in dysentry case. e.g., throat swab in pharyngitis.

Discuss the general considerations in specimen collection.

A.2 General considerations

Improper specimen and poor specimen quality, may result in misdiagnosis and inappropriate antimicrobial therapy. The following are some of the considerations in collection of the sample.

- Specimens should be collected before initiating antimicrobial.
- Provisional diagnosis should be mentioned in the requisition form, so that appropriate diagnostic processing can be started.
- While collecting sample, restrict contamination with indigenous flora. In reality, most specimen collection sites get colonized, with varying quanta (quantities) of commensal microbial flora. For instance; the flora of the oropharynx contaminates sputum, the surface (cutaneous) wounds get colonized with the skin flora and endometrial specimens (collected through the endocervix) get contaminated with the cervical and vaginal flora.
- The timing of the specimen collection is important, as if you collect serum sample in first week of a enteric fever case, the result is likely to be reported as negative.
- The specimens likely to be containing highly infectious microbes should be appropriately labelled, along with the biohazard symbol.

Discuss the aspects of 'choosing right specimen collection'.

A.3 *Choosing the right specimen:* In many critical cases, choosing a right specimen could make a difference between successful and failed therapy. For instance, in case of a severe pneumonia, relying on sputum sample and avoiding an invasive sample; as bronchoalveolar lavage could result in a missed diagnosis and a failed therapy. Similarly when attempting to isolate respiratory viruses, nasopharyngeal aspirate is preferred over nasopharyngeal swab, as swabs may not collect enough cells. For the same reason faecal sample (about 2 gm) is preferred to faecal swab, as the latter may contain inadequate amount of material.

For bronchoalveolar lavage sample (used in cases of pneumonia), specimen quality validation depends on presence of alveolar macrophages.

Scraping, conjunctival swab, and vesical fluid samples are used in cases of vesicular rash, conjunctivitis and genital infections, respectively. Specimen quality validation depends on presence of epithelial cells.

Discuss the role of sensitivity and specificity of a test in choosing a correct laboratory test. Give example.

A.4 *Role of sensitivity and specificity of a test in choosing the correct test:*

Ideally the test should have high sensitivity and specificity (if not 100% sensitivity and specificity), however this is not always possible in practice. So one should be able to understand the limitation of a performed test with reference to its claimed sensitivity and specificity. A highly sensitive test means that there is a high probability, that the test would be positive; in the presence of the pathogen. A highly specific test means that there is a high probability of the test being negative; in the absence of the pathogen.

An example can help the student to understand the concept.

Lets say four new tests are under evaluation for diagnosis of tuberculosis. If these tests are run for 10 cases, out of which 7 have tuberculosis and 3 do not have tuberculosis. The results of the tests throw light on their utility:

- If one test type reported all the TB infected individuals as positive and the 3 non-infected individuals as negative, then the test would be categorized as highly (100%) sensitive and highly (100%) specific.
- If second test type reported all the TB infected individuals as positive but also labelled the two non-infected cases as positive, the test would be categorized as still being highly sensitive, but having low specificity.
- If third type of test could pick up only four of seven infected individuals as positive, but did not give any of the non-infected individuals as positive, then the test would be said to have low sensitivity but high specificity.
- If fourth type of test could pick up again only four of the seven infected individuals, but also labelled positive two of the non-infected cases, then the test would be said to have low sensitivity and specificity.

Discuss the general considerations, while transporting samples for microbiological processing.

A.5 **Transport:** The specimen has to be so transported, that it prevents death of the relevant organisms and the over growth of the unwanted organisms..

All specimens for bacterial specimens should be transported immediately to the laboratory. If the transport time to the laboratory requires more than 2 hours, then holding medium (transport medium) may be used or the specimen can be refrigerated. For specimens, where the transport period exceeds 24 hours, holding media (transport media or refrigeration) may not be appropriate techniques. It should be noted that small volumes of specimen (less than 1 ml) are more prone to drying and loss of the pathogens.

H.influenzae gets lysed by exposure to low temperatures, so CSF, genital or eye specimens in which one expects to isolate this organisms, should never be refrigerated. Some other organisms; as *N.meningitidis, S.pneumoniae* are also sensitive to low temperature. Some anaerobes and other organisms as; *N.gonorrhoeae* are fragile and exposure to ambient conditions can affect their viability.

Discuss the aspect of sample transportation, when viral diagnosis is suspected and viral processing needs to be undertaken.

A.6 **Transportation of samples** (when viral diagnosis is suspected and viral processing needs to be undertaken).

- Viral viability* can be affected in transportation, hence appropriate transport medium is required for many samples. One should not go with the impression that viruses are 'inanimate' physical particles and can be transported carelessly.
- The specimens should be transported at the earliest to the laboratory. If delay of more than 1 hour but less than 24 hours is anticipated, then sample other than blood should be maintained at 4°C. For delay longer than 24 hours, specimens may be frozen.
- Many types of commercial viral transport media (VTM) are available. They contain protein to stabilize the virus, antibiotics to minimize (prevents) bacterial and fungal growth and buffers to control pH. VTM is used for respiratory samples, swabs (as conjunctival, vesicle and genital) and tissue specimens. This medium is not required for blood and fluids; as CSF, urine, pleural fluid, amniotic fluid etc.

* Viability is not required for antigen or nucleic acid assays (tests).

Discuss the collection and transportation aspects of samples, when mycotic diseases are suspected.

A.7 **Collection** (when mycotic diseases suspected)

This aspect is being adressed separately, as mycological diagnosis is often missed and misdiagnosed. To make an accurate fungal diagnosis, it is important that a correct sample is taken appropriately. Details see Mycology section pgs. 524-525.

Central Nervous System Infectious Disease/ Syndromes with Special Reference to Meningitis

The great thing, then in all education, is to make our nervous system our ally, instead of our enemy. — *William James*

God may forgive our sins, but your nervous system won't. — *Alfred Korzybski*

Let's begin the study of this electrical ! system with core aspects of this system; to be followed by a clinical case based study.

Classify the central nervous system infectious syndrome.

A.1

Brain	**Meninges:** *Meningitis*
• Encephalitis*	• Acute purulent
• Brain abscess◊	• Aseptic (symptoms of meningitis, but failure to grow bacterial agent)
Spinal cord • *Myelitis*** – usually associated with aseptic meningitis and sometimes encephalitis	• Chronic (insidious onset with progression of sign and symptoms, over a period of time) **Nerves** • *Neuritis* (polyneuritis)***

Describe the collection and transport aspects of specimens with reference to infectious diseases of the central nervous system.

A.2 Sample/specimen (in encephalitis/meningitis)

1. CSF
2. Sera (acute and convalescent)
3. Brain biopsy (rarely; when *H.simplex* virus suspected and antiviral therapy contemplated)
4. CT guided aspiration in brain abscess, if indicated
5. Blood (for culture)
6. Pharyngeal, nasopharyngeal and rectal swabs (can help provide indirect evidence)

Collection-CSF

(a) *Amount:* 1 ml for routine culture and 5-10 ml for mycobacterial or fungal cultures.

(b) *Technique:* The site is disinfected with an iodine based preparation. The LP needle is inserted with the stylet at L3-L4 or L4-L5 interspace. When it reaches the subarachnoid space, the stylet is removed and appropriate amount of fluid is collected into sterile screw-cap tubes (tight fitting).

Transport

The sample can be transported at room temperature for bacterial culture studies. It should never be refrigerated for these studies, even if delay is likely. It should be kept at room temperature, as many bacterial pathogens; as *N.meningitidis, S.pneumoniae* and *H. influenzae* are sensitive to low temperature and can get lysed at this temperature. For virologic studies the sample should be frozen at –70°C in a deep freezer. Large amount is required for isolation of these agents.

*Encephalitis is a predominantly viral disease in contrast to ◊brain abscess, which is predominantly bacterial in origin and arise due to spread of infection from infected sites; as cardiac valves, mastoid sinuses and middle ear.

**Myelitis: An important example of it is poliomyelitis, which refers to selective destruction of anterior horn cells in spinal cord and/or brain stem, with the hall mark of asymmetric flaccid paralysis.

***Polyneuritis is an inflammation of several peripheral nerves at the same time.

Classify the infectious agents causing meningitis.

A.3 Organisms causing meningitis

Pyogenic Meningitis	Chronic Meningitis
• *Streptococcus pneumoniae*	• *Mycobacterium tuberculosis*
• *Hemophilus influenzae*	• *Cryptococcus neoformans*
• *Neisseria meningitidis*	• *Coccidioides immitis*
• Gram-negative bacteria including *Elizabethkingia meningoseptica*	• *Histoplasma capsulatum*
• *Streptococcus agalactiae*	• *Blastomyces dermatidis*
• *Listeria monocytogenes*	• Candida spp.
• Staphylococcus spp.	• Other fungi
• Leptospira spp.	• Nocardia spp.
Aseptic Meningitis	• Actinomyces spp.
• Naeglaria spp.	• *Treponema pallidum*
• Acanthamoeba spp.	• Brucella spp.
• *Viruses	• Salmonella spp.
• *Toxoplasms gondii*	• *Toxoplasma gondii*
• *Angiostroglyloides cantonensis*	• *Taenia solium*
	• *Entamoeba histolytica*
	• *Paragonimus westermanii*
	• *Strongyloides stercoralis*

*Viruses	
Neurotropic	**Non-neurotropic**
• Poliovirus	• Mumps virus
• Coxsackie A & B virus	• Measles virus
• Echovirus	• HHV-2 [Varicella zoster virus]
• Lymphocytic choriomeningitis virus	• HHV-1 and 2 [Herpes simplex virus]
• Arboviruses	• HHV-4 (Infectious mononucleosis virus)
	• Post-small pox vaccination

Common etiological agents of meningitis; according to age

Age	Common etiological agent/s
Neonates	*Streptococcus agalactiae, Escherichia coli* and other Gram-negative bacilli, *Listeria monocytogenes*
<6 years	*Hemophilus influenzae* type b
>6 years	*Neisseria meningitidis, Streptococcus pneumoniae*

Clinical Case Based Study 1

A 30 year man, Satish presented with weakness of the left side of body and loss of speech for the last 2 weeks. Contrast enhanced CT scan of the brain revealed a large roundish lesion in the parietal lobe.

What is your clinical diagnosis?

A.1 The case is most *likely* having a space-occupying infective cerebral lesion. The case is *unlikely* to have a cerebrovascular accident, as the case is a young man with no history of hypertension or chronic disease; as diabetes.

What is your differential diagnosis?

A.2 The brain abscess could be pyogenic, tubercular fungal or nocardial in origin. The parasitic causes could be cysticercosis or toxoplasmosis. The lesion could also be a neoplasm.

What investigations would be desirable in this case?

A.3 The relevant investigations would be blood culture and CT guided aspiration of the lesion. (if necessary).

How would you manage this case?

A.4 The long term management of the case would depend on the aspirate characteristics. If the aspirate appears as pus, presumptive antimicrobial therapy could be started and the antimicrobials be modulated; if necessary, according to the results of pyogenic culture and susceptibility.

Reference: Other related cases, see. Meningitis (p. 205), Epidemic typhus (p. 348) and Cryptococcosis (p. 348).

3 Cardiovascular System Infection with Special Reference to Endocarditis, Bacteremia/ Fungemia and Myocarditis

Let's keep the body's heart rhythm in harmony with the nature.

'Blood may be thicker than water, but love is thicker than blood.' — ***Goldie Nash***

Let's begin the study of this 'non-stoppable beat!' system with core aspects of this system; with brief mention of myocarditis, detailed elaboration of infective endocarditis and septicaemia, to be concluded with three clinical based studies.

Classify the infectious disease syndromes of the cardiovascular system. Define bacteremia, fungemia, SIRS, septicaemia, sepsis, severe sepsis and septic shock.

A.1

Heart (cardiac)	Vascular system
• *Pericarditis* (infection of pericardium)	• Intravascular system—Arteritis (infection of the arteries)
• *Myocarditis* (infection of myocardium)	• Thrombophelbitis (infection of the veins)
• *Endocarditis*-acute*, subacute** (infection of endocardium)	• Blood - Septicaemia (bacteremia/fungemia/viremia/parasitemia).

NB: In clinical practice, these terms includes infections and inflammatory disease of these sites.

*Infection by highly virulent microbes on previously normal heart.

**Infection by less virulent microbes (organisms) on previously diseased heart.

Certain terms

- *Bacteremia:* It is defined, as the presence of cultivable bacteria in the blood. This may be transient and inconsequential, if it is of physiological category.
- *Fungemia:* It is defined as the presence of cultivable fungi in the blood. This is often a clinical significant finding.
- *Systemic inflammatory response syndrome (SIRS)*: This term has originated on the ground that systemic responses, occurs in response to stresses; as infection (local or diffuse), which can be defined using clinical and laboratory findings. It is defined as the presence of two of more of the following:
  - Temperature >38°C or <36°C
  - Heart rate >90 beats/min
  - Respiratory rate >20 breaths/min
  - WBC >12,000 cells/mm^3 or <4,000 cells/mm^3, or >10% immature (band) forms.
- *Septicaemia:* It is a clinical term, which indicates signs of infection in the patient, who is having organisms (microbes) and/or their toxins in blood.
- *Sepsis:* SIRS that has a proven or suspected microbial etiology.
- *Severe sepsis:* Sepsis with one or more clinical signs of dysfunction; for instance low blood pressure and/or urine output.
- *Septic shock:* It is defined; as sepsis with hypotension that requires pressor therapy, despite administration of adequate fluids.
- *Pyaemia:* It is septicaemia with metastatic infection as abscesses.

Enumerate the etiological agents of myocarditis.

A.2 **Myocarditis:** In most cases with this entity, no definite cause can be established. However, almost any type of microbe (organism) is capable of causing myocarditis. Viruses are key infectious agents in causing this entity. Myocardial involvement has been seen in several viral outbreaks.

- *Viral:* Coxsackie A and B, Echo viruses, polio, non-polio enteroviruses, adenovirus, Mumps, Influenza A and B.
- *Bacterial: C. diphtheriae*, C. perfringens, N.meningitidis, Rickettsia prowazekii R. rickettsii, O. tsutsugamushi*
- *Fungi:* Aspergillus spp., Candida species, Blastomyces spp., *H. capsulatum*
- *Parasites: Trypanosoma cruzi, T. gambiense, Trichinella spiralis, Toxoplasma gondii, Toxicara canis*

*Myocarditis is one of the causes of death in diphtheria cases.

Discuss the term 'Infective endocarditis' (I.E.).

A.3 (a) The term **infective endocarditis** is currently used and is preferable to bacterial endocarditis, as other agents; besides bacteria (as chlamydiae), fungi and even viruses can also cause this syndrome. The term I.E. refers to infection of cardiac valves and endocardium by microbes. The entity of cardiac valve endocarditis can be categorized into native (original) valve endocarditis and prosthetic (artificial/implanted) valve endocarditis. The latter can be categorized into early onset (within 2 months of surgery) or late onset.

In the past, I.E. was classified as acute or subacute. This classification was based on the progression of the untreated diseases. This differentiation is of clinical interest and the differences are depicted in the table 16.3.1.

Table 16.3.1: Characteristics of acute and subacute endocarditis

Acute endocarditis	Subacute endocarditis
• Occur on previously normal heart	• Prior valvular disease exists
• Caused by highly virulent organisms; as *S.aureus, S. pyogenes, S. pneumoniae, N. gonorrhoeae*	• Mostly by 'viridans streptococci' (which are less virulent)
• Follows fulminant course with high fever and systemic toxicity	• Follow slow indolent course with low grade fever and vague symptoms
• High morbidity and mortality, despite treatment	• Most cases recover

Clinical entities; as post-operative endocarditis, which follows commonly prosthetic valve replacement and endocarditis in intravenous drug users (skin being the commonest source of infection) exist.

Enumerate the etiological agents of I.E.

A.3 (b) **Etiological agents of I.E.**

• Streptococci	• Fungi
– 'Viridans' (most common)	– *C. albicans*
– Enterococci	– Aspergillus spp.
– Others	• Others
• Staphylococci	– *C. psittaci*
– *aureus*	– Viruses
– Coagulase negative	– 'HACEK' group
• Gram negative aerobic bacilli	
– *E. coli*	
– Others	

Enumerate the specimens to be collected for diagnosis of I.E. Discuss in detail the blood collection procedure, blood culture technique and other techniques utilized in diagnosis of I.E.

A.3 (c) **Specimens**

1. Blood
2. Serum (for serologic procedures)
3. Valvular tissue (rarely, postoperative or after autopsy)

Procedure of blood collection

(i) Disinfection principles in collection, same as in blood culture technique

(ii) *Number* of blood samples: At least three blood culture sets (each set has classically an aerobic and an anaerobic bottle) should be obtained in the first 24 hours. More specimens may be necessary, if the patient has received antimicrobials in the preceding few weeks. The advantage of collecting these in a few minutes, is that antimicrobial therapy can begin early.

The basis of this recommendation, is that the bacteremia may be intermittent and may be of low grade (majority of cases have <100 colony forming units/ml).

Techniques in diagnosis and recommendation of treatment

1. Blood culture (most important).
2. *Echocardiography:* It helps in visualization of vegetations and valve changes. Transoesophageal echocardiography is considered to be more sensitive than the conventional transthoracic echocardiography in the detection of intracardiac vegetations. One limitation with this technique is high interobserver variability of echo in interpretation of images.
3. Various serologic procedures have role in diagnosis of culture negative endocarditis cases. It substantiates diagnosis of entities; as fungus, Chlamydia etc. causing I.E.
4. Cardiac catheterization with quantitative blood cultures (aids in localizing vegetations).
5. Direct fluorescent antibody technique, electron microscopic techniques on endocardial tissue (which has been removed surgically) to demonstrate etiological; agents as Chlamydia, Coxiella etc.
6. MIC and MBC must be determined for usual antimicrobials and doses accordingly adminstered, to ensure that relapse of infection may not occur.
7. Serum bactericidal test – SBT peak titres of 1:64 of greater may be sought for effective therapy in bacterial endocarditis.

Blood culture

In case the laboratory has a manual blood culture system, then inoculated blood culture bottles are incubated for at least 1 week at 37°C. Subcultures can be made onto solid media, on indication of growth in the liquid medium or performed routinely according to a schedule.

In laboratories equipped with an automated blood culture systems as 'Bactec', subcultures are performed onto the solid media, when the system signals positive for presence of growth (Fig. 16.3.1).

Although blood culture is a key investigation, one must be aware of an entity as "culture negative endocarditis". As the name indicates, these are cases who have infective endocarditis, but the culture result, does not yield any significant growth. Blood culture can be negative in 10-20% cases of infective endocarditis cases.

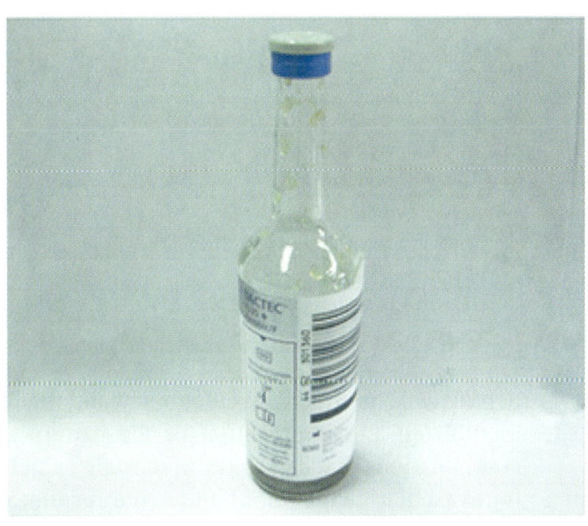

Fig.16.3.1: Blood culture bottle (used in automated systems)

The reasons include:

(i) Infections caused by difficult to culture organisms; as *Coxiella burnetii* and Chlamydia spp.
(ii) Fastidious organisms; as nutritionally deficient streptococci, which require pyridoxal hydrochloride for improved growth.
(iii) Recent antimicrobial intake by the patient, which can inhibit or destroy the incriminating organisms.

Describe the technique of the antibiotic susceptibility to be followed for isolates from the I.E. cases and the importance of it.

A.3 (d) Antibiotic susceptibility tests

It needs to be emphasized that qualitative antimicrobial testing techniques, performed on the isolated organisms, provide inadequate information and quantitative susceptibility techniques; as MIC and MBC must be performed. The drugs that are tested should preferably have bactericidal activity. The administration of antimicrobials, based on the result of these tests would help to sterilize the infected lesion and prevent the lesion activity. 'Viridans' streptococci are highly sensitive to penicillin. Determination of synergistic combination of antimicrobials can be useful. Clinically the relevant drugs have to be administered for prolonged periods of many weeks to be effective.

Mention the preventive aspects in Infective endocarditis (I.E.).

A.3 (e) Prevention (in I.E.)

As Bacteremia can result, after performance of some surgical procedures in susceptible cases. So prophylactic antimicrobial administration is recommended in them. These include procedures; as dental extractions, gastrointestinal procedures; as endoscopies, obstetric and gynaecological procedures; as D&C and genitourinary procedures; as urethral catheterization. Besides a good dental hygiene is an asset, as these areas harbour high concentrations of bacteria and simple routine activity; as brushing of teeth can also result in bacteraemia.

NB: Anaemic is present in almost all cases of I.E. (70-90%)

Classify the etiological agents responsible for causing septicaemia. Mention about the risk factors for septicaemia.

A.4 Septicaemia (can be resulting from bacteremia, fungemia, viraemia or parasitemia)

Etiological agents	
Bacteremia	**Fungemia**-(fungi in blood)
Aerobic bacteria	• Candida species
Gram negative bacilli	• *B. dermatitidis*
• Salmonella species (as Typhi, Paratyphi A)	• *H. capsulatum*
• *E. coli*	• *Cryptococcus neoformans*
• Klebsiella spp.	• Aspergillus spp.
• Brucella spp.	• Others
Gram negative cocci	**Viremia** (viruses in blood)
• *N.meningitidis*	• HIV
Gram positive cocci	• Many viruses circulate in peripheral blood at some stage of disease
• *S.aureus*	**Parasitemia** (parasites in blood)
• *S.pneumoniae, S. pyogenes, E. faecalis*	• In RBCs – Plasmodium spp.
Gram positive bacilli	– Babesia spp
• *Listeria monocytogenes*	• In WBC – Leishmania spp.
Anaerobic bacteria	– Toxoplasma spp.
• Bacteriodes species (esp fragilis)	• In Plasma/serum: microfilaria
• Clostridium spp.	
• *Fusobacter necrophorum*	

NB: Almost any organism can be incriminated

Septicaemia is a medical emergency and requires management in an intensive care unit. Besides antimicrobial therapy, monitoring and intervention of the cardiovascular, respiratory and renal systems may have to be performed. The complications that can result in mortality; include acute renal failure, haematological failure (as DIC, i.e., disseminated intravascular coagulation) and acute respiratory failure (as acute respiratory distress syndrome). For these reasons, a technique that can result in an early and specific diagnosis can be life saving for the patient.

For risk factors of septicaemia (see, Table 16.3.2).

Table 16.3.2: Risk factors of septicaemia

Factor	Examples
• Immature immune system	• Neonates
• Generalized disease	• Diabetes mellitus • Malignancy
• Pre-existing localized infection	• Localized abscess; as skin • Upper urinary tract infection • Lower respiratory tract infection
• Break of mucosa/skin integrity	• Burns • Leg ulcer • Surgical wound
• Invasive procedure	• Intravascular catheter • Urinary catheter • Prosthetic implant; as artificial hip joint

Enumerate the non-culture methods utilized in diagnosis of septicaemia.

A.5 (a) The advantage of the non-culture methods, is that they give rapid diagnosis, however few of these are non-specific in nature; as limulus amoebocyte lysate assay and antibiotic susceptibility pattern cannot be known from this category of tests. It includes:

(i) Molecular detection tests; as PCR etc.

(ii) Antigen detection kits for demonstration of *S.pneumoniae, N. meningitidis, H. influenzae*, Candida spp. and some others. Commonly latex agglutination technique is used

(iii) *Gas liquid chromatography* to detect metabolites of some microbes; as *M. tuberculosis* and some anaerobes.

(iv) *Limulus amoebocyte lysate assay:* It is based on the ability of this lysate to gelify in the presence of endotoxin (lipopolysaccharide) in blood. This test is highly sensitive, as it can detect a fraction of a nanogram quantity of endotoxin.

(v) Procalcitonin assay.

Decribe the blood culture technique including the collection technique with a mention of the automated blood culture system.

A.5 (b) Blood culture technique (principles)

- *Collection of sample*
  - Disinfect hands (medical technologist/nurse), using any good hand rub or soap and water
  - Glove your hands
  - Disinfection of the (skin) puncture site, before withdrawing blood is important, otherwise one may get a false positive (contaminants) blood culture result.
- *Sample:* Blood from a venepecture site and/or from an intravascular line. Arterial blood offers no advantage over venous blood in the isolation of pathogen.
- *Time of drawing blood:* Any time for most microbes, as bacteremia is more or less continuous. However if periodicity in fever is present, then may draw sample prior to peak of temperature.
- *Amount of blood:* The amount of blood to be inoculated into the blood culture bottle varies with age (see table 16.3.3). This is based on the observation that small children usually have greater number of bacteria in their blood in comparison to adults, hence less quantity is required for analysis.

Table 16.3.3: Recommended blood to be inoculated into blood culture system, based on age

Age (in years)	Volume in one bottle (in ml)
<2	1
2-5	4
6-10	6
>10	10

- *Type of blood culture bottles:* Depending on the clinical picture, any combination of bottles may be used as aerobic/anaerobic/fungal/Mycobacterial/others.
- *Blood culture system:* It can be categorized into two types, namely; *manual* and automated system. In the former, one has to visually or otherwise look for microbial growth indications in the blood culture bottle and then perform subculture onto solid media for isolation of microbes. In the *automated* system, the fluorescent/colorimetric/radiometric sensors are present in the bottle, which detects the growth in the inoculates bottles. The obvious advantage of this system is that, it can signal (detect) the growth at the earliest and can save vital time, for the appropriate intervention in the patient.
- *Period of incubation*

  The bottles should be incubated for at least a week. This period can be increased to many weeks, depending on the type of organism expected to be isolated; for instance in fungi, brucella, mycobacteria, leptospira and 'HACEK' group of organisms. (H-Haemophilus spp., A-*Aggregatibacter actinomycetemcomitans*, C-*Cardiobacterium hominis*, E-*Eikenella corrodens* and K-*Kingella kingae*.)
- *Transportation*

  Blood culture bottles (inoculated with blood) can be kept at room temperature (25°C) till they are transported to the laboratory. These should never be refrigerated (inoculated ones), as the low temperature would impede the recovery of the microbes. The transporation time of these bottles to the laboratory should be ideally less than 2 hours.

Outline the preventive strategies with reference to septicaemia.

A.6 Prevention

It is worth investing in this approach, as it can cut down the exorbitant cost management of an intensive care unit and can reduce the morbidity and mortality in a case

(i) Rapid diagnosis and treatment of infective foci; as a lung abscess.

(ii) Appropriate use of prophylactic antimicrobials, as before an invasive gastrointestinal procedure.

(iii) Aseptic care and proper usage of indwelling devices.

(iv) Proper infection control policies in the hospital and especially in ICUs, neonatal units and OTs, including hand hygiene.

Integrated Clinical Case Based Study 1

A 35 year old male, Shabudin, presented with fever (temperature of 39°C). Physical examination revealed bilateral crepts, heart rate of 96 beats/minute and respiratory rate of 23 breaths/min. Blood culture did not yield and organism.

What is your presumptive diagnosis?

A.1 Systemic inflammatory response syndrome (SIRS)

His condition deteriorated over the next three days. A repeat blood culture yielded growth of *S.pneumoniae.* Bronchoaleolar lavage revealed gram positive cocci in pairs (on staining), but culture did not reveal any growth.

What is the current diagnosis?

A.2 (a) Sepsis due to *S.pneumoniae*

What was the risk factor in the case under discussion?

A.2 (b) Resipiratory tract infection

What is the likely cause of sepsis?

A.3 Pneumonitis due to *S.pneumoniae*

Could his clinical deterioration have been prevented?

A.4 If this case had been investigated adequately and received presumptive antimicrobial therapy in the initial stage, clinical worsening in this case could have been curtailed.

Integrated Clinical Case Based Study 2

A forty-five years woman, Savita presented with right upper quadrant pain of 1 day duration. Ultrasound examination of the abdomen revealed multiple echo-dense areas consistent with diagnosis of cholecystitis with cholelithiasis.

What sample from the case can be helpful in the diagnosis and treatment?

A.1 Bile can be collected under ultrasound guidance or by some other technique. It can be cultured and antimicrobial susceptibility test performed, if indicated. However, the administration of the antimicrobial need not wait for the laboratory report.

She was started on ampicillin and gentamicin. After one day, however her condition deteriorated. She becames drowsy and her BP dropped to 80 mm/40 mm Hg. Bile culture revealed growth of *S.aureus*. Blood culture gave positive signals after 4 hours of incubation in the automated blood culture system.

What is the clinical diagnosis?

A.2 The case has developed septicaemia following cholecystitis.

Could the deterioration of this case have been prevented?

A.3 The case should have been initiated on presumptive antimicrobials at first contact, without waiting for the investigation results.

Integrated Clinical Case Based Study 3

A 35 year old man, Sanjay presented with low grade fever and weakness for the past 14 days. History revealed that he had cardiac prosthetic valve since 10 years and a tooth extraction two months back. Physical examination revealed a pansystolic murmur and no other signs of any other disease.

What is the likely clinical diagnosis?

A.1 Infective (subacute) endocarditis (I.E.).

What is the commonly followed criteria used for diagnosis of I.E.?

A.2 'Modified Duke' criteria for diagnosis of endocarditis. It has major and minor criteria, which are utilized in the making the diagnosis.

What is the most important microbiological investigation, that can be of relevance in this case (of I.E.)?

A.3 **(a)** Blood culture

What radiological investigation, is often employed for diagnosing I.E.? Mention the typical findings.

A.3 **(b)** Echocardiography, can reveal vegetations on the cardiac valves and endocardium

What would be the most likely microbe to be isolated from this case (of I.E.)?

A.4 'Viridans' streptocci

What category of antimicrobial susceptibility test should be performed to obtain a cure of the case? Explain.

A.5 Quantitative category of antimicrobial susceptibility tests; as MIC and MBC. The administration of antimicrobials based on the result of these tests, would help to sterilize the infected lesions and prevent relapse.

Could this infection have been prevented, if the dentist had elicited proper history?

A.6 If the dentist had elicted the positive history of cardiac prosthetic valves from this case, then prophylactic administration of antimicrobials, before the extraction of tooth could have prevented the infection in the heart.

Discuss the preventive aspects in I.E.

A.7 See pg. 566, A.3(e)

Reference: Other related cases

- FUO – Case (p. 327)
- Septic shock – (p. 86)

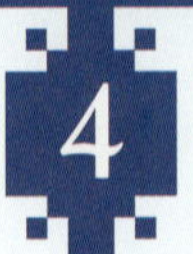

4 Respiratory Tract Infections with Special Reference to Sore Throat (Pharyngitis/Tonsillitis, i.e., Upper Respiratory Tract Infection) and Pneumonia (Lower Respiratory Tract infection)

'They say the lung branch out like trees. Trees give off oxygen. Let's keep the respiratory diseases in check to let all the mankind maintains the vital paO2 levels, without reliance on the artificial oxygen equipment.'
— Anonymous

'Coughing in the theater is not a respiratory ailment. It is a criticism'.
— Alan Jay Lerner

Let's begin a study of this 'rejuvenating–oxygenating' system with core aspects of this system, to be concluded with two clinical based studies on upper and lower respiratory system. Hoping to keep the microbial stressors in control and be always 'prana' saturated.

Classify the infectious disease syndromes of the respiratory tract anatomically.

A.1 (a) **Upper respiratory tract**

(a) Nasal mucosa – Rhinitis

(b) Nasal passage

- Rhinoscleroma (chronic granulomatous infection of nasal passage, including the sinuses and occasionally the pharynx and larynx)

(c) Pharynx and tonsil

- ΔPharyngitis and tonsillitis (sore throat)**

(d) Sinus

- Sinusitis

Middle respiratory tract♦

(a) Epiglottis – epiglottitis

(b) Larynx – laryngitis

(c) Bronchi – bronchitis

(d) Bronchiole – bronchiolitis

♦For discussion purposes considered to comprise of epiglottis, surrounding aryepiglottic tissue, larynx, trachea and bronchi

Lower respiratory tract -Alveolar spaces (incld supporting structures and terminal bronchioles)

Lung parenchyma – PneumoniaΘ
– Lung abscess***

**Sore throat – It is described as a condition, where the mucus membrane of throat is inflamed, due to an infection.

ΔPharyngitis: Acute pharyngitis is described as a triad of sore throat, fever and pharyngeal inflammation.

Θ Pneumonia: It may be described as a lung parenchymal inflammation, accompanied with consolidation of the lung. It can be categorized into acute and chronic categories.

*** Is a complication of pneumonia, in which organisms cause localized destruction of lung

NB: Most cases of pharyngitis are due to viral infections.

Enumerate the etiological agents of sore throat.

A.1 (b) Etiological agents: A 2b., p. 572

Specimens: See A.2 (a), p 571

Enumerate the specimens to be collected for diagnosis of upper respiratory tract infection (sore throat).

A.2 (a) For sore throat

- Throat swab
- Nasopharyngeal swab (better than T/S, for isolation of viruses)

Enumerate the specimens to be collected for diagnosis of lower respiratory tract infection (pneumonia).

A.2 (b)

Table 16.4.1: Specimens in LRT1

Non invasive	Invasive
• Sputum	• Bronchial washing (taken during bronchoscopy, from upper airway)
• Induced sputum (if patient does not expectorate)	• Bronchoalveolar lavage
• Gastric aspirate (in children, who swallow their sputum)	• Fine needle aspiration of material from involved lung with/without bronchoscopy
	• Percutaneous transtracheal aspirate
	• Open lung biopsy (rarely)

Describe the collection techniques for samples required in the laboratory diagnosis of upper respiratory tract infection (sore throat).

A.3 (a) Collection

Throat swab

The patient is explained the need and procedure of the test. He is made to sit on a stool and asked to tilt his head back and close his eyes. The throat is well illuminated, tongue is depressed with a tongue depressor and the patient asked to say 'Ah'. The throat (including the tonsillar and inflamed area) is swabbed from side to side with a swab and placed in the culture tube to be transported (procedure done with gloved hands).

Nasopharyngeal swab

(i) *Pernasal technique*

As the name indicates, a small dacron swab or a flexible, fine shafted swab is introduced into the posterior nasopharynx through the anterior nares. The swab is swabbed slowly for few seconds (5-6) to absorb secretions. Calcium alginate swab is used, when suspecting pertusis infection.

(ii) *Postnasal technique*

A technique exists to reach the posterior nasopharynx through the oral cavity.

- Nasopharyngeal aspirate: An appropriate catheter is introduced into the nasopharynx and material may be aspirated with a syringe.

Describe the collection techniques of samples required in the laboratory diagnosis of lower respiratory tract infection (pneumonia).

A.3 (b) Sputum (not saliva)

Types:

(i) *Expectorated:* The patient is asked to rinse the mouth with water to minimize oral flora. Then, is instructed to cough, so as to produce a lower respiratory specimen, which is collected in a sterile container.

(ii) *Induced:* This process is initiated, when the patient is not able to expectorate naturally. The patient is first asked to rinse his mouth. Then the patient is made to inhale about 20 ml of sterile saline, using a nebulizer. The specimen is then collected and labelled as induced sputum, as it resembles saliva and can be rejected mistakenly by the laboratory, as an unacceptable specimen.

Acceptability (adequacy)

A good expectorated sputum sample represents lower respiratory tract specimen and should not get contaminated with upper respiratory tract secretions, such as saliva. An acceptable sputum sample will have less than 10 squamous epithelial cells and preferably more than 25 polymorphonuclear leucocytes per low-power field (10X).

- *Time of collection and number:* For routine bacterial diagnosis, sputum collected anytime is acceptable. However for mycobacterial and fungal diseases, first early morning specimen is desirable. For mycobacterial and fungal diseases, three consecutive first morning specimens are recommended.

Bronchoalveolar lavage

During bronchoscopy, sterile fluid is introduced into the alveolar spaces of a portion of lung of interest, which is then aspirated back for analysis. In the past, this procedure was described as 'liquid lung biopsy'.

About 40-80 ml of fluid is required for quantitative analysis of this specimen. Quantitative cultures may help to assess the significance of the isolates, i.e., indicate if the isolate is a pathogen or a commensal.

Mention about the transportation aspect of clinical samples collected for respiratory tract infection (to the microbiology laboratory).

A.4 Transportation

Throat swab: *Pike's medium* (blood agar with crystal violet) in tube can be used for transporting throat swab.

Stuart's medium (buffered semisolid after containing sodium thioglycollate as reducing agent) can also be used for transportation.

The transportation can be performed at room temperature, preferably within 2 hours to the laboratory.

Nasopharyngeal swab: This specimen is used in the diagnosis of *B.pertusis, C.diphtheriae, N. gonorrhoeae, N. meningitidis, S.pyogenes* (carrier).

The specimen may be directly inoculated onto the media on bedside or transported in appropriate media at room temperature to the laboratory, within two hours of collection.

Sputum: This sample should be transported within two hours to the laboratory, however for a delay up to 24 hours, it may be stored at 4°C in a refrigerator.

Bronchoalveolar lavage (BAL): it should be transported to the laboratory within 2 hours, but it may be kept at 4°C, if a delay upto 24 hours is expected.

Enumerate key bacterial pathogens which cause typical pneumonia.

A.5 (a) *Streptococcus pneumoniae, Haemophilus influenzae.*

Enumerate key bacterial pathogens which cause atypical pneumonia.

A.5 (b) *Chlamydophila pneumoniae, Bordetella pertusis, Mycoplasma pneumoniae and Legionella pneumophila*

Integrated Clinical Case Based Study 1

A 4-year old boy, Ashu presented to a general physician; with complaints of sore throat, irritability and aversion to feeds. Oral examination revealed an inflamed throat. The child gave a history of having a common cold, two week back.

What disease has the child likely had two weeks back? Mention its presentation.

A.1 (a) The child had rhinitis, which is essentially an infection of the nasal mucosa. It presents as rhinorrhoea (nasal discharge) and sneezing.

Which are the etiological agents of rhinitis?

A.1 (b) Adenovirus, Rhinovirus, Coronavirus, Parainfluenza virus, Influenza virus, Respiratory syncytial virus and Coxsackie A are the key etiolgical agents. Fungi and bacteria are rarely implicated in this entity.

What is the clinical importance of rhinitis?

A.1 (c) As mostly this disease is caused by viruses, it is not amenable to specific therapy. However the disease is self limiting.

Many cases of sore throat may be a continuum of nasal mucosa infection.

What is the role of laboratory testing in diagnosis of rhinitis?

A.1 (d) Laboratory testing is usually done only in severe cases, atypical cases and in investigating outbreaks.

What is sore throat?

A.2 (a) Sore throat is essentially an acute infection of the tonsils and/or pharynx.

What etiological agents cause sore throat?

A.2 (b)

- ***Bacteria:*** *C.diphtheriae, Streptococcus pyogenes*, Streptococcus group C and G, *H.influenzae, Bordetella pertusis, Lepotrichia buccalis.*

- ***Viruses:*** Adenoviruses, HHV-4 (EBV) and Coxsackie A.
- ***Fungi:*** *Candida albicans*

Why is it important to take a throat swab?

A.3 It is important to know, if the sore throat is due *Streptococcus pyogenes,* as it can result in catastrophic sequelae; as RHD. It is important to treat this infection. This agents can only be determined by culturing the throat swab or performing a rapid antigen assay on an extract from the throat swab.

Four weeks later the child presented with a discharge from the right ear.

What complication, the child has had?

A.4 Otitis media.

What sample can be taken in a case of Otitis media? Mention the test that can be performed on it?

A.5 The middle ear discharge in the ear canal can be taken with a swab and cultured.

Integrated Clinical Case Based Study 2

A 35 year old male, Parikshit presented to the medical emergency with complaints of fever, breathlessness and productive cough. Physical examination revealed pulse rate of 130/minute and respiratory rate of 38/minute. His chest examination revealed dullness to percussion in right midzone. Chest radiography revealed infiltrates in the right middle zone. Blood gases revealed low PaO_2 level (arterial partial pressure of oxygen). Gram stain of the sputum revealed plenty of pus cells (3+) and mixed bacteria. Sputum culture revealed growth of coagulase negative staphylococci and *Klebsiella pneumoniae*.

What is the clinical diagnosis

A.1 Community acquired pneumonia

What findings in this case indicate, that the case is having a severe disease?

A.2 Increased breathing rate, pulse rate, fever presence, cough with expectoration and reduced paO_2 levels; indicate a severe clinical case.

How do you explain finding of mixed bacteria on gram stain and mixed growth on culture.

A.3 (a) The sputum collected by the patient and sent to the laboratory, has got contaminated with the oropharyngeal flora of the patient.

Which organism is likely to be pathogen of the two isolates? Enumerate key etiological agents of pneumonia.

A.3 (b) *Klebsiella pneumoniae* is likely to be the pathogen. See A.5a,b, pg. 572.

How can the quality of sputum be assessed for culture?

A.4 See A.3 (b), pg. 571-572

For which organism antimicrobial susocptibility test should be performed? Explain.

A.5 Antimicrobial susceptibility test should be performed for *Klebsiella pneumoniae,* as it is likely to be the pathogen in this case. Coagulase negative Staphylococci is likely to represent the commensal flora.

5 Gastrointestinal Infectious Disease with Special Reference to Diarrhoeal Disease

'All diseases begin in the gut'. **— Hippocrates**

Digestion is quickly shut down during stress...The parasympathetic nervous system, perfect for all the calm, vegetative physiology, normally mediates the action of the digestion. Along comes stress: turn off parasympathetic, and forget about digestion'. **— Robert M. Sapolsky**

Let's begin a study of the gastrointestinal system infectious diseases with the core aspects of the system to be followed by references of five integrated clinical based studies (including one of virology). Hoping to keep the microbial stressors in control to have a life full of gastronomic delights.

Classify gastrointestinal infectious disease syndromes.

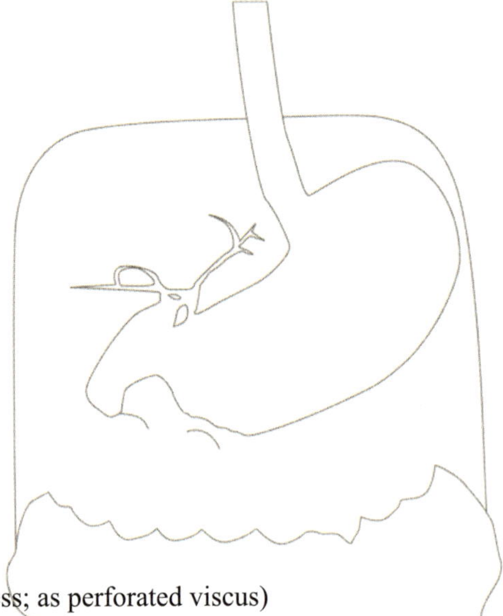

A.1 Classification

- **Stoma**
  - Stomatitis (inflammation of stoma)
- **Stomach**
  - Peptic ulcer (ulcerative lesions)
- **Stomach/small intestine to large intestine**
  - *Gastroenteritis*Δ
    - o Diarrhoea□
    - o Dysentry◊
    - o Food poisoning*
- Peritoneum
  - *Peritonitis*
    - o Primary
    - o Secondary (Is secondary to some underlying process; as perforated viscus)

Δ*Gastroenteritis:* It may be defined; as its name indicates, an inflammation of the mucus membrane of the stomach and intestine, often accompanied with alteration in the stool character with clinical symptoms; as abdominal pain.

□*Diarrhoea:* It may be defined as an increase in the frequency, volume (amount) or fluid of the stool is an individual.

◊*Dysentry:* It may be defined; as the presence of blood and/or mucus in stool, often accompanied with $^{\Delta}$tenesmus.

ΔFeeling of incomplete evacuation despite empty colon

**Food poisoning:* It may be defined; as an illness acquired due to ingestion of food containing microbes, microbial toxins or chemicals. It often presents; as acute diarrhoea with or without vomiting.

NB: *Traveller's diarrhoea:* It is an acute diarrhoeal disease observed occasionally in visitors from foreign countries, during their stay in the developing countries.

Classify the etiological agents which cause stomatitis and peritonitis.

A.2 Stomatitis (inflammation of oral cavity)

- *Bacterial:* Spirochetes, Fusobacterium spp.
- *Fungal:* Candida spp.

- *Others* (as dissemination from remote sites; as disseminated histoplasmosis)
- *Viral*
  - Herpes simplex, Coxsackie A,
  - Measles, HHV-3 (chicken pox)
  - Enterovirus (as hand and mouth disease)

Peritonitis (inflammation of peritoneum)

Table 16.5.1: Etiological agents in Peritonitis

Primary- in children	**In adults**
• *S.pneumoniae*	• *E. coli (commonest)*
• *S. pyogenes*	• *S. pneumoniae*
• *M.tuberculosis*	• *M. tuberculosis*
• Coliforms	• *N. gonorrhoeae*
• Staphylococci spp.	• *C. trachomatis* (In sexually active young women)
Secondary (in sequel to some underlying process in abdomen; as perforated viscus, so etiological agent depends on the pathologic process).	

Classify the etiological agents of:

(a) Diarrohea ***(b) Food poisoning*** ***(c) Dysentry***

A.3 (a)

Table 16.5.2: Diarrheagenic agents

Bacterial	**Viral**
• *E. coli* (EPEC, ETEC)	• Rota, Echo, Polio, Coxsackie
• *Vibrio cholerae,*	• Adenovirus, Norwalk, Calcivirus
• Salmonella spp, other than Typhi and Paratyphi A as, Typhimurium, Enteritidis	• Astrovirus, Coronavirus
• Salmonella Typhi, Paratyphi A, B and C (during early stages of infection)	**Parasitic**
• *S. aureus* (after treatment with broad spectrum antibiotics)	• *G. lamblia, Cryptosporidium parvum*
• *Campylobacter jejuni*	• Microsporidia and Cyclospora spp.
• *Plesiomonas shigelloides*	• *F. hepatica, F. buski*
• Providencia spp.	• *C. sinensis, P. westermanii*
• Aeromonas spp. (rarely)	• Helminths (rarely)
• Edwardsiella spp. (rarely), Proteus spp. (doubtful)	**Fungal**
• *P. aeruginosa* (doubtful)	• *C. albicans* (after treatment with antibiotics)
• In immunosuppressed (any organism)	• Miscellaneous (not due to microorganisms)

(b) **Food poisoning**

Table 16.5.3: Etiological agents for food poisoning

Infective
• All Salmonellae except Typhi, Paratyphi A & B
• *Clostridium perfringens* type A (In U.K., a common agent, due to meat being a common ingredient in food)
• *Vibro parahaemolyticus* (In Japan, a common agent due to common marine food consumption)
Toxic
• *Staphylococcus aureus* (enterotoxin produces strain belonging to phage group III or phage type 42D)
• *B.cereus*

(c) **Dysentry**

- *Bacterial: E.coli* (EIEC, EHEC), Shigella spp., *C.perfringens* (type C)
- *Protozoal: E.histolytica, Balantidium coli, Cystoisospora belli*
- *Helminthic: S.japonicum, S.mansoni*
- *Viral:* none

Enumerate the samples to be collected in a diarrohea/food poisoning case.

A.4 **(a)** Samples (in diarrhoeal/food poisoning disease)

1. Stool 2. Rectal swab 3. Vomitus 4. Food sample 5. Serum

Describe the collection procedure of stool and rectal swab. Comment on their transportation.

A.4 **(b)** **Collection of these samples**

- **Stool:**

  The liquid/non-formed/bloody/pus/mucus part* is preferred over a formed (normal) stool fraction for sampling and collected into a clean, (not necessary to be sterile) leak-proof, wide mouth container. Three samples preferably on consecutive or alternate days can be processed. This approach could be especially useful in detecting parasitic infection, where the ova/cysts are being excreted intermittently in varying quantas.

- **Rectal swab:**

  A swab is inserted about 2-5 cms beyond the anal sphincter. It is rotated gently to swab the anal crypts. A properly sampled swab should get stained with faeces. A stool specimen is preferable to a swab specimen, as a tiny amount of sample gets sampled with a swab specimen. The swab may be transported as such or in the transport medium to the laboratory.

  NB: Stool specimen from patients admitted in hospital for >3 days is not accepted by some laboratories.

  * These fractions represent pathologic part of the stool likely to be in contact with infected intestinal mucosa.

Transportation

The stool specimen without any holding (transport) medium should be transported to the laboratory within 1 hour at room temperature. In case; a delay is likely, the stool specimen can be kept at 4°C for less than 24 hour.

In case, Cary Blair medium is used for holding, the specimen can be kept at room temperature for ≤24 hours.

Buffered glycerol transport medium can also be used for transportation.

References: Cases related to GIT-Diarrohea (p. 261), Dysentry (p. 264), Food possoning (p. 271) and viral diarrohea (p. 402)

Urinary Tract Infection

- **Leave a legacy of life. Be an organ (kidney) donor.**
- **'Do not think of organ (kidney) donations as part of yourself to keep a total stranger alive. It's really a total stranger giving up almost all of them, to keep a part of you alive'.**

— Anonymous

Let's begin the study of this 'continuously filtering system' with core aspects of the system, to be followed by three clinical case based integrated studies. Hoping that the knowledge allows the specialized filtration in the body to continue unimpededly till the end.

Outline the infectious disease syndromes of the urinary system.

A.1

Upper urinary tract
- Kidney (including pelvis) → *pyelonephritis*

  Ureter → *Ureteritis*

Lower urinary tract
- Bladder → *cystitis*
- Urethra →
  - *Urethritis*
  - *Urethral syndrome* (abacterial cystitis)

Enumerate the common etiological agents causing urinary tract infection (UTI).

A.2 Etiological agents

E. coli. (most common), Klebsiella spp., Proteus spp., Pseudomonas spp., *E. faecelis*,

S. pyogenes, *S. aureus*, Coagulase negative Staphylococcus spp., *Staphylococcus saprophyticus*, Leptospira spp, Mycoplasma spp, Mycobacterium spp, Chlamydia spp, anaerobic organisms and Candida spp.

Describe the techniques to obtain samples for diagnosis of upper and lower tract infection. Mention also the transportation principles of urine samples to the microbiology laboratory.

A.3 Technique to take samples

For upper UTI

- *Ureteric catheterization:* Urine is taken from ureter (not urethra), If the sample has organisms, it indicates upper UTI.
- *Fairlay technique:* Fairlay *et al.* 1971 presented a technique to differentiate upper UTI from lower UTI.

  According to it, a Foley's catheter is introduced into bladder and all urine is collected, which represents sample I. Then an antibiotic; as neomycin and 'Elase' (combination of two enzymes, fibrinolysin and deoxyribonuclease) is introduced into the bladder for about 30 minutes. The bladder is then emptied and washed with 2 litres of sterile saline. This represents sample II. A further three samples are collected at intervals of 10 minutes, which represent samples III to V. Interptretation is done on the basis of the bacterial counts in the different samples. If five times bacterial counts are seen in the samples III to V in comparison to the sample II, upper UTI is indicated.
- *Renal biopsy*

For Lower UTI

- *Midstream urine:* This as the name indicates involves collection of the middle part of the passed out urine for purposes of processing of the urine; with the initial part of the urine being discarded. This is a optimal method,most often used. It involves no risk to the patient.

  In males, the prepuce is retracted and glans penis is cleaned with wet cotton. The first part of the urine is discarded and the middle part is collected in a sterile container aseptically.

In females, anogenital toilet is performed and cleaning is performed using soap and water. Non irritating antiseptics as chlorhexidine is recommended for vulval cleaning. Here again; the first part of the urine is discarded and mid part is collected.

- *Urethral catheterization:* This technique is indicated in the anaesthetized patients and comatose patients. In the past, this method was used to avoid contamination of the urine, while collection for culture, but it led to urinary tract infection in 2% of cases, even under ideal conditions
- *Suprapubic aspiration:* This technique is indicated in infants, from whom satisfactory specimen may be difficult to obtain and in patients with equivocal counts on several occasions.

  In it, when the bladder is distended, suprapubic skin is aseptically prepared and sterile needle is thrust in the bladder for collection of the urine.

  In interpreting the report of sample collected by this sample, it should be noted that urethral contamination is avoided and few bacteria isolated by this technique are considered significant.
- *3 glass test:* First 5 ml represents urethral sample. Second 10 ml of urine represents urinary bladder sample. Third sample after bladder emptying and prostatic massage, represents prostatic sample

Transport of specimen: It is important to inoculate the urine sample onto media immediately, as a semi quantitative count of the organisms is to be reported. If this is not possible, then the urine can be refrigerated at 4°C, for no more than 18hrs. It should be noted that urine is a good culture medium, for many microbes and growth can occur, if urine is kept at room temperature.

Interpretation of results:

Urine is sterile, when formed, but gets contaminated when passes out of distal urethra. So it is important to differentiate between urinary tract infection and contamination. According to Kass (1956), following criteria are to be used

(i) Count of more than 10^5 bacteria per ml indicate active UTI (significant)

(ii) Count between 10^4-10^5 bacteria per ml, indicate doubtful significant.

(iii) Count less them 10^3 bacteria per ml, no significance

Integrated Clinical Case Based Study 1

A 23-year old Delhi intern, Shitij presented to the medical emergency with fever and acute pain in the lumbar region radiating to the groin

What is your clinical diagnosis?

A.1 The case is likely to have acute pyelonephritis (upper urinary tract infection). The presentation of fever in the case is a likely pointer to an infectious lesion in the case.

What could be the reason of acute pain?

A.2 Renal stones are common in the Northern India including Delhi. The acute pain in the case, could be due to ureteric colic, caused by dislodgement (displacement) of a renal stone.

Ultrasound performed on the case revealed renal stones. Microscopy of the unspun (uncentrifuged) urine revealed 25 leucocytes per high power field and occasional epithelial cells. Gram stain of the uncentrifuged urine revealed 4 bacilli per oil immersion field.

What do the findings of of urine examination and gram staining of urine indicate?

A.3 These indicate a significant pyuria and bacteriuria and suggest a clinical diagnosis of an upper urinary tract infection.

What is the significance of the presence of epithelial cell findings in the urine?

A.4 The presence of an occasional epithelial cell indicate a minor contamination of the urinary sample by perineal flora, during urine collection.

What impact the finding of the renal stone would have on the treatment of this case?

A.5 The presence of renal stones imply that the renal stones should be removed to prevent relapse of UTI and antimicrobial therapy should be prolonged (probably more than 2 weeks) to ensure eradication of the infective foci.

Culture of the urine revealed a growth of the *E.coli* with a 10^5/cfu (colony forming units) per ml of the urine. The isolate is resistant to Ampicillin and Trimethoprim.

What is your interpretation of the findings?

A.6 The *E.coli* isolate is likely to represent the etiological agent of the renal infection and is unlikely to represent a perineal contamination, which may occur during urine collection. A properly collected repeat urine culture with identical (similar) findings would confirm the probable diagnosis.

Could you comment on the possible source of the bacterial isolate in this case?

A.7 The *E.coli* isolate has most likely arisen from her perineum and resulted in an ascending infection. The presence of the renal stones with their occasional dislodgement could cause stasis of urine in the urinary tract, leading to bacterial proliferation with urine acting as a good medium for bacterial growth.

Clinical Case Based Study 2

A 70 year old man, Ziaudin presented with increased frequency of micturition and burning pain on micturition

What is the clinical diagnosis?

A.1 Lower UTI (most likely cystitis)

What could be a likely factor responsible for precipitating his illness?

A.2 **(a)** Benign hypertrophy of prostrate is a common ailment in the elderly males.

What physical examination would help in detecting the precipitating factor in this case?

A.2 **(b)** Rectal examination to look for enlargement of the prostrate. Ultrasound of the lower abdomen can confirm the findings.

What sample should be taken from this case? Mention the microbiological test to be performed to confirm the clinical diagnosis?

A.3 Midstream urine with microbiological culture performed on the sample.

What do you understand by 'pre-analytical problems' with reference to laboratory diagnosis of UTI?

A.4 Collection and transport of the urine sample, plays a key role in the correct diagnosis of UTI. This is so, as urine itself is a good culture medium and the microbes can grow in it affecting the colony count of the specimen; if delay in processing occurs.

The case is administered antimicrobials, but does not respond and on the contrary develops fever.

What could be the cause of the resulting fever?

A.5 The case could have developed sepsis, secondary to cystitis.

What is the likely reason of the case not responding to antimicrobials?

A.6 **(a)** The case is likely to have an obstruction in the lower urinary tract leading to stasis of urine, promoting infection in the region.

What surgical intervention may be indicated in this case?

A.6 **(b)** Prostatectomy, if the case is having BHP.

Can urinary tract infections be prevented? If so, explain.

A.7 Yes in many situations. Correction of the pre-existing urinary tract pathology; as renal stones or BHP may reduce the incidence of UTIs. Some authorities recommend low dose of antimicrobial therapy to prevent recurrent UTIs. Post-coital ('honeymoon cystitis') in women can be minimized by urination, immediately after coitus.

Integrated Clinical Case Based Study 3

A 23- year old female, Rekha presented with left flank pain, fever chills and rigor. Physical examination revealed left costovertebral angle tenderness. Urinalysis revealed >30 WBCs/high power field, 4-6 RBCs/HPF and 4+ bacteria

What is the provisional clinical diagnosis?

A.1 The case is likely to have upper urinary tract infection (most likely pyelonephritis), evident from clinical findings of fever and pain in left costovertebral angle and urinary microscopic findings including pyuria, haematuria (presence of RBCs in urine) and bacteriuria (presence of bacteria in urine).

Is it unusual for this case to be of female sex? Enumerate the reasons for UTIs to be more frequent in women than men.

A.2 No, UTIs are more common in females than males. The reasons include short urethra, proximity of urethral opening to anus and physiological conditions; as pregnancy; which can predispore to UTI.

Which microbiological test can confirm the diagnosis?

A.3 Urine cultured by semiquantitative/quantitative technique.

What instructions should be given to the patient for collection of the urine sample? Explain the importance of these instuctions.

A.4 Proper collection of urine is vital in the diagnosis of UTIs. The reason is that urine is a sterile specimen, when formed but gets contaminated, while passing out through the distal urethra. So contamination of the urine sample is to be minimized.

In both the sexes, the person is asked to give a 'mid-stream urine' with the idea that the initial part of urine representing urine in contact with distal urethra and/or perineum (in female) is not used for culturing this specimen

Details (A.3, pg. 577-578)

Why is it important to culture urine within a few hours of its collection?

A.5 (a) Urine sample is a good growth medium. So, if urine is not analyzed within 1-2 hours, the organisms in urine (derived from distal urethra) can multiply many times and give rise to falsely increased organisms count in urine.

If this is not possible, what intervention should be done?

A.5 (b) So; if the urine sample processing is likely to be delayed for more than few hours, then it should be refrigerated in an attempt to inhibit the organism multiplication.

Why is urine sample, cultured semiquantitatively/quantitatively?

A.6 Very few samples are cultured semiquantitatively or quantitatively. Urine is one of these samples to be processed so. Such processing becomes necessary, when one has to differentiate between colonization of a site and infection of that site. In diagnosis of UTI, it is important to differentiate between colonization of distal urethra and infection of lower/upper urinary tract. Quantitating the organisms level in urine aids this distinction.

What is the importance of differentiating upper UTI from lower UTI?

A.7 The pathogenesis and management of upper and lower UTI is different, so it is important to categorize a UTI case. Various techniques are available to do differentiate these entities.

During her hospitalization, BP dropped to 100/50 mmHg, pulse rose to 150/min and respiratory rate rose to 35/min.

What complication has likely occurred in this case?

A.8 The case is likely to have developed sepsis, stemming from the UTI.

While performing antimicrobial susceptibility of the organism isolated from urine, why are some of the antimicrobial disc used, have higher antimicrobial concentration than the usual used ones?

A.9 Many of the antimicrobials are concentrated in urine, so for their testing, higher antimicrobial concentration discs are to be used in comparison to the routine discs (used for serum correlations).

Genital Tract Infection

'Man continues to be the only 150 pound nonlinear servomechanism that can be wholly mass-produced by unskilled labour'.
— Ashley Montagu

'The flower is the poetry of reproduction. It is an example of eternal seductiveness of life.'
— Jean Giraudoux

The microscopic study of the private parts should not be hindered any way and one should be able to find all hidden microbes, capable of causing havoc. The study of this section, begins with a study of the core aspects of this section; including classification of agents, specimens to be collected, their collection technique and transport. References of clinical based integrated studies are referenced at the end of the section. Hoping the 'proliferating' mechanism remains in our control!

Outline the lesions that occur in the genital tract.

A.1 Lesions on genital sites

• *Infectious* – Venereal – Non-venereal (non sexually transmitted)	• *Non-infectious* – Traumatic NB: AIDS is an STD, but causes no genital lesion

Classify the sexually transmitted diseases (STDs) according to etiological agents and associated syndromes.

A.2 (a) Classification:

Table 16.7.1: Sexually Transmitted Diseases, according to etiological agent and associated syndrome

	Disease/Syndrome		
Pathogens	**Males**	**Both**	**Female**
Viruses • Human herpes, virus 1 & 2 • Hepatitis B virus • Hepatitis A virus • Human Papillomavirus • Human Immunodeficiency virus • HHV-5 (CMV)	• Cancer of penis (some cases)	Primary and recurrent herpes, neonatal herpes • Hepatitis • Condyloma acuminatum • Acquired immunodeficiency syndrome • Congenital infections	• Cervical dysplasia, vulvar cancer
Chlamydiae *Chlamydia trachomatis*	• Urethritis, epididymitis, proctitis	• Lymphogranuloma venereum	• Urethral syndome, bartholinitis, salpingitis and sequelae
Mycoplasmas • *Ureaplasma urealyticum* • *M. hominis*	• Urethritis -	- -	• Postpartum fever, bartholinitis

Contd.

Contd.

Bacteria			
Neisseria gonorrhoeae	Epididymitis, prostatitis, urethral stricture	Urethritis, proctitis, pharygitis, disseminated gonococcal infection	Cervicitis, endometritis, salpingitis, and (infertility, ectopic pregnancy, recurrent salpingitis)
			–
- *Treponema pallidum*	–	- Syphilis	–
- *Haemophilus ducreyi*	–	- Chancroid	–
- *Klebsiella granulomatis*		- Granuloma inguinale (donovanosis)	
- Shigella spp.	–	- Enterocolitis	
- Campylobacter spp.		- Enterocolitis	–
	–		–
- Group B streptorocci	–	- Neonatal sepsis and meningitis	–
Protozoa		- Amebiasis	
- *Trichomonas vaginalis*	- Urethritis, Balanitis	- Giardiasis	- Vaginitis
- *Entamoeba histolytica*			
- *Giardia lamblia*			
Fungal			
- *C. albicans*	-Balanitis	–	- Vulvovaginitis
Ectoparasites			
- *Phthirus pubis*	–	- Pubis lice infection	–
- *Sarcoptes scabiei*	–	- Scabies	–

NB: STDs need not be occurying only on genital site

Classify the STDs according to the anatomical sites infected.

A.2 (b) According to the anatomical site involved

In male
• *Genital Skin*
– Vesicular: Human Herpes virus 1 and 2
– Ulcerative: *T. pallidum*, Human Papilloma virus
Male internal genital organs – testis – Orchitis – *N.gonorrohea, Chlamydia* spp., Mumps and others
– *Prostrate- prostatitis* – Any bacteria that can cause urinary tract infection
– *Epididymis* – *Epididymitis* – *N.gonorroheae, Chlamydia* spp. and others

In Female	
• *Genital skins/introitus*	• *Cervix:*
– Vesicular: Human Herpes virus 1 and 2	– Cervicitis – Human Herpes viruses 1 & 2
– Ulcerative: *T. pallidum*	*N. gonorrohoeae*
Human Papilloma virus	*C. trachomatis*
N. gonorrhoeae	• *Cervix to endometrium and contiguous pelvic structures:*
H. ducreyi	– Pelvic Inflammatory disease (includes endometritis, salpingitis and tuboovarian abscess)-
Klebsiella granulomatis	Mixture of coliforms and/or anaerobes
• *Vagina:*	*C. trachomatis*
– Vaginitis – *Trichomonas vaginalis* (protozoan)	*N. gonorrhoeae*
C. albicans	
Gardnerella vaginalis (Bacterial vaginosis)	
N. gonorrhoeae	

NB: Bubos may form in inguinal region, after certain genital infections.

NB: Some genital lesions, which are non-sexually transmitted; include folliculitis, tuberculosis, tularemia and histoplasmosis

Enumerate the specimens to be collected in males and females for the laboratory diagnosis of STDs.

A.3 (a) Specimens:

In male:	In Female:
(i) Urethral secretion (ii) Prostratic secretion (iii) from lesion on external male genitalia; as chancre on glans penis	(i) Urethral secretion (ii) Cervical lesion (iii) Endometrial tissue and secretions (iv) Cul-de-sac fluid (v) Products of conception (vi) Lesions on external female genitalia; as labia

Describe the collection procedures of samples required in diagnosis of STDs.

A.3 (b) Collection:

In Male

(1) *Urethral secretion/swabs (male)*: A small swab about 2-4 cm is inserted into the urethral lumen and rotated a few times. It is left in the lumen for a few seconds (about 2-4) to facilitate absorption of secretion.

(2) *Prostatic secretions*: The urethral meatus is cleaned with soap and water. A finger is inserted per anus to massage the prostrate. The fluid expressed through urethra is collected on a sterile swab.

NB: Urine can also be collected after prostratic massage (discarding initial urine).

(3) *Lesion on external male genitalia:* The lesion is cleaned with sterile saline and the lesions on surface may be scraped with sterile scalpel blade, if necessary. The base of the lesion should be firmly pressed to express the fluid, before the sterile swab is used to collect the specimen. A similar procedure is utilized to collect such samples, from lesions of female genitalia.

In Females

(1) *Urethral secretion (in female):* The collection should be done at least one hour, after the patient has urinated. The periurethral area is washed with soap and water. The process can be followed by disinfecting with Povidone Iodine. A small swab about 2-4 cm is inserted into the urethra, rotated few times before leaving it in the lumen for a few seconds to facilitate absorption of secretion.

(2) *Cervical secretion:* The cervix is visualized using a speculum. Lubricant use is discouraged, as it may interfere with results of reporting. Any cervical secretions at the cervical os should be removed with a swab (discarded). Using a new swab, the endocervical canal is sampled.

(3) *Cul-de-sac fluid:* The fluid is aspirated

(4) *Endometrial tissue and secretion:* This can be collected while doing dilation and curretage procedure.

Describe the transport considerations of samples required in diagnosis of STDs.

A.3 (c) Transport of specimens:

For these specimens, generally swab can be used to transport the specimen to the laboratory. The transport time should be preferably less than 2 hours and the temperature should be room temperature. However, the swab can be stored at room temperature for < = 24 hours.

For cul-de-sac fluid and endometrial secretions, anaerobic transport medium to be used.

Modified stuart's medium or Amie's charcoal medium at room temperature should be used (for agents of STD, as these are fragile).

For samples likely to contain Chlamydia and Mycoplasma, sucrose buffer with antibiotics (gentamicn, amphotericin and vancomycin) can be used to transport the specimen.

Reference: Cases related to genital tract–syphilis (p 299, 302), P.I.D (p 354) and genital herpes (p 408).

8 Anaerobic Infections

'The large majority of those infectious microbes, that cause us so much illness and pain are anaerobic.....a big word that means that they live and proliferate best in an environment, where there is little or no oxygen'. — **Fd Mc Cabe**

'One man's food, may be poison to another'. — **Anonymous**

Anaerobic infections can occur in almost any site but the diagnosis of these infections is a challenge from sites, where commensal anaerobic organisms flourish; as the oral cavity and the GIT. The fundamental aspects of these infections including diagnosis and management are covered in the following two integrated clinical based studies.

Integrated Clinical Case Based Study 1

A 30 year man, Faizal complained of nausea and pain in right upper abdomen. Examination revealed mild fever. Ultrasound examination revealed a small hepatic abscess. The abscess was aspirated and was foul smelling. It was cultured aerobically and anaerobically, but no growth occurred aerobically. The gram staining of the isolated colonies, which grew anaerobically, revealed gram negative bacilli.

What is the differential diagnosis of this case?

A.1 The differential diagnosis includes liver abscess, biliary disease (including gallstone disease), pancreatitis and acute pyelonephritis.

What are the indications that hint that this case, is likely to have an anaerobic infection?

A.2 (a) The pus is foul smelling, microscopic examination of pus revealed microbes but no growth occured on aerobic incubation.

What are the other general clues that indicate an anaerobic infection?

A.2 (b) The clues/indications of anaerobic infections are:

History:	***Appearance:***
• Dental manipulation	• Foul smelling discharge
• Gastrointestinal surgery/anorectal manipulation	• Gas in tissue
• Road trauma associated with muscle necrosis	• Black discoloration
• Septic abortion	• Necrotic tissue/gangrene
• Animal bite (even human)	• Sulphur granules
Site of lesion:	**Clinically:**
• Proximal to mucosal site	• Sterile aerobic cultures
• Septic thrombophelbitis	• Repeated use of broad spectrum antibiotics (and no response)
	• Infection related to malignancy or other tissue destroying disease
	• Subcutaneous crepitus
	• Deep abscesses (as empyema, appendicular abscess)
	• Infection related to use of aminoglycosides

What are the possible anaerobes that can be incriminated in this case?

A.3 (a) Since the gram staining has revealed gram negative bacilli, the pathogens could be *B. fragilis,* Prevotella, spp., Porphyromonas spp., Fusobacterium spp. or Mobiluncus spp.

Describe Mobiluncus spp.

A.3 (b) Mobiluncus is a gram variable bacillus, curved and motile. *M. mulieris* and *M. curtisii* along with *G. vaginalis* are incriminated in bacterial vaginosis. Presence of clue cells and vaginal pH of more than 4.5 is indicative of bacterial vaginosis.

What are the common diagnostic criteria for Bacteriodes melaninogenicus?

A.3 (c) *B. melaninogenica,* when cultured on blood agar produces black colored colonies, the color is due to a hemin derivative. These cultures, when exposed to U.V. light, produce a characteristic red fluorescence.

Which is the most likely pathogen involved in this case?

A.3 (d) *B. fragilis* is the most likely pathogen in this case, as it is responsible for more than 80% of intraabdominal infections.

What are the microscopic, metabolic and virulence features of B. fragilis?

A.4 The microscopic and metabolic features are depicted in table on pg. 256 and *B. fragilis* has a number of virulence factors, which contributes to their pathogenicity. It has fimbriae, which act as adhesins and a capsule; which is antiphagocytic to PMNs.

How do you identify B. fragilis?

A.5 *B. fragilis* can be cultivated on standard media anaerobically. The identity of the isolate is confirmed using various parameters; including gas liquid chromatography. The isolate is susceptible to metronidazole but not to penicillin.

Which antimicrobials would be effective in this case?

A.6 (a) Metronidazole/Ampicillin-sulbactam can be given orally/intravenously (parenterally). Penicillin and clindamycin are usually effective against anaerobes excepting Bacteriodes spp., where resistance to these agents has been reported.

Why is antimicrobial susceptibility testing routinely not put up for anaerobic isolates?

A.6 (b) Resistance of anaerobes to antimicrobial agents is not a major issue. Also, the antimicrobial tests for anaerobes require standardization and can be performed only in reference laboratories.

Mention a category of antimicrobials ineffective in anaerobes?

A.6 (c) Aminoglycosides are usaully ineffective.

Integrated Clinical Case Based Study 2

Shahid, a forty year man was diagnosed of having pancreatic abscess. The pus is collected by CT guided aspiration. Microscopic examination of the pus revealed gram positive cocci and gram negative bacilli. No growth occurred, when cultured on standard media incubated aerobically.

Give reasons for no growth occuring from the specimen, despite microscopic evidence of organisms.

A.1 (a) One of the reasons could be that the case was receiving antimicrobials, which could have resulted in lysis of bacteria; resulting in no growth. Ideally, all specimens should be collected before administration of antimicrobials. Secondly, the specimen was cultured only aerobically and not anaerobically, so the possible anaerobic pathogens in the specimen could not he cultivated.

Why do anaerobic organisms die on exposure to oxygen?

A.1 (b) The anaerobes lack some enzymes; as catalase, peroxidise, and superoxide dismutase, which are normally present in aerobes. Due to this, certain metabolites; as hydrogen peroxide and others, which can be toxic to these organism, do not get inactivated.

How do you explain anaerobes flourishing in human body (which is well oxygenated)?

A.1 (c) First of all, not all anaerobes are obligate anaerobes. Secondly, there are oxygen deficit sites in the body; as sebaceous glands (skin), gingival crevices (gum) and lumen of gut and urogenital tract, where anaerobes proliferate.

Is the presence of two types of organisms from a clinical specimen a usual finding? Explain the possibilities of the presence of such a combination.

A.2 (a) Mostly a single organism is involved in causing an infective lesion, however in anaerobic infections, involvement of polymicrobial flora is common. In abdominal pathology, two or more organisms are often involved in the pathogenicity. A mixture of aerobic and anaerobic organisms causing abdominal pathology is often seen. It is also possible that one of the two isolated organisms may be a commensal or a contaminant.

What are some of the characteristics of anaerobic infections?

A.2 (b) Firstly; the anaerobic infections are frequently polymicrobial. Secondly; the anaerobes are mostly derived from patients own normal flora excepting some environmental clostridia. Thirdly; patient to case transfer of infection is rare except in *Clostridium difficile* infections.

Describe the pathogenesis of anaerobic infections.

A.2 (c) The determinants of pathogenicity of anaerobic infections is obscure. These are part of the normal flora of man. So the isolation of anaerobe from a clinical sample may not incriminate it to be a pathogen. These organisms can survive and proliferate in the body in a number of sites. In fact these organisms outnumber the aerobic organisms in the gut, by a ratio of thousand to one.

These organisms are likely to act as opportunistic pathogens, when body resistance is lowered; especially at sites outside their normal habitat. The most important factor favouring multiplication of anaerobes is lowering of Eh (oxidation potential). This gets lowered, when there is decreased blood supply to tissue often associated with necrotic tissue. Once the conditions become optimal for the anaerobes, different virulent toxins and enzymes; as proteases get expressed which contribute to their pathogenicity.

Mention the common methods used to obtain an anaerobic environment, to culture anaerobic bacteria.

A.3 (a) Conventionally the *McIntosh and Filde's* anaerobic jar (Fig. 1.6.1a,b; p. 46) is used, in which the principle of displacement and combustion of oxygen is utilized, using hydrogen stored in large cylinders. The combination of oxygen with hydrogen is catalyzed by palladium (alumina pellets coated with palladium). A successful creation of anaerobic reaction is denoted by creation of vacuum (noted on meter with a reading of -15 mm Hg). The environment is supplemented with addition of 10% CO_2. The cultures are incubated at 37°C for 24-48 hours. The system requires expertise but the distinct advantage is that precise environment in the jars, can be made by varying the concentration of gases.

In small labs, anaerobic conditions can be provided in the jars, using commercial 'Gas Pak' kits. The pack kit consists of sodium borohydride, cobalt chloride (catalyst), sodium bicarbonate and citric acid. On addition of water to this pack, hydrogen gas is released, which reacts with oxygen in the jar. The special jar is made of polycarbonate. The system is expensive but the advantage is that this system, can be used in a small laboratory; where gas cylinders and pumps are not available. However the disadvantage of the system is that the concentration of gases cannot be altered. Large reference labs have anaerobic cabinets, in which anaerobic conditions are provided and manipulations can occur from outside in the system.

What are the indicators that can be used during anaerobe culture, that indicate that anaerobiosis was maintained during the incubation period?

A.3 (b) These include:

(i) *Chemical:* It is often methylene blue, which is colorless in reduced conditions and blue in oxidized condition.

(ii) *Physical:* In a system, where as Mc Intosh and Filde's apparatus is used, development of vacuum after introduction of gases is indicative of development of anaerobic condition.

(iii) *Biological:* If growth occurs in the plate having an aerobic organism, it indicates absence of anaerobic condition in the system. A known anaerobe is also put in the system. If it grows, it indicates the presence of anaerobic conditions in the system.

Which samples are unsuitable for anaerobic culture and why?

A.3 (c) Samples; as nasotracheal aspirate, sputum, faeces and urine are unsatisfactory for anaerobic culture, as the anaerobes isolated from these sites are likely to represent normal anaerobic flora.

Enumerate anaerobes constituting normal flora of man.

A.3 (d) Normal anaerobic flora of man

Anaerobe	Skin	Mouth & nasopharynx	Intestine	Vagina
Gram positive cocci		++	++	++
Gram negative cocci		++	+	++
Bifidobacterium spp.		+	++	+
Propionibacterium spp.	++			
Actinomyces spp.		+		
Clostridium spp.			++	
Bacteriodes fragilis			++	
P.melaninogenica		++	+	++
Fusobacterium spp.		++	+	
Spirochaetes		+		

How can pus be transported to laboratory for anaerobic culture with minimal exposure to oxygen?

A.4 (a) Pus can be transported in anaerobic transport media. These include PRAS (pre-reduced anaerobic sterilized) transport medium, a commercial system or Robertson cooked meat medium. If no special media is available, aspirated pus can be transported in syringe with needle plugged in a cork.

What precautions need to be taken (generally), when taking sample for anaerobic culture?

A.4 (b) Normal resident flora is to be avoided during sample collection.

Enumerate the common anaerobic gram positive cocci of medical importance.

A.5 (a) The commonly encountered are Peptococcus spp., and Peptostreptococcus spp.. The uncommon ones are Coprococcus spp., Ruminococcus spp. and Sarcinia spp.

Classify non sporing anaerobes of medical importance.

A.5 (b) Classification of nonsporing anaerobes

Cocci	
Gram positive cocci	Peptococcus spp., Peptostreptococcus spp.
Gram negative cocci	Veilonella spp., Acidaminococcus spp., Megasphaera spp.
Bacilli	
Gram positive bacilli	Eubacterium spp., Lactobacillus spp., Bifidobacterium spp., Propionibacterium spp., Mobiluncus spp., Actinomyces spp.
Gram negative bacilli	Bacteriodes spp., Prevotella spp., Porphyromonas spp., Fusobacterium spp., Lepotricha spp.
Spirochaetes	Treponema spp.

Enumerate common anaerobic infections.

A.5 (c)

Table 16.8.1: Common anaerobic infections

Infection site and type	**Implicated anaerobes**
Central nervous system	
Brain abscess	Peptostreptococcus spp., *B. fragilis*
ENT	
Chronic sinusitis,Otitis media, Mastoiditis,	Fusobacterium spp.
Oral cavity and allied structures	
Ulcerative gingivitis, Dental abscess, Jaw abscess	Fusobacterium spp., Lepotrichia spp, Actinomyces spp & others
Respiratory system	
Bronchiectasis, Aspiration pneumonia, Lung abscess, Empyema	Anaerobic cocci, Fusobacterum spp., *P. melaninogenica*
Abdominal system	
Hepatic abscess, Ischiorectal abscess, appendicitis, Peritonitis	*B. fragilis*, Anaerobic cocci
Female genital system	
Tubo-ovarian abscess, Bartholin abscess, Septic abortion, Puerperal sepsis	*Prevotella melaninogenica* , Anaerobic cocci, *B. fragilis*, *C. perfringens*
Skin and underlying structures	
Sebaceous cyst (infected), Cellulitis, Breast ulcer, Gangrene	Peptostreptococcus spp., Peptococcus spp, *B. fragilis*, *Prevotella melaninogenica*

Is the administration of antimicrobial sufficient to resolve the infection in this case?

A.6 No, an abscess can not resolve without surgical intervention, as incision and drainage. Antimicrobials play a part of 'sterilization' of the lesion.

Reference is placed here of other clinical case based studies that focus on anaerobic diseases pgs. 240-249, chapter 11-16 of Section 5.

9 Assessment/Examination Questions

Chapter 1

1. Explain giving an example; the importance of choosing a right sample, in making a correct diagnosis. A3., p. 559
2. Explain giving an example, the importance of the concept of sensitivity and specificity of a test, in the interpretation of the test. A4., p. 559-560
3. Discuss the aspects to be considered in transporting samples, when a viral diagnosis is suspected. A6., p. 560
4. Discuss the aspects to be considered in transporting samples, when a fungal diagnosis is suspected. A 7., p. 560
5. Describe the sample collection techniques, when fungal diagnosis is suspected. Discuss the aspects to be considered in sample collection A 7., p. 560

Chapter 2

1. Enumerate the agents causing pyogenic meningitis, aseptic meningitis and chronic meningitis. Discuss the laboratory diagnosis of acute pyogenic meningitis. A2., p. 561, pg., 205
2. Enumerate the common agents causing meningitis, according to age of the case. A 3., p. 562
3. Enumerate important microbes causing meningitis that would get lysed, if the CSF sample was by mistake kept in the refrigerator by the technologist/nursing personnel. A2., p. 561
4. What technique can give a rapid bed side diagnosis (in few minutes) of the common etiological agents of meningitis in the CSF. A 5a., p. 567
5. Describe aseptic meningitis and tuberculous meningitis. A 3., p. 562

Chapter 3

1. Define the terms Bacteremia, fungemia, septicaemia, sepsis, severe sepsis and septic shock. A1., p. 563
2. Define Systemic inflammatory response syndrome and mention its importance. A1, p. 563
3. Define Infective endocarditis (I.E.). Enumerate the common agents causing Infective endocarditis. Tabulate the differences between acute and subacute endocarditis (SABE). A 3a,b,., p. 564
4. Describe the blood collection procedure utilized in a case of suspected I.E. Discuss the laboratory diagnosis of I.E. emphasizing the techniques utilized including the blood culture. Outline the preventive strategies in I.E. A 3c., p. 564-565, A3e., p. 566.
5. Enumerate the etiological agents causing septicaemia. Describe the laboratory diagnosis with a special emphasis on the blood culture technique (principles). A4., p. 566, A 5 a,b., p. 567, 568

Chapter 4

1. Define the terms sore throat, pharyngitis and pneumonia. Ala., p . 570
2. Enumerate the etiological agents that cause sore throat. How is throat swab and nasopharyngeal swab collected and transported to the laboratory? What is the indication of collecting the nasopharyngeal swab? A 1b., p. 571; A3a, p. 571, A4., p. 572
3. Describe the laboratory diagnosis of sore throat (upper respiratory infection). Case 1., p. 572 and p. 571
4. Enumerate the etiological agents that cause acute pneumonia. Mention two key specimens to be collected, their procedure of collection and transport to the laboratory. Comment upon the acceptability criteria of sputum. A 5a,b., p. 572, A2b., p. 571; A3b., p. 571
5. Describe the laboratory diagnosis of acute pneumonia with special reference to pneumococcal pneumonia. Case 2., p. 573 + Linkages (p. 196)

Chapter 5

1. Enumerate the causes of acute gastroenteritis (diarrohea). How do you proceed to make the diagnosis in the laboratory. A 3a-c., p. 574-575, A4a,b., p. 576 and linkages section 6
2. Enumerate causes of dysentery. Describe the laboratory diagnosis of this entity with special reference to bacillary dysentery (Shigellosis)? A3c., p. 576 and pg. 264
3. Name the various agents that cause food poisoning. Describe the laboratory diagnosis of bacillary dysentry with special reference to Salmonella gastroenteritis. A 3b., p. 575, pg. 271
4. Describe Viral diarroheas, Traveller's diarrhea and Food–borne botulism. A 3a., p. 575, A1., p. 574, pg. 261, 271, 402

Chapter 6

1. Classify Urinary tract infections (UTI) based on the anatomical site of involvement. A 1, A2., p. 577
2. Enumerate the samples required for diagnosing of lower UTI. Mention the procedure of their collection. How is lower UTI differentiated from upper UTI and mention the importance of differentiating the two entities. A 3., p. 577-578
3. Enumerate the common etiological agents incriminated in lower UTI. A2., p. 577
4. Discuss the importance of proper urine collection in diagnosis of UTI. Explain the importance in processing the urine sample within a few hours and culturing the sample quantitatively/semiquantitatively. A3., p. 578, A4., p. 579, A 5a., p. 579 A6., p. 580
5. Describe the laboratory diagnosis of UTI. Case 1-3., p. 578-580

Chapter 7

1. Classify sexually transmitted diseases according to (a) etiological agent and associated syndrome and (b) according to anatomical site of involvement. A 2a,b., p. 581-582
2. Enumerate the samples to be taken in the male and female genital tract infections and describe the technique of the collection. A 3a,b., p. 582-583
3. Describe LGV, NGU, Donovanosis and Vulvovaginal candidiasis. p. 354, 208, 319, 321, 324, 545

Chapter 8

1. Enumerate anaerobes constituting normal flora of man. A 3d., p. 586
2. Classify bacteria causing anaerobic infections with special reference to non sporing anaerobes. A 5b., p. 587
3. Enumerate common anaerobic infections due to them. A5c., p. 581
4. What are the indications/clues that a clinical case might be having an anaerobic infection. A 2a,b., p. 584
5. Enumerate some characteristics of anaerobic infections. Describe pathogenesis of anaerobic infections. A 2b,c., p. 586
6. Describe the microscopic, metabolic, virulence factors and laboratory diagnosis of *Bacteriodes fragilis*. A4, 5., p. 585, A 5bc., p. 587
7. Describe (a) Mobiluncus spp. (b) *Prevotella melaninogenica* (c) Anaerobic cocci (d) Propionibacterium spp. A3b-A6, p. 585; A5, pg. 587
8. (a) Why are some samples unsuitable for anaerobic culture? Explain. A 3c., p. 586
   (b) What precautions need to be taken (generally), when taking sample for anaerobic culture? A 4b., p. 587
   (c) Mention the common methods used to obtain an anaerobic environment to culture anaerobic bacteria. What indicators during culture, ensure that anaerobiosis was maintained? A 3a,b., p. 586
9. Discuss the laboratory diagnosis of infections caused by non sporing anaerobes. Case 1 and 2., p. 584-587
10. Describe antimicrobial treatment for anaerobic infections. A 6a, 6c., p. 585

Section XVII: Applied Microbiology

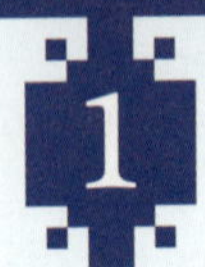

1 Normal Human Flora

– **We are inhabited by as many as ten thousand bacterial species; these cells outnumber those which we consider our own by ten to one, and weigh, all told, about three pounds the same as our brain. Together, they are referred to as our microbiome—and they play such a crucial role in our lives that scientists have begun to reconsider, what it means to be human.**

— Michael Specter

– **'Bacteria lives in unbelievable mixtures of hundreds or thousands of species. Like on your teeth there are 600 species of bacteria every morning. This trend also continues for other systems; as gut and the respiratory system'.**

— Bonnie Bassier

Student cartoon four
—**Priya Singh**

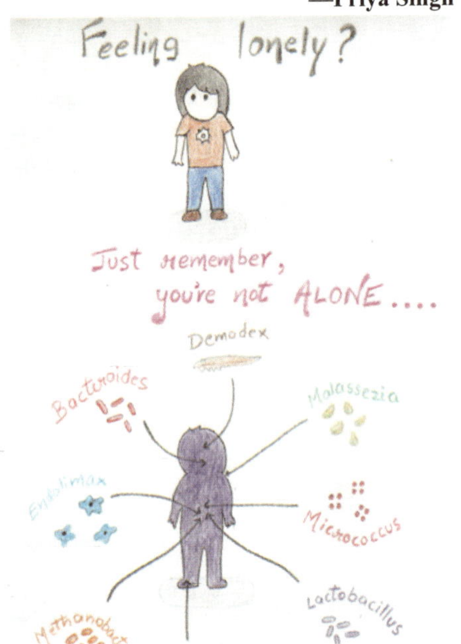

Let's study this aspect

When does man acquire the normal flora*?

A.1 The healthy fetus 'in utero' is free from microorganisms, until the placental separation occurs.

So the human get exposed, at birth to microorganisms. Within a few hours after birth, the oral and the nasopharyngeal flora develops. Within a few days, the flora in the intestine develops.

*In latin, refers to goddess of flowers, from "flos' flower.

What is the source of the normal human flora?

A.2 Initially it depends on the infants contact. These include the flora of the mother's genital tract (during delivery of the foetus, it has to pass through it, to outside), the skin and the respiratory flora of the medical personnel; including nurses and relatives, who handle the baby and to the organisms present in the environment.

Do the characteristics of the normal flora change in the infant?

A.3 Yes, in the first few days of life, the infant usually acquire, whatever organisms it gets exposed to it. This occurs, as there are no organism competitors. Such flora remains for a short while and is called *transient flora*. However, as the infant grows, its exposure to person and different environment increases. Gradually a flora, gets to become (sort of) fixed at different sites of the body. This is the flora, which is best adapted at a particular site and is called the *resident flora*.

Are there sites in body, which are devoid of normal microbial flora?

A.4 The key body fluids, blood (occasional physiological low-level bacteremia), cerebrospinal fluid, urine (before coming in contact with terminal urethra), pleural fluid, pericardial fluid, internal organs and body systems (except GIT) are sterile. This information is important because any organisms isolated from sample of these sites collected aseptically, indicate infection.

Which body system has the highest concentration and maximum variety of microorganisms? Mention their distribution.

A.5 Gastrointestinal tract. Oesophagus has transient flora of oral cavity. Stomach has few organisms because of presence of hydrochloric acid and enzymes. Small intestine has scanty organisms, except for terminal ileum; where the flora resembles that of colon, which has the highest concentration

Name a clinical condition that arises, as a result of undeveloped normal flora.

A.6 Infants usually have incomplete (undeveloped) colonic flora. If they consume articles; as honey, which have spores of *C. botulinum*, these can germinate in the colon, due to lack of competition from other flora and cause botulinum toxin production, which can present as infant botulism (in extreme case; paralysis and death). In adults, the spores of *C.botulinum* may not be able to germinate.

What are the factors that determine the nature of normal flora? Mention the importance to study them.

A.7 Numerous variables; as nutrient availability, pH, oxidation-reduction potential, substances; as bile, lysozyme; can affect the local physiologic and ecologic conditions, which may determine the nature of the flora. The exact role of these factors is difficult to determine; as the flora is complex, including the interaction between the microbial populations and the human body.

We have to live with the normal flora, but we should know how to manipulate the conditions to bring back the optimal flora composition, when it deviates (shifts). Also ideally in future, we should be able to manipulate the flora in dangerous conditions to desirable ones; for instance in a neonatal unit, where there is an outbreak of methicillin resistant *S.aureus* (MRSA), we should be able to colonize the patients with safer 'flora' microorganisms.

How best can the relationship of the microbes of the normal human flora and the human body be described as?

A.8 It can be best described as symbiotic (most of the times). The microbes benefit by getting a niche for existence, nutrients for their existence and site to throw waste. The man gets a lot of benefits, the chief being that the flora prevents the pathogens, from colonizing the region by providing competition.

What are the key benefits, man gets from normal human flora?

A.9 (i) Protection from pathogens.

(ii) The microbes appear to stimulate the reticuloendothelial system and the immune system of man, as a result of which the immune system gets well developed and functional. Endotoxins released by the organisms, can initiate the alternate complement pathway. This inference also follows from the fact that *gnotobiotic animal* (germ free animals), those that are delivered (born) and raised (grown) under completely aseptic conditions, have poorly developed R.E. system and immune system. Such animals, when shifted to normal environment from sterile environment, succumb (die) soon to the infection.

(iii) Synthesis of vitamin B group and vitamin K (though the amounts, finally made available to the body except; for vitamin K, mayn't be significant)

(iv) Colonic fermentation of polysaccharides; as acetate, propionate and butyrate, which can be used as sources of carbon and energy. This amount mayn't be significant, with the current diet, being rich in meat and refined food but deficient in plant fiber.

(v) Bacteriocins produced by some organisms, benefit the host by inhibiting some pathogens.

What are the conditions, in which the typical microflora of a region changes (shifts) its composition? Mention the consequence of such changes?

A-10a(i) In vaginal tract, when the normal flora changes from a predominantly gram positive (having lactobacilli) to a predominantly gram negative one; including *Gardnerella vaginalis.*

A disease develops called *bacterial vaginosis*, characterized by a discharge with fishy odor.

(ii) Patients taking certain antibiotics; especially broad spectrum one; as ampicillin, cephalosporins and fluoroquinol -ones; can have tremendous increase of an organism called *Clostridium difficile,* which is normally present in low numbers. This can cause a fatal condition called *pseudomembraneous colitis*.

(iii) *Candida albicans,* which is a minor component of the small intestine, can proliferate to large number and cause diarrhoea, in some patients on antimicrobials.

(iv) In some patients, the flora of the gums due to poor hygiene changes; from one of being predominantly gram positive to being, predominantly; gram negative. This induces mucosal inflammation which can lead to *tooth loss*.

What are the condition, in which breech of the human defense, make the normal flora, organisms invade the human body and cause disease?

A.10b (i) Actinomyces can invade the oral cavity during tooth extraction and cause cervicofacial actinomycosis.

(ii) *Streptococcus 'viridans'* can invade the blood during dental manipulation and cause bacterial endocarditis.

(iii) During gastrointestinal surgery; as of colon, the anaerobes (normal) can invade the blood and present as bacteraemia and initiate septicaemia.

(iv) Viral infection of the respiratory system can make *S.pneumoniae* [commensal in some] invade the lung and cause pneumococcal pneumonia.

(v) *S. mutans* in condition of poor hygiene can cause dental caries

(vi) Coagulase negative staphylococci can colonize the i/v catheter, which can later on act as source of bacteremia

What are the key detrimental effects the human flora (microbiome), can have on the host?

A.10c(i) If the clinical samples taken for diagnosis of infected cases are not collected properly and get contaminated with normal flora, a false positive diagnosis or a wrong diagnosis could be given, e.g., blood sample from a suspected septicaemia taken, if gets contaminated with coagulase negative staphylococci of skin (proper disinfection not performed), pseudobacteremia diagnosis would occur, e.g., sputum sample of suspected bacterial pneumonia get contaminated with *S. pneumoniae* of pharyngeal flora, would give false diagnosis of bacterial pneumonia.

(ii) If the individual becomes immunocompromised due to any cause; for instance as malignancy or AIDS, the normal human flora can become pathogenic

e.g., *Candida albicans* in AIDS can cause severe oral lesions and candidemia.

e.g., premature babies have to kept in sterile incubators, as they cannot fight against the infections by normal flora.

e.g., cases to undergo bone marrow transplantation (have their immune system suppressed because of irradiation), have to be given sterilized foods, besides other precautions.

(iii) Organisms outside their normal habitat, can act as pathogens.

e.g., faecal *E.coli* (in perineal area acts as normal flora) can ascend the urethra and cause lower and upper urinary tract infection.

e.g., organisms of perineal area and vaginal area can ascend the genital tract of the female, after delivery (birth) or abortion and present as *endometritis* or *salpingitis*.

(iv) Can act as source of genetic material, which may be transferred to pathogens, e.g., R-plasmid (carrying resistance to antibiotics and other agents).

(v) Penicillinase producing organisms can interfere with antimicrobial therapy.

(vi) In patients with anatomical defects; as multiple blind-ended diverticula, flora of the small intestine (normally has scanty growth), becomes heavily colonized with anaerobes, which deconjugate bile salts (required for absorption of fat and fat soluble vitamins), resulting in malabsorption.

(vii) Inflammatory bowel disease, chronic wound infection and obesity have also been associated with alteration of human mcrobome.

Table 17.1.1: Key flora at various sites

• **Skin** (including distal urethra and anterior nares (proximal), as flora is derived from neighbouring skin)	• **Small intestine**
– *S. epidermidis*	– Scanty (except for terminal ileum)
– *Propionibacterium acnes*	Consisting of
– Other CONS	o Lactobacilli spp.
– Corynebacterium sps	o Bacteriodes spp.
– 'Viridans' streptococci	o Enterobacteriaceae
– *Malassezia furfur*	**Small intestne** has low microbial load (10^3 organisms per ml), higher levels of 10^5–10^7 organism per ml, may indicate abnormality of the digestive system; as achlorhydria or malabsorption syndrome.
• **Conjunctiva**	• **Large intestine**
– *Corynebacterium xerosis*, *S.epidermidis*, Moraxella spp, Non haemolytic streptococci	During breast feeding
• **Mouth**	– Bifidobacterium (predominantly)
'Viridans' streptococci	– Lactobacilli

Contd.

Contd.

– *S. epidermidis*	Other periods
– 'Viridans' streptococci	Predominantly anaerobes as
– Neisseria spp.	– Bacteriodes spp.
– Anaerobes	– Peptostreptococci
– *C. albicans* (occasionally)	– Lactobacillus spp.
• **Gums**	– Clostridium spp.
– Bacteriodes spp.	– Enterobacteriacae (minor constitutent)
– Fusobacterium spp.	• **Vagina**
– Actinomyces spp.	Prepuberal and postmenopausal
– Other anaerobes	– Members of the perineal skin regions (gets a component of large intestine)
– *Trichomonas tenax*	Postpubertal (before menopause)
• **Throat**	– Lactobacillus spp.
– Oral organisms	– Bifidobacterium spp.
– Transient carriage of *S. pyogenes*, *S. pneumoniae*	– Streptococcus spp.
– *N. meningitidis*	– Yeasts as *C. albicans*
– Haemophilus spp.	
• **Oesphagus**	
– Transient oral flora	
• **Stomach**	
– Scanty and variable flora of food and upper respiratory tract	
– *H. pylori* [microbe can became opportunistic pathogen]	

Body fluids as blood, CSF, urine (when formed), peritoneal, pleural, pericardial and internal organs as uterus, bladder, sinuses, middle ear and body systems (except GIT) are sterile.

Mention the key normal human flora at various sites.

A.11 The key flora on important sites is depicted in table 17.1.1.

Skin: On the surface, skin consists essentially of the dead epithelial cells, but deeper it has multiple layers of cells containing ducts of hair follicles, sebaceous and sweat glands, which add complexity to the environment. Their activity is responsible for the variability in the skin flora. Generally skin has a dry surface and is slightly acidic, these discourage the growth of many pathogenic bacteria. The flora is most abundant on moist areas of the skin; such as axillae, perineal and space between toes. *S. epidermidis* and Propionibacterium spp. are prevalent all over the skin. *P. acne* is an obligate anaerobe (however some strains are aerotolerant) present especially in the deeper layers of the skin, it has been implicated in acne. Hence the anti-acne cream contain antimicrobials.

One of the problems these days is the biofilm formation on i/v catheters and other catheters by *S. epidermidis*. These can have dangerous consequences, as their prolonged usage can give rise to localized and systemic infection. To counter this, some manufacturers are making antimicrobial coated catheters but surprisingly the organisms are developing resistance to these. Two fungi, namely Malssezia and Candida can be part of the flora in some individuals. The flora at sites, as anterior nares and distal urethra, is derived from neighouring skin.

Conjunctiva: Normally the conjunctiva culture gets a scanty growth of *S.epidermidis* and Corynebacterium spp. (non-pathogenic). The low count is because of the repeated flushing by tears with its high lysozyme (contains antimicrobial enzyme) content. Sometimes other pathogens; as *S. aureus* or *S pneumoniae* colonize this site, in which case they need to be treated, before the case has to undergo an eye surgical operation.

Oral cavity: Most of the organisms are facultative and strict anaerobes. The concentration of organisms in it is very high, for instance; saliva has a mixed flora of about 10^8 organisms per millilitre. This is one of the reasons, why human bites (oral) may cause mixed severe infection with severe morbidity and is difficult to treat.

Nose: The proximal part of nose has essentially the same organisms; as found in the adjoining skin. However, one organism that is carried in about one third of the human population *is S.aureus*. This is critical, as *S.aureus* from nose may colonize skin of other or transfer to food and cause food poisoning. Carriage of *S.aureus* (especially drug resistant;

MRSA) is critical in the medical personnel, as it could result in nosocomial infections of the patients especially with compromised functions. Treatment of the nasal carriers of *S.aureus* (drug resistant) in medical fraternity is critical.

Throat: The key organisms found in it are depicted in table 17.1.1. One concern here is of the transient carriage of pathogens; as *S.pneumoniae* or *N.meningitidis,* which can at times, when host's resistance is low, invade the body and cause localized and fatal systemic infections.

GIT: Many individuals carry asymptomatically *H. pylori* in their stomach, the carriage rate being higher in the developing countries than in the developed world. It is debatable whether to put this organism into the normal flora category, through many carry this organism asymptomatically.

The colon carries the most prolific flora in the body with the concentration exceeding 10^{10} organism/per gram of contents. More than 90% of the organisms are anaerobes including *C.perfringens,* which may occasionally contaminate the OT and cause havoc.

Vagina: The flora of it varies with age; as glycogen gets deposited in vaginal epithelial cells under influence of oestrogen hormones, gets metabolised to lactic acid by lactobacilli. The lowered vaginal pH of 4-5 inhibits many other bacteria.

Mention about the human microbiome project?

A.12 It was a five year project launched in 2007, to analyze the genetic composition of microbial population of healthy adults. It identified the microbes by sequencing the 16S ribosomal genes. Gene content of all organisms was found by sequencing the whole genome.

What are Probiotics?

A.13 These are microbes that can improve the functioning of the normal flora. They are usually gram positive bacteria and include Lactobacillus spp., Bifidobacterium spp. and yeast; *Saccharomyces boulardi*.

2 Vehicles and Vector (Including Zoonoses and Bacteriological Examination of Water)

– **'When there is an influenza threat, drop everything and focus on risks from influenza pandemics. When SARS spreads, focus on unknown respiratory diseases. This approach helps to quell public concern, but it's a hugely inefficient way to deal with future risks'.**

— Nathan Wolffe

Let's study the vehicle and vector aspects in this context with four clinical based integrated studies

Integrated Clinical Case Base Study 1

A sample of water *from a newly installed home water purification system (Aquaguard)* is to be tested for its quality. Many water purification systems are available in the market and each one claims to be the best.

Why it is important to test the quality of water to be consumed?

A.1 (a) Effective tests are necessary to evaluate the effectiveness of drinking water treatment procedures carried out by domestic houses and municipal bodies in a city. These tests are of immense public health importance, as the inability to detect the ineffectiveness of the treatment procedures, can lead to serious disease outbreaks.

Tabulate the bacterial flora of water.

A.1 (b) See table 17.2.1

Table 17.2.1: Bacterial Flora of Water

In natural water	Micrococcus spp., Serratia spp., Fusobacterium spp., Pseudomonas spp., Alcaligenes spp., Acinetobacter spp., Chromobacterium spp.
In water with washed soil	*Enterobacter aerogenes, E. cloacae, B. subtilis, B. megaterium, B. mycoides*
In *sewage water-intestinal bacteria	- *E. coli, Enterococcus faecalis, C. perfringens, S. Typhi, V. cholerae* - *Proteus spp., Clostridium spp., Nocardia spp.*

*Other bacteria are sometimes present as result of decomposing organic matter activity

What are the diseases transmitted by water?

A.2

Table 17.2.2: Diseases spread by water

Bacterial	**Helminthic**	**Viral**
• Cholera	• Roundworm infestation	• Hepatitis A (viral hepatitis)
• Enteric fever	• Threadworm infestation	• Hepatitis E (viral hepatitis)
• Shigellosis (dysentery)	• Whipworm infestation	• Rotavirus diarrhoea
• Diarrhoea (gastroenteritis) due to:	• Hydatid disease	• Poliomyelitis
E. coli	• *Guineaworm disease	**Protozoal**
Yersinia enterocolitica	• Fish tapeworm infestation	• Amoebiasis
Campylobacter fetus	• Schistosomiasis^	• Giardiasis
• Legionellosis • Leptospirosis (Weil's disease) • Tularemia		*due to aquatic Cyclops ^due to snail

NB: In a hospital setting, contaminated water may enter the respiratory system (as during suction) and result in pneumonia.

The cases (1-4) have been contributed by Dr. Ravleen K. Bakshi (MD-Community Medicine)

What is the general principle of microbiological tests, to test the infectious agents that may be present in water?

A.3 Microbiological examination offers the most sensitive test for detection of recent and potentially dangerous faecal pollution. The demonstration of pathogenic bacteria; as Shigella species in a water sample would constitute a direct proof of water impurity but such tests are not technically feasible; as these tests have to rely on very small number of pathogenic bacteria. Instead; we rely on demonstrating test organisms; as *E.coli* (coliforms) in water, as an evidence of water contamination. This organism is chosen, as it is present in large numbers in the intestine and is easily cultivable. The presence of this organism in water, indicates faecal contamination of water from human or animal sources.

The coliform group of lactose-fermenting gram-negative bacilli usually demonstrated in this test, can be categorized into two groups. The *typical* (or faecal) group has organisms as *E.coli*; which are commensals of the intestine. The *atypical* group (e.g., Klebsiella spp.) has organisms, derived from soil and other inanimate sources. The presence of *E.coli* in water, usually indicates recent faecal contamination, as these perish in water in few day or weeks, after exiting the animal intestine.

The tests usually performed in the bacteriological examination of water include (i) presumptive coliform count (ii) differential coliform test and (iii) plate count (enumeration of bacteria). In the *presumptive coliform count test*, varying quantities of water an inoculated to bile lactose peptone water tubes with an indicator for acidity. The presence of acidity and gas in the tubes indicate growth of coliform bacilli. This test is so named, as it is based on the *presumption* that each tube showing fermentation is due to coliforms.

The *differential coliform test* is done to ascertain that the coliform bacilli detected in the presumtive test is *E.coli*. This test is based on the ability of the *E.coli* to produce gas in the medium at 44°C and the inability of the atypical coliform bacilli to do so.

In the *plate count*, the water sample is usually subcultured onto media at 22°C and 37°C to isolate the coliform organisms. Organisms growing best at 22°C indicate saprophytes of water and soil; whereas those growing best at 37°C are mainly of parasitic nature.

What is the general requirement to perform microbiological examination of water?

A.4 Single strength MacConkey fluid medium, Double strength MacConkey fluid medium,

Durham's tubes, Pipettes (sterile), Incubator, McCrady's table (for most probable number).

Describe the procedure of a commonly used test for testing the quality for water?

A.5 With sterile graduated pipettes add, (i) 50 ml quantity water (to be tested) to 50ml double strength medium, (ii) five 10 ml water quantities each to five 10 ml strength solutions, (iii) five 1 ml quantities each to 5ml single strength solutions.

- Incubate at 37°C for 48 hrs.
- Examine for acid production and gas production in durham's tube. Record your findings (for presumptive coliform count test). Use the McCrady's table for interpretation.
- If any of the tubes above show positive reaction, subculture the tubes to fresh single strength MacConkey medium and incubate at 44°C for 24 hrs (if yield gas, taken as confirmation for *E.coli*).

Outline a classification system commonly used to grade the water.

A.6 One classification of drinking water according to bacteriological tests is depicted in the table 17.2.3.

Table 17.2.3: Gradation of water

Class	Grade	Presumptive count (per 100 ml)	E.coli count (per 100 ml)
I	Excellent	0	0
II	Satisfactory	1-3	0
III	Suspicious	4-10	0
IV	Unsatisfactory	>10	0, 1 or more

Integrated Clinical Case Based Study 2 (Bacteriology of Air)

A newly constructed neurosurgery OT in Fortis hospital, New Delhi is to be tested for its air quality, before it can be operationalized.

What does the quality of air in the Operation theater complex depend on?

A.1 The quality of air in an operation theatre complex is of utmost importance. The bacterial content of it depends on various factors; as human movement, temperature, humidity, surrounding environment and other conditions. Microorganisms in the air consist essentially of aerobic spore bearer bacilli, Achromobacter spp., Sarcinia spp. and Micrococcus spp.; besides molds.

What test is commonly performed to assess the quality of OT air?

A.2 The *slit sampler method* can be performed, which overcomes the limitations of the *settle plate method.* It sucks in air from the environment at a particular rate and causes the suspended particles to impinge on the surface of the agar plate, which on incubation forms colonies. These colonies can be counted.

Describe the procedure of the slit sampler method?

A.3 The lid of the blood agar plate is removed. One cubic foot volume of the OT air is directed onto it, through a slit 0.25 mm wide. The plate is rotated mechanically, so as to allow the organisms to distribute out evenly on the medium. The plate is incubated at 37°C for 48 hrs. The number of colonies are counted and bacterial count per cubic feet of air is estimated.

What is the recommended level for air quality in the OTs?

A.4 The acceptable microorganisms count in a routine surgical OT is 10 per cubic feet and in a neurosurgical OT is 1 per cubic feet of air.

What is the limitation of the Settle plate method?

A.5 This method is simple but measures only the rate of deposition of large particles from air and not the total number of large and small bacteria carrying particles suspended in it.

In it, the open plate of culture plate is exposed for specific period and then incubated at 37°C for 24 hrs. The number and type of colonies are recorded.

Integrated Clinical Case Based Study 3 (Zoonoses and vectors)

A 35 year old spinster, Mrs William maintained a dog, as pet for the last five years. Recently she developed a 'ring worm' skin infection on the right forearm (due to *Microsporum canis*)

What other infections, can she develop, as a result of her association with dog?

A.1 The human diseases associated with dog include:

Bacterial – Anthrax

Viral – Rabies (bite)

Fungal – Dermatophytosis (some)

Protozoal – Leishmaniasis (in some geographical areas)
– Amoebiasis (in some geographical areas)
– Trypanosomiasis

Helminthic – Toxocariasis (by *T. canis*)
– Hydatid disease (dog tapeworm)
– Fasciolopsiasis (by *F.buski,* large/giant liver fluke)

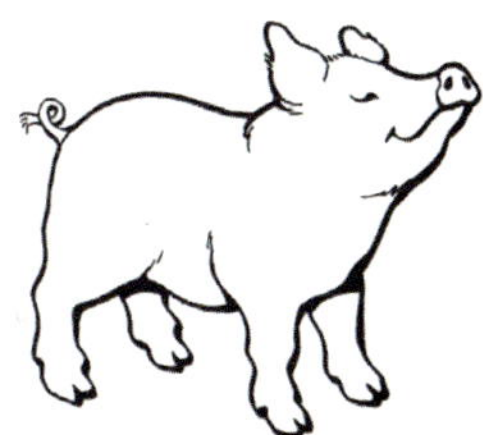

Mention the mode of transmission of the above infections.

A.2 The mode of infection of these entities is varied as Dermatophytosis occurs by contact with animal/animal product, rabies by dog bite and Hydatid disease by ingestion of egg.

Can human contract infections from other pets; as cats, birds and animals; as cows and pigs reared for meat? Mention the infections.

A.3 (i) Yes, with cat and birds the commonly acquired infections include Toxoplasmosis and Psittacosis (Ornithosis), respectively.

(ii) From the cow the human infections that can be acquired include:

Bacterial: Salmonellosis, Brucellosis, *M. bovis* infection, Leptospirosis.

Viral: Cowpox, Orf

Parasitic: Taenia saginata, *Fasciola hepatica* infection

(iii) From the pig, the human infections that can be acquired include *Taenia solium* (including cysticercosis), *Balantidium coli* and *Fasciolopsis buski.*

Enumerate the disease, man can contract from rodents?

A.4 From the rodents, the human infections that can be acquired are

Bacterial: S.Typhimurium, *Y.pestis* (plague), *F.tularensis* (Tularemia), Leptospira spp. (Leptospirosis), Borrelia spp. (Borreliosis), *R. typhi* (mooseri), *R. akari* and *O. tsutsugamushi*

Viral: Lassa fever (by Arenavirus), Haemmorrhagic fever with renal syndrome, Encephalitis, Hantavirus infection (including Hantavirus pulmonary syndrome) and Omsk haemorrhagic fever.

Define zoonoses: Classify them according to (a) life cycle and mode of transmission (b) Reservoir host, (c) Etiological agent.

A.5 Zoonoses are diseases essentially of animals that can be transmitted to man. These can be classified according to three categories.

I. According to the life cycle of the infecting organisms		
(1) ***Direct zoonoses:***		
• Transmitted from infected vertebrate to susceptible host (man) by contact, with fomite or mechanical vector • Agent goes little or no propagation changes or developmental change e.g. rabies, anthrax, brucellosis		
(2) ***Cyclozoonoses:***		
• Requires more than one vertebrate host but no invertebrate host to complete life cycle of th agent e.g. Taenasis, Echinococcosis		
(3) ***Metazoonoses:***		
• transmitted biologically by Invertebrate host • In the invertebrate agent, the agent multiplies or develops or both and there is always an extrinsic incubation period. E.g., Arboviruses, Schistosomiasis, Leishmaniasis, Plague		
(4) ***Saprozoonoses:***		
• Have both vertebrate host & non animal development site or reservoir eg. Various forms of larva migrans		
II. According to reservoir host		
1. *Anthropozoonoses:* infections transmitted to man from lower vertebrate animals eg rabies, plague, arbovirus 2. *Zooanthroponoses:* infections transmitted from man to animal 3. *Amphixenoses:* Infection maintained in both man & animal and transmitted in either diirection, e.g., Salmonellosis		
III. According to etiological agent		
(1) **Bacterial**		
	Disease	**Etiological Agent**
	• Tuberculosis	• *M.tuberculosis, - M. bovis*
	• Salmonellosis	• Salmonella spp.
	• Brucellosis	• *B.abortus, B.suis, B.melitensis*
	• Anthrax	• *B.anthracis*
	• Glanders	• *Pseudomona mallei*
	• Leptospirosis	• *L.interrogans*
	• Plague	• *Y. pestis*
	• Relapsing fever	• Borrelia spp.
	• Tularemia	• *F.tularensis*
Rickettsial		
	• Endemic typhus (murine typhus)	*R. mooseri*
	• Scrub typhus	*O. tsutsugamushi*
	• Q fever	*C.burnetti*
Chlamydial		
	Psitaccosis	*C.psittaci*
Fungal		
	Dermpatophytosis Ringworm)	Microsporum spp. e.g., *M. canis* Tricophyton spp. e.g., *T. verrucosum*
	Deep mycoses	Cryptococcosis
Viral		
	• Rabies	Rhabdovirus
	• Arbovirus infections as KFD, Yellow fever	Arboviruses
	• Influenza	Influenza virus
	• J.E.	J.E. virus
	• Poxvirus infections	Cowpox virus
Protozoal		
	• Amoebias	*E. histolytica*
	• Balantidiasis	*B.coli*
	• Leishmaniasis	*L.donovani*
	• Toxoplasmosis	*T.gondii*
	• Trypanosomiasis	*T.cruzi*
Helminthic		
	• Hydatid disease	*E.granulosus*
	• Taeniasis	*T.solium*
	• Trichinosis	*T.spiralis*
	• Schistosomiasis	Schistosoma spp.
	• Guinea worm	*D.medinensis*
	• Ancylostomiasis	*A.duodenale*
Arthropod borne		
	• Scabies	Sarcoptes spp.
	• Tunga infection	*Tunga penetrans*

What are some of the factors that have led to resurgence of the zoonotic diseases?

A.6

(i) Deforestation and increased area brought under farming and other activities.

(ii) Change in life style; including trekking, adventure sports and increased travel.

(iii) Increase in life span of population and individuals with immunocompromised status, making them susceptible to new infectious agents

(iv) Change in the molecular profile of the microbes, as acquisition of new virulent genes

What are emerging zoonoses?

A.7 In the last few decades, many new human diseases have been linked to animal reservoir; as Verotoxigenic *E. coli* gastroenteritis, Campylobacter enteritis, Lassa fever and Cryptosporidiosis. These may be designated as emerging zoonoses. It is possible that in the future, many new diseases may be recognized that are of zoonotic origin.

Mention the principles utilized in diagnosis of zoonoses.

A.8 Initially, it is important to elicit a history of animal contact or its products. The occupation of the person, the travel history and the extracurricular activities of the person can also be helpful.

It is important to realize that a diagnosis has to be made both in the animals and man. The techniques include the standard ones including the appropriate specimen collection, gross examination, culture (isolation), serological, immunological and molecular analysis. The tests would depend on the tentative diagnosis, that would have been made in the case.

Enumerate the arthropod vectors and the diseases (including zoonoses) transmitted by them.

A.9 The various arthropod vectors and the transmitted diseases are:

(a) FLIES

(i) *House fly*–Enteric fever, gastroenteritis, dysentery (shigellosis) and cholera

(ii) *Black fly* (Simulium)–Filaria (Onchocerca)

(iii) *Deer fly* (Chrysops)–Filaria (Loa loa), Tularemia

(iv) *Horse fly* (Tabanus)–Anthrax (in cattle and horse), Rinderpest (viral disease) and Trypanosomiasis

(v) *Sandfly* (Phelbotomus)–Kala azar, Orietal sore (*L. tropica*), Sandfly fever

(vi) *Tsetse fly* (Glossinia)–Sleeping sickness

(b) MOSQUITO

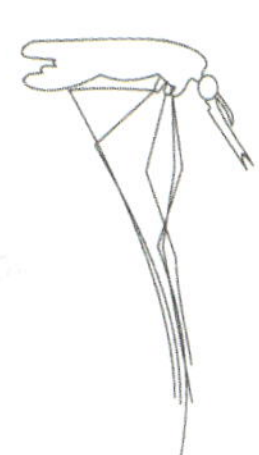

(i) *Aedes*–Chickengunya, Dengue, Yellow fever, Filaria (not in India), Rift valley fever

(ii) *Anopheles*–Malaria, Filaria (*B. malayi,* not in India), Chittor virus

(iii) *Culex*–Filaria, Japanese encephalitis, Chitoor, Sathuperi, Sindbis, Umbre, West Nile

(iv) *Mansonoides*–Filaria (*B. malayi*), Chickengunya fever

(c) FLEA

(i) *Cat flea* (*Ctenocephalides felis*)–*Dipylidium caninum*

(ii) *Human flea*–Cestode infection, *P. irritans*

(iii) *Rat flea (Xenopsylla)* –*Bacterial*-Plague, Endemic typhus (R. typhi), Shigellosis,
–*Helminthic*-**H.diminuta, H. nana, Dipylidium caninum*

(iv) *Sand flea*–Chiggerosis (mite larva-chiggers scrub)

* Rat tapeworm (*H. diminuta*) infrequently seen in man

(d) LOUSE

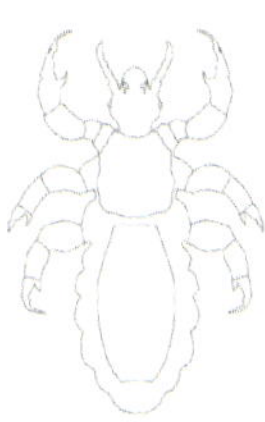

(i) *Head louse*–Epidemic typhus, mechanical irritation

(ii) *Body louse*–Epidemic typhus, Trench fever, Relapsing fever, Dermatitis

(iii) *Pubic* (pthrus)–mechanical irritation

(e) MITE (also called Acari)Δ

Δ Acari (or Acarina) are taxon of arachnids that contains mites or ticks

(i) *Chicken mite* (*Dermanyssus gallinae*)–St. Louis encephalitis

(ii) *Itch mite* (*Sarcoptes scabei*)–Scabies

(iii) *Trombiculid mite*–Scrub typhus, R.pox

(f) CYCLOPS
- –*Dracunculus medinensis* (Guinea worm)
- –*Diphyllobothrium latum* (fish tapeworm)

(g) TICK

(i) *Bacterial*–Relapsing fever (Ornithodoros), Lyme disease (Ixodes, *Ambylomma, Dermacentor*), Tularemia (Dermacentor, Ambylomma))

(ii) *Rickettsial*–Indian Tick Typhus, Rocky mountain spotted fever (Dermacentor, Ambylomma)), Q fever.

(iii) *Parasitic*–Babesiosis (Ixodes)

(iv) *Viral*–Kyasnur forest disease (Haemaphysalis, Ixodes), Russian spring summer encephalitis (Ixodes), Colorado tick fever, Omsk haemmorhagic fever, Crimean Congo haemorrhagic fever

(h) SANDFLY

Viral–Chandipura

Parasitic–Kala azar, Orietal sore, Sandfly fever

(i) REDUVID BUG

Chagas disease

NB: Rhipicephalus bursa (is one of the tick) is involved in CCHF, others are also involved.

Integrated Clinical Case Base Study 4 (Diseases transmitted by blood)

A thirty year old young executive, Shri Rajnath has been asked to donate blood for his father, who is to be operated the next day. He is trying to arrange one unit of blood through a commercial donor, whose health antecedents are not clear.

Explain to the patient's relative, the importance of blood donation by close relatives.

A.1 He should be explained that the purpose of the blood transmission is to provide nutrition and vitality of all types to the recipient, hence the transfused blood should be of the best kind and should be free of all infectious agents. It should be communicated to him that the best of the tests, cannot guarantee, that a tested blood is devoid of all infectious agents; even if tested negative for the infectious agents.

What pathogens can be transmitted by blood?

A.2 Organisms that can be transmitted through blood transfusion, are depicted in table 17.2.4.

Table 17.2.4: Pathogens transmissible by blood transfusion

Viruses	Parasites	Bacteria	Fungi
ΔHepatitis B virus	Δ*Plasmodium spp.*	Δ*Treponema pallidum*	Aspergillus spp.
ΔHepatitis C virus	*Toxoplasma gondii*	*Brucella abortus*	Penicillium spp.
Hepatitis D virus	*Trypanosoma cruzi*	Proteus species	Hormodendrum spp.
ΔHIV 1 & 2	*Wuchereria bancrofti*	*E.coli*	
ΘHTLV I, II	*Brugia malayi*	Klebsiella species	
Hepatitis A virus	*Loa loa*	Micrococcus spp.	
HHV-5 (CMV)*	*Leismania donovani*	Enterobacter spp.	
HHV-4 (EB)*	*B.microti*	*Salmonella Cholerasuis*	
Parvovirus		Pseudomonas species	
Ebola virus		*Staphylococcus epidermidis*	
Lassa virus		*R.rickettsii*	
◊West nile encephalitis virus			
Yellow fever virus			

* Generally blood transfused is not tested for CMV and many other viruses, so the risk of their transmission remains.

Δ In India, these pathogens are tested before blood transfusion.

Θ Testing is mandatory in many countries before blood transfusion.

◊ Trial of its testing was initiated in U.S. in 2003.

Healthcare Associated Infections–HAIs (HAP)

- The Center for disease control (CDC) estimates that there are 2 million cases of HAI per year. Treatment cost for HAI in the USA can reach $4.5-11 million annually. Of these two million HAI cases, the CDC estimated 20,000 patients die from HAI complications.

  — ML

- 'It is not a fact that people must get hospital-acquired infections. The goal ought to be the prevention of every single hospital-acquired infection.'

  — Marc P. Volarka

Let's study this important aspect of HAIs as two integrated clinical based studies.

Integrated Clinical Case Base Study 1

A 70 year old male, Shehnaz, got admitted to a neurology ward for neurological problems including loss of memory. At time of admission, his other systems including pulmonary did not reveal any abnormality. After 3 days of admission, he complained of breathlessness, purulent sputum and chest radiography revealed infiltrates (pneumonia) in the right upper lung.

What is the clinical diagnosis of the above case?

A.1 (a) Hospital acquired pneumonia (HAP) - also termed as nosocomial infection.

If this case had been on mechanical ventilation before he developed pneumonia, what would have been the diagnosis?

A.2 (b) Ventilator associated pneumonia

How do you define hospital associated pneumonia?

A.2 (a) *Hospital associated pneumonia is defined;* as a pulmonary infection that occurs in a patient, who has been hospitalized and occurs after 48 hours of admission. This time limit has been set so as to exclude the presentation of infection in a case, which one might be incubating at the time of admission.

How do you define HAIs?

A.2 (b) *Hospital associated infections* are known by various names; as health care associated infection, nosocomial infection and hospital acquired infection. It is defined, as an infection developed by patient, in a hospital (usually after 48 hours of admission) which was neither present, nor in the incubation period at time of admission.

Enumerate the common HAIs and microbes associated with them.

A.3 (a)

Table 17.3.1: Common types of Health associated Infections and implicated microbes

Health associated Infection	Microbes
Urinary tract infection (commonest)	*E. coli,* Klebsiella spp., Proteus spp. and others (including Candida spp.)
Respiratory tract infection	*S. aureus*, Klebsiella spp., Enterobacter spp., Serratia spp., *E. coli*, *P. aeruginosa*, Acinetobacter spp., *L. pneumophila*. Respiratory viruses as measles and others
GIT infections	Salmonella spp., Shigella spp., *C. difficile*, Viruses as Rotavirus, Coxsackie and others.
*Surgical site infections**	*S. aureus*, *P. aeruginosa*, *E.coli*, Enterococcus spp., Coagulase negative Staphylococci, *C. perfringens*, *C.tetani*.
Blood stream infection; as septicaemia	Coagulase negative Staphylococci, *S. aureus*, Enterococcus spp., Klebsiella spp., Serratia spp. and Candida spp.

*Are defined as infection that develops at the surgical site within 30 days of surgery.

What are the possible modes for acquisition of pneumonia in this case? Enumerate the microbes associated with nosocomial infection.

A.3 (b) The case could have the pneumonia due to aspiration of endogenous flora; as *S.pneumoniae, S. aureus* etc. or due to exogenous hospital acquired microbial flora. The latter could be due to inhalation of droplets (aerosol) generated by other patients (including staff) or aspiration of oropharyngeal flora of the medical staff (with which they are colonized).

Microbes associated with nosocomial infections	
Gram Positive bacteria	***Gram Negative bacteria***
• *Staphylococcus aureus*	• *Escherichia coli*
• *Streptococcus pyogenes*	• Citrobacter spp.
• *Staphylococcus epidermidis*	• Klebsiella spp.
• *Streptococcus pneumoniae*	• Serratia spp.
• *Clostridium difficile*	• Enterobacter spp.
• *Clostrdium perfringens*	• Proteus spp.
• *Clostridium tetani*	• Pseudomonas spp.
	• Legionella spp.
Viruses	***Fungi***
• Hepatitis B	• *Aspergillus spp.*
• Hepatitis C	• *Candida albicans*
• Hepatitis D	
• HIV	***Parasites***
• Herpes viruses	• *Toxoplasma gondii*
• Cytomegalovirus	• *Entamoeba histolytica*
• Influenza virus	• *Pneumocystis jirovecii*
• Enteroviruses	• Cryptosporidium spp.

Categorize the sources of the infection in HAIs.

A.3 (c) The sources of infections can be placed into two categories, namely endogenous and exogenous source.

- *Endogenous source:* The majority of HAIs are endogenous in origin, i.e., the patient's own microbial flora invades the patient's body, during surgical procedures (including instrumentation).
- *Exogenous source:* The source for this hospital environment include hospital staff and other patients
  - Hospital environmental source includes inanimate objects; as walls, medical instruments; as endoscopes.
  - Hospital staff can be staff nurses carrying microbes; as methicillin resistant *S. aureus*

Enumerate the modes of transmission in HAIs.

A.3 (d)

Table 17.3.2: Modes of transmission of hospital acquired infections

Contact transmission	
- Direct contact	Skin to skin contact between susceptible host and an infected colonized personnel, often healthcare worker
- Indirect contact	Involves contact of a susceptible host with contaminated inanimate objects, such as dressings and instruments; as endoscope
Inhalational mode	
- Droplet transmission (droplets of >5 μm, travel short distances usually <3 mts)	- Droplets generated from infected person; while coughing, sneezing and even talking, expelled into environment - Is a key mode of transmission for agents; as meningitis, diphtheria, RSV and others

Contd.

Contd.

- Aerosol transmission (airborne droplet nuclei usually, <-5 μm, remain suspended in the air, travel long distances)	More effective mode of transmission than droplet transmission - Is a key mode of transmission for Legionella, *M. tuberculosis,* Measles virus and others
Other modes	
- Oral route	As water, food
- Parenteral route	By disposable syringes/needles

What specimens can help to find the aetiology of the pneumonia in this case?

A.4 (a) These include sputum (induced sputum, if the patient is not expectorating), endotracheal aspirates or sampling of distal airways with specimens; as broncheoalveolar lavage. These samples would be assessed microscopically to assess the inflammatory cells, bacterial flora and cultured using semi-quantitative and quantitative techniques.

How reliable is tracheal aspirate; as a representative specimen of pneumonia?

A.4 (b) If the case is on mechanical ventilator, tracheal aspirate specimens from such cases, may not be representative of lower respiratory tract, as it could be contaminated with microbial flora from upper airways.

What are the risk factors for development of nosocomial pneumonia?

A.5 The risk factors include extremes of age (as elderly), severe illness, heavy smoking, existing cardiopulmonary disease, surgical operation (chest/abdomen), decreased gastric acidity (encourages microbial proliferation in gastric fluid; which may be aspirated), decreased level of consciousness (which can predispose to aspiration), presence of equipment; as nasogastric tube, colonization of patient by potential pathogens (predisposed by prior antibiotic therapy) and reduced host defense mechanisms.

What is ventilator associated pneumonia?

A.6 (a) It is defined; as an pulmonary infection that occurs in a hospitalized patient more than 48 hours, after endotracheal intubation and mechanical ventilation.

Describe diagnostic approach in laboratory diagnosis of HAIs.

A.6 (b) The laboratory diagnosis requires good understanding of the type of HAI (see A.3b), source of the infection (A.3c) and modes of transmission of HAIs (A.3d). The samples from the patient and hospital would depend on the above scenario.

What could be the measures that could have been adopted to prevent the HAP episode in this case?

A.7 The patient could be encouraged to maintain proper posture, that would discourage aspiration and initiate oral cavity care at least 6 times a day. The hospital staff should have practiced hand hygiene before and after patient care, changed gloves between patients and procedures and used decontaminated equipment.

Integrated Clinical Case Based Study 2

A panicky intern, Dr Nivetha reported to the AIDS counsellor with history of needle stick injury from a HIV positive case, while drawing blood from the case. Subsequently investigations indicated her to have become a victim of occupational HIV infection.

Which are the key infections that can be transmitted with needle (syringe) stick injury?

A.1 (a) The infections that can be transmitted primarily include HIV, hepatitis B, hepatitis C.

In India, how many cases of occupational HIV transmission to Health Care Workers (HCWs) have been reported?

A.1 (b) There is no case of occupational HIV reported. However, that should not be construed that no such cases have occurred, as many such cases get reported even in the developed countries, where the general implementation of infection control is more rigorous. No reporting of case in India, might indicate poor documentation and investigation.

How many such cases have been reported in US?

A.1 (c) In USA (in 2001), 57 cases of occupational HIV transmission to health care workers (HCW) were reported. All these cases; except one had documentation of HIV antibody seroconversion in temporal association with discrete HIV exposure.

What are the transmission rates of HIV, HBV and HCV, after percutaneous exposure of infected blood?

A.2 The transmission rates 'after percutaneous exposure of infected blood for HIV, HBV and HCV are 0.05-0.4%, 9-30% and 3-10% respectively. This implies a greater transmissibility of hepatitis B and C viruses than HIV despite greater morbidity and mortality caused by HIV infections than hepatitis B and C viruses.

Which precaution, if had been implemented in this case, could have prevented her from being infected?

A.3 (a) Standard precautions (universal precautions), if had been implemented could have prevented her from getting infection.

When were 'universal precautions' guidelines published?

A.3 (b) 'Universal precautions' were published in 1987 and in the same year, this term was coined.

What was the basis of these precautions?

A.3 (c) These precautions followed the recommendation of the Centre for Disease Control in 1985, that blood of all patients should be regarded as infectious. They followed the emergence of HIV/AIDS in 1985.

When did the 'universal precautions' get replaced by 'standard precautions'?

A.3 (d) (i) In 1996, the 'Standard precautions' replaced the 'universal precautions'.

Why did this replacement occur?

A.3 (d) (ii) The *standard precautions* are more comprehensive than *universal precautions.* They are based on the principle that every person should be considered as potentially infectious and susceptible to infection. It considers blood, body fluids (as cerebrospinal fluid, pleural fluid), secretion (except sweat), non-intact skin mucous membranes of all patients to be potentially infected with various pathogens; especially HIV and HBV. The 'universal precautions' were to be observed, when any sample that was to be handled could be tinged with blood.

What is the basis of the standard precautions?

A.3 (d) (iii) Most people with blood borne viral infections; as HIV and HBV, do not have any symptoms and occasionally cannot be picked up by laboratory tests. Therefore precautions and specific personnel protective equipment are to be used by the medical personnel, whenever the possibility of exposure to any of the body fluid exists. The equipment includes gloves, masks, goggles (eye protection) and gown to produce a barrier between the medical personnel and the infectious fluid of the patient. Hand hygiene is essential before and after contact with the potential infected fluids and after change of protective gear.

These precautions avoid the cumbersome disease-specific isolation precautions.

Describe the Infection Control Policy.

A.3 (e) See A.5a and A.5b

Is there a possibility of reverse flow of infection, i.e., from the medical personnel to the patient?

A.4 (a) Yes

How many such cases have been reported?

A.4 (b) Three cases are on record where the transmission of the HIV infection occurred form the providers of medical services to the patients. The infection providers included one dental surgeon, one orthopaedician and one nurse.

Describe the preventive aspects in reference to health care associated infections.

A.5 (a) For prevention of HAIs, the essential aspect is to block their transmission. To implement it, every healthcare institution must have a functional Infection control committee (details see A.5b)

The infection can be controlled by:

(i) *Reducing the microbial load* in the hospital: This can be addressed by focusing on environmental cleaning. This entails cleaning of the environmental surfaces by various means including physical means; as scrubbing with water and detergent. This process reduces the microbial load, so this process must precede the disinfection protocols.

(ii) *To reduce the transmission* of microbes amongst *hospital personnel*: The categories amongst this would include from patient to patient and hospital personnel to patient. An important route is also from patient to hospital personnel to patient (i.e., hospital acts as a vector).

(iii) *Minimizing the spread* of infection from *inanimate objects*; as linen, instruments and other articles. To enforce this aspect, an effective Central sterile supply department (CSSD) needs to be in place in the hospital.

A core activity that needs to be implemented is the Standard precautions. This concept has been presented in this case (see A3). The following aspects need an emphasis.

1. Hand hygiene (see A5c)
2. Personnel protective equipment (PPEs): This aspect has been presented in A3(iii). To reinforce, gloves must be worn, whenever there is a possibility of contact with body fluids; including non-intact skin and contaminated equipment.

3. Safe injection practices; including installation of needle destroyers.
4. Implementation of disease specific precautions-It includes compliance of respiratory hygiene (as covering mouth/nose while coughing), contact precautions and separating/cohorting patients.

Describe Hospital Infection Control Committee (***HICC).***

A.5 (b) A functioning HICC is the key to the hospital infection control and prevention in a hospital.

Constitution: Medical Superintendent (usually Chairperson), HOD–Microbiology (usually secretary), HODs of clinical departments, Infection control nurses, Members from various sections as CSSD, pharmacy, CPWD (Central public work department) and others.

Functions (Mandate):
- Formulation and implementation of the hospital *infection control policy*
- HAI surveillance-This work is essentially carried out by the Infection Control nurses (ICNs), who gather the data from the patient records and are involved in the sample collection. From the information gathered, the rates of surgical site infections (SSIs) catheter associated urinary tract infection (CA-UTI) and other parameters in the hospital can be estimated.
- Development of antibiotic policy for the hospital
- Outbreak detection, control and prevention
- CMEs for various categories of hospital staff

The HICC meets at regular intervals and as when required to meet any emergency.

Describe Hand Hygiene.

A.5 (c)
- **Need:** Hand colonized with microbes have been known to be involved in many infectious disease outbreaks in nurseries, neonatal units, ICUs and other hospital settings. This is because hands of medical personnel can be transiently infected with pathogenic microbes, from infected cases and environment and these agents can then be transferred to other patients. Therefore, effective hand hygiene can be a cornerstone in keeping the nosocomial infection rate at a minimum.
- **Types of skin flora:** Normal human skin is colonized with microbes, the total aerobic bacterial count ranging from 1×10^6 colony forming units (CFU/cm^2 on the scalp) to 1×10^4 (CFUs/cm^2 on the forearm. The microbial flora of the skin consists of *transient* and resident microbes. The former; consists of recent contaminants that can survive for only a limited periods. The *resident microbes* survive and multiply in the superficial epidermis.
- **Techniques:** Broadly they can be categorized unto three categories, as depicted in the table 17.3.3.

Table 17.3.3: Hand hygiene techniques

	Routine	Alcoholic hand rub	Surgical hand wash/hand scrub
Water usage	+	Dry hand required	+
Duration of contact with hygiene product	Minimal	Minimal (should cover all surfaces)	More time (few minutes), depends on recommendation from product manufacturer
Anatomical parts involved	Hands	Hands	Hands, wrist and forearms
Drying process	With clean towel	Occurs naturally by exposure to environment	With sterile towel

- **Indications:** Five moments for hand hygiene have been recommended in a health care setting by WHO, namely:
  (i) Before touching a patient
  (ii) Before a procedure
  (iii) After a procedure
  (iv) After touching a patient
  (v) After touching a patient surrounding

  The routine hand wash should be used, when hands are soiled. If hands are visibly soiled, alcohol based rub should not be used.
- **Procedure:** This aspect has been dealt in table 17.3.3. It should be ensured that the five types of hand movements are incorporated.

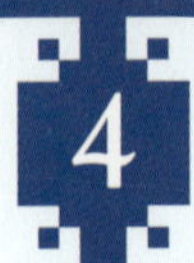

Biomedical Waste Management

- 'Water and air, the two essential elements on which all life depends, have become global garbage cans'. — Anonymous
- 'It makes a big difference to recycle. It makes a big difference to use recycled products. It makes a big difference to reuse things, to not use the paper cup and each time you do that's a victory'. — Emily Deschanel
- 'I do not want to protect the environment'.
  I want to create a world, where the environment does not need any protection'. — Formahilin

Let's understand the motto of the Biomedical waste management rules and how these are to be implemented. These are of paramount importance to all health providers and punishable under law, if not adhered to. The rules have undergone major changes in March 2016, after their first notification in 1998. Let's study this aspect with a clinical vignette based study.

A hepatitis B outbreak occurred in Modasa, North Gujarat (India), affected over 125 people and 49 people succumbed to the infection in early 2009. Investigations revealed that doctors had re-used syringes contaminated with the viruses. The medical practitioners were arrested under IPC (Indian penal code) for culpable homicide not amounting to murder.

What aspect of the clinic, if had been handled adequately could have prevented this outbreak?

A.1 Management of the biomedical waste. In this episode, the needles were not destroyed and the syringes were not disinfected and appropriately disposed.

When did the biomedical waste (VMIV) rules of India come into existence?

A.2 (a) The biomedical waste rules came into effect, as the biomedical waste (management and handling) rules on 27th July 1998. They were implemented by the Ministry of Environment and Forests, Government of India.

When did the new BMW rules come into being?

A.2 (b) The new BMW rules came into being on 28th March, 2016. The changes were made to implement the rules more effectively and improve the collection, segregation, treatment and disposal of bio-medical waste.

What is the area of domain of the BMW rules?

A.2 (c) These rules are applicable to every hospital, nursing home or clinic, which generates biomedical waste.

What is the motto and principle of these rules?

A.2 (d) The motto of these is to minimize the infection risk to medical personnel and preserve the earth for future generations. The principle is to segregate the waste at source; prior to treatment and then effectively treat it.

What is the scheme of segregating the waste, according to the BMW management rules (2016)?

A.3 The waste is to be separated at the point of separation into various types with reference to its category (Table 17.4.1). The principle is that the majority of the waste (as much as 80 percent) is non hazardous and can be easily discarded in the municipal bin and does not need any treatment, if it does not get mixed with the infectious waste. However; if it does get mixed not only it adds to the cost of the waste management but also increases the hazardousness.

What are the advantages of segregating the waste?

A.4 The advantages are that it minimizes biomedical waste, as the general waste as paper, unused food gets separated from it. It reduces cost expenditure of the hospital and reduces risk of hazards to health workers, scavengers and general communities.

What is the schedule 1 of the of biomedical waste rules (2016)?

A.5 According to the Schedule 1 (modified in March, 2016), only four biomedical waste categories exist, namely yellow, red, white and blue. The motto of reducing the number of categories is to simplify the process for health-care workers. The categories of biomedical waste (adapted) are depicted in table 17.4.1.

Table 17.4.1: Biomedical waste segregation as per 2016 rules

Category	Type of waste	Type of bag or container to be used	Treatment and disposal options
Yellow	(a) Human anatomical waste	Yellow colored non-chlorinated plastic bags	Incineration/Plasma pyrolysis/Deep burial
	(b) Animal anatomical waste	-	-
	(c) Soiled waste (as dressings, cotton swabs)	-	-
	(d) Expired or discarded medicines	Yellow colored, non chlorinated plastic bags	Returned to manufacturer for incineration/ encapsulation/plasma pyrolysis at >1200°C
	(e) Chemical waste	Yellow colored, non chlorinated plastic bags	Incineration/plasma pyrolysis/encapsulation in hazardous waste treatment
	(f) Chemical liquid waste	Separate liquid system leading to effluent treatment system	After resource recovery, the chemical liquid waste shall be pre-treated, before mixing with other waste water
	(g) Discarded linen, mattresses, bedding contaminated with body fluid	Non-chlorinated, yellow plastic bag or suitable packing material	Non-chlorinated chemical disinfection followed by incineration or plasma pyrolysis
	(h) Microbiology, Biotechnology and other clinical laboratory waste as blood bags, lab cultures etc.	Autoclave safe plastic bag or container	Pretreat to sterilize with non chlorinated chemicals on site; as per NACO guidelines
Red	Contaminated waste (recyclable) Wastes generated from disposable items; as tubings, bottles, catheters, urine bags vacutainers (with needles cut)	Red colored, non chlorinated plastic bags or containers	Autoclaving/Hydroclaving/Micrwaving followed by shredding or mutilation. Treated waste to be sent to authorized recyclers.
White (translucent)	Waste sharps including metals; as needles, scalpels etc.	Puncture proof, leak proof, tamper proof containers	Autoclaving/dry heat sterilization followed by shredding/mutilation/encapsulation into metal container or concrete. Final disposal to iron foundries or designated concrete sharp pit
Blue	• Glassware • Metallic body implants	Card-boxes with blue colored marking	Disinfection/autoclaving/Microwaving/ Hydroclaving. Finally sent for recycling

Describe the techniques to treat biomedical waste?

A.6 The following techniques are often used to treat the infected waste

(i) *Incineration:* Many large hospitals install a double chambered incinerator to deal with the solid infected waste.The waste is burnt in the primary chamber with temperature of approximately 800°C, while the secondary chamber has a temperature of 1000°C. The combustion of the gases occurs in the secondary chamber, where the gases are sucked into it, by the negative pressure. The process converts the waste into ash, which is about the tenth of the original volume.

The advantage of this technique is that almost all type of solid waste can be dealt by this machine except PVC plastics, which release toxic gases; as dioxins and furans, if incinerated. The incinerator system can be installed only in big hospitals and the released gases may be injurious to the community.

(ii) *Autoclaving:* It is a technique often used to treat the waste. Prevaccum autoclaves are often used, where the load is on the higher side.

(iii) *Microwaving:* It is a useful technique to sterilize small amount of waste at the point of generation. Microwaves produced by the system raise the temperature in the system to approximately 98-100°C for a particular cycle time and disinfect the load.

(iv) *Hydroclaving:* It is another technology, using steam for sterilizing of the load.

(v) *Plasma technology:* It is a recent efficacious technology, but expensive. Plasma is considered to be the fourth state for matter.

(vi) *Chemical treatment:* Various chemicals; as sodium hypochlorite are used for the disinfection.

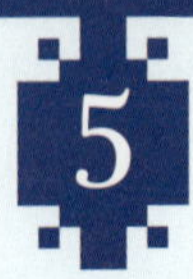

Bioterrorism

– **'Innovation is a good thing. The human condition-put aside bioterrorism and a few footnotes –is improving because of innovation'.** **— Bill Gates**

Let's see how medical technology can be applied to make the world a safe place to live.

An integrated clinical based study has been discussed at pg. 223, in section 5.

Enumerate the bioterrorism diseases/agents.

Classification of Bioterrorism diseases/agents:

Anthrax (*Bacillus anthracis*)
Botulism (*Clostridium botulinum*)
Brucellosis (Brucella spp.)
Cholera (*Vibrio cholerae*)
Cryptosporidiosis (Cryptosporidium spp.)
Eastern equine encephalitis
Ebola Haemorrhagic fever (Ebola virus)
Escherichia coli infection (*E.coli* O157:H7)
Glanders (*Burkholderia mallei*)
Hantavirus pulmonary syndrome (Hantavirus)
Lassa haemorrhagic fever (Lassa virus)
Marburgh haemorhagic fever (Marburg virus)
Melidiosis (*Burkholderia pseudomallei*)
Plague (*Yersinia pestis*)
Psittacosis (*Chlamydia psittaci*)
Q fever (*Coxiella burnetii*)
Salmonellosis (Salmonella spp.)
Small pox (Variola major)
Tularemia (*Francisella tularensis*)
Typhus fever (*Rickettsia prowazekii*)
(*Adapted from CDC site*)

Drug Resistance

- **No action today (on drug resistance)**
- **No cure tomorrow.**

7th April, 2011. World Health Day

Let's study first the fundamental aspects of this problem to be followed by two integrated clinical based studies.

Act !

And make a better tomorrow for the new generation. !!

Student cartoon 5
-Ramiya George

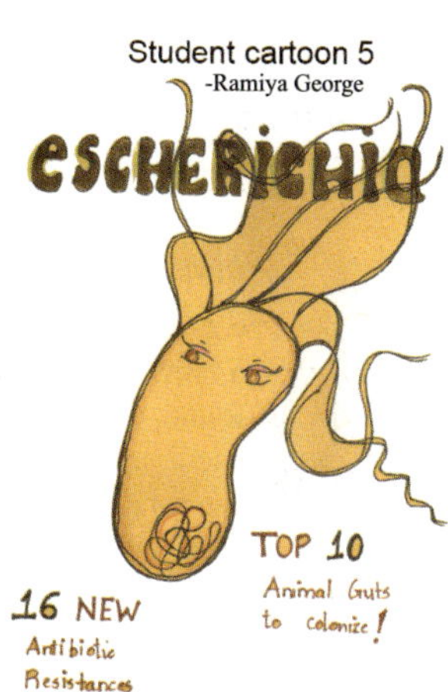

Why is it that so much emphasis is given on the rational usage of antimicrobials?

A.1 It will prevent the widespread sensitization of the population with resulting hypersensitivity, rashes, blood dyscrasias, cholestatic jaundice, development of drug resistance, drug f ailure and other disorders. It will prevent the problem of replacement of normal flora of the body with drug resistant organisms, that can cause disease (superinfection). It can also prevent the replacement of the drug sensitive organisms of the hospital flora with drug resistant organisms.

On what factors does drug resistance depend on?

A.2 (a)

The factors in drug resistance can be classified and are depicted in the flow diagram

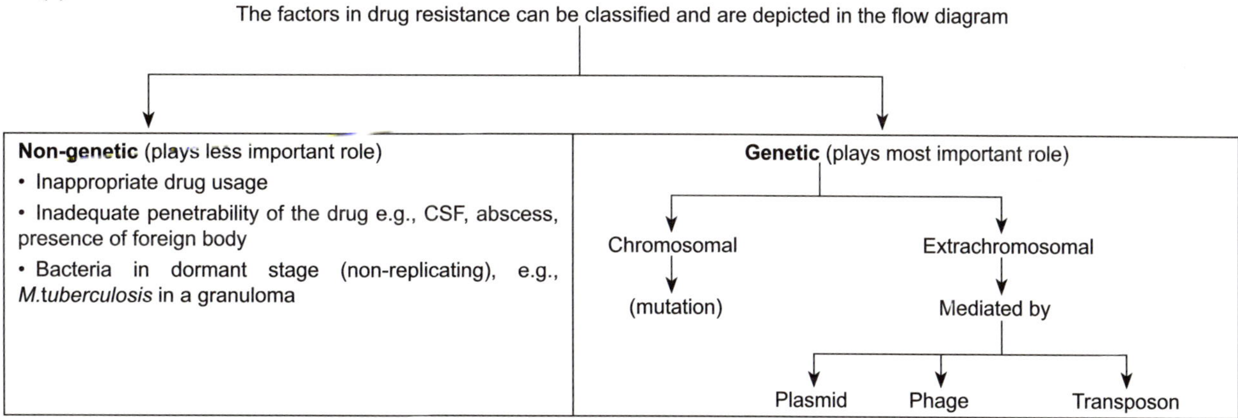

How can drug resistance be categorized?

A.2 (b)

– *Innate/inherent resistance/primary resistance*- some bacteria always resistant to some antimicrobials (e.g., *Pseudomonas aeruginosa* always resistant to PnG

– *Acquired resistance* → as result of genetic change

Give some examples that clearly depict that the euphoria that was generated, after the introduction of antibiotics in 1940s, was shortlived.

A.3 (i) In *S.aureus,* 'wild' type, penicillin resistant strains started appearing in the human beings, even before the introduction of penicillin at a frequency of about 3% or less. Exorbitant usage of penicillin (in hundreds of tons every year) caused an increase of the penicillin resistant *S. aureus* isolates to a current figure of about 85% resistance. This organism is currently resistant to many other antimicrobials also.

(ii) For gonorrhoea, before the 1930s, no effective treatment was available. Then sulphonamides were introduced for treatment of this disease. They were successful for some years, before resistance started getting developed to it. Then penicillin was available, which was effective in the treatment of this disease; besides tetracycline. Resistance started occurring to penicillin, but it could be overcome with high doses of penicillin for many years, till β-lactamase producing gonococcal strains started appearing in 1970s. This necessitated the administration of spectinomycin to treat gonorrhoea, but resistance to even this antimicrobial forced the health personnel to look for alternatives.

(iii) Sulphonamides; which were uniformly used for prophylaxis and treatment for meningococci till 1962, lost the usefulness, after the sulphonamide resistant meningococci proliferated.

(iv) Penicillin resistant pneumococci started appearing after 1963 (till then the organism was uniformly susceptible to PnG).

Describe the mechanisms of drug resistance.

A.4 For an antimicrobial to have its action, it must enter the microbe and bind to appropriate receptor, whether in the cell wall, cell membrane, nucleic acid or others receptors. The different mechanisms of drug resistance in microbes are categorized into:

I. Production of enzymes that inactivate/destroy the drug before it attaches to the receptor in the microbe.

Following are the mechanism by which the bacterial enzymes destroying the structure of the antimicrobial or making it functionally inactive,

e.g., various types of β-lactamases (penicillinases) can destroy the β-lactam ring of various penicillins (penicillinases of *S.aureus,* which are usually plasmid mediated, but spread by transduction). One group of specific β-lactamases occasionally found in some enterobacteriaceae members are termed extended-spectrum β-lactamases (ESBLs), as they confer on the bacterium the additional ability to hydrolyze the β-lactam of 3rd generation cephalosporins; as cefotaxime, ceftazadime or aztreonam. Further examples exist.

e.g., Aminoglycoside modifying enzyme, by some gram negative bacteria, as acetyltransferases, phosphotransferases, nucleotidyltransferases; which acetylate, phosphorylate or adenylate, respectively the various aminoglycosides, making them inactive.

e.g., Chloramphenicol resistant gram negative bacteria (as S. Typhi), due to synthesis of acetyltransferase, which acetylates the chloramphenicol and inactivates it (mediated by plasmid.).

II. Alteration in cell wall/cell membrane of microbes

Structural changes can occur in it, which can prevent the antimicrobial to act on these sites or prevent their entry into the bacterium.

- Vancomycin resistance in gram positive cocci, is due to structural peptide change in peptidoglycan of cell wall e.g., vancomycin resistance in enterococci (increasingly reported).
- Alterations in pores (porins) of some bacterial membrane, by changes of proteins, which can hinder the antimicrobial transfer across the membrane, making them resistant to some antimicrobials.

  e.g., resistance to certain quinolones, tetracyclines and aminoglycosides has occurred by this mechanism.
- Some enterococci have natural permeability barrier to aminoglycosides. This can be partly overcome by a simultaneous administration of a cell wall active drug; as penicillin G. It could act by altering the synthesis of structures of the outer membrane.

III. Altered drug receptors targets (changes in number/affinity of drug receptor)

If the bacterial receptor, where the antimicrobial has to bind (attach), gets altered, then the binding of the antimicrobial to the bacterium cannot occur, hence resistance to antimicrobial can occur. This can occur due to mutation or by acquiring of new genes from the outside by the microbe

- Erythromycin resistance is caused by bacterial enzyme (plasmid mediated), which methylate the ribosomal RNA (bacterial), altering the structural target and preventing the drug to bind to the receptor. Aminoglycoside resistant bacteria develop, as a result of structural alteration on the 30S subunit of ribosome, preventing drugs attachment.
- Resistance to penicillin (both low level and high level) in *S.pneumoniae*, occurs due to alteration of some penicillin binding proteins (PBPs) (mediated by chromosomal mutation)
- Resistance to quinolones (e.g., Ciprofloxacin in S.Typhi) is due to structural change in bacterial DNA gyrase, as a result of chromosomal mutation, which prevents the drug from acting on these enzyme.
- *M. tuberculosis* develops resistance to rifampicin, due to mutation in the gene coding DNA dependent RNA polymerase.
- Methicillin resistance in *S.aureus,* is related to alteration in the binding proteins in the cell wall.

IV. **Altered metabolic pathway**

Some microorganisms develop an altered metabolic pathway, as a result of mutation, that bypasses the reaction inhibited by the drug

e.g., some sulphonamide resistant bacteria, donot require extracellular PABA.

Drug dependence: certain organisms are not only resistant to a drug but require it for growth. e.g., streptomycin-dependent meningococci, when injected into mice, progressive fatal disease results, only if the animals are treated simultaneously with streptomycin.

How does drug resistance transfer from one microbe to another?

A.5 Organisms initially displayed resistance only to one antimicrobial. In late 1950s (1954) in Japan, concept of multiple drug resistance took firm ground, with occurrence of an epidemic of *S.dysenteriae*. Isolates of *S.dysenteriae* were found resistant to four antimicrobials; namely tetracycline, chloramphenicol, streptomycin and sulphonamides. Surprisingly, similar drug resistance (of resistance to four antimicrobials) pattern was also seen in *E.coli* of the gut flora of the persons affected by the epidemic. The multidrug resistance in *S.dysenteriae* was postulated to have been acquired by acquisition of plasmid and transposons having genes of antimicrobial resistance from bacteria of other genera (unlikely to have arisen by chromosomal mutation).

The various processes involved in transfer of drug resistance among bacteria include

Transduction: Plasmid DNA enclosed in a bacteriophage (bacterial virus), transferred to another bacterium of the same species.

e.g., β-lactamase enzyme in *S.aureus*

Transformation: Naked DNA transferred from one cell of a species to another cell, altering its genotype.

Conjugation: A unilateral transfer of genetic material between bacteria of same or different genera occurs during a conjugation process. Genetic transfer by conjugation is known to exist amongst all genera of family entrobacteriaceae and other genera; as Pseudomonas. Clinical evidence suggests that transfer of drug resistance can occur in the gastrointestinal tract of man. Such resistance is widespread and is associated with extensive oral antibiotic therapy.

Transposition: A transfer of short DNA sequences occurs between plasmid and a portion of the bacterial chromosome (in a bacterium) or between one plasmid and another. Transposons (jumping genes) are non-replicating (depend on the host cell for replication) pieces of DNA 2000-20,000 bp in size and can jump between within one plasmid, between plasmid and the chromosome and also within the chromosome. The discovery of the transposons provided the basis for the rapid spread of resistance genes throughout the diverse bacterial kingdom.

Hopping of transposons accounts for the spread of resistance to organisms, that are otherwise unable to support the replication of the plasmid; originally harbouring the resistance gene. This process accounted for the spread of β-lactamase genes from plasmid of enteric bacteria to Haemophilus and Neisseria spp.

Spontaneous mutation occurs with a frequency of 10^{-7}-10^{-12} and this is an infrequent cause of emergence of clinical drug resistance in a given patient. However chromosomal mutants resistant to rifampicin occur with a high frequency (about 10^{-5}) and consequently treatment of bacterial infections with rifampicin alone usually fails.

Natural selection for drug resistant forms frequently occur in various natural habitats, hospitals, laboratories and in body of man.

Name infectious diseases, that have emerged because of antimicrobial resistance component.

A.6 (i) Multidrug resistant *M.tuberculosis* (including XDR-TB)

(ii) Multidrug resistant S.Typhi

(iii) Drug resistant *Plasmodium falciparum* (including malaria resistant to artemisinin combination therapy - ACT)

Drug resistance has complicated treatment of:

- *N. gonorrhoeae, S. pneumoniae, S. aureus* infections

What do you understand by cross-resistance (parallel resistance) in the field of antimicrobials? Mention its implications.

A.7 *Cross resistance* in antimicrobials imply that if a microorganism displays resistance to one anti-microbial, it is also (high probability) resistant to other related antimicrobials. It is also described as resistance in a microbe to two or more similar antimicrobials via a common mechanism.

The implication of this concept is in reporting of antibiotic susceptibility report. If an organism shows resistance to one specific type of antimicrobial, then other related classes of antimicrobials, can also be predicted to be resistant, e.g., an isolate of *S. aureus* which is resistant to ceftazadime, is also likely to be resistant to cefuroxime.

The importance of this concept is also in the management of patients. For instance, if there is clinical failure with an antimicrobial in the treatment of a case, it is not advisable to administer related antimicrobials in the case.

Most of the times when we talk of resistance in a microorganism, it is implied that the microorganism, which was previously susceptible to the action of the antimicrobial, is now not susceptible to it.

What are the various factors that have lead to increased spread of drug resistance in microbes? Discuss their role.

A.8 These should be clearly understood, as then the factors that can lead to control are effectively implemented. The role of the environment that leads to spread of resistance, should also be understood, so that steps can be taken to minimize the spread of resistant strains in the environment. One should be aware of the conditions that can lead to the organism colonizing an individual and cause spread from one person to another. As is well known that overcrowding, inadequate ventilation and sanitation can lead to increased transmission of the resistant organism, so the following measures can be taken to minimize cross-infection.

- Standard hand-hygiene procedures to minimize the spread of resistant organisms.
- Use of containment isolation procedures for critical patients and those infected with resistant organisms.
- Minimization of environmental contamination.
- Epidemiological monitoring of resistant organisms in wards and critical care areas.
- Minimize drugs release in the hospital environment, which also encourages development of drug resistant organisms.

It is said that colonization of new cases with drug resistant organisms is to be minimized. Administration of an antimicrobial to a patient can increase this possibility. This is because the suppression of the susceptible strains amongst the normal flora, would encourage the resistant organisms to proliferate; as they would face less competition for nutrition and space from susceptible strains that otherwise would have competed Fig. 17.6.1.

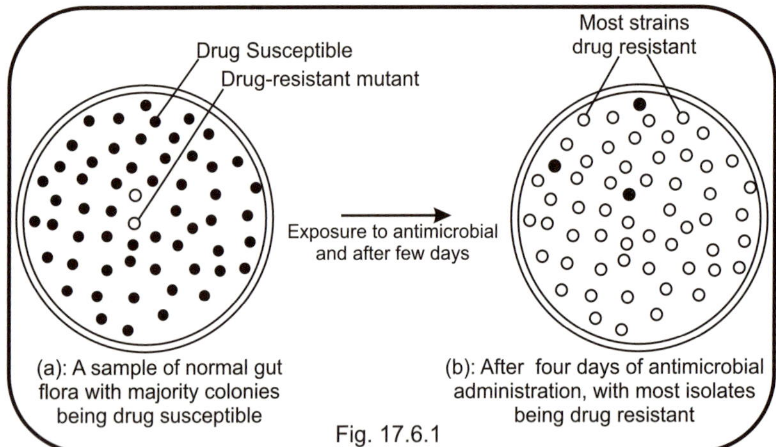

Fig. 17.6.1

Assume a case harbours, as a very small part of his intestinal flora, a strain of *E.coli* carrying a plasmid with genes encoding resistance to chloramphenicol, tetracycline, streptomycin and trimethoprim and develops dysentery with *S. flexneri,* which is susceptible to all common antimicrobials. If he gets treated with chloramphenicol, most of the normal flora (excluding multidrug resistant strain of *E. coli*) and the Shigella gets destroyed, with multidrug resistant *E.coli* strains becoming a predominant one in the individual. Further plasmid transfer can occur between resistant *E.coli* and some surviving shigella strains, resulting in the latter acquiring the drug resistance genes. The latter in future can multiply and cause a relapse of dysentery, with a shigella strain that would be multidrug resistant. Many enteric gram negative bacilli have become multiresistant to as many as 15 agents. The resistant strains are often found in a very small proportion of members of a species (before the introduction of an antimicrobial) and their frequency greatly increases with usage of antimicrobial.

Other factors that can minimize the above transition, is usage of antimicrobials according to the susceptibility pattern of the infecting isolate (wherever feasible) and preferable usage of narrow rather than broad spectrum antimicrobials. The latter are usually used, when aetiology of infection is not known. For this reason, antimicrobials should not be used for causes, where benefit may be minimal; as in a common cold (where aetiology is mostly viral)

Another factor that encourages development and colonization of drug resistant organisms in a host (human) is **inadequate** *dosage* and *duration* of an antimicrobial. Many patients and even the medical personnel are to be blamed for this practice of discontinuing the antimicrobial, once the symptoms disappear (Fig. 17.6.2). The compliance in taking the complete course of the antimicrobial must be ensured. This would result in the eradication of the concerned organism from the body and prevent the masking of serious infections; without eradicating them.

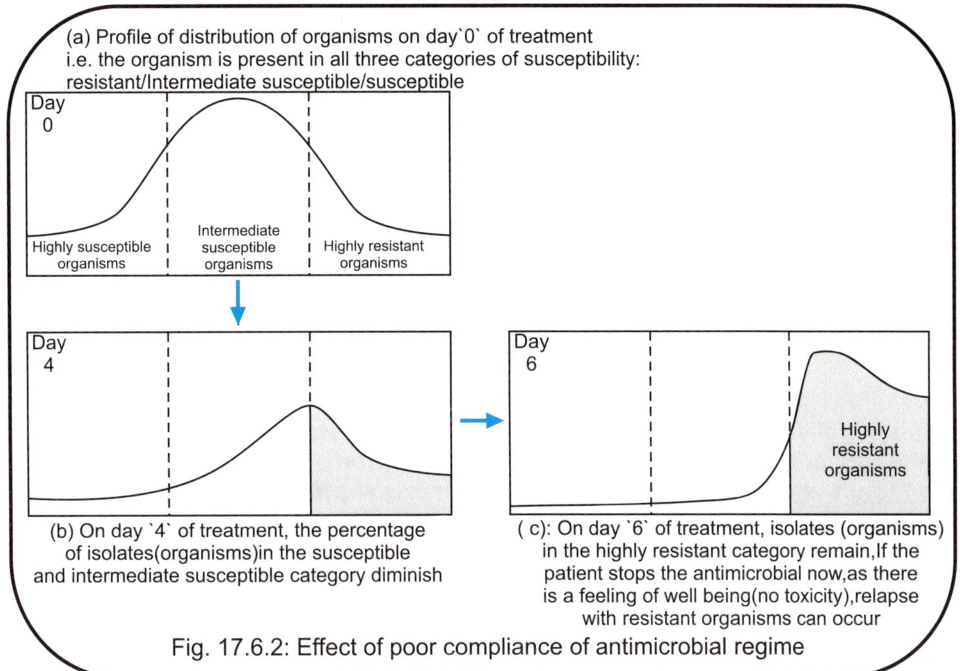

Fig. 17.6.2: Effect of poor compliance of antimicrobial regime

Massive use of antimicrobial agents in numerous fields; as farming, veterinary and medical front leads to significant *environmental pollution* with the antimicrobial agents getting excreted for prolonged periods in the faeces and urine of the consumers. Such a scenario disturbs the ecological balance and promotes antibiotic resistance.

What are the factors that can control drug resistance?

A.9 It has been well established from many studies that the prevalence of antibiotic resistant strains is generally proportional to the extent of usage of a particular antibiotic in the area. A notable exception to this rule [concept],is *Streptococcus pyogenes* that has failed to become resistant to penicillins, though some evidence of tolerance has been seen The reduction of usage of the particular antimicrobial has resulted in the reduction of the proportion of resistant isolates (to that antimicrobial) in many studies, though not exactly to the pre-antibiotic period. There is also a vicious cycle that operate in the environment, in which treatment with one antimicrobial, though successfully manages one infectious episode; leaves behind few organisms resistant to that antimicrobial. The next infectious illness may require a newer antimicrobial. The above cycle may be repeated, in which the organism may keep developing resistance to the newer antimicrobials.

Another strategy to control the antimicrobial resistance, is to condemn and stop the practice of *lacing the animal feed* with antimicrobials; as penicillin, tetracycline and fluoroquinolones, with aim of decreasing (animal) intestinal infections and increasing the animal growth rate. This practice resulted in selection of drug resistant strain in the animals; which ultimately make their way into humans

Other measures

- Inappropriate usage of antimicrobials for surgical prophylaxis should be discouraged.
- Second line antimicrobials should be reserved for serious infection
- Over the counter sale, of antimicrobials (without proper prescription), prevalent in many Asian and other countries should be stopped
- Right combinations as:
  - β-lactam drug + β lactamase inhibitor
  - Synergistic combination (Trimethoprim + Sulfamethoxazole) (Penicillin + aminoglycoside) should be encouraged.
- New drug discovery to be encouraged (a new drug to come into market may take about 10 years, after undergoing 4 phases of clinical trial)

– Newer approaches; as developing drugs, based on quorum sensing, intercellular signalling compound, to be encouraged.
– Programmed cell death or inhibitors and antisense drugs to be exploited in the development of new antimicrobials.

To manage the optimal usage of antimicrobials in a medical institution or a bigger region, an *antibiotic policy* should be formulated by key medical personnel. The idea is to have the availability of an antibiotic formulary and antibiotic guidelines for treatment of general and specific infections. Practices as electronic auditing should be encouraged, so as to monitor the trends of antimicrobial usage. Specific practices; as periodic change of antimicrobials for treatment of infections may play a minor role. This practice may help in decreasing the emergence of resistant bacteria in the environment.

Integrated Clinical Case Based Study 1

A thirty year old housewife, Santosh with pulmonary tuberculosis (left apical lung cavity) was started on Anti-tubercular treatment (ATT). She started feeling well, after a course of 1 month of therapy and discontinued the treatment. After 2 months, her initial symptoms reappeared, she restarted the therapy, to discontinue it once again; after two months of therapy. She presented again to the medical OPD, after four months in a worsened condition. Currently; she is not responding to the administered regime of ATT.

What is likely diagnosis?

A.1 **(a)** The case is likely to have multidrug resistant tuberculosis. MDR-TB is defined as a form of tuberculosis, in which the bacteria that are causing the disease are resistant to at least INH and Rifampicin, two of the first line (most effective) drugs used in treatment.

How can the diagnosis of MDR-TB be microbiologically proved?

A.1 **(b)** This entity is difficult to be microbiologically proved, as classically, it requires a successful isolation of the bacterium from the clinical sample and then performing a mycobacterial drug susceptibility testing to demonstrate the drug resistance.

What key factor led to her current problem?

A.1 **(c)** Non compliance to antituberculous treatment (ATT) regime occurying twice at a gap of a few weeks.

What are the likely reasons for M.tuberculosis isolates to become drug resistance in this case?

A.2 Although *M.tuberculosis* can naturally acquire drug resistance by spontaneous mutation, for most of the drug resistance, man can be made responsible. The drug resistance arises due to preferential selection of naturally occurring resistant mutants, due to inadequate drug regimens. The common reasons for this scenario are non-compliance by the patient (i.e., not adhering to the treatment regimen), inadequate regimen prescribed by the physician and poor quality of drugs.

What is the expected prevalence of MDR-TB in India?

A.3 The expected prevalence (based on many surveys) is approximately 3% amongst new cases and 12-18% in re-treatment cases.

What strategies can be used to minimize the development of drug resistance in M.tuberculosis?

A.4 The TB control programme emphasizes many components. An optimal leadership in the form of good policies and plans have to be provided. Adequate health financing of the programmes has to be provided. The health workforce has to be adequate and trained regularly. Good quality drugs especially rifampicin have to be made available, which should have good bio-availability. Practices as over the counter sale of anti-TB drugs have to be curtailed.

What is Extensively drug resistant tuberculosis [XDR-TB] and TDR-TB? Mention one reason to be scared over the development of this entity.

A.5 The WHO Global Task Force: defines XDR-TB as tuberculosis caused by strains with resistance to rifampicin and isoniazid in addition to any fluoroquinolone and at least one of the three following injectable drugs: capromycin, kanamycin or amikacin.

Totally drug resistant (TDR-TB) is defined as Tuberculosis caused by *M. tuberculosis* strains with resistance to all first line drugs (INH, Rifampicin, Pyrazinamide and Streptomycin) and second line drugs (as ofloxacin, Kanamycin, PAS, ethionamide and other)

The XDR-TB is life threatening to the individual, as very few drug options are available to treat the case. The drugs used in controlling this infection, are expensive. These resistant strains are known to circulate from case to contacts.

Describe the conventional anti-tubercular susceptibility tests?

A.6 **(a)** (i) *Absolute concentration method*-A number of media containing varying concentrations of drug are inoculated with the test strain only, the minimum inhibitory concentration is estimated to various drugs.

(ii) *Resistance ratio method:* Two sets of media(often LJ medium) are inoculated ,one set with the test strain and the other with the standard strain of known sensitivity (often H37Rv strain of *M. tuberculosis*). The minimum inhibitory concentration (MIC) is defined, as the lowest concentration of the drug that inhibits the growth, reading taken after 3weeks of incubation. A strain is considered susceptible, if the ratio of MIC (test)/MIC (control) is 1-2 and resistant; if the ratio is 8 or more.

(iii) *Proportion method:* Strains in a population can have varying degrees of susceptibility, so here average susceptibility is estimated. A strain is considered as resistant, if ≥1% grows in the presence of drug (colonies counted).

What are their limitations?

A.6 (b) These antimicrobial susceptibility techniques are time consuming and can take few weeks, before results are available.

Enumerate and describe the newer anti-tubercular susceptibility tests.

A.6 (c) (i) BACTEC 460 (radiometric)

(ii) BacT/ALERT (colorimetric, estimating carbon dioxide production)

(iii) MGIT (fluorometric)

(iv) GenoType MTBDR plus (multiplex PCR and DNA hybridization assay)

(v) Chemiluminescence (luciferase reporter mycobacteriophage technology)

For details of these techniques (See. A 6b, c., p. 235)

Integrated Clinical Case Based Study 2

An outbreak of multi-drug resistance Salmonella Typhi occurred in India, which peaked in 1992-93 *(Prakash and Pillai 1993)*. There are a number of lessons to be learnt from this episode.

What was the mechanism of drug resistance in this outbreak?

A.1(a) This was as a result of plasmid mediated S.Typhi strain, which carried the plasmid with drug resistance genes to many antimicrobials. The strains varied to the pattern and size of the plasmid, they carried. Many of these strains had antimicrobial resistance genes to 'ACSuST' and were resistant to all these antimicrobials; namely ampicillin, chloramphenicol, sulphonamide, streptomycin and tetracycline.

Enumerate the differences between mutational and transferable drug resistance

A.1(b) See table 17.6.1.

What were the likely reasons for this outbreak to have arisen?

A.2 One of the apparent key reasons for this outbreak, was the misuse of chloramphenicol. This drug was used excessively and empirically by private practitioners for treating all types of fevers and gut infections; as diarrhoea. This drug was cheap and effective. No kind of microbiological testing; as culture and antimicrobial susceptibility testing was done on majority of the cases, where this antimicrobial was adminstered.

What change occurred in the S. Typhi phage type patterns in India, after this outbreak?

A.3 After this outbreak, MDR S. Typhi phage type E1 emerged, as the most prevalent S.Typhi strain outnumbering all other phage types as O and A that were prevalent then.

What change occurred globally in the treatment of enteric fever in areas, where this drug resistant strain of S.Typhi became prevalent?

A.4 In the areas, where MDR S. Typhi phage type E1 were prevalent, quinolone group of drugs; as ciprofloxacin became the drug of choice for typhoid fever; replacing chloramphenicol.

Could this outbreak of drug resistant S. Typhi in 1992-93 have been prevented?

A.5 This outbreak could have been prevented, if the antimicrobials especially chloramphenicol had been judiciously used, i.e., there had been a rational use of antimicrobials.

Table 17.6.1: Differences between mutational and transferable drug resistance

Mutational drug resistance	Transferable drug resistance
Resistance due to mutation	Resistance due to gene transfer
Involves one drug at a time	Multiple drugs involved
Low degree resistance	High degree resistance
Can be prevented by combination of drugs	Can not be prevented by combination of drugs
Resistance does not spread	Spreads to same or different genera
Mutants may be defective	Not defective

Antimicrobial Susceptibility Tests

One of the key contributions of the Clinical Microbiology laboratory is the generation of the antibiotic susceptibility reports for the admitted and the OPD case. Requisitioning an appropriate type of susceptibility test is of paramount importance. Let's understand the intricacies of this technology with the help of an integrated clinical based study.

Integrated Clinical Based Study 1

A 40 year man, Kailash was diagnosed to be having infective endocarditis. The echocardiography revealed vegetations on the aortic valve and blood culture revealed growth of 'viridans' streptococci (*S.sanguis*).

What category of antimicrobial susceptibility test would you like to perform on the isolate obtained from the above case? Explain.

A.1 (a) A quantitative antimicrobial susceptibility; such as e-test (MIC test) would be desirable in this case. This case is having a critical infection of the heart and it is important that adequate concentration of the antimicrobial be achieved at the affected site to eradicate the infection.

What is the role of empirical and definitive therapy in this case?

A.1 (b) Ideally, the identification of the infectious agent causing the disease and its antibiotic susceptibility pattern should be available before antimicrobial therapy is initiated. However this is mostly not feasible

Rational antibacterial therapy can be categorized; as initial *empirical therapy*; which is usually on clinician's judgement and is a 'blind' therapy. This is usually followed by a *specific/definitive treatment*, which is usually based on antibiotic susceptibility test report. The definitive therapy is usually initiated, if it the susceptibility report is in contradiction with the initial treatment being given. For example; Cefotaxime is being administered to this case but the antibiotic susceptibility report, reported it in the resistant category, then the treatment is changed. In the absence of an antibiotic susceptibility report, the clinician can switch over to another drug, if the patient does not seem to be responding to the initial drug, after adequate observation time is over.

What are the antimicrobial susceptibility tests trying to achieve?

A.1 (c) The tests help to predict the effectiveness of the antimicrobial drugs inside the body (i.e., 'in vivo').

Is antimicrobial susceptibility testing required for all isolated pathogens?

A.1 (d) It is required for most pathogens, except some organisms such as group A streptococci (which are uniformly susceptible to penicillin). Most anaerobes (except Bacteriodes) are also uniformly susceptible to penicillin.

How does one choose the antimicrobials to be included for testing in a susceptibility test?

A.1 (e) These depend on the clinical entity, identity of the isolated microorganism and the body site from where pathogen is isolated (different body sites; as urine, blood etc. have different drug concentration).

What do the terms susceptible, intermediate susceptible and resistant in an antimicrobial susceptibility report convey?

A.1 (f) *'Susceptible'* implies that the organism is readily inhibited by the concentrations of antimicrobial attainable in the blood or urine (in the case of those agents, only active in the urinary tract) with doses appropriate for treatment of uncomplicated systemic infections, caused by the infecting organism. The infection responds (mostly) to the normal dosage of the antimicrobial.

'Resistant' implies that organism is not inhibited by normally attainable drug levels. The infection is unlikely to respond to the usual dosage of antimicrobials. *'Intermediate susceptible';* implies range to antimicrobial, should be specially studied, if therapy with that agent has to be used. This category implies two situations, in which these

drugs can be used. One, if the antimicrobial can be used at a higher dosage because of low toxicity of the drug. Two, if the antimicrobial is concentrated at focus of infection, e.g., urine.

Resistance and susceptibility are not always absolute. For example, relatively non-toxic antimicrobial agents; such as penicillin or cephalosporin can be administered in massive doses and may thereby inhibit some pathogens that would normally be considered as resistant 'in vitro'.

How can the antimicrobial susceptibility tests be classified?

A.2 (a) There are several classifications. One classification can be according to the *type of microorganisms* being tested, namely- antibacterial, anti TB, antifungal, antiviral and antiparasitic tests. Antibacterial and antituberculous tests are the commonest antimicrobial susceptibility tests, especially the former. Antituberculous tests are mostly performed only in reference laboratories, where provision of isolation and containment exist. Antiviral and antiparasitic susceptibility tests are less developed and available only in few laboratories.

Another classification is based on the type of the tests being performed; either *classical or automated.* In the former; the procedures are laborious and usually follow the 18 hour incubation period. In the latter, as the name indicates, test requires minimum labour and the incubation format is usually short. Some systems provide results in a few hours (3-6), while for slow growing organism it may require 2 days.

Another classification is one the basis, whether the tests are of *qualitative or quantitative* nature. In the former, the report only tells, whether the microorganisms is resistant, intermediate susceptible (moderately susceptible) or susceptible. In the latter category test, report considers quantitative aspects. These tests belong to dilution category. The two important tests in this category are the MIC and MBC. The dilution series can be in broth (broth dilution method) or agar based (agar dilution method). The broth dilution tests can be macrodilution or microdilution (in microtiter plate) based. The former are cumbersome and now outdated. One of the advantages of performing the broth dilution technique is that the same tubes, can be used for determining the MBC. Semi-automated and automated methods are also available commercially.

Epsilometer test (E test) is a recently developed strip diffusion test to determine the MIC of the microorganism to antimicrobials. It was developed by Ann Bolstrom from Sweden. It is 5 cm long plastic strip, one surface of it is marked with MIC reading scale and the reverse side contains predefined exponential grade of the antimicrobial.

Describe the evolution of the antimicrobial susceptibility tests?

A.2 (b) For many years, after the second world war, the newly discovered antimicrobials were considered as 'wonder drugs', so much so that Paul Ehrlich, even coined the term 'Magic bullets', so there was no need of any antimicrobial susceptibility tests. However; as the time progressed, increased antimicrobial resistance started getting reported and the need of such tests was felt. Initially these tests caused a lot of confusion, as the many variables in the tests were not standardized and the different laboratories reported the same tests differently.

What are the indications of performing the qualitative antimicrobial susceptibility tests?

A.2 (c)
(i) All cases; where pathogenic organisms are isolated.
(ii) In immunocompromised/immunodeficient individuals, these tests may have to be performed, even when commensal organisms are isolated.
(iii) For identification of some microbes, as bacitracin sensitivity; for identification of group A streptococci.
(iv) In epidemiologic studies, to study the trends of antimicrobial susceptibility.

Describe the technique of qualitative antimicrobial susceptibility tests.

A.2 (d) Most of the qualitative antibiotic susceptibility techniques are disc diffusion tests, based on making a lawn culture of the test organism and then allowing the drug from the filter disc impregnated with antibiotic to diffuse into the agar medium at a rate dependent on its physical and chemical characteristics. The plates are then incubated overnight. At some particular distance from each disc, the antibiotic is diluted to the point that it no longer inhibits microbial growth. The diameter of the zone of inhibition of growth is dependent on numerous factors; including susceptibility (MIC) of the organism, growth rate, disc concentration and diffusibility of the antimicrobial. The diameters of the zone of inhibition obtained with different antimicrobials are measured and converted to categories; as susceptible/resistant/intermediate susceptible by references to a standard table.

The ideal inoculum after overnight incubation gives uniform semi-confluent growth. The density of microbes usually used to make inoculum is of density, that corresponds to approximately 10^8 cfu/ml, by comparing its turbidity with that of 0.5 McFarland opacity standards.

The medium usually used is Mueller Hinton medium for most bacteria.

Control strains of *E.coli* and *Staphylococcus aureus,* American type culture collection (ATCC) or National Culture Type Collection (NCTC) are used for CLSI/ Kirby-Bauer and Stoke's methods, respectively. These strains act as controls for the test and help in the validation of the performed test.

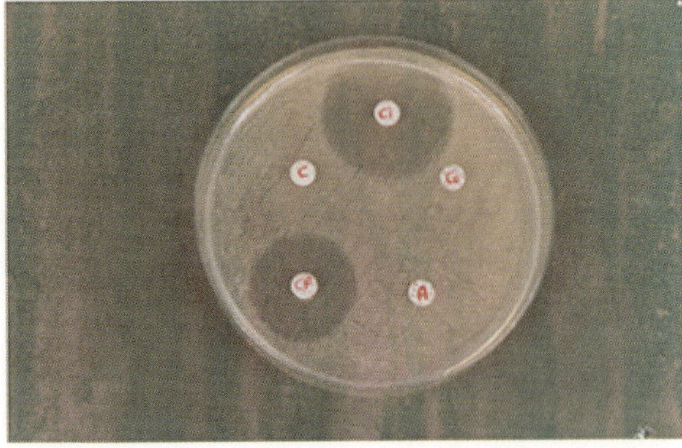

Fig. 17.7.1: CLSI disc diffusion antibiotic susceptibility test

Mention the principle of reporting in Kirby-Bauer/CLSI technique.

A.2 (e) In the Kirby-Bauer/CLSI method (Fig. 17.7.1), the control strain is not inoculated on the same plate as the test strain and the zone of inhibition for each antibiotic is determined and compared to standard values for each bacterial type. The organism is considered to be susceptible to an antibiotic, if the zone of inhibition is equal to or larger than the predetermined zone for that antibiotic.

Describe the Stoke's method for antimicrobial susceptibility testing.

A.2 (f) *Stokes method* involves comparison of zones of growth inhibition of test strain to control strains and then interpreting them (Fig. 17.7.2). The central (middle) one-third of the plate has the test bacterium inoculated, while the upper and lower one-third of the plate has the control bacterial strain inoculated. In the modified Stokes' method, disc diffusion test (method), the positions of the test and control bacterial strains are reversed. If the zone of the inhibition of the test strain is equal to or more than that of the control strain, it indicates susceptibility to that antibiotic.

If the zone of inhibition of the test strain is less than 3 mm, it indicates resistance to that antibiotic.

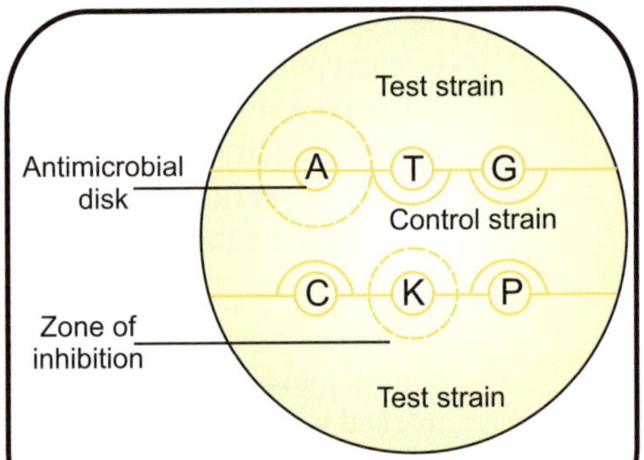

Test strain
Antimicrobial disk
A T G
Control strain
C K P
Zone of inhibition
Test strain

Fig. 17.7.2:Modified Stokes antibiotic susceptibility test

If the zone of inhibition of the test strain is less than that of the control stain but the difference between the two is more than 3mm, it indicates intermediate susceptibility to that antibiotic. However; if the difference between the two is less than 3 mm, it indicates susceptibility to that antibiotic.

What are the limitations of the qualitative antimicrobial susceptibility tests?

A.2 (g) The disc diffusion methods are not valid for:

(i) Slow growing organisms and fastidious organisms

(ii) Antimicrobials which have poor diffusion characteristic, e.g., polymyxin must be interpreted cautiously

(iii) Where quantitative and bactericidal information is required

(iv) Less effective for anaerobic organisms

Mention about the internal/external quality control of antimicrobial susceptibility tests and the role of the CLSI recommendations?

A.2 (h) *Internal quality* control denotes a set of procedures undertaken by the medical and laboratory personnel (including paramedical) for continuously and concurrently assessing the laboratory conditions and thereby ensuring accurate results.

External quality assessment is a system of objectively assessing the laboratory performance by an external agency. The aim of this assessment is to improve the internal quality control.

CLSI stands for Clinical Laboratory Standard Institute, USA. The recommendations given by this institute include detailed steps that are to be followed to perform antimicrobial susceptibility tests and to interpret them.

As we know the testing of the antimicrobial activity 'in vitro' can be affected by numerous factors; as pH of medium, composition of media, size of inoculum of testing microorganisms etc. Different laboratories in a region and across different countries should follow one methodology, so that uniform antimicrobial susceptibility data becomes available for monitoring local and international trends in antimicrobial susceptibility. If this does not occur, then incorrect clinical reporting and confusion in the scientific literature would occur.

What are the indications of performing the quantitative antimicrobial susceptibility tests?

A.3 (a) (i) In critical infections, where it is important that the adequate concentration of the drug is achieved at the infection site, e.g., infective endocarditis

(ii) When qualitative antimicrobial susceptibility report indicates an organism to be intermediate susceptible to an antimicrobial (equivocal results are obtained with qualitative antimicrobial susceptibility tests)

(iii) When the administered drug is toxic and where the therapeutic and toxic level are quite close (narrow therapeutic zone), e.g., aminoglycosides.

(iv) Infections in compromised individuals (in the absence of host defence factors), which require bactericidal activity of the antimicrobial; where elimination of infecting organism may not occur

(v) Where minor degree of antimicrobial resistance is to be determined

What do you understand by 'Inhibitory quotient' and 'Therapeutic index'?

A.3 (b) *Inhibitory quotient:* It is the ratio of average drug peak achievable level at clinical site (from where organism isolated) to MIC.

The drugs with lowest human toxicity should be chosen. The concept of *therapeutic index* deals with this aspect, which is defined as the ratio of a drug toxic dose to its minimum effective dose. The closer these two figures are to each other, greater is the potential for toxic drug reaction. For instance; an antimicrobial with a therapeutic index of 2(10 µg/ml toxic dose/5 µg ml), is a safer choice than that one with a therapeutic index of 1.2(10 µg/ml/8 µg/ml)

Describe the concept of MIC and MBC.

A.3 (c) **Minimum Inhibitory Concentration(MIC)** – It is the lowest concentration (or the highest dilution) of the antimicrobial agent that inhibits growth of a microbe, which may be detected as lack of visual turbidity (in liquid medium) (Fig. 17.7.3). This information helps in determining the smallest effective dosage of an antimicrobial and in providing a comparative index against other antimicrobials.

If the MIC of the antimicrobial being tested to the microorganism is much above the achievable level of antimicrobial at the required site, the microorganism is said to be *resistant.*

The clinical importance is that, it is the minimal concentration of the antibiotic that must be achieved at the site of infection to inhibit the growth of the microorganisms. By knowing the MIC/MBC (minimum bactericidal concentration) values and the levels of the antimicrobial that may be achieved in body fluid; such as urine, the clinician can select the appropriate antimicrobial, dosage schedule and the route of administration.

In *broth microdilution (MIC) method*, a sterile plastic microdilution tray containing various concentrations of antimicrobial agents is taken. It is inoculated with standardized suspension of test bacteria and incubated overnight at 37°C, followed by observation. The basic broth microdilution MIC panel utilizes cation-adjusted Mueller-Hinton broth. For full range MIC testing, five to eight concentrations representing a therapeutically achievable range for each agent are usually tested. *Breakpoint MIC* testing represents a modification of microdilution MIC, testing in which generally one to three concentrations of each agent are tested.

Minimum Bactericidal Concentration (MBC): It is the lowest concentration that can kill 99.9% of microorganisms or the lowest amount of antimicrobial agent that allows less than 0.1% (or kills more than 99.9%) of the original inoculum to survive; as judged by subculture (Fig. 17.7.3). Such a definition is taken, as it very difficult to measure, when exactly 100% lysis occurs. It determines the ability of the antimicrobial agent to kill the bacteria. When an antibiotic's MBC is at least 32 times greater than MIC, the organism may be *tolerant* to that drug. This test can be performed by subculturing the broths from the wells showing no growth and doing a CFU/ml count.

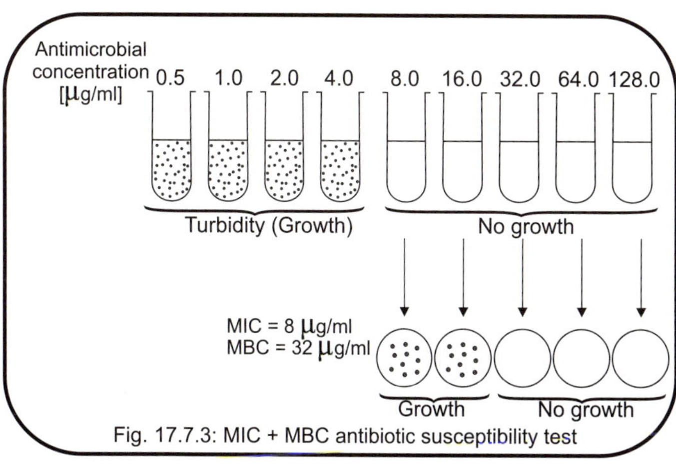

Fig. 17.7.3: MIC + MBC antibiotic susceptibility test

Describe the E test.

A.3 **(d)** E test see A.2(a)

What is clinical break point?

A.4 A *breakpoint* represents the concentration of an antimicrobial that separates population of microorganisms. *Clinical* breakpoint implies the concentration that can be achieved clinically and separate the susceptible from the resistant organism population.

In the past, a safety margin of 8-10 times the MIC of the relevant drug at the site of infection, was considered desirable to ensure successful treatment of the infection.

Why were such high levels of antimicrobial recommended?

A.5 There were a number of reasons:

(i) Increase of serum proteins can lower concentration of antimicrobial.

(ii) Level of the antimicrobial at the actual site of infection may be lower than from the site (mostly serum), from where the concentration of the antimicrobial is being tested.

e.g., the concentration of the antimicrobial at the wound site may be lower than the serum, where the antimicrobial needs to act.

(iii) Tissue inhibitors can decrease the efficacy of the antimicrobial (as can inactivate antimicrobial).

Currently to establish breakpoint, pharmacodynamic data are given emphasis.

The antimicrobial susceptibility report of an isolate from a case was susceptibe to cefotaxime but resistant to penicillin. However; inadvertently when penicillin was administered to the case, the case was able to resolve the infection. Explain this episode (i.e., the discrepancy of the 'in vitro' penicillin resistant report).

A.6 The activity of antimicrobial 'in vivo' is more complex and unpredictable than 'in vitro'. The patients defense systems can come into 'play' and use the limited antimicrobial activity of the drug to overcome the infection.

If the antimicrobial susceptibility report of Streptococcus spp. isolated from a case read as susceptible to cefotaxime. However the case was not able to resolve the infection, on optimal administration of this antimicrobial. Explain this episode (i.e., the discrepancy of the 'in vitro' cefotaxime susceptible report)

A.7 It can occur due to the following conditions

(i) Antimicrobial not reaching the site of infection, e.g., does not reach effectively the cerebrospinal fluid in CNS infections.

(ii) Concentration at site, where antimicrobial is required is less than, where assessed.

e.g., tissue levels of antimicrobial are less than in the serum, whose drug concentrators are usually analysed.

(iii) Inhibitors of drug are present at the inflammation site

(iv) Patients defense are compromised, so microorganism after inhibition, regrow; after antimicrobial is tapered off.

(v) Few resistant cells (microorganisms) do not get analyzed in the test.

(vi) Infection is caused by multiple microorganisms, some of which are resistant to the drug.

What do you understand by therapeutic drug monitoring?

A.8 *Therapeutic drug monitoring (antimicrobic assays):* This is required clinically, when toxic drugs are being administered and is usually performed by rapid immunoassay technology. In the past, biological techniques (bioassays) were mostly used.

While performing these, it is important to know if more than one antimicrobial is being used to treat a patient, so that a procedure is employed to ensure that the antimicrobial under consideration gets measured; for example, if amikacin level are to be measured in the presence of penicillin, a β-lactamase preparation can be added to inactivate the penicillin.

What do you understand by primary disc diffusion test?

A.9 *Primary Disc diffusion tests* are performed directly on clinical specimens; as urine, instead of the usual technique of performing on pure cultures of bacteria. Such approaches are not recommended, as they can give erratic results, due to difficulty, especially in standardization of the sample inoculum. However in critical cases, this procedure may be performed to get some clue for the initiation of the antimicrobial therapy.

What is antimicrobial stewardship programme?

A.10 It is a program recommended by CDC in 2014 to be implemented by all acute care hospitals. This programme can result in improved quality of patient care, reduced adverse effects, improved quality of patient care, improved patient safety, reduced treatment failure and reduced antibiotic resistance.

The key elements of this program include leadership commitment, accountability, drug expertise, action tracking, reporting and education.

Microbial Typing Technique

Efforts have been for a long time in Europe to eliminate Measles, by an effective vaccination programme. However this has not been possible, due to importation of Measles from neighbouring countries. In 2011 in Norway, four outbreaks of measles were reported by measles viruses of genotypes B3, D4 and D9 *(Eurosurveillance 2012)*.

Microbial typing is an important technique that helps to study of outbreaks, detect the index case and delineate other parameters. Let's study this technology.

What are the indications of microbial typing; especially strain typing?

A.1 To investigate outbreaks, which could be occupying in *hospitals, cities or even across countries (in pandemics), e.g., of MDR S. Typhi, Avian Influenza, Food poisoning, Cholera etc. Without performing strain identification by genotyping method, it is not possible to declare an outbreak.

The study would help to track the path of the outbreak and may help in determining the point source of an outbreak. If the latter can be found, the outbreak can be controlled and it could be prevented in the future.

*examples of hospital outbreaks could be bacterial (Klebsiella, Serratia) and viral (RSV, measles) in a neonatal or an intensive care unit.

When do you suspect an outbreak to have occured?

A.2 When the frequency of isolation of a pathogenic microbe outnumbers the usual baseline recovery rate.

e.g., The isolation number of methicillin resistant *Staphylococcus aureus* (MRSA) in a particular ward is 40 in a particular month in comparison to 5 from the same ward in the previous year in the same month.

e.g., the number of *Salmonella* Typhi isolated from India in 2007 is 10,000 in comparison to 6,000 in 2006.

What do you understand by 'index case'?

A.3 The *index case* is the first patient that indicates the existence of an outbreak. Earlier case may be found and are labelled as *primary secondary*, *tertiary* etc. "Patient zero" was used to refer to the index case in the spread of HIV in North America.

How do you classify the typing methods for microbes?

A.4 The techniques can be categorized into two broad groups, namely *phenotypic* based methods and *genotypic* based methods as depicted in the table 17.8.1.

Table 17.8.1: Typing Methods for microbes

Phenotypic based methods	Genotyping based methods
• Serotyping (using antisera) • Biotyping (using biochemical and other methods) • Antibiogram (pattern of an isolate according to antibiotic susceptibility testing) • Bacteriophage typing (pattern produced by phage application) (Fig. 17.8.1) • MLEE (Multi-locus enzyme electrophoresis) – whole cell protein is subject to electrophoresis in starch gel and then exposed to chromogenic substrate for detection of enzymatic activity	• General – plasmid finger printing • **Restriction enzyme based** - Restriction fragment length polymorpism (RFLP) - REA of plasmid DNA - Pulse field gel electrophoresis (PFGE) - Ribotyping **PCR based** – random amplification of polymorphic DNA (RAPD) - Rep PCR (Repetitive) - Amplified fragment length polymorphism (AFLP) • DNA sequencing

What are the attributes of a good typing method?

A.5 (i) High typeability (i.e., high percentage of strains should come in a category of being typeable)

(ii) Reproducibility (i.e., on repeating the test, same results should be obtained)

(iii) High discriminatory power (i.e., should be able to distinguish strains, which are closely related)

(iv) Easy to perform
(v) Clear interpretation
(vi) Criteria should be there and should be easy to interpret
(vii) Cost should be low

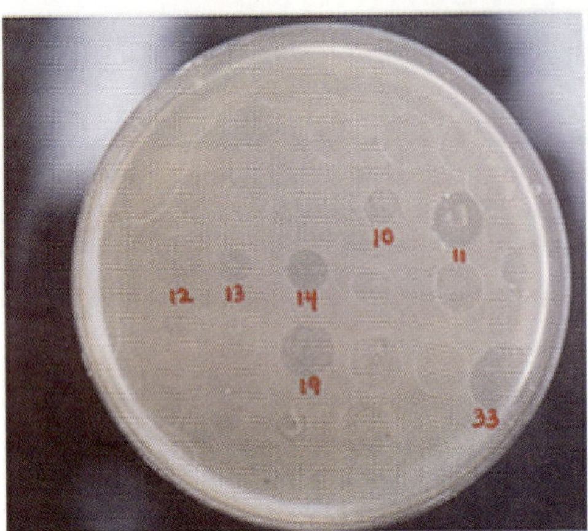

Fig.17.8.1: Phage typing for S. Typhi(E1 phage type)

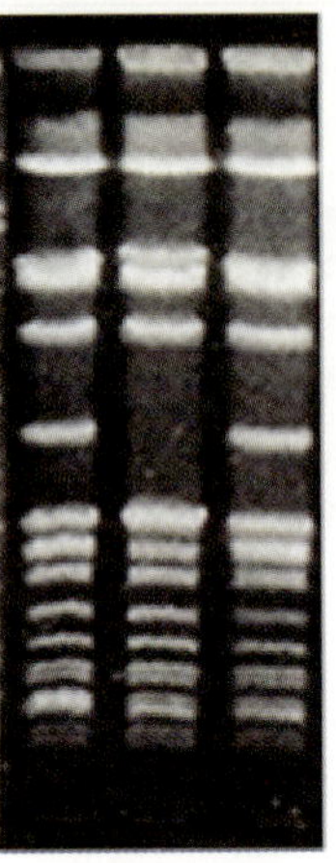

Fig.17.8.2: Pulse field Gel Electrophoresis profile

What are the advantages of the genotypic based methods over the phenotypic based typing methods?

A.6 (i) High discriminatory power at genetic level
(ii) High typeability and reproducibility
(iii) Helpful in evolutionary studies

What a the general advantages of the phenotypic based over the genotypic based typing methods?

A.7 (i) Ease of performance (ii) Low cost

Give a clinical example to show the importance of microbial typing at the strain level

A.8 **(a)** For three days consecutively in March 2011, more than five Klebsiella spp. strains were isolated daily from the blood of the neonates, from a neonatal unit of Kalawati Saran Children Hospital. This is in contrast to the highest isolation rate of Klebsiella spp. from blood in the month of February 2011, being less than two in a single day. This situation would be termed; as a bacterial outbreak in the neonatal unit and would call for an investigation of the outbreak, which would include typing of the strains, isolated from the various samples of the neonatal unit.

How can strain typing help in the management of the outbreak (mentioned above)?

A.8 **(b)** The important thing that the hospital epidemiologist/clinical microbiologist has to answer in this situation is, if the Klebsiella strains from the neonatal unit have arisen from a single point source or are different strains having arisen from multiple sources. The strain typing data can help to identify the possible source of infection, find its cause and lead to its eradication. The breakdown in the neonatal infection practices that would have lead to this outbreak could be addressed and prevented in future.

Mention one test based on phenotypic and genotypic based technique.

A.8 **(c)** – Klebocin typing (e.g., of phenotypic based typing technique)
– Ribotyping (e.g., of genotypic based typing technique)

Describe common genotypic based typing techniques

A.9 (i) **Plasmid fingerprinting:** the numbers and sizes of the plasmids present in an isolate, may provide critical information.

(ii) **Restriction enzyme analysis of chromosomal DNA:** In this technique, the chromosomal DNA of the strain to be typed is isolated; using standard protocol and then subjected to restriction endonucleases (which cuts the DNA at specific sites). Subsequently the lysates (product obtained, after lysis by restriction enzymes) are subjected to gel electrophoresis, the comparison of the strains is done by the pattern of the bands. A molecular marker (of a known strain is also run), which helps to find the molecular weight of the bands the test strains. The largest fragment will migrate slowest in the gel and will cluster close to the well, in which the sample was loaded. If gross differences are not detectable in the isolates on image analyzer (gel documentation system), a *scanning densitometer* can be used to locate and quantitate the bands.

This test is based on the principle that bacterial chromosome of the strains contains some regions that are variable and other regions that are highly conserved. The difference in nucleotide sequence of the variable regions, could be reflected in the restriction endonuclease patterns of chromosomal DNA, when the fragments are resolved on agarose gel. The pattern of the bands produced on the gel are called *restriction fragment length polymorphism (RFLPs)*. The limitation of this technique, is that sometimes different strains cannot be differentiated by this test and sometimes too many bands are produced in the technique, which make the analysis difficult.

(iii) **Ribotyping**

This test is based on the principle, that genes (DNA) encoding ribosomal RNA amongst different strains vary and would be reflected in this test.

In this test, first the restriction endonuclease analysis of the chromosomal DNA is performed on agarose gel; followed by transfer of the DNA fragments to a membrane (such as nitrocellulose/nylon). Subsequently DNA probes (radio labelled or enzyme labelled) are used to target the genes of ribosomal RNA. Hybridization reactions visible, as small number of bands (usually 2 to 10) reflect the RFLPs of the region. The latter procedure of using DNA probes, as a hybridization reaction, after blotting DNA from gel to a membrane, is known as *Southern blotting*.

(iv) **Pulse-field gel electrophoresis (Fig. 17.8.2)**

This technique is a modification of the technique of the REA of chromosomal DNA (RFLP analysis), in which many of the limitations of that technique are overcome. It is considered as a gold standard for typing of many microbes. The technique is named, after the use of pulsed electrical field across the agarose gel, that subjects the large DNA fragments to varying voltage, from varying angles (often pole reversal); at different time intervals. In this technique, such restriction enzymes are used, which have few (rare) restriction sites on the genomic DNA, so that only few (about 10 to 20) DNA fragments, which are large in size, often varying 10-1000 Kb are produced. Same or highly similar band profile, indicate identical or closely related strains.

Give examples of elementary phenotypic based typing techniques.

A.10

Table 17.8.2: Phenotypic based typing techniques

Technique	Microbes, where utilized
Antibiogram or Resistogram	*Staphylococcus aureus, Staphylococcus epidermidis, Clostridium difficile, Pseudomonas aeruginosa,* Salmonella spp., Proteus spp.
Biotyping	*Haemophilus influenzae, Escherichia coli,* Klebsiella species
Phage typing	*S. aureus,* Salmonella spp.
Bacteriocin typing	*P. aeruginosa* (Pyocin typing), Klebsiella (Klebocin typing)

Describe Bacteriocin typing.

A.11
- **Historical:** In the early twentieth century, specific substances produced by *E. coli* active against the other strains of same species were detected. The name 'colicin' was given to this substance. Subsequently such substances were found to be produced by other bacteria, and then the name coined was 'bacteriocin'.
- **Characteristics:** Bacteriocin is a protein like substance (antibiotic like) produced by one bacterium, which is capable of killing some strains of the same species. This characteristic has an application in the typing of some bacteria. Bacteriocin; especially pyocins have some structural resemblance to phages. The synthesis of bacteriocin is affected by colicinogenic factors, which are episomal in nature.
- **Applications:** The bacteriocins have been used in the typing of the following bacteria, namely Pseudomonas (pyocin typing), Klebsiella (Klebocin typing) and *E. coli* (colicin typing).
- **Procedure:**
  - Test strain streaked on the center of the culture plate.
  - Subsequently standard indicator strains of same species inoculated at right angles to the original inoculum.
  - Plate incubated and pattern of inhibition of standard indicator strains documented.
  - Interpretation carried out

- **Step 5:** Host cells containing recombinant DNA to be *selected*, on the basis of specific property conferred by the vector and identifying the transformed cell that contains the recombinant gene of interest.

  A challenge that remains at this stage, is that only a low percentage of host cells are transformed genetically. The *first* challenge is to identify, which of the bacteria have become infected by the vector. One trick sometimes used is to ensure that the plasmid carry a gene; for drug resistance to a particular antibiotic and incorporate that antibiotic to the culture medium, in which the host cells are grown (cultivated). Only those host cells would be able to grow in such a medium, which have incorporated the drug resistance genes in them. The *second* challenge is that one has thousands of bacteria (host cells), each one of which may be carrying a very tiny part of the total genome of the organism under study. How to find out, which of these host cells has the gene of interest to us? One of the techniques employed to identify the recombinant DNA clones is the Southern blot hybridization, named after Dr. Edward Southern, who developed this technique. Briefly in this technique, the suspected colonies are replica plated onto a filter paper, the nucleic acid in the colonies is denatured by exposure to alkali, followed by exposure to specific labeled DNA probes, which would identify (give a positive result) the colony containing the gene of interest.

- **Step 6:** Manufacture of gene products, namely proteins; which the gene codes

  Sometimes the gene is cloned to produce large amounts of protein, for instance the human insulin gene. In such a case, it is important that the gene of concern is placed exactly next to an appropriate control system. For the expression to occur, the cloned gene must contain the appropriate start and stop signals for the transcription and translation. So, the RNA polymerase of the host must recognize the promoter region of the cloned gene and transcribe DNA. Also, the ribosomal binding site must be recognized by the ribosome of the host.

  mnemonic for steps (of Lucknow student) – **'तोड़ो, काटो, जोड़ो, ठोको और नंबर बढ़ाओ'**

Enumerate the steps involved in the HBV vaccine synthesis.

A.4 See chapter 9, section 12, A4C, pg. 425-426

Describe the applications of genetic engineering technology (including gene therapy).

A.5 **Applications of genetic engineering** (recombinant DNA technology):

1. **Production of hormone**

   (a) *Human growth hormone (Somatotropin):* Used in treatment of growth disorders. It was the first protein made by *E. coli* through genetic engineering in 1977. The hormone has only fourteen amino acids, so a stretch of forty-two bases could code for this protein. It is used to treat a rare human disease called 'pituitary dwarf' caused by the failure of the pituitary gland to manufacture this hormone. Previous to the availability of this recombinant hormone, this hormone was procured from human pituitaries in post-mortem rooms by a tedious chemical technique. Such a limited and expensive product also had the limitation of getting contaminated by endotoxin and also the fear of transmitting prion mediated diseases; as Creutzfeldt-Jakob disease.

   (b) *Human insulin:* It is used to treat diabetes (IDDM). Previous to the availability of the recombinant insulin, this product was procured from slaughtered cattle and pigs. This process not only raised ethical issues, but the product also led to *insulin resistance and allergic reactions. The current business of manufacturing recombinant insulin is a thriving business.

   *Because of production of anti-insulin antibodies, as product was of foreign origin.

2. **Pharmaceutical products** (other than hormones and vaccines):

Protein	Use
Factor VIII^	Haemophilia
Factor IX	Christmas disease
Erythropoietin	Anaemia
Tissue plasminogen activator	Treat CAD and dissolve clot
Interferon-α	Chronic hepatitis B infection, HCV infection, some malignancies (as Kaposi Sarcoma, CML, hairy cell leukemia)
Interferon-β	Helpful in Multiple sclerosis
Interferon-γ	Chronic granulomatous disease.
Interleukin 2	Immunodeficiencies

Contd.

Contd.

Tumor necrosis factor	Cancers
Epidermal growth factor	Heal wounds
Bone growth factor	Heal fractures and treat osteoporosis
Monoclonal antibodies	See Section 2, pg. 119
Antibiotic	Infections (increased yield by techniques employing this technology
α1-antitrypsin	Emphysema

^Previous to the availability of the recombinant molecule, these products would be prepared from the fresh human blood by steps involving a series of fractionation, so there was always the fear of HIV, HBV and HCV transmission.

3. **Vaccines◊:**

Type	Use
Hepatitis A	Prevent hepatitis A
Hepatitis B	Prevent hepatitis B (recombinant vaccine)
AIDS subunit vaccine	In phase trial

◊ Deoxyribonucleic acid (DNA) vaccines represent a newer approach in vaccines. Here plasmid DNA is injected into muscle/skin cells, which is later expressed and acts as immunogen.

4. **In diagnosis:**

- Enzymes; as cholesterol oxidase– cholesterol metabolism disorders
- DNA probe
- RNA probe

Identifying microbes, genetic diseases; as cystic fibrosis and Duchenne muscular dystrophy and prenatal diagnosis of genetic defects.

5. **Gene therapy:**

This is one of the most exciting applications of genetic engineering, where a missing or a defective gene could be replaced with a healthy gene in the adult human cell, egg or sperm. Once the technique is developed and standardized, it would go a long way at least in treating, if not curing the genetic disorders. There are two basic approaches to this therapy, namely *germline therapy* and somatic cell therapy. In the former, fertilized egg is provided with a copy of the desired (correct) relevant gene and reimplanted into the mother. If the procedure is successful, the gene would be present in all the cells and optimally expressed.

The *somatic cell therapy* involves removal of the cells which are to undergo this treatment, performing the technique and placing them back in the body. The approaches applied commonly for gene delivery include transfection (infection with phage having the desired gene) and retrovirus infection. In a successful application, there would be a homologous recombination between the chromosomal gene (of the target cell) and the gene introduced into the cell by different means (vectors), so chromosome is replaced by the correct gene from the vector. This approach has been successful in cystic fibrosis, in which a fully functional copy of the 'cftr' gene is delivered to human cells.

Another disease for which clinical trials have occurred is *severe combined immunodeficiency* (SCID), in which the gene for the enzyme adenosine deaminate is defective. The derangement of this gene can debilitate the immune system.

Other diseases, where this approach could be effective include hemoglobinopathies (thalassemias), Hemophilia A and B, Duchenne's diseases dystrophy and lysosomal storage diseases.

6. **Applications in industry/agriculture** (i.e., other than medical)

By the process of genetic engineering, a class of microbes known as *genetically modified microorganisms* (GMOS) have been produced, some of which have novel applications. For instance; recombinant bacteria have been created, which can clean oil spill (in seas), there are viruses; which can act as insecticides and there are bacteria (*Pseudomonas syringae*), which can prevent frost damage to crops.

In India three Bt (*Bacillus thuringiensis*) crop species (cotton, corn and potato) have been commercialized with benefits to farmers (although controversy exists about its usage and safety).

Mention about personal genome service.

A.6 (a) **Personal genome service:** A saliva swab or a skin swab is swiped on a device and all the genomic data appears on computer screen, which can help know one's genomic make up (read half million points on genome). It relies on microarrays, that can detect lakhs of SNPs (single nucleotide polymorphisms) in DNA and make comparison.

It can help know one's susceptibility to diseases and help getting a specifically suited drug for ailments (instead of one drug suiting all)

Mention briefly about nanotechnology.

A.6 (b) **Nanotechnology:** It refers to anything engineered down to nanometer (a billionth of a meter). It provides the ability to isolate and manipulate single atoms. MIT engineer; K. Eric Drexler coined this term in the mid-80s. The technology enabled cheaper and faster medical diagnostics, newer therapeutics and novel methods of drug delivery (e.g., targeted delivery of anticancer drug).

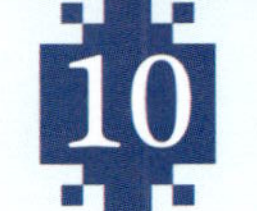

Vaccines

– **'Childhood vaccines are one of the greatest triumphs of modern medicine.Indeed parents whose children are vaccinated no longer have to worry about their child's death or disability from whooping cough, polio, diphtheria, hepatitis and a host of other infections'.**

— Ezekiel Emanuel

Let's study the BACTERIAL vaccines organized in a tabular fashion..

Bacterial Vaccine Types	Composition		Indications	Route & Dosage Schedule	Mechanism	Effectiveness	Adverse Effects	Contraindication/Special Precaution
Pneumo-coccal	• Monovalent composed of single Serotype • 23 valent 23 serotype (most prevalent) • Heptavalent protein (7 serotype) conjugated to protein	Capsular polysac-charide	Those at increased risk • adults > 65 years old • adults & children > 2 yrs. with chronic disease of Heart, Lung, Diabetes, alcoholism, asplenia & sickle cell disease; • immunocompromised individuals for ex-ample with Hodgkin's disease, lymphoma, multiple myeloma, AIDS	Parenteral s/c or i/m 25 µg/ml of each type	Antibodies elicited against the different serotypes, opsonizes the bacteria, which are then more efficiently phagocytosed. Also effective in children below 2 years	Immunity appears after few weeks of vaccination & lasts for 5 years, Boosters not considered necessary. Some studies, efficacy of >90% in reducing invasive pneumococ-cal disease. Reduction also in Otitis media & penicillin resistant pneumococcal strains	- Local reaction: swelling redness, pain - General: Fever, rarely neural disorders as Guil-lain Barre syndrome, anaphylaxis (rarely)	- Acute febrile illness - Severe reaction; as neurological or anaphylactic to any component of vaccine - Pregnancy, Children less than 2 yrs. age (unsatisfactory response as is a polysaccharide component) -Malignancies; as lymphomas
Meningo-coccal	• Bivalent A,C • Tetravalent A-C-Y-W135 • Conjugate protein polysaccharide tetravalent vaccine	*Capsular Polysac-charide (50 µg of each antigen)*	Population at risk during outbreak (children above 2 years, below this age the vaccine is poorly immunogenic) All pilgrims to Mecca for Haj	parenteral i/m	Antibodies elicited, opso-nizes bacteria, which are readily phagocytosed	Immunity appears within few days of vaccination & lasts for 3 years. Boosters are mandatory after 3 years Cost is a limiting factor in use Effective also in children below 2 years (conjugate vaccine)	Local: Swelling, redness, pain Systemic: rarely anaphylaxis	-Allergic severe reaction to dry natural rubber - Acute febrile illness - Children <2 years of age, unless conjugate vaccine
Diphtheria	• Toxoid (25Lf) • Other forms • In combination with per-tusis & tetanus (DPT) • Future: CRM197 (Cross reacting material) recom-binant, vaccine, (synthetic antigen)	Diphtheria Toxoid	Routine in Immunization programme	parenteral, i/m Chil-dren 3 doses starting at 6 weeks of life • Booster at: 18 months and 5 years	• Does not eliminate carriage of organism (*C. diphtheriae*) in pharynx or skin • Antibacterial antibody is of no significance • Immunity depends solely on the presence in blood & intestinal fluid of an IgG anti-toxin which forms an antigen - antibody complex, which prevents the toxin from binding to target cell. This complex is readily phagocytosed	Nearly 100% Schick conversion rate	Children, Allergic-hyper-sensitivity (a) Type I (b) Delayed Adults: Same as in paediatric except that incidence & sever-ity is far greater in adult population	No special contraindication except that should be restricted after 6 yrs. older children as are more likely to be sensitized to diphtheria antigens, thus offering a higher rate of adverse effects

Contd.

Contd.

Tuber-cular	• Bacillus calmette Guerin (attenuated *M. bovis* strain) • New vaccine candidates include recombinant BCG Protein & DNA vaccines	Strain subcultured 239 times in glycerol-bile-potato medium over a period of 13 years	• Routine in Immunization programme • Revaccination at school entry or those who are tuberculin negative • All family contacts of open tuberculin cases, if tuberculin negative • Community wide vaccination of all individuals with tuberculin reaction to 5 T.U. of P.P.D. of less than 5 mm after 72 hrs. In India BCG manufacturered in Guindy, Tamil Nadu	i/d (intradermal at birth or immediately after (in India)	Specific cell mediated responses (beneficial)	• Efficacy has varied in different trials from 0% protection (Chingleput, South India) to 80% (1935, North America) • Benefits: Disease, when occurs is mild. Severe disease forms, as miliary tuberculosis avoided	• Papule at site of vaccination may ulcerate due to inadvertent s/c infection or excessive dosage • Adenitis lupoid type of localized lesion • Widespread dissemination of injected organism, anaphylactic reaction (rarely)	• Acute febrile illness • Generalized eczema (vaccination can be given during remission) • Septic skin condition at site of vaccination
Leprosy	• B.C.G alone • B.C.G. + heart killed *M.leprae* • Mycobacterium W • ICRC (Indian Cancer Research Centre, Bombay) • Currently 'Leprovac', marketed by Cadila Ltd.		• Useful in prophylaxis of contacts • Useful in Lepromatous cases	• i/d • i/d 3-4 times at of interval of few months	• Cross reactivity with *M.leprae* • Mycobacterium is a fast growing saprophyte (non-pathogen) mycobacterium of the soil which cross-reacts with M.leprae	• Good lepromin conversion rate, which varies with different vaccines		
Tetanus : Toxoid : Serum	• <25 Lf toxoid in single + preservative + aluminum & calcium compounds as adjuvant • Available as single vaccine or Double (DT.PT) or triple (DPT) or Quadruple (DPT+polio)	Tetanus Toxoid	• To children as part of immunization schedule • Pregnant women • Individuals who have suffered injury suspected to be contaminated with tetanus spores • Non-immune individuals • Workers with greater than usual risk of injury; as military personnel	• i/m or s/c 3 doses + booster • 2 doses • Usually one booster • 3 doses at 0,1 & 6-12 months & then booster at 10 yrs.	IgG antitoxic antibodies are formed after vaccination, which are present in the blood & extravascular fluids. These can neutralize the toxin, which is released locally, in lymph & blood (by the bacteria) before it becomes fixed to the ganglioside in the nervous system. Vaccination during pregnancy (5th & 8th month) results also in the enhancement the response of these infants to subsequent immunization. In tetanus there is no natural immunity following disease or sub-clinical infection (but natural attack of pertusis confers immunity)		• Local: Swelling, redness & pain up to 10 days after injection • Systemic: Pyrexia, headache, malaise, myalgia, urticaria, acute anaphylaxis, peripheral neuropathy, elevated IgE levels • Frequent boosters may be associated with local arthrus type & urticarial reactions.	• GBS < 6 weeks, after previous dose • History of arthrus type hypersensitivity after previous dose of TT containing vaccine.

Contd.

Contd.

Typhoid	• T.A • T.A.B • Ty21a (Typhoral) • V_i (Typhim)	Has killed organisms of S. Typhi & S. Paratyphi A (phenol or acetone inactivated) Is live attenuated strain (mutant of S.Typhi 21a, which lack galE gene, as well as Vi antigen Vi polysaccharide antigen based	High risk	• i/m one dose • oral 3-4 doses preferably taken one hour before food on alternate days with cold/ lukewarm water • parenteral 1 dose	With live attenuated strain which lacks gal E & Vi antigen gene, cellular & secretory IgA response in the intestinal tract is initiated/ latter prevents infection (strain is mutant developed by genetic manipulation, which takes UDP-galactose - 4-epimerase, the enzyme responsible for incorporation of galactose into cell wall lipopolysaccharide. Elicits IgG Vi antibody (poorly immunogenic in infants)	• 64-72% - 3 years (for typhoral)	Nausea, vomitting & diarrhoea, (local), and systemic side-effects • Interferes for screening for serum Vi antibody (for V: vaccine) • 'Typhim Vi' given only after 2 years of age • 'Typhoral' indicated after 6 years of age	Like those of any live vaccine (for Ty21a) Precaution: (1) time gap of 2 weeks between oral polio vaccine & Ty21a (2) Minimum gap of 12 hours between administration of vaccine & mefloquine, as may inhibit replication Vaccine not licensed for Children <18 months, as there may be sub-optimal response in their age group
Plague	Killed vaccine (modification of original Haffkine vaccine)		High risk group: Field workers as ecologists, geologists in area known to have plague: Lab personnel working with infected material. In outbreak limited role (even vaccinated persons with adequate level titre must be given prophylactic antibiotic	Farenteral s/c - two doses at interval of 4 weeks - boosters g ven every 6 months	Mediated by circulating antibodies directed against Fraction 1 (i.e. capsular antigen in *Y.pestis,* which stimulates antibacterial immunity) As a consequence, vaccination reduces the risk of infection spread from rat to man by fleas (bubonic plague) but it's effect against airborne infection (primary pneumonic plague) is unknown	• Protection is 50% fir 3-6 months • Immunity appears 5-7 days after vaccination • May not give protection against air borne pneumonic plague	Erythema, induration at injection site, fever, headache, malaise, lymphadenopathy	
Cholera	• Killed, whole cell (heat killed, phenol preserved) prepared from *V cholerae* type Ogawa & inaba • B subunit & whole cell cholera consists of purified B subunit from cholera toxin & formalin/heat inactivated classical & El tor *V. cholerae* of Inaba & Ogawa serotype rBS_WCV (Dukoral or Colorvac) CVD 103_HgR (Mutacol or Orochol)	Utilizes recombinant B Subunit with whole cell vaccine Oral live attenuated (lack gene for cholera toxin) Live attenuated	Individual of all ages who live in high risk areas, during cholera outbreaks, Travellers to endemic areas	• S/c parenteral 2 doses at intervals of 4-6 weeks orally • 3 dose • Two oral dose immunization regimen 10-14 day apart	• Elicits high blood level of vibriocidal antibodies of IgG class. Small amount of the antibody may reach gut. • Vaccine is prepared from classical biotype, but carries equal protection against Eltor biotype • Significant rise in serum vibriocidal antibodies & antitoxin levels	Limited protection for few months • Variable • Transient protection in children • High cost of oral vaccine because of acid sensitivity of B subunits vaccine administered together with NaHCO3, citric acid, buffer solution to ensure adequate neutralization of stomach acidity for preservation of vaccine, while passing through stomach, recombinant technology reduces produc-tion cost, varying protection rates	Local: Transient redness, swelling, pain General: Headache, pyrexia, reaction	
H. influenzae	• H.influenzae type b polysaccharide vaccine. Combinations available • Diphtheria toxoid conjugated vaccine • Tetanus toxoid conjugated		Routine, especially for High risk children • Children and adults with sickle cell anemia • Splenectomized patients, Hodgkin's disease, Lymphoblastic Leukemia	Parenteral - 2 doses at gap of 1-2 months children > 18 months	Type b is used, as, 90% of infections are caused by it, combination may be used	Good protection	Local - slight reaction, elevation of temperature	• Severe allergic reaction after previous dose • Severe acute illness

Contd.

Contd.

Anthrax - In Man - In Animal	• Protective antigen (PA) adsorbed on aluminum hydroxide (alum precipitated toxoid) • rPA (recombinant Protective antigen) is a current approach • Spores of a nonvirulent strain (Sterne vaccine)		Individuals likely to be exposed to anthrax	i/m, 3 doses at intervals of 6 weeks & 6 months parenteral, single injection	• Antibodies to PA have a protective role probably by blocking binding of lethal factor to cell surface • Immune response against spore, which is an infective form	Booster dose may be administered after 1 year, Effective for a year		• Severe allergic reaction after previous dose • Severe acute illness
Pertusis	• Whole cell pertusis vaccine • Acellular pertusis (using recombinant technology)	Smooth, encapsular, virulent, phase I strain of *B pertusis* (Killed) having 3 principal, agglutinogens is used Contains predominantly FHA, agglutinogens and inactivated PT.	Routinely in immunization programme	• Parenteral given with Diphtheria and Tetanus. • Three doses at intervals of 4-6 weeks, 6 months of age • Boosters at 1½ and 4 years	• Vaccine induced immunity is mediated partly by circulating IgG antibody which reaches respiratory sercetion, the latter opsonizes the bacteria, which are easily phagocytosed. • C.M.I. confers long-term protection	Good protection (Approximately 90%)	Local swelling and redness, Fever, Shock, Encephalopathy, convulsion	• Febrile seizure • Epilepsy,progressive neural disorder • severe reaction to previous dose as, convulsion

VIRAL VACCINES

Disease	Composition	Dose/Route/ Schedule	Indications	Mechanism	Efficacy	Adverse	Contraindication
Papilloma	• Quadrivalent HPV vaccine (types 6, 11, 16 and 18) • Bivalent (types 16 and 18)	• i/m • Three doses • First dose at 9 years, second after 2 months, third after 6 months • Three doses i/m	• To reduce incidence of cervical cancers and anogenital warts • Males aged 9-26 years may be adminstered quadrivalent vaccine to reduce incidence of anogenital warts	Papilloma viruses are not cytocidal but they cause proliferation. Only some Papilloma viruses associated with cancer Generation of type specific neutralizing antibodies	Goal is to prevent the infection that causes cancer An average of 15 years may pass between the acquisition of the papilloma infection and the development of cancer Majority of people with papilloma infection may never develop the disease	Local reaction	
Chicken Pox	• Live attenuated *Oka strain for Varicella-zoster virus, obtained by propagation of virus in MRC5 human diploid cell culture (each dose of the reconstituted vaccine contains not less than $10^{3.3}$ plaque forming units of the attenuated Varicella-zoster virus. Trace antibiotics (to ensure sterility during preparation), Stabilizers * Strain named Oka after the boy, whose vesicular fluid used for the vaccine strain derivation	s/c age : 12 months to 12 yrs -> single dose : 13 years & above -> two doses at an interval of 6-10 weeks	• Healthy subjects (varicella susceptible) from the age of 12 months onwards • Susceptible healthy close contacts to reduce the risk of transmission to high-risk patients (including parents, siblings of high risk-patients, paramedical & other personnel) • Immunompromised children e.g. with low TLC counts • Healthy adults(who are at increased risk e.g. teachers of young children, military personnel	Induction of the cell mediated immunity ◊	• In one study, over all seroconversion rate was >98%	• Mild • Fever • Papulovesicular eruption • Breakthrough varicella (varicella developing more than 42 days after immunization, is mild response with lesser skin lesions) Δ No adverse effect associated, however avoid salicylates for 6 weeks after varicella vaccine because of association between salicylate use and Reye syndrome	• During pregnancy (although congenital varicella not reported) • Allergy to vaccine component (it has no preservative or egg • Steroid therapy • Avoid pregnancy for 3 months after immunization • Postpone in patients suffering from acute, severe febrile illness • In subjects with total lymphocyte count <1200mm³ or presenting other evidence of lack of cellular immune response • Intake of salicylatesΔ • Steroid *therapy
Small Pox (now eradicated)	• Suspension of live vaccinia virus grown on different agents (freeze dried vaccine)	i/d, dose may be repeated after 5 yrs. to boost immunity	• W.H.O. maintain a large stock of the vaccine to be deployed, if necessary in the future (as small pox) has been eradicated • High risk individuals as those in labs where this virus is maintained	• Production of neutralizing, complement fixing & other antibodies occur but no correlation between these antibodies & protection from infection	-	• Generalized vaccina • Eczema vaccinatum • Post vaccinial encephalitis (rarely) • Other	Those of live viral vaccines applicable here

Contd.

Contd.

Hepatitis B	• Plasma derived (inactivated by formalin/ heat/urea & pepsin) Previously this was the only antigen source, as virus could not be cultivated. Asymptomatic healthy carriers who had high titres of HBsAg were used as source, The particles were separated, purified & finally treated with inactivating agent, which inactivated HBV and any other virus present in the serum • DNA recombinant (is produced from HBsAg derived from *Saccharomyces cerevisiae* into which plasmid containing the gene for HBsAg subtype adw has been inserted. The purified HBsAg is inactivated by treating with formalin.	i/m (In haemophilia patients I/d or s/c route may be considered) • Merck vaccine 1 dose - 20μg/ml of HBsAg protein • Doses 0,1 & 6 month Pre-exposure Post-exposure to assess Half (approx) dose adminstered in children and double dose in immunologically impaired Hepatitis B immunoglobuluin if indicated)	• Medical staff - all those who are exposed to carriers, patients & clinical material infected with hepatitis B • Clinical condition • Infants(HBsAg negative) borne to hepatitis B positive mother • Haemophiliac patients on renal dialysis (negative for HBsAg and antiHBs • Persons with specific behaviour Male homosexuals, individuals with multiple sexual partners or with HBV cases Drug addicts Sexual contact of hepatitis B carriers	• HBV enters by break in the skin or the mucosa, where it can be easily neutralized by the antibody produced against HBsAg. This antibody combines with the surface antigen on envelope of virus. The resulting immune complex readily undergoes phagocytosis	• 80-95 %conversion or efficacy in preventing infection • No role if individual is HBsAg or antibody positive to above • If person has had hepatitis B Vaccine, must have anti_HBs levels of more than 10 I.U./ml to provide protection • If levels are lower than this, booster dose is recommended • Assess antibody status 6 weeks post vaccination, if no response, revaccinate	• Transmission of viruses & other infective agents as HIV, HCV, if ineffective inactivation in plasma derived vaccines • Local - swelling, redness • General - pyrexia, malaise, fatigue, headache, myalgia, arthralgia, rashers	• Acute febrile illness • Severe reaction to previous administration of HBsAg • Not pregnancy • Persons hypersensitive to yeast
Rotavirus	_Rhesus_human reassortant tetravalent vaccine (RotaShield)	orally	Goal of rotavirus vaccine is to immunize a significant children population and decrease rota virus associated hospitalization and mortality	Increased local immunity	Protection rate varied in various studies	Vaccine WITHDRAWN because of vaccine associated intussusception in vaccines	
	Rotateq (Merck) (pentavlent, atlenuated types of G1, G2, G3, G4 and G9	• Oral • Three doses	For children who are prone	• Increased local immunity		• Diarrohea, vomiting, and others	• History of hypersensitivity to any vaccine component • History of SCID (severe combined immunodeficiency disease) • History of intussusception
Influenza	Influenza strains are isolated worldwide,are characterized and evaluated with reference to the antibodies present in the population. On the basis of these information, the WHO recommends the composition of vaccines for use in forthcoming winter. Grown in embryonated egg for 2-3 days, after which allantoic fluid is harvested & inactivated by formalin or BPL. Influenza types A & B are usually included, as are clinically significant & involved in epidemics.						
	Killed - contains whole virus particles inactivated & purified as detailed above (usually contain 3 prevalent strains, two most recent of A types (as H1N1 & H3N2) and one most recent type B.	• i/m or s/c • Primed adult - single dose (person who had one or more natural infections in the past) • Children (4-13 yrs.) may need 2 doses	• Individuals with chronic disease of heart or lungs • Institutionalized patients with chronic medical conditions (high risk group) • Patients with Diabetes, mellitus, renal failures, anaemia, immunosuppression • Healthy individuals older than 65 yrs • Travel to Southern hemisphere during April to September	• Administration of vaccine results in substantial blood level of anti H haemagglutinin) & anti N (neuramindase) antibodies of IgG class. Anti H antibodies help to prevent absorption of virus into receptor sites on respiratory epithelium while Anti N antibodies reduce dissemination of the virus & hence severity of disease (Influenza is not an invasive infection & remains localized on	• Vaccine is effective when given one month before exposure to virus is expected (usually autumn) • Vaccine has no effect in limiting the outbreak, once it has occurred • Confers about 60% (in unprimed) to 80% (in primed) for one yr. • Many assumed vaccine failures are actually false negative results (other respiratory	Acute exacerbation of Guillain -Barre syndrome, multiple sclerosis etc., as occurred in 1976 in U.S., when vaccination was discontinued	• Acute febrile illness • Hypersensitivity to egg (hen) or polymyxin • Severe reaction to previously administered influenza vaccine

Contd.

Contd.

			• Also travel to Northern hemisphere • Medical personnel as physicians and nurses, who might transmit infection to those at high risk	Respiratory tract. Immunity following disease is therefore due to local abs of sIgA type)	pathogen) - Does not prevent infection but can prevent disease (this fact was demonstrated in early 1940s, when inactivated preparations were used)		
	Split vaccine - contains virus particles inactivated & purified as above. It is further disrupted with detergents & organic solvents to remove lipids.	• Parenteral	This vaccine may be of lower antigenicity & less reactogenicity in children				
	Subunit - contains haeagglutinins & neuraminidase antigens, chemically separated from other non-immunogenic components	• Parenteral					
	• Live attenuated vaccine (Ts mutant vaccine, approved by US, FDA)	• By aerosol spray or intranasal (Fig. 17.10.1) spray		• Can grow at lower temperature of the nasopharyngeal mucosa (32 -34°C) but not in lungs. Stimulates the production of local sIgA antibodies and other antibodies	92% protection in children (one study)		• Very safe, can be administered even to cases having egg hypersensitivity • History of GBS within 6 weeks of previous dose
	• Cell culture co-infected with cold adapted attenuated virus and wild type virus, reassorted virus progeny (designated as cold adapted, CA)						
Measles	Edmonston Zagreb (live attenuated) strain is used on human diploid cells, can be combined with Mumps & Rubella vaccines (original virus was isolated from a child named Edmonston)	Single dose i/m or deep s/c • In developed countries, vaccine administered after 15th month because few cases seen during 1st year of life • In developing countries, W.H.O. has recommended at 9 months (single dose) because cases occur earlier but sero-conversion following vaccination between 6-8 months is <85%, so if vaccination given earlier 2 doses would be required & also maternal antibody could inactivate the vaccine	• recommended for children all over the world. No upper age limit, however immunization of adults is seldom required, as these subjects are likely to have developed natural immunity	Measles virus enters the respiratory tract & in short time is carried into blood & other organs & tissues (primary Viremia) Post-vaccination circulating antibodies can neutralize extracellular virus locally or during primary viremia phase. Antibody reacts with virus antigen & the immune complex activates complement and is easily phagocytosed High levels of population immunity would be required to eliminate the circulation of the measles virus	Seroconversion seen in at least 95% of susceptible individuals Effective antibody level seen to remain for more than 10 yrs. Needle free vaccine delivery can improve the vaccine compliance	*Local:* rash, slight fever *Systemic:* convulsion encephalopathy S.S.P.E Children sensitive to egg may have allergic reaction but not to the one which is raised in human diploid cell vaccine May exacerbate tuberculosis	• Acute febrile illness • Immunodeficiency & malignancy • Pregnancy & 3 months before conception • Within 3 weeks of administration of another live virus vaccine, but may be administered simultaneously at different site • Severe sensitivity to egg or antimicrobials in vaccine (as neomycin)
	Schwartz Moraten (live attenuated measles strain isolated from chick embryo tissue culture)						

Contd.

Contd.

Mumps	Jeryl Lynn strain (live attenuated) grown in chick embryo cell line	• Single dose • i/m • After 12 months	Recommended to children	Similar mechanism as in Measles	• Seroconversion in at least 97% of children • Exact duration of protection not known but probably lasts 15 years	*local* - swelling, redness, pain *General* - fever, urticaria, parotitis, rarely orchitis encephalitis *Adverse* - haemolytic uremic syndrome, deafness, Guillain Barre syndrome	• Acute febrile illness • Immunodeficiency & malignancy • Pregnancy & 3 months before conception • Within 3 weeks of administration of another live virus vaccine, but may be administered simultaneously at different site • Severe sensitivity to egg or antimicrobials in vaccine (as neomycin) • Children less than 1yr may have maternal antibodies, which can interfere with immune response
MMR	1000 TCID 50 Measles virus (Schwartz strain) 5000 TCID 50 (at least) Mumps virus (Urabe or Zagreb or Jereyl Lynn 1000 TCID 50 (atleast) Rubella virus (Wistar RA 27/3)						
Rabies_In Man	• Semple's sheep brain vaccine (sheep brain infected with modified rabies virus & inactivated with phenol • BPL vaccine Above vaccine with beta propiolactone (BPL) as inactivating agent • Nervous tissue vaccines (**discontinued**, due to neurological complications, due to myelin presence)	• Deep s/c into overlying or underlying muscle • ideal site is Anterior abdominal wall • Primary course is 10 injections (additional boosters in class II & III wound)	• Biting animal is a wild one or rabid or a stray dog or cat • The biting animal presents with clinical sign & symptoms of rabies • The animal is proven (positive by lab) for rabies or suspected of being rabid, even though lab tests fail to confirm • Following handling of animals diagnosed as rabid, where abrasions of skin have been contaminated with saliva	• Specific adequate antibodies produced in blood, which neutralizes the virus, which would travel from the wound site to the central nervous system	-	• *Local* - pain, redness • *Systemic* mild - fever, headache, generalized urticaria, shock, Neuroparalytic complication (encephalitogenic)	• Allergy to nervous tissue component • Avoid in person with convulsions
	Non Neural Egg vaccine-i)Duck egg -ii)Chick embryo						
	Tissue culture based (i) HDCV (human diploid cell vaccine) Virus is raised in human cell (WI 38) _HDCV (ii) Purified chick embryo cell vaccine (PCEC)_raised in chicken fibroblast cell culture (Rabipur) (iii) Purified vero cell vaccine (PV RV) (Verorab)	• i/m • Pre-exposure 0, 7 & 28 days + one booster at interval of 1-3 yrs. • Post-exposure 5 + one booster (0, 3, 7, 14, 30 & 90) NB: Day 'O' in schedule reflects the day, when first dose of vaccine is administered (Not the day of dog bite)	Same as above, but as vaccine is safe, given also in pre-exposure situations : Lab staff handlers of virus : Veterinarian : Animal handlers : Wildlife officers & Taxidermist	• Similar	Immunity persists for 3-5 yrs. (titre of 0.5 I.u./ml or more is considered, as protective)	General - fever, headache Allergic : type I & type III hypersensitivity reaction, : Neural complication (rare as Guillain Barré)	More safe than above (injection given at deltoid rather than gluteal since adminstration at the latter site associated with vaccine failure as probably not adequately absorbed)
	Subunit vaccines (Surface glycoprotein based, experimental stage)						
In Animals	Tissue culture vaccine inactivated by BPL, adsorbed on aluminum hydroxide	i/m single dose booster at 1-3 year intervals	Pets, as dogs				

NB: Importance of live attenuated vaccines is that they can prevent infections in comparison to other category of vaccines, which can only decrease complications.

Δ Generally a person who can eat eggs or other products is safe for administration of an egg based vaccine. If vaccine is to be given to a person with egg hypersensitivity, perform desentization of eggs before administration.

Contd.

Contd.

Hepatitis A (single serotype, despite existence of multiple viral genotypes)	Formalin inactivated preparation of virions (HM 175 strain of HAV) grown in human fibroblasts or monkey kidney cell lines, absorbed to alum as an adjuvant	• i/m (parenteral) • 2 doses(one month apart) & one booster after 6 months	• In endemic areas to local residents, if risk of acquiring infection high, Malnourished, sewage workers, sexually active, homosexual men, i/v drug users • Those at increased risk of fulminant liver disease, as individuals with chronic liver disease due to hepatitis C virus • All children above 2 years of age if very high prevalence rate of infection(under 2years of age vaccine not approved) • Visitors to prevalent areas, where prevalence high	Circulating antibody produced is highly protective against symptomatic hepatitis A infection. High cost of the vaccine limits the ability of the vaccine to control the disease	good immune response in 99% of vaccines lasting some years (according to one study)	local	Pregnancy
Poliomyelitis OPV (oral)	Sabin: Mixture of 3 types (monovalent) of attenuated polioviruses, $MgCl_2$ (stabilizer), less than 25µl of each of the antibiotics namely Streptomycin, neomycin and indicator (Phenol red) *(attenuated through rapid passage on monkey kidney cell & purified through plaque processing Pink color is due to phenol red (pH indicator 6.6-8.0). If after partial use color of the vaccine changes from pink to red or yellow,it is sign of bacterial contamination	Orally, three doses + one booster along with DPT($1^{1/2}$ yrs) May booster at school entry & then additional booster Type1>300,000 TCID50 Type 2>100,000 TCID 50 per 2drops Type3>300,000TCID50	• In the National immunization schedule • Universal immunization program • Ring polio immunization • To cover all children ---- years of age in radius of to 5 km, surrounding the index case, urban areas and at least 5000 children in a rural areas as a containment measures (2 doses at one month interval) • As part of the polio eradication programme (GPEI)	The vaccine passes along the alimentary tract to ileum where it enters & multiplies in the cells of epithelium & in lymphoid tissue of lamina propria. The virus (strain) then travels to mesentric lymph nodes & possibly between 2nd & 5th day after vaccination excreted in the faeces for as long as 3 weeks, process stimulates sIgA (local) & IgG (specific)	- Many studies have shown seroconversion in almost 100% recipients (after 5-7 doses). Seroconversion after 3 doses in some studies was 60%. That's the reason, why >5 does required - Humoral antibody has been seen to persist after 15 yrs of vaccination - prevents reinfection with wild virus	- vaccine associated paralysis in recipient (VAPP) (one in two million doses) - vaccine associated paralysis in contacts (one in 3 million doses)	- Acute febrile illness - severe diarrhoea & vomiting - sensitivity to antibiotics in vaccine - Immunodeficiency & malignancy - Pregnancy - Severe reaction to previous vaccination - 3 weeks before or after the administration of normal immunoglobulin
In pulse polio programme followed since 2000 AD, all children <5years given, 2 doses of pulse polio every year till age of 5 years							
The aim is to totally eliminate the wild virus from the community							
Eradication is polio is defined as absence of clinical poliomyelitis _Zero Polio							
Global polio eradication initiative (GPEI) - to eradicate polio worldwide by 2018							

Contd.

Contd.

IPV-Salk (inactivated polio vaccine)	• Contains 40, 8 & 32 D units respectively of type 1, 2 & 3 in each dose	• Parenteral i/m • Same as above	• Used in few countries for routine immunization eg. Sweden & Netherlands • In persons over 18 yrs (preferred because risk of live vaccine associated paralysis slightly higher in adults) • Those in whom live virus vaccine contraindicated	• The antigen stimulates IgG production in the serum virus is neutralized as it enters the blood stream, so preventing involvement of nervous system) • Does not induce detectable level of sIgA in gut	• Produces significant antibody responses in >95% of vaccines	• Local • Systemic	
Dengue	CYD_TDV (Sanofi Pasteur)	Phase 3 clinical testing including in India done	Persons living in endemic areas Travellers to endemic areas				
	Live attenuated, Primary monkey kidney cell raised (tetravalent)	Three doses on 0/6/12 month schedule in 9-45 years age group					
	DENV_4 chimera			30 nucleotides removed to attenuate the virus			
Yellow fever (YF)	17 - D Vaccine (live attenuated) (cultivating live attenuated 17-D strain in specific pathogen free chicken embryonated egg, especially Avian leukosis free. 17D vaccine virus differs from the wild virus parent at multiple sites but the precise molecular basis for attenuation is not understood	• s/c or i/m (in adults and children above 6 months) • Single dose booster after 10 years		• Travel to endemic areas (International travel requirement) • In endemic areas (all people above 6 months old) including Tropical areas of Africa and Americas	YF is a vaccine prevetable illness Future priority is to make vaccine more safe and expand YF vaccine coverage	• Fever and headache (rarely occur between 4 & 7th post vaccination day) • Rarely Encephalitis (severe) risk in children below 4 months) • Rarely syndrome characterized with multiple organ failure	• Acquired or congenital immunodeficiency • Acute febrile illness • Infants below the age of 6 months unless risk of infection is high • Severe sensitivity to egg protein • Pregnancy (if risk of Y.F. to mother outweighs the small risk of infection to foetus, then can give the vaccine) • Within 3 weeks from adminstration of another live virus vaccine, but may be adminstered simultaneously at another site • History of neurological disorder • Immunosupressive therapy (wait for 1 month, after t/t is over)
Japanese encephalitis	• Formalin inactivated vaccine derived from brain of suckling mice, prepared at C.R.I. Kasauli (not in National immunization schedule)	• s/c • Two doses at interval of 7-14 days • A booster may be given few months after primary immunization • Revaccination may be done at 3yrs	-	• In endemic areas • Prior to anticipatory outbreaks (about 1 month)	• Immunity develops at least one month after 2nd injection, so give 1 month prior to anticipated outbreak	• *Local:* swelling, pain • *Systemic:* fever, headache, chills, malaise	• Person suffering from high fever, illnesses of heart, liver, Diabetes, malignancy & convulsion • Avoid in pregnancy
Kyasanur Forest disease	Inactivated vaccine, manufactured at C.R.I., Kasauli (H.P.)	-	-	• In endemic areas			

Contd.

Contd.

Rubella	• live attenuated strain (derived from RA-27/3 vaccine strain) • this vaccine is often combined with Mumps & measles & administered at least 1000 PFU (plaque forming units) • In MMR in combination 1000 TCID (1000 median tissue culture infective doses	Combined MMR vaccine i/m at 15 months to both sexes or 9-12 months (earlier vaccination, prior to it gives varying proportion of failure, owing to presence of maternal antibody) • Exclusive rubella component to women of childbearing age, with no evidence of immunity • In Austria & some other European countries approval is to vaccinate only pre-puberty 14 years age (approach has the disadvantage that disease incidence not reduced in young children & such non-immune individuals could contract rubella during pregnancy from ill children	• Objective is to prevent fetal infection & consequent congenital rubella syndrome (CRS) Rubella occurs early in pregnancy and risk of fetal infection and CRS is high in the first eight gestational weeks	- The American approach is to interrupt transmission, so vaccine recommended to all children at 15 months of age. Vaccine strain elicits high titre of circulating antibody & local secretion of sIgA in nasopharynx. These antibodies neutralize virus, which may be extracellular (locally or otherwise during viremic phase) This approach could eliminate the circulation of wild type rubella virus within population & more successful in preventing congenital rubella & reducing disease morbidity)	• Not clear as to how long protection lasts	• Local: pain, redness • General: Fever, sore throat, rashes, lymphadenopathy, rarely thrombocytopenia & neural problems (joint pains, neuropathy)	• Congenital or acquired immunodeficiency • Pregnancy • Recent (within three months) administration of immunoglobulin • Other as for any live vaccine • Post-pubertal female shouln't become pregnant for at least 3 months after vaccination (although no evidence that virus can cause defect in foetus)
HIV	Trials of many potential vaccines are in progress include : recombinant, envelope based : cocktail vaccine : core protein e.g., gp-120 vaccine hybrid virus vaccine e.g., Modified Vaccinia Ankara vector vaccine e.g., Clade B Adenovirus _HIV _gag vector vaccine e.g., Multiclade (A,B,C) prime_boost	- Phase trial in National Aids research Institute, India		• Some attempt to prevent infection • Some attempt to prevent disease • Antibodies generated against significant molecules & cell mediated immunity help the individual		-	-

Live atlenuated vaccines (Usually single dose) sufficient	**Killed Vaccines** (Usually multiple doses required	**Toxoid Based**
BCG	Pneumococcal	Diphtheria
Dukoral (For cholera)	Meningococcal	Tetanus
Ty21a (for enteric)	TAB (Typhoid)	
Varicella	'Typhim' (Typhoid)	
Rotateq (for rotavirus)	Plague	
Ts mutant (for influenza)	Hib (*Haemophilus influenzae*)	
MMR	Anthrax	
Yellow fever	Influenza	
	Salk	
	HAV, HBV	
	Rabies, J.E.	

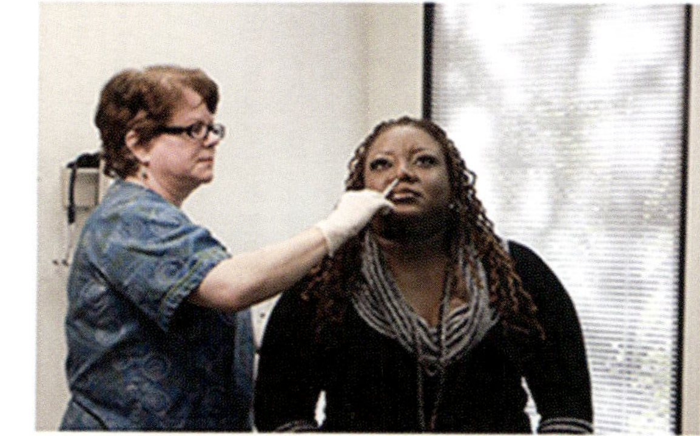

Fig. 14.6.1: Intranasal Vaccine Adminstration: A nurse administering a flu vaccine into the right nostril and thereby into the patient's nasal cavity. The nurse's hands are gloved, avoiding the possibility of cross-contamination

Courtesy: Douglas Jordan/CDC

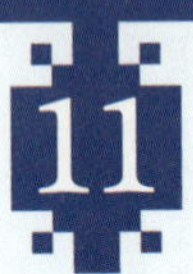

Emerging and Re-Emerging Diseases

Over 30 new infectious diseases, have been detected worldwide in the last three decades. Epidemics have been caused by the emerging and re-emerging infections world-wide. The gravity of the scenario can be gauged by the fact, that the 2009 H1N1 influenza outbreak was declared an emergency in the USA. Recommendations need to be formulated for these diseases, for an effective response to be instituted.

Let's study these emerging and re-emerging infections

What do you understand by emerging and re-emerging infectious disease? Give examples.

A.1 **Emerging infectious disease** have been defined, as infectious disease; whose incidence has increased during the last two decades and threatens to increase. It includes newly appearing infectious diseases, caused by newly identified microorganisms or known infections spreading to new geographic area (Table 17.11.1). These lists could vary nationally and internationally.

Re-emerging infectious diseases are disease, which were once major health problems but have reappeared after a significant decline in their incidence, as a result of antimicrobial resistance to known agents or breakdown in public health measures. Many infectious disease specialists consider this to be a subcategory of emerging diseases.

e.g., in 1990- diphtheria reemerged in the states of the new Soviet Union, in 1991-epidemic cholera reappeared in South America and in 1994-plague reappeared in Surat (India).

It is very important to recognize these in the population, so that the public health authorities can quickly act to any new threats and minimize the morbidity and mortality, besides the economic loss. For instance, the outbreak of plague in Surat (India) in 1994 caused an estimated loss of $1 billion to $2 billion in commerce.

Give an example of an emerging disease, in which an ecological factor has been found to be instrumental in its causation and control of that factor minimized the disease emergence.

A.2 Legionnaire's disease

Enumerate new infectious diseases (and their etiologic agents) that have been identified since 1973.

A.3 It is amazing that new etiologic agents and infectious disease continue to be discovered. These are depicted in table 17.11.1.

Table 17.11.1: Emerging diseases since 1973

Year	Agent	Disease
1973	Rotavirus	Infantile diarrhoea
1975	Parvovirus B19	Fifth disease
1976	*Cryptosporidium parvum*	Acute enterocolitis
1977	*Legionella pneumophila*	Legionnaire's disease
1977	*Campylobacter jejuni*	Enteritis
1977	Hantaan virus	Haemorrhagic fever with renal disease
1977	Ebola virus	Ebola haemorrhagic fever
1980	Human T cell lymphotropic virus (HTLV-1)	T-cell lymphoma or leukemia
1981	Toxin-producing strain of *Staphylococcus aureus*	Toxic shock syndrome
1982	*Escherichia coli* 0157:H7	Hemolytic uremic syndrome Hemorrhagic colitis
1982	*Borrelia burgdorferi*	Lyme disease
1982	HTLV-II	Hairy cell leukemia
1983	*Helicobacter pylori*	Gastric ulcer
1983	Human immunodeficiency virus-1 (HIV-1)	AIDS
1985	HIV-2	AIDS (milder disease)
1985	*Enterocytozoon beineusi*	Chronic diarrhoea
1986	*Cyclospora cayetanensis*	Persistent diarrhoea

Contd.

Contd.

1986	Bovine spongiform encephalitis agent (Prion)	Bovine spongiform encephalopathy (in cattle)
1988	Human herpes virus – 6 (HHV-6)	Roseola subitum
1988	Hepatitis E	Hepatitis E (enterically transmitted)
1989	*Ehrlichia chaffeensis*	Human ehrlichiosis
1989	Hepatitis C	Hepatitis C (parenterally transmitted)
1991	*Tropheryma whipplei*	Whipple's disease
1991	Guanarito virus	Venezuelan haemorrhagic fever
1992	*Vibrio cholerae* 0139	Chlolera (new strain associated with epidermics)
1992	*Bartonella* (Rochalimaea) *henselae*	Cat scratch disease, Bacillary angiomatosis
1993	Sin Bombre virus	Hantavirus pulmonary syndrome (adult respiratory distress syndrome)
1994	Sabia virus	Brazilian haemorrhagic fever
1995	Human herpes virus-8 (HHV-8)	Kaposi sarcoma (in AIDS)
1997	*Influenza virus (H5N1)	'Avian' Influenza
2001	Human Metapneumovirus	Respiratory infections
2002	West Nile virus	Acute flaccid virus
2003	SARS Coronavirus	Severe acute respiratory syndrome

* First time man infected with avian influenza strain. Controlling the outbreak required culling (killing) more that 1 million chickens in the local market and sanitization of place. Pandemic could have occurred, as man had no exposure to H5N1 subtype, so no immunity.

What is the importance of studying the emerging and re-emerging infectious diseases?

A.4 See last para A.1

Is man likely to win a battle against the infectious diseases?

A.5 Microbes have survived ecologic changes for millions of years, due to their rapid rate of replication and ability to adapt; using processes of mutation, genetic recombination and other processes. Man has come much later in the time frame. In the early 1970s, there was a hope that infectious diseases would not be public health issue, due to the success with antimicrobials and vaccines. But, a conquer is unlikely, with a truce being a likely reality.

What is the foundation of all public health programmes?

A.6 Adequate infection surveillance in the population to detect the new cases at the earliest.

What are some of the factors that have led to emerging and re-emerging infectious diseases?

A.7 *One* of the important factors has been the rapid urbanization, which increases the population density and puts more individuals at risk of disease.

Second; is the ecological changes that have occurred due to many reasons; as encroachment of forest areas. One example of it has been the fatal Hantavirus infectious in humans, due to their encroachment of the forests with rodents, in whom Hantaviruses were harmlessly present.

Third has been introduction of new technology in many fronts; as increased usage of air conditioner, increased air travel and commercialization in food industry. Lapse in the procedure in a food industry at a single point; as use of contaminated beef, can effect a large population.

Fourth are the changes in the microbial genome; including development of antimicrobial resistance. *Last* is the breakdown of the public health measures.

Section XVII: Applied Microbiology

12 Assessment/Examination Questions

Chapter 1

1. Discuss the concept of normal flora. What are the conditions, in which the typical microflora of the region changes its composition? Mention the medical consequences of such changes. A1 (P 590-591), A10a, b (P 591-592)
2. Describe pseudomembranous colitis. A 10aii (P 591)
3. Why is it important to study the factors that determine the nature of normal flora? A 7 (P 590)
4. What are the conditions, in which breech of the human disease, make the organisms of the normal flora invade the human and cause disease? A10b (P 591-592)
5. Describe normal flora of skin, mouth & respiratory tract, gastrointestinal tract and genitourinary tract. All (P 593-594)

Chapter 2

1. Describe bacterial flora of water. A 1b (P 595)
2. Enumerate the diseases transmitted by water. A 2 (P 595)
3. Describe the technique of bacteriological examination of water. A3-A6 (P 596)
4. Describe presumptive coliform count and differential coliform count. A3 (P 596)
5. Describe the techniques used to perform bacteriological examination of water. A 3 (P 596)
6. Describe the techniques used to monitor quality of air of the O.T. A 2-A5 (P 597)
7. Describe bacteriology of air. Case Study-2 (P 596-597)
8. Enumerate the diseases transmitted by pets (including animals reared for meat) namely dog, cat, pigs and birds to man. A1, A3 (P 597)
9. Define zoonoses. Classify them according to (a) etiological agent (b) direction of transmission and (c) life cycle and mode of transmission. A 5 (P 598)
10. Enumerate the organisms that are transmitted by blood. A 2 (P 600)
11. Enumerate the diseases transmitted by rodents to man. A4 (P 597)
12. Enumerate the diseases transmitted by the following arthropod vectors, namely; Flies (House fly, Black fly, Deer fly, Horse fly, Sandfly and Tsetse fly), Mosquitos (Aedes, Aopheles, Culex and Mansonoides), Flea (Cat flea, Human flea, Rat flea and Sandfly), Lice (Head louse,body louse and pubic louse), mite (?Chicken mite. Itch mite and Trombiculid mite), Cyclops, Tick, Sandfly and Reduvid bug. A 9 (P 599-600)

Chapter 3

1. Define Healthcare associated infection (hospital acquired infection/nosocomial infection). What are the common type of these infections. Enumerate the microbes implicated in them. Mention the sources of them and their modes of transmission. A 2b, A3a (P 601-602)
2. Mention the measures used to control infections in a health care setting. A 7 (P 603) and see related case
3. Describe Infection control policy. A 5a, b (P 604-605)
4. Describe Hand hygiene and personal protective equipment. A5c (P 605), A 5a(P 604)
5. Discuss the diagnosis of hospital acquired infections. A 6b(P 603)
6. What was the basis of the 'universal precautions'? A3c(P 604)

7. What are 'Standard precautions'? When did the universal precautions get replaced by the standard precautions? Why did this replacement occur? A 3d(i-iii) (P 604)

Chapter 4

1. What is the scheme of segregating the waste according to the BMW 2016 rules? A 3(P 606)
2. What is the motto and principles of the BMW rules? A 2d (P 606)
3. Describe the types of biomedical waste. A 5 (P 607)
4. Describe the techniques to treat the biomedical waste. A6 (P 607)

Chapter 6

1. Enumerate the differences between mutational and transferable drug resistance. Table 17.6.1 (P 615)
2. What are the factors that have led to spread of drug resistance in microbes? Discuss their importance. A 8 (P 612-613)
3. Why is that so much emphasis is given on appropriate and rational usage of antimicrobials? A1 (P 609)
4. Discuss the factors that can control drug resistance. A2a(P 609)

Chapter 7

1. How are antimicrobial susceptibility tests classified? A 2a(P 617)
2. What are the indications of performing the qualitative antimicrobial susceptibility tests? A 2c(P 617)
3. What are the indications of performing the quantitative antimicrobial susceptibility tests? A 3a (P 619)
4. Describe Stokes disc diffusion method and Kirby–Baeur disc diffusion method. A 2f, A2b, A2e(P 618)
5. Describe minimum inhibitory concentration (MIC) and minimum bactericidal concentration (MBC). A 3c(P 619)

Chapter 8

1. What are the indications of performing microbial typing? A1 (P 621)
2. Classify the phenotypic and genotypic typing techniques. A4 (P 621)
3. Describe Bacteriocin typing. All (P 623)
4. When is an outbreak suspected? A2 (P 621)

Chapter 9

1. Mention the principles and applications of genetic engineering. A1-A5 (P 624-627)
2. What is gene cloning? Enumerate the steps involved in it? A 2a, A3 (P 624-625)
3. Describe restriction endonucleases. A2b (P 624-625)
4. Describe gene therapy. A5 (Point 5, P 627)

Chapter 10

1. Describe the composition,indications, mechanism, mode of administration, adverse effects and contraindications of the following bacterial vaccines namely pnemococcal, meningococcal, tubercular, leprosy, tetanus, typhoid, cholera, H. *influenzae*, pertusis, and plague. See table at P 629-632
2. Describe the National immunization schedule in existence in India.
3. Describe live attenuated vaccines, Killed vaccines and toxoids. P 639
4. Define passive immunization. Describe the role of antisera in it. A 5 (P 104), A1-A5 (P 134)
5. Enumerate the live viral vaccines. P 639
6. Describe the following antiviral vaccines namely IPV, small pox, chicken pox, hepatitis B, Rotavirus, Influenza, Measles and Rubella. See Table of P 633-639

Chapter 11

1. Explain the concept of emerging and re-emerging diseases. Give examples. A1 (P 640)
2. Enumerate new infectious diseases and etiological agents, that have been identified since 1973. A3 (P 640-64)
3. What are some of the factors that have led to the emerging and re-emerging diseases? Mention the importance of studying these diseases. A 7 (P 641), A1 (P 640)

Internet Resources

– **The internet is becoming the town square for the global village of tomorrow.** **— Bill Gates**

The current generation keeps learning even when on the move. Keeping this in perspective, this section has been incorporated. The reliance of the undergraduates on the conventional references as a resource for learning is diminishing. The section has included some key internet references, which would be useful to the undergraduate medical student pursuing a course in medical microbiology.

The sites have been compiled by *Dr Charu Jain*, Junior Consultant, ESIC, Faridabad.

General Microbiology and Bacteriology

1. http://micro.magnet.fsu.edu/ – The website features an extensive collection of images obtained by different types of microscopes .
2. https://www.microbiologysociety.org/ – Largest learned microbiological society in Europe
3. http://microbiologyonline.org/ – This inspirational online resource supports the teaching and learning of microbiology in the classroom across the key stages.
4. https://www.asm.org/ – The American Society for Microbiology (ASM), the world's oldest and largest life science organization.
5. http://www.sciencephoto.com/ – The website provides images and clips using high resolution microscopes making complex concepts easy to comprehend.
6. https://www.microbes.info/news/ – Microbes info is a free access internet web site designed to bring useful and interesting microbiology informational resources and attempts to reduce the clutter of information on the internet
7. http://www.sfam.org.uk/ – SFAM is the oldest microbiology society in the UK, serving microbiologists around the world.
8. http://microbiology.washington.edu/ – The website is of University of Washington, Department of Microbiology, having various undergraduate and post graduate courses involving microbiology.
9. http://www.microbeworld.org/ – MicrobeWorld is an interactive multimedia educational outreach initiative from the American Society for Microbiology that promotes awareness and understanding of key microbiological issues.
10. http://www.medscape.com/ – Medscape is the leading online global destination for physicians and healthcare professionals worldwide, offering the latest medical news and expert perspectives; essential point-of-care drug and disease information; and relevant professional education and CME.
11. http://www.microbeworld.org/history-of-microbiology – Compilation of important events in the field of microbiology.
12. http://www.history-of-the-microscope.org/ – All the information on microscopes including history.
13. http://www.generalmicroscience.com – Good collection of notes and powerpoint of various aspects of clinical and laboratory microbiology
14. https://bact.wisc.edu/ – The website of the University of Wisconsin-Madison, Department of Bacteriology for students.
15. http://myplace.frontier.com/~dffix/medmicro/ – Douglus Fix has created a website with the purpose of providing notes for easy understanding for students
16. http://www.infectioncontroltoday.com/ – Infection Control Today addresses the most pertinent infection prevention principles and practices for healthcare professionals.
17. http://www.microbiologynetwork.com/ – The website provides consultation and quality assurance training to various medical personnel.
18. https://www.ncbi.nlm.nih.gov/taxonomy/ – The link provides taxonomical aid for the right placement of various microorganisms
19. http://www.meningitis.org/ – At Meningitis Research Foundation (MRF), the vision is of a world free from meningitis and septicaemia.
20. https://www.dnalc.org/ – The mission of the DNA Learning Center is to prepare students to thrive in the gene age.
21. http://vaccines.org/ – The Vaccine Page provides access to up-to-the-minute news about vaccines and an annotated database of vaccine resources.
22. http://www.dnavaccine.com – The website has been a central resource in the fields of DNA vaccinology.
23. http://www.ivi.int/ – The International Vaccine Institute (IVI) is dedicated to vaccines and vaccination for global health.
24. https://www.niaid.nih.gov/ – NIAID scientists study all aspects of infectious diseases, from bench to bedside.
25. http://www.isid.org/ – The Society is dedicated to developing partnerships and to finding solutions to the problem of infectious diseases across the globe.
26. http://www.idsociety.org – The Infectious Diseases Society of America (IDSA) promotes work relating to infectious diseases.
27. http://www.microrao.com/index.html – Its an online resource on medical microbiology designed for both UG and PG students.
28. http://www.fightbac.org/ – The Partnership for Food Safety Education develops and promotes effective education programs to reduce foodborne illness risk for consumers.
29. http://www.biotech.wisc.edu/ – The University of Wisconsin Biotechnology Center is committed to maximizing the benefits of biotechnology research.

Virology

1. http://www.virology.net/ – Has link to all the relevant virology websites including viral images.

2. http://virology-online.com/ – Designed as a study aid for students on virology including examination questions.
3. http://www.ihv.org/ – The Institute of Human Virology provides the latest information on all aspects of HIV.
4. http://www.virology-education.com/
5. https://www.ncbi.nlm.nih.gov/genome/viruses/ – This resource provides viral and viroid genome sequence data and related information
6. https://microbewiki.kenyon.edu/index.php/Viral_Biorealm – Microbewiki is a free wiki resource on microbes and microbiology.
7. http://www.asv.org/ – The American society for virology promotes discussion and collaboration among virologists.
8. http://influenza.nhri.org.tw/ATIVS/ – Deals with influenza surveillance.

Mycology

1. http://www.mycology.adelaide.edu.au/ – This website helps in identification and management of human and animal fungal infections.
2. http://mycology.net/ – The website is an Internet Portal for Scientists on Diversity of Fungi
3. http://www.aspergillus.org.uk/ – The Aspergillus website is a worldwide comprehensive resource providing detailed information about Aspergillosis.
4. https://eportal.mountsinai.ca/Microbiology//mig/index.shtml – MicroWeb Mycology Image Gallery has some of the best educational images including comments.

Parasitology

1. http://parasites-world.com/ – Has a nice collection of images for understanding parasites including historical details.
2. https://www.cdc.gov/dpdx/az.html – CDC site offers laboratory diagnositic aids for the parasites of public health importance.
3. http://www1.udel.edu/mls/dlehman/medt372/index.html – The University of Delaware collection of images of intestinal / extraintestinal parasites.
4. http://atlas.or.kr/about/index.html – Web Atlas of Medical Parasitology.
5. http://amsocparasit.org – The American Society of Parasitology site.
6. http://malaria.org/ – Compilation of information on malaria diagnosis and management.

Immunology

1. https://www.hiv.lanl.gov/content/immunology/ – The HIV molecular immunology database.
2. http://www.immunologylink.com/ – The Immunology Link is an immunology, cell biology, biotechnology, and molecular biology research resource.
3. http://www.immunologyclinic.com/CaseIndex.asp – The link is of the fifth edition of Essentials of Clinical immunology book by Helen Chapel, Mansel Haeney, Siraj Misbah and Neil Snowdwn. (Format is of case studies/ MCQs).

Practical and laboratory skills

1. http://www.asmscience.org/VisualLibrary.
2. https://www.microbiologyinpictures.com – The site has images of commonly used culture media with growth of microorganism.
3. http://feeds.feedburner.com/asm – A podcast is rich media, such as audio or video, distributed via RSS. Feeds like this one provide updates, whenever there is new microbiology content on the popular websites.
4. www.microeguide.com – The Micro eGuide is designed to provide basic instruction on laboratory safety, microbiological skills and laboratory equipment.
5. http://www.cellsalive.com/toc_micro.htm – CELLS alive! represents 30 years of capturing film and computer-enhanced images of living cells and organisms.
6. http://www.microbiologyinfo.com/ – Microbiology Notes on Microbiology theory and practical.
7. http://www.scienceprofonline.com/instructors-corner/instructors-corner-vmc.html – Science Prof Online offers developed biology courses for the Virtual Microbiology Classroom.
8. http://microbiologyonline.org/students – This interactive section especially designed for students to explore the secret world of microbes.
9. http://commtechlab.msu.edu/sites/dlc-me/ – It's a digital learning center for microbial ecology.
10. http://microbiologyonline.org/what-s-new/videos – The link provides YouTube videos for various microbiological techniques.

Other important websites of key global organisations

1. www.who.int – The World Health Organization (WHO) is a specialized agency of the United Nations that is concerned with international public health.
2. www.nlm.nih.gov – The National Library of Medicine (NLM), on the campus of the National Institutes of Health in Bethesda, Maryland, is the world's largest biomedical library.
3. www.fda.gov – The Food and Drug Administration (FDA or USFDA) is a federal agency of the United States, Department of Health and Human Services.
4. https://www.cdc.gov/ – The Centers for Disease Control and Prevention, Atlanta, USA- site.
5. https://www.atcc.org – American Type Culture Collection is the premier global biological materials resource and standards organization for production, preservation, development, and distribution of standard reference micrbes, cell lines, and other materials.
6. http://www.webmd.com/ – Provide personalized multi-media interactive educational experiences .
7. https://www.epa.gov/ – The link is of U.S. Environmental protection agency, whose purpose is to protect human health and the environment
8. http://www.clinicaltrials.com/ – ClinicalTrials.com is a comprehensive resource for medical research studies (clinical trials).
9. http://www.searo.who.int/india/en/ – World Health Organization (WHO) is the United Nations' specialized agency for Health (Indian link).

Indian

1. http://naco.gov.in/ – National AIDS Control Organization is a division of the Ministry of Health and Family Welfare that provides leadership into HIV/AIDS control.
2. http://nvbdcp.gov.in/ – Directorate of National Vector Borne Disease Control Programme (NVBDCP) is the central nodal agency for the prevention and control of vector borne diseases.
3. http://nicd.nic.in/ – National Centre for Disease Control, India. National centre of excellence for the control of communicable diseases.
4. http://www.nii.res.in/ – The National Institute of Immunology (NII) is committed to advanced research with a view to understand body's defense mechanisms for developing modalities of immune system manipulation, that can intervene disease processes.
5. http://mohfw.nic.in/ – Ministry of Health & Family Welfare's official website, GOI.
6. http://nlep.nic.in/ – The National Leprosy Eradication Programme, of Health and Family Welfare, Govt. of India.
7. www.nhp.gov.in – The Ministry of Health and Family Welfare, Government of India has set up the National Health Portal in pursuance to the decisions of the National Knowledge Commission, to provide healthcare related information to the citizens of India.
8. http://idsp.nic.in/ – This web portal is for online reporting under Integrated Disease Surveillance Programme (IDSP) for all States and UTs.
9. http://www.icmr.nic.in/ – The Indian Council of Medical Research (ICMR), New Delhi, the apex body in India for the formulation, coordination and promotion of biomedical research.
10. http://www.dhr.gov.in/ – Department of Health Research (DHR) aims at modern health technology to introducing innovations into public health service through health systems research.
11. http://nrhm.gov.in/ – National Rural Health Mission (NRHM) is an Indian health program for improving health care delivery across rural India.
12. http://www.tbcindia.nic.in/ – About tuberculosis control in India.
13. http://www.igib.res.in/ – CSIR-Institute of Genomics & Integrative Biology (IGIB) is a premier Institute of Council of Scientific and Industrial Research (CSIR), engaged in national research in the areas of genomics, molecular medicine, bioinformatics, proteomics.
14. http://www.nabh.co/ – National Accreditation Board for Hospitals & Healthcare Providers (NABH) is a constituent board of Quality Council of India, to establish and operate accreditation programme for healthcare organizations.
15. http://www.nabl-india.org – National Accreditation Board for Testing and Calibration Laboratories (NABL) under the aegis of DST, GOI for laboratory accreditation through third-party assessment for formally recognizing the technical competence of laboratories.
16. http://ctri.nic.in/Clinicaltrials/login.php – The Clinical Trials Registry- India (CTRI), hosted at the ICMR National Institute of Medical Statistics (NIMS), is a free and online public record system for registration of Indian clinical trials.

Microbiology news and events

1. https://phys.org/biology-news/microbiology/
2. https://www.nytimes.com/topic/subject/microbiology
3. https://www.sciencedaily.com/news/plants_animals/microbiology/
4. http://apps.who.int/globalatlas/default.asp

Books

1. https://archive.org/ – The website provides a large collection of medical and non medical books available for download.
2. https://www.ncbi.nlm.nih.gov/books/NBK7627/– Site has a comprehensive textbook of microbiology and a concise review text under General Concepts
3. http://textbookofbacteriology.net/ – This textbook has course modules on microbiology.
4. http://www.roitt.com – Site for the classic book of Immunology.
5. http://www.macmillanlearning.com/catalog/static/whf/kuby/ – This Web site is designed to help students review key concepts through interactive exercises and learning tools.
6. http://minst.org/library.htm – The Mednansky Institute online library acquires classic scientific books which are reviewed and commented upon for educational purposes.
7. http://www.microbiologybook.org/ – Covers second year medical student course on microbiology.
8. http://www.ccmhmtschool.org/uploads/docs/color-atlas-of-diagnostic-microbiology.pdf – The link is of color atlas of diagnostic microbiology with relevant information for students.
9. http://highered.mheducation.com/sites/0072437316/student_view0/index.html – The link is online learning centre with chapter wise information

Social networking sites

1. On Facebook – American Society for Microbiology, Rao's Microbiology, Microbiology Research Society, Microbiology Today and Science Updates.
2. Blogs

   http://thunderhouse4-yuri.blogspot.in/

   http://www.virology.ws/

   http://scienceblogs.com/aetiology/ – Aetiology by Tara C. Smith (@aetiology): "Discussing causes, origins, evolution, and implications of disease and other phenomena."

   http://labrat.fieldofscience.com/ Life of a Lab Rat ("occasional insights into the life of a lab rat") and Lab Rat ("Exploring the life and times of bacteria") by S. E. Gould (@labratting).

   https://rybicki.wordpress.com/ ViroBlogy by Ed Rybicki (@edrybicki): "Up-to-date Virology-related posts, mainly for students at the University of Cape Town".

Index

C

W

X

Y

Z